THE NEUROBIO

C000132943

Trust is essential for establishing and maintaining cooperative behaviors between individuals and institutions in a wide variety of social, economic, and political contexts. This book explores trust through the lens of neurobiology, focusing on empirical, methodological, and theoretical aspects. Written by a distinguished group of researchers from economics, psychology, human factors, neuroscience, and psychiatry, the chapters shed light on the neurobiological underpinnings of trust as applied in a variety of domains. Researchers and students will discover a refined understanding of trust by delving into the essential topics in this area of study outlined by leading experts.

FRANK KRUEGER is Professor of Systems Social Neuroscience in the School of Systems Biology at George Mason University, USA. As a psychologist, physicist, and neuroscientist, he has authored or co-authored approximately 170 publications in scientific journals and has been cited as an expert in the national news media and television such as *The New York Times*, *New Scientist*, *The Economist*, and *PBS News Hour*.

THE NEUROBIOLOGY
OF TRUST

EDITED BY

FRANK KRUEGER

George Mason University

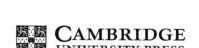

CAMBRIDGE
UNIVERSITY PRESS

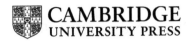

Shaftesbury Road, Cambridge CB2 8EA, United Kingdom

One Liberty Plaza, 20th Floor, New York, NY 10006, USA

477 Williamstown Road, Port Melbourne, VIC 3207, Australia

314–321, 3rd Floor, Plot 3, Splendor Forum, Jasola District Centre, New Delhi – 110025, India

103 Penang Road, #05–06/07, Visioncrest Commercial, Singapore 238467

Cambridge University Press is part of Cambridge University Press & Assessment,
a department of the University of Cambridge.

We share the University's mission to contribute to society through the pursuit of
education, learning and research at the highest international levels of excellence.

www.cambridge.org
Information on this title: www.cambridge.org/9781108726702

DOI: 10.1017/9781108770880

First published 2022
First paperback edition 2022

A catalogue record for this publication is available from the British Library

ISBN   978-1-108-48856-3   Hardback
ISBN   978-1-108-72670-2   Paperback

PART V NEUROPATHOLOGICAL LEVEL OF TRUST

16   Trust and Psychotic Disorders: Unraveling the Dynamics
     of Paranoia and Disturbed Social Interaction   389
     Imke L. J. Lemmers-Jansen and Anne-Kathrin J. Fett

17   Trust and Personality Disorders: Phenomenology,
     Determinants, and Therapeutical Approaches   430
     Stefanie Lis, Miriam Biermann, and Zsolt Unoka

18   Trust and Lesion Evidence: Lessons from Neuropsychology
     on the Neuroanatomical Correlates of Trust   464
     Hannah E. Wadsworth and Daniel Tranel

Index   492

Figures

1.1	The payoffs (outcomes) in a trust-relevant situation	*page* 17
1.2	The dyadic model of trust in relationships (Simpson, 2007)	20
2.1	Trust game from Kreps (1990)	38
2.2	Trust game from Camerer and Weigelt (1988)	40
3.1	Major trust scenarios in a digital world	56
4.1	Human, environmental, and automation-specific variables interact to influence human trust in automated systems	78
5.1	Conceptualization of trust behavior	103
6.1	Effects of the induction of specific incidental emotions on trust	129
6.2	Brain networks involved in trust decisions	137
7.1	Iterative trust game with partners varying in terms of closeness (computer, stranger, and close friend)	167
8.1	Schematic formation of trustworthiness impressions guiding trust behavior	187
8.2	Brain regions involved in trust learning	194
10.1	Illustration of a trust game	238
10.2	Illustration of economic theory-predicted neural outcomes	241
15.1	Structure of the oxytocin receptor gene	373
15.2	Structure of the arginine vasopressin receptor 1A gene	377
16.1	The development of trust across repeated interactions	403
16.2	Brain regions tested in region of interest analyses during the trust game	413
16.3	Outcomes of the whole brain analyses, showing reduced activation in psychosis	414
18.1	The trust game	467
18.2	A photo of the insular cortex in left hemisphere	469
18.3	Illustration of the amygdala	475
18.4	The role of the amygdala in trust	477

Tables

3.1 Trusting beliefs in interpersonal relationships and
corresponding trusting beliefs in human–
technology relationships   *page* 65

3.2 Major neuroscience studies on computer-mediated
human–technology interaction with a focus on trust
and mentalizing   67

9.1 Dissociating trust and distrust as psychological constructs   222

10.1 Outcome-based trust and belief-based reciprocity,
evidence from neuroscience literature   256

11.1 Overview of studies that examined the effect of age
on the neural mechanisms of trust   280

12.1 Comparison between task-based and task-free
neuroimaging approaches   302

16.1 Participant characteristics and trust measures of the
reviewed studies   391

16.2 Behavioral findings and symptom correlations in the
reviewed studies on trust in psychosis   397

16.3 Neuroimaging studies on trust in psychosis   408

Contributors

AIMONE, JASON A., Department of Economics, Baylor University, Waco, TX, USA

BELLUCCI, GABRIELE, Department of Computational Neuroscience, Max Planck Institute for Biological Cybernetics, Tübingen, Germany

BIERMANN, MIRIAM, Institute of Psychiatric and Psychosomatic Psychotherapy, Central Institute of Mental Health, Medical Faculty Mannheim, Heidelberg University, Heidelberg, Germany

BOSE, DEVDEEPTA, Division of Humanities and Social Sciences, California Institute of Technology, Pasadena, CA, USA

BRUDNER, EMILY G., Department of Psychology, Rutgers University, Newark, NJ, USA

CAMERER, COLIN, Division of Humanities and Social Sciences, California Institute of Technology, Pasadena, CA, USA

CHANG, LI-ANG, Center for Research in Experimental Economics (CREED), Amsterdam School of Economics, University of Amsterdam, Amsterdam, The Netherlands

CHIU, PEARL H., Fralin Biomedical Research Institute at VTC, Virginia Tech, Roanoke, VA, USA

DELGADO, MAURICIO R., Department of Psychology, Rutgers University, Newark, NJ, USA

DREHER, JEAN-CLAUDE, Laboratory of Neuroeconomics, Institut des Sciences Cognitives Marc Jeannerod, Centre national de la recherche (CNRS), Lyon, France

ENGELMANN, JAN B., Center for Research in Experimental Economics (CREED), Amsterdam School of Economics, University of Amsterdam, Amsterdam, The Netherlands

FARERI, DOMINIC S., Gordon F. Derner School of Psychology, Adelphi University, Garden City, NY, USA

FAROLFI, FEDERICA, Center for Research in Experimental Economics (CREED), Amsterdam School of Economics, University of Amsterdam, Amsterdam, The Netherlands

FETT, ANNE-KATHRIN J., Department of Psychology, City, University of London, London, United Kingdom

HAAS, BRIAN W., Department of Psychology, University of Georgia, Athens, GA, USA

HANCOCK, PETER A., Department of Psychology, University of Central Florida, Orlando, FL, USA

KAPLAN, ALEXANDRA D., Department of Psychology, University of Central Florida, Orlando, FL, USA

KAROUSATOS, ALEC J., Department of Psychology, Rutgers University, Newark, NJ, USA

KING-CASAS, BROOKS, Fralin Biomedical Research Institute at VTC, Virginia Tech, Roanoke, VA, USA

KIRSCH, PETER, Department of Clinical Psychology, Central Institute of Mental Health, Medical Faculty Mannheim, Heidelberg University, Heidelberg, Germany

KRABBENDAM, LYDIA, VU Amsterdam, Amsterdam, The Netherlands

KRUEGER, FRANK, School of Systems Biology, George Mason University, Fairfax, VA, USA

LAUHARATANAHIRUN, NINA, Department of Biomedical Engineering, Department of Biobehavioral Health, Pennsylvania State University, State College, PA, USA

LEE, MARY R., Intensive Community Mental Health Recovery Services, Washington, DC, USA

LEMMERS-JANSEN, IMKE L. J., Department of Psychosis Studies, Institute of Psychiatry, Psychology & Neuroscience, King's College London, London, United Kingdom

LI, FLORA, Economics Experimental Laboratory, Nanjing Audit University, Nanjing, China

LIS, STEFANIE, Institute of Psychiatric and Psychosomatic Psychotherapy, Central Institute of Mental Health, Medical Faculty Mannheim, Heidelberg University, Heidelberg, Germany

MACARTHUR, KEITH, School of Modeling, Simulation, and Training, University of Central Florida, Orlando, FL, USA

NISHINA, KUNIYUKI, Kochi University of Technology, Kochi City, Japan

RIEDL, RENé, University of Applied Sciences Upper Austria and Johannes Kepler University Linz, Austria

SANDERS, TRACY L., Transportation Innovation Center, The MITRE Corporation, McLean, VA, USA

SHOU, QIULU, Brain Science Institute, Tamagawa University, Machida, Tokyo, Japan

SIJTSMA, HESTER, Vrije Universiteit Amsterdam, Amsterdam, The Netherlands

SIMPSON, JEFFRY A., Department of Psychology, University of Minnesota, Minneapolis, MN, USA

TAKAGISHI, HARUTO, Brain Science Institute, Tamagawa University, Machida, Tokyo, Japan

TRANEL, DANIEL, Department of Neurology (Division of Neuropsychology and Cognitive Neuroscience), Carver College of Medicine, University of Iowa, Iowa City, IA, USA

UNOKA, ZSOLT, Department of Psychiatry and Psychotherapy, Semmelweis University of Medicine (SOTE), Budapest, Hungary

VEERAREDDY, APOORVA, School of Systems Biology, George Mason University, Fairfax, VA, USA

VIETH, GRACE, Department of Psychology, University of Minnesota, Minneapolis, MN, USA

VOLANTE, WILLIAM G., Department of Psychology, University of Central Florida, Orlando, FL, USA

WADSWORTH, HANNAH E., Department of Neurology (Division of Neuropsychology and Cognitive Neuroscience), Carver College of Medicine, University of Iowa, Iowa City, IA, USA

WU, YAN, Department of Psychology, College of Education, Hangzhou Normal University, Hangzhou, China

YAN, ZHIMIN, Department of Clinical Psychology, University of Konstanz, Konstanz, Germany

Abbreviations

ACC	anterior cingulate cortex
ACE	adverse childhood experience
AEMT	autobiographical emotional memory task
amPFC	anterior medial prefrontal cortex
AP	affective psychosis
ASD	autism spectrum disorder
AVPR1A	arginine vasopressin receptor 1A
BA	Brodmann area
BOLD	blood oxygen level-dependent
BPD	borderline personality disorder
CARA	constant absolute risk aversion
CASA	computers are social actors
CEN	central-executive network
CRRA	constant relative risk aversion
dACC	dorsal anterior cingulate cortex
DBT	dialectical behavior therapy
DCM	dynamic causal modeling
DG	dictator game
dlPFC	dorsolateral prefrontal cortex
DMN	default-mode network
dmPFC	dorsomedial prefrontal cortex
DRD4	dopamine D4 receptor gene
DSM	Diagnostic and Statistical Manual
dSTR	dorsal striatum
EEG	electroencephalography
EP	early psychosis
ESM	experience sampling method
FC	functional connectivity
FCDM	functional connectivity density mapping
FEP	first episode psychosis

fMRI	functional magnetic resonance imaging
FSL	FreeSurfer FMRIB Software Library
GCM	Granger causality mapping
HAI	human–automation interaction
HC	healthy controls
ICA	independent component analysis
IPL	inferior parietal lobule
ITU	International Telecommunication Union
IU	international units
lPFC	lateral prefrontal cortex
MAP	minimum acceptable probability
MBT	mentalization-based therapy
MCC	middle cingulate cortex
MDMA	3,4-Methyl-enedioxy-methamphetamine
MIP	mood induction procedures
mPFC	medial prefrontal cortex
MPH	methylphenidate
OFC	orbitofrontal cortex
OR	opioid receptor
OXT	oxytocin
OXTR	oxytocin receptor gene
PANAS	positive and negative affect schedule
PCC	posterior cingulate cortex
PD	personality disorder
PDG	prisoner's dilemma game
PE	prediction error
PGG	public goods game
PPI	psychophysiological interaction
PTSD	post-traumatic stress disorder
RL	reinforcement learning
ROI	region of interest
RSFC	resting-state functional connectivity
rTPJ	right temporoparietal junction
RWN	reward network
SAN	salience network
SES	socioeconomic status
SLC6A4	serotonin transporter gene
SPM	statistical parametric mapping
ST	schema therapy
STR	striatum

STS	superior temporal sulcus
TAG	take advice game
tb-fMRI	task-based fMRI
tf-fMRI	task-free fMRI
TG	trust game
ToM	theory of mind
ToS	threat of shock procedure
TPJ	temporoparietal junction
UG	ultimatum game
vlPFC	ventrolateral prefrontal cortex
vmPFC	ventromedial prefrontal cortex
vSTR	ventral striatum
VTA	ventral tegmental area
WEIRD	western, educated, industrialized, rich, and democratic
WL	warm liking
WVS	World Values Survey
μ-OR	mu opioid receptor

Introduction

Since the early days of humankind, trust has been an essential factor for establishing and maintaining cooperative and mutually beneficial interpersonal relationships with strangers, friends, family members, etc., impacting our social interactions across all aspects of our private and public lives in a wide range of social, economic, and political contexts. Portraying a social dilemma, trust can be conceptualized as a trustor's investment of resources (e.g., money, time, energy) into another party (i.e., a trustee) that encompasses uncertainty regarding the benefits of reciprocation in the future, thus opening up the possibilities for deceiving and cheating in human society. These interpersonal trust decisions – ranging from small (e.g., trusting that a stranger provides you with a correct route description) to large (e.g., trusting your spouse to be faithful) transactions – are imperative for shaping our social lives and have cascading positive and negative consequences. When people trust each other, society is more inclusive and accessible, economic transactions are facilitated, and feelings of well-being prosper (Rothstein & Uslaner, 2005; Simpson, 2007; Zak & Knack, 2001). For example, the current unprecedented pandemic of COVID-19 has highlighted the significance of trust in regulating our social lives. We not only trust our political leaders to tell the truth about the impact of this virus but also that others take the necessary precautions (e.g., social distancing, wearing face coverings, limiting unnecessary contact, self-isolation and quarantining in the case of an infection) to slow the spread of the virus.

Over the last few decades, scholars from a variety of academic fields, including economics, sociology, psychology, human factors, and more recently neuroscience, have delved into the phenomenon of trust both theoretically and empirically (e.g., Rousseau et al., 1998; Swan et al., 1999). These endeavors revealed that trust is a multidimensional construct shaped by various factors at the behavioral, psychological, and neurobiological levels; however, no agreement yet exists about a unified definition of trust across disciplines. The dispute about defining trust is based on essential questions such as whether trust is considered as a belief, an intention, or a behavior (Jones & Shah, 2016). Trust as a belief refers to the evaluation of the partner's trustworthiness by observing, interpreting, and attributing their ability, benevolence, and integrity (Mayer et al., 1995), leading to a positive anticipation toward the behavior of the trustee (Hardin, 2001; Rousseau et al., 1998; Sapienza et al., 2013). Trust as an intent stresses the trustor's willingness to be vulnerable toward the trustee's actions (Jones & Shah, 2016), whereas trust as an action indicates that the trustor has to rely on the trustee to perform an anticipated action (Elster, 1998; Fehr, 2009). Essentially, the type of definition determines how trust is examined from a neurobiological perspective and what methodologies can be implemented to measure it – crucial determinates for developing a neurobiological framework of trust. Although an excess of definition for the conception of this phenomenon exists (Seppanen et al., 2007), the identification of common psychological components (motivation, affect, cognition) across explanations allows a working definition of trust across disciplines to be formulated (Krueger & Meyer-Lindenberg, 2019, p. 92): "Interpersonal trust encompasses a psychological state in which a trustor is willing to be vulnerable to the risk of betrayal (affect) based on the expectation (cognition) regarding the action of a trustee that will produce some anticipated reward (motivation) due to reciprocation in the future."

The neuropsychological mechanisms of trust have been explored during the last 20 years, but a conceptual framework that assimilates isolated findings into a neuropsychological model of trust is nevertheless outstanding. The objective of this book is to provide an overarching neurobiological framework of trust that serves as a common root for the broad and multidisciplinary community of trust research. Although other books exist on the topic of trust, previous projects focused either on the trust research in other selected academic fields (e.g., sociology, psychology, politics, and economics) (Bachmann & Zaheer, 2013; Lange et al., 2017; Uslaner, 2018; Zmerli & Meer, 2017) or research methods of trust (e.g., qualitative and quantitative methods) (Lyon et al., 2015). For the first time, this book provides a comprehensive collection of the most pressing, relevant, and timely topics of the neurobiology of trust research – focusing on theoretical, methodological, and empirical aspects – to explore a conceptual neurobiological framework of trust. The book offers a more integrative collection compared with previous descriptive neuroscience reviews (Fehr, 2009; Riedl & Javor, 2012; Tzieropoulos, 2013) and neuroimaging meta-analyses (Bellucci et al., 2017; Bellucci et al., 2018) on trust.

This unique book will provide invaluable insights for several readers across multidisciplinary fields, including economics, psychology, neuroscience, human factors, and psychiatry, who are looking for reflection, discussion, and inspiration in the research field of the neurobiology of trust. This book is of value to anyone who is planning interdisciplinary research on the neurobiological basis of trust – open for discovering new and promising research avenues. Moreover, it serves as reference material on trust and provides a stimulating starting point for future queries and for teaching research-based multidisciplinary courses on trust and related topics. Finally, the book is of interest for practitioners, policymakers, and laypersons who want to inform themselves about the neuropsychological mechanisms of trust based on curiosity and pertinence.

This book gathers together a distinguished group of noted scholars and researchers from diverse backgrounds, including economics, psychology, human factors, neuroscience, and psychiatry, to shed light on the neurobiological underpinnings of trust in one essential volume. The contributions of the prominent and highly respected experts will advance the field by asking new research questions that will potentially lead to a refined understanding of trust and, therefore, to essential novel developments for future research on trust (Krueger & Meyer-Lindenberg, 2020). The volume aims to achieve an overarching neurobiological framework of trust, one that highlights the benefits and challenges across empirical, methodological, and theoretical aspects of the current state of trust neuroscience research across disciplines. Given that certain neural structures are associated with distinct psychological (motivational, affective, cognitive) functions, functional neuroimaging studies – especially implementing functional magnetic resonance imaging (fMRI) studies, as discussed throughout this book – will help shed light on the underlying processes or psychoneurobiological mechanisms that may give rise to trust behavior.

Each of the 18 chapters is written by leading senior scholars – paired with junior scholars – who are the most recognized experts in their fields. Each chapter provides an overview about the current status at different psychoneurobiological levels of trust, summarizing controversies, problems, and challenges that the trust community must tackle in the near future to fulfill the request for an overarching psychoneurobiological framework of trust. The volume offers chapters on the *fundamental, neuropsychological, neurocharacteristic, neuromolecular, and neuropathological levels* of trust with an up-to-date research review, that are based on a coherent organization. Each chapter reviews both seminal and current key findings that are relevant to each of the psychoneurobiological levels of trust research: emphasizing essential foundations, presenting theoretical accounts, and suggesting future research questions.

I.1   Fundamental Level of Trust

The chapters covering the ***fundamental level of trust*** present a comprehensive overview of relevant definitions, concepts, and measurements of both the propensity and dynamics of interpersonal trust behavior in key research fields of trust, including psychology, economics, human factors, and digital technology. Within *psychology*, theoretical and empirical work on interpersonal trust has shown that experiencing higher levels of trust, particularly early in life, with close people can pave the groundwork for happier, more functioning adult relationships. In ***Chapter 1*** – *Trust and Psychology: Psychological Theories and Principles Underlying Interpersonal Trust* – Jeffry A. Simpson and Grace Vieth review major theories of interpersonal trust and deliver a representative overview of recent trust research in the field of psychology on how, when, and why trust develops, is maintained, and sometimes disintegrates between people. The authors provide a dyadic model of trust that integrates key principles to understand how trust operates in different types of relationships, including strangers, coworkers, family members, friends, and romantic partners.

In *behavioral economics*, trust as a type of strategic decision making is modeled mathematically in the language of game theory and explored empirically in both laboratory and field experiments. Devdeepta Bose and Colin Camerer explore in ***Chapter 2*** – *Trust and Behavioral Economics: Exploration of Trust Based on Game Theory* – the role of trust in easing economic transactions between two parties (e.g., individuals, firms), covering both seminal and recent research. They demonstrate how the utilization of the trust (investment) game (and assorted variations) – grounded in a game-theoretic approach – can improve our understanding of how trust affects the underlying dynamic in dyadic transactions, relationships at the societal level, and macroeconomic growth.

With the increasing use of digital technologies, determining whom to trust has changed when dealing with digital technology, because we communicate with other people less face-to-face but more often via the Internet (e.g., Zoom) or engage with technological artifacts (e.g., autonomous vehicles). ***Chapter 3*** – *Trust and Digitalization: Review of Behavioral and Neuroscience Evidence* – by René Riedl examines the growing use of digital technologies and their foremost implications on how trust and trustworthiness should be conceptualized in a digital world. The author contrasts four interaction scenarios – including a technology-free human–human interaction, a computer-mediated human–human interaction, a direct human–technology interaction, and a computer-mediated human–technology interaction – and integrates theoretical and empirical studies based on behavioral and neurophysiological findings.

While trust is often intellectualized as relationships among people, the rise of automation – ranging from simple decision aids to artificial intelligence systems – requires a reconceptualization of trust between humans and automated systems. In ***Chapter 4 – Trust and Human Factors: Foundations of Trust in Automation*** – Tracy L. Sanders, Alexandra D. Kaplan, Keith MacArthur, William G. Volante, and Peter A. Hancock review the latest research in stressing an emerging demand that humans (biological agents) and automated systems (artificial agents) have to work together to accomplish a larger goal in the foreseeable future. Highlighting differences between human–human trust (i.e., relying on the morals and motivations of the human trustee) and human–automation trust (i.e., lacking internal motivations and acting on its programming), the authors introduce a three-factor model grounded in the multidisciplinary field of human factors (concerned with the human aspects of engineering) – incorporating the human trustor, the automated trustee, and the environment – which helps to conceptualize trust in automation and ensures appropriate trust calibration between both types of agents.

I.2 Neuropsychological Level of Trust

The chapters covering the ***neuropsychological level of trust*** provide an overview about the psychological components of trust – including risk, emotion, reputation, and learning – and its underlying neural signatures. Trust can be seen as an investment of resources in another person or group that involves a degree of risk (i.e., uncertainty) as to whether such an investment may be reciprocated or provide future benefits. In ***Chapter 5 – Trust and Risk: Neuroeconomic Foundations of Trust Based on Social Risk –*** Nina Lauharatanahirun and Jason A. Aimone discuss how interpersonal trust behavior can be seen as a decision based on social risk in a microeconomic system where another person or group is the primary source of uncertainty. The authors discuss how functional neuroimaging studies play a pivotal role in disambiguating the contribution of preferences and beliefs (e.g., risk preferences, betrayal aversion) to the neurobiological mechanisms of trust behavior.

Emotions can have a direct and indirect impact on the psychological processes that enable trust decisions during social interactions. *Chapter 6 – Trust and Emotion: The Effects of Incidental and Integral Affect –* by Federica Farolfi, Li-Ang Chang, and Jan B. Engelmann provides an overview about the behavioral, psychological, and neuroeconomic research that investigates the influence of positive and negative affective states on trust behavior. The authors explain how both incidental (unrelated to the trust decision) and integral (contemplating features of the trust decision) emotions (positive, negative) can impact trust behavior and stress the significance of the role of emotions in learning to trust from past experiences.

The reputation of a partner (i.e., a belief about a person's trait characteristics) is a central indicator that can be utilized to predict whether that partner can be trusted in familiar or novel social environments. Emily G. Brudner, Alec J. Karousatos, Dominic S. Fareri, and Mauricio R. Delgado review in *Chapter 7 – Trust and Reputation: How Knowledge about Others Shapes Our Decisions –* fundamental and current neurobiological findings on how trustworthiness reputations are developed and how reputational information from indirect sources interacts with these direct experiences, driving trust behavior. They discuss the neurocomputational mechanisms involved in forming rapid, perceptual-based trustworthiness impressions, moment-by-moment reputation learning through direct experience, and reputations shaped by a wide array of social experiences and long-standing, established relationships.

Learning whether to trust or distrust other partners in social interaction is a vital skill in building social relationships. In *Chapter 8 – Trust and Learning: Neurocomputational Signatures of Learning to Trust –* Gabriele Bellucci and Jean-Claude Dreher examine the neuropsychological mechanisms on how social information about others (i.e., social characteristics, psychological traits) functions as central determinants and predictors of trustworthiness impressions and trusting behaviors. Looking at neuroimaging evidence, the authors examine the learning dynamics and computational mechanisms that determine how people integrate social information about others to update their trustworthiness beliefs and revise their trusting behaviors.

I.3   Neurocharacteristic Level of Trust

The chapters on the **neurocharacteristic level of trust** give a summary about the distinctive neural signatures of trust in comparison to distrust and reciprocity as well as related to demographic factors such as age and gender and dynamics of measurement such as task-based vs. task-free trust. How people form concepts about trust and distrust in their minds is still a matter of debate in different scientific disciplines. ***Chapter 9*** – *Trust and Distrust: Key Similarities and Differences* – by Brian W. Haas summarizes the neuropsychological literature across a range of disciplines on what constitutes trust and distrust. The author seeks to develop a cohesive model of the neurobiological basis for trust vs. distrust and elucidating its neuropsychological mechanisms holds the central potential of improving the way people communicate with one another and are able to work effectively within groups.

As trust and reciprocity are associated with prosocial behavior, positive reciprocity often exhibits very similar neurobehavioral signatures to trust, making it particularly difficult to distinguish between these two psychological concepts. In ***Chapter 10*** – *Trust and Reciprocity: The Role of Outcome-Based and Belief-Based Motivations* – Flora Li, Pearl H. Chiu, and Brooks King-Casas review potential motivations that drive trust (characterized by vulnerability or risk) and reciprocity (characterized by positive reciprocity) – two closely linked concepts that are ubiquitous within cooperative exchange – incorporating economic theory with neuroscientific findings. The authors examine whether internal preferences over monetary distributions (outcome-based) and expectations about others' intentions (belief-based) may contribute to trust or reciprocate behaviors.

Being present from a very young age, the influence of individual characteristics on the development of trust is a prerequisite for forming and maintaining stable, satisfying relationships across the lifespan. In ***Chapter 11*** – *Trust and Demographics: Age and Gender Differences in Trust and Reciprocity Behavior* – Hester Sijtsma and Lydia Krabbendam summarize the research on age and gender differences in trust and reciprocity that show important changes over the lifetime. The authors explore developmental trajectories from childhood, through adolescence, to adulthood of trust and reciprocity behavior with a focus on the influence of individual characteristics on its underlying neural correlates, including brain regions related to mentalizing, reward, and learning.

Over the past two decades, an increase in task-based and task-free (resting-state) fMRI studies have been observed that explored the conjoint psychological function of brain regions working together as large-scale networks in producing individual differences in trust behavior. In ***Chapter 12*** – *Trust and Brain Dynamics: Insights from Task-Based and*

Task-Free Neuroimaging Investigations – Yan Wu and Frank Krueger compare the commonalities and dissimilarities between task-based fMRI and task-free (resting-state) fMRI approaches for studying trust at the group as well as individual level. They explore how these two approaches can make unique contributions in our understanding of the psychoneurobiological underpinnings of the motivational, affective, and cognitive components of trust and its underlying large-scale domain-general networks.

I.4   Neuromolecular Level of Trust

The chapters on the ***neuromolecular level of trust*** provide an overview about neuropeptides, psychopharmaca, and genes associated with changes in trust behavior. The neuropeptide hormone oxytocin has been found in many kinds of species ranging from invertebrates to mammals to regulate social cognition and behavior, including trust behavior. In ***Chapter 13*** – *Trust and Oxytocin: Context-Dependent Exogenous and Endogenous Modulation of Trust* – Zhimin Yan and Peter Kirsch review the association of oxytocin with interpersonal trust, looking at exogenous administration of oxytocin as well as its endogenous and genetic levels. The authors explore the plethora of studies that have investigated the context-dependent neuropsychological effects of oxytocin on intention to trust, behavior of trust, and mental disorders.

Psychopharmacological drug manipulations create causal mechanisms for selectively stimulating or blocking target neurotransmitter receptors known to modulate brain networks engaged in trust behavior. In ***Chapter 14*** – *Trust and Psychopharmaca: Neuromodulation of the Signaling Pathways Underlying Trust Behavior* – Mary R. Lee, Apoorva Veerareddy, and Frank Krueger review studies that combined the trust game or trust ratings with pharmacological agents to act as neuromodulators such as opiates, monoamine neurotransmitters (e.g., serotonin, dopamine), and pharmacologic agents such as 3,4-Methyl-enedioxy-methamphetamine (MDMA) in the neural signaling pathways underlying trust behavior. The authors further point out shortcomings in the present psychopharmacological research approach and offer guidance for future interdisciplinary research on the psychoneurobiological underpinnings of trust.

To determine which specific gene is associated with trust, researchers look at twin studies or genetic polymorphisms of specific genes to examine mechanisms of heritability and genetic variation in producing individual differences in trust behavior. In ***Chapter 15*** *– Trust and Genetics: Genetic Basis of Trust Behavior and Trust Attitude* – Qiulu Shou, Kuniyuki Nishina, and Haruto Takagishi review neurogenetic investigations to answer the question about the heritability of trust. The authors explore twin studies and examine the relationship between trust measures and polymorphism of some specific genes –oxytocin receptor gene, arginine vasopressin receptor 1A, dopamine D4 receptor gene, and serotonin transporter gene – to reveal the genetic basis of trust behavior and trust attitude.

I.5 Neuropathological Level of Trust

The chapters on the ***neuropathological level of trust*** present a summary about how trust behavior is impaired in mental disorders such as psychotic disorders and personality disorders and lesion evidence from patients leading to problems in interpersonal and social functioning. Isolating the underlying neuropsychological underpinnings of trust in healthy people can possibly help us to learn more about trust impairment as documented in the neuropathology of psychotic disorders. In ***Chapter 16*** *– Trust and Psychotic Disorders: Unraveling the Dynamics of Paranoia and Disturbed Social Interaction* – Imke L. J. Lemmers-Jansen and Anne-Kathrin J. Fett debate theoretical accounts considering motivational, affective, and cognitive aspects of disturbed trust in psychosis, looking at findings that either employed the trust game or trustworthiness ratings of faces. The authors summarize findings related to baseline and trust dynamics in terms of first-episode and chronic patients as well as individuals at high risk for psychosis who show impairment in brain regions associated with theory of mind and reward processing.

Psychopathological descriptions, diagnostic criteria, and experimental studies show an impairment of trust due to traumatization during childhood and adolescence across the spectrum of different personality disorders (e.g., borderline personality disorder or BPD). Stefanie Lis, Miriam Biermann, and Zsolt Unoka provide in ***Chapter 17*** *– Trust and Personality Disorders: Phenomenology, Determinants, and Therapeutical Approaches* – an overview of the definition, classification, and methodological approaches used to study trust as one domain of interpersonal functioning in personality disorders, focusing on BPD. They also discuss trust as a target concept in psychotherapeutic and pharmacological interventions as an improvement for treatment options for this domain of interpersonal dysfunction.

Research about brain activation during trust decision in the healthy brain has shown several brain regions involving different networks; however, a causal involvement of these regions for specific trust components is often unknown but can be determined by studying lesions in human subjects due to stroke, etc., in specific trust-related brain areas. *Chapter 18 – Trust and Lesion Evidence: Lessons from Neuropsychology on the Neuroanatomical Correlates of Trust* – by Hannah E. Wadsworth and Daniel Tranel gives an overview about lesion studies in patients with damage to the insula, amygdala, and prefrontal cortex, known to be associated with the motivational, emotional, and cognitive processes of trust behavior. They describe how different types of trust may change when each of those regions is damaged, followed by how these rare findings can inform our understanding of the neuroanatomical signatures of trust.

In summary, the compilation of those chapters will accelerate, expand, and advance the existing status about the neurobiological mechanisms of trust, enabling the incorporation of research findings into a conceptual neurobiological framework of trust. Each chapter illustrates the shortcomings of the existing research methods and addresses unanswered questions that can shape future interdisciplinary research for a deeper understanding of the neuropsychological signature of trust, addressing also institutional and intercultural trust besides interpersonal trust. Looking into the future, as the transdisciplinary research for a neurobiology of trust matures, the knowledge presented in this volume can expectantly be used to advance our understanding of trust, helping not only to identify objective biomarkers for disease diagnostic specificity and novel treatment strategies for mental health disorders (often characterized by mistrust in social relationships) but also to advocate for a more trusting and inclusive society.

References

Bachmann, R., & Zaheer, A. (2013). *Handbook of advances in trust research.* Edward Elgar.

Bellucci, G., Chernyak, S. V., Goodyear, K., Eickhoff, S. B., & Krueger, F. (2017). Neural signatures of trust in reciprocity: A coordinate-based meta-analysis. *Human Brain Mapping*, 38(3), 1233–1248. https://doi.org/10.1002/hbm.23451

Bellucci, G., Feng, C., Camilleri, J., Eickhoff, S. B., & Krueger, F. (2018). The role of the anterior insula in social norm compliance and enforcement: Evidence from coordinate-based and functional connectivity meta-analyses. *Neuroscience Biobehavioral Review*, 92, 378–389. https://doi.org/10.1016/j.neubiorev.2018.06.024

Elster, J. (1998). Emotions and economic theory. *Journal of Economic Literature*, 36(1), 47–74. www.jstor.org/stable/2564951

Fehr, E. (2009). On the economics and biology of trust. *Journal of the European Economic Association*, 7(2–3), 235–266. https://doi.org/10.1162/JEEA.2009 .7.2-3.235

Hardin, R. (2001). Conceptions and explanations of trust. In K. S. Cook (Ed.), *Trust in society* (pp. 3–39). Russell Sage Foundation. http://www.jstor.org/ stable/10.7758/9781610441322.5

Jones, S. L., & Shah, P. P. (2016). Diagnosing the locus of trust: A temporal perspective for trustor, trustee, and dyadic influences on perceived trustworthiness. *Journal of Applied Psychology*, 101(3), 392–414. https://doi.org/10 .1037/apl0000041

Krueger, F., & Meyer-Lindenberg, A. (2019). Toward a model of interpersonal trust drawn from neuroscience, psychology, and economics. *Trends in Neurosciences*, 42(2), 92–101. https://doi.org/10.1016/j.tins.2018.10.004

(2020). Editorial: Towards a Refined Understanding of Social Trust (T-R-U-S-T). *Frontiers in Human Neuroscience*, Article 14:305. https://doi.org/10 .3389/fnhum.2020.00305

Lange, P. A. M. v., Rockenbach, B., & Yamagishi, T. (2017). *Trust in social dilemmas*. Oxford University Press.

Lyon, F., Möllering, G., & Saunders, M. N. K. (2015). *Handbook of research methods on trust* (2nd ed.). Edward Elgar.

Mayer, R. C., Davis, J. H., & Schoorman, F. D. (1995). An integrative model of organizational trust. *Academy of Management Review*, 20(3), 709–734. https://doi.org/10.2307/258792

Riedl, R., & Javor, A. (2012). The biology of trust: Integrating evidence from genetics, endocrinology, and functional brain imaging. *Journal of Neuroscience Psychology and Economics*, 5(2), 63–91. https://doi.org/10 .1037/a0026318

Rothstein, B., & Uslaner, E. M. (2005). All for all: Equality, corruption, and social trust. *World Politics*, 58(1), 41–72. https://doi.org/10.1353/wp.2006 .0022

Rousseau, D. M., Sitkin, S. B., Burt, R. S., & Camerer, C. F. (1998). Not so different after all: A cross-discipline view of trust. *Academy of Management Review*, 23(3), 393–404. https://doi.org/10.5465/amr.1998.926617

Sapienza, P., Toldra-Simats, A., & Zingales, L. (2013). Understanding trust. *The Economic Journal*, 123(573), 1313–1332. https://doi.org/10.1111/ecoj .12036

Seppanen, R., Blomqvist, K., & Sundqvist, S. (2007). Measuring inter-organizational trust: A critical review of the empirical research in 1990–2003. *Industrial Marketing Management*, 36(2), 249–265. https://doi .org/10.1016/j.indmarman.2005.09.003

Simpson, J. A. (2007). Foundations of interpersonal trust. In A. W. Kruglanski & E. T. Higgins (Eds.), *Social psychology: Handbook of basic principles* (pp. 587–607). The Guilford Press.

Swan, J. E., Bowers, M. R., & Richardson, L. D. (1999). Customer trust in the salesperson: An integrative review and meta-analysis of the empirical literature. *Journal of Business Research*, 44(2), 93–107. https://doi.org/10.1016/S0148-2963(97)00244-0

Tzieropoulos, H. (2013). The trust game in neuroscience: A short review. *Social Neuroscience*, 8(5), 407–416. https://doi.org/10.1080/17470919.2013.832375

Uslaner, E. M. (2018). *The Oxford handbook of social and political trust*. Oxford University Press.

Zak, P. J., & Knack, S. (2001). Trust and growth. *The Economic Journal*, 111(470), 295–321. https://doi.org/10.1111/1468-0297.00609

Zmerli, S., & Meer, T. W. G. v. d. (2017). *Handbook on political trust*. Edward Elgar.

PART I

Fundamental Level of Trust

CHAPTER I

Trust and Psychology
Psychological Theories and Principles Underlying Interpersonal Trust

Jeffry A. Simpson and Grace Vieth

I.I Introduction

Trust: "confidence that [one] will find what is desired [from another] rather than what is feared."

(Deutsch, 1973, p. 148)

As indicated in this well-known quote, trust involves the delicate balance of people's brightest hopes relative to their darkest fears. Being able to trust partners is often a prerequisite to developing and maintaining stable, satisfying relationships across the life span. Indeed, several major theories, including attachment theory (Bowlby, 1969) and Erikson's (1963) theory of psychosocial development, are based on the premise that experiencing higher levels of trust with close others, particularly early in life, can lay the groundwork for happier, better-functioning relationships in adulthood. Moreover, evolutionary theorists have proposed that psychological mechanisms associated with the expression and detection of trust evolved in humans given the need to assess the intentions of others well and accurately (Tooby & Cosmides, 1996).

While there have been pockets of important theoretical and empirical work on interpersonal trust within the field of psychology, much remains unknown about how, when, and why trust develops, is maintained, and sometimes unravels. Why, therefore, has trust received relatively modest attention within psychology? There are several probable reasons. First, trust is a complex, multidimensional construct, which makes it challenging to operationalize, measure, and interpret in many instances. Second, trust is likely to assume differential importance in different types of relationships (e.g., friendships, work relationships, and romantic relationships) and at different stages of their development. Third, trust develops and changes in situations that are often challenging to study, such as in "strain-test"

Corresponding author: Jeffry A. Simpson (simps108@umn.edu).

situations (Holmes, 1981). In strain-test situations, one person is highly dependent on their partner, but the actions that would promote an individual's own best interests are at odds with those that would benefit their partner. If, for example, John desperately needs Amanda's help to achieve an important personal goal and Amanda gladly helps, even though providing help impedes an important goal that she wants to accomplish, Amanda has "passed" a strain test, which should lead John to trust her more.

In this chapter, we first review several theoretical accounts of interpersonal trust and identify some of the key principles that anchor our current understanding of trust within the field of psychology. Next, we describe a dyadic model of trust informed by these theories that integrates many of these principles. Following this, we provide a representative overview of recent research on trust within the psychological literature, revealing how it operates in different types of relationships (e.g., with strangers, coworkers, family members, friends, and romantic partners). We conclude the chapter by suggesting some future directions in which research on trust might head.

1.2   Theories and Principles of Trust

Over the years, interpersonal trust within the field of psychology has been conceptualized in two basic ways. Most early work adopted a dispositional (person-centered) view of trust in which it was presumed to be reflected in a person's global attitudes, beliefs, and expectations about the extent to which other people tend to be reliable, cooperative, or helpful in various social contexts (e.g., Deutsch, 1973; Rotter, 1971). Conceptualizations and measures of trust, however, became more partner- and relationship-focused in the 1980s (e.g., Holmes & Rempel, 1989; Rempel et al., 1985). According to this interpersonal (dyadic) viewpoint, trust reflects the psychological orientation of an actor (the truster) toward a specific partner (the trustee) with whom the actor is interdependent to some degree (i.e., the truster needs the trustee's help to obtain valued resources or good outcomes). What makes trust challenging to investigate is that it contains three components (e.g., "*I* trust *you* to do *X*"; Hardin, 2003). Trust, in other words, depends on properties of the self (I), the specific partner (you), *and* the current situation (to do X).

Consistent with these ideas, Kramer and Carnevale (2001) claim that trust entails a set of beliefs, expectations, and attributions that a partner's future actions will benefit one's own best interests consistently across time,

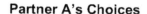

Partner A's Choices

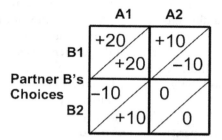

Figure 1.1   The payoffs (outcomes) in a trust-relevant situation.

especially in situations in which a person needs to rely on their partner to achieve important goals and outcomes. These types of trust-relevant situations often launch two psychological processes: (1) feelings of vulnerability and (2) anticipating how the partner will behave. Particularly when a partner consistently supports and facilitates what is best for an individual instead of what is best for themselves, *both* partners – but particularly the person who benefits – should trust one another more. In addition, trust should be greater when (1) both partners' self-interested outcomes are closely aligned with those that would be best for their relationship and/or (2) both individuals are confident that their *partner* will do what is best for their relationship, even when the partner's self-interests differ.

Employing principles from interdependence theory (Kelley & Thibaut, 1978; Thibaut & Kelley, 1959), Kelley and his colleagues (2003) propose that the proper degree of trust to be placed in a partner can be ascertained more accurately in certain types of situations, especially in trust-relevant situations. Trust-relevant situations, which also include "stag hunt" and "assurance" experimental paradigms within game theory (see also Chapter 2), usually contain high levels of interdependence (i.e., each partner's thoughts, feelings, and actions are strongly affected by the other), a mixture of rules that promote coordination and exchange (which maintain interdependence between partners in the relationship), and partners experiencing moderately corresponding (i.e., similar) interests (see Kelley et al., 2003). A prototypical trust-relevant situation examined within the psychological literature is shown in Figure 1.1. In this situation, trust typically increases when relationship partners repeatedly make A1/B1 (i.e., mutually beneficial) decisions that repeatedly result in the most reward for *both* partners.

Payoffs above the diagonal in each cell are for partner A; those below the diagonal are for partner B. If both partners choose option 1 (e.g., they work together on a difficult but important task, shown in the A1/B1 cell), each partner receives 20 units of benefit because the task gets done and partners spend time together. If both partners select option 2 (neither works on the task, indicated by the A2/B2 cell), neither partner receives benefits because nothing gets done. If partner A chooses option 2 (not to work on the task: A2) but partner B chooses option 1 (works solo on the task: B1), partner A benefits by 10 units because progress is made on the task, but partner B experiences a loss of 10 units because they must do all of the work. The reverse pattern exists when partner A chooses A1 (to work on the task) and partner B chooses B2 (to not work on the task). Most trust-relevant situations have three unique properties. First, cooperative behavior on the part of both partners (A1/B1) always yields better outcomes than when partners do not cooperate (A1/B2 or A2/B1). Second, the best outcome always occurs when both partners make the cooperative choice (A1/B1). Third, cooperative choices are risky; if one's partner makes a noncooperative choice, making a cooperative choice generates the worst possible outcomes for the exploited individual.

To date, the bulk of empirical research on trust within the psychological literature has been guided by dispositional or interpersonal approaches. Much of the dispositionally focused work has confirmed that people who are more insecurely attached or have lower self-esteem tend to trust their relationship partners less on average (see Simpson, 2007). Most of the interpersonally focused work has revealed that trust is higher when individuals believe their partners are committed to the relationship, have benevolent intentions toward them, and possess pro-relationship goals and motivations. Trust also tends to be higher when partners display pro-relationship transformations of motivation by translating their initially negative feelings about the potentially destructive actions of their partners into constructive responses that benefit the partner or the relationship. These transformed reactions often result in self-sacrificial or accommodative behaviors that serve to maintain or improve the relationship. Moreover, the development of trust typically involves a process of uncertainty reduction whereby individuals shift from being confident in their partner's general predictability (e.g., "I know what my partner will do in this situation") to having confidence in their partner's pro-relationship values, motives, goals, and intentions (e.g., "I know that my partner will do what's best for me and/or our relationship in this situation"; see Holmes & Rempel, 1989).

Recent, broad reviews of the interpersonal trust literature within psychology (e.g., Dunning et al., 2019; Simpson, 2007; Van Lange, 2015) have identified a set of core principles of interpersonal trust, several of which emerge from the research discussed above:

1. Trust develops primarily in response to social interaction experiences with others, including people in one's social networks and exposure to media.

2. It is adaptive to regulate, monitor, and change the amount of trust placed in others.

3. People frequently underestimate how trustworthy other people are, but they report being willing to place trust in others at least initially, including strangers (see Dunning et al., 2019; for exceptions, see also Chapter 2).

4. Individuals determine how much they can trust their partners by observing whether they display transformation of motivation in *trust-diagnostic* situations, such as in trust-relevant, stag-hunt, or strain-test situations where partners can make decisions that go against their own self-interest and support the best interests of their partner and/or relationship.

5. Although trust-diagnostic situations occasionally occur in everyday life, individuals may enter or create trust-diagnostic situations to test whether their current level of trust in their partner is justified.

6. Individual differences associated with attachment security versus insecurity and high versus low self-esteem (among other variables) can affect changes in trust over time in relationships. For example, people who are securely attached or have higher self-esteem tend to report higher levels of trust and increases in trust more often in their relationships.

7. Neither the level nor the trajectory of trust in relationships can be fully understood without considering the dispositions and actions of *both* relationship partners.

1.3 The Dyadic Model of Trust in Relationships

A dyadic model specifying how several of these core principles interrelate and operate during social interactions is shown in Figure 1.2. The dyadic model of trust in relationships (Simpson, 2007) contains two basic components: normative components (shown in the boxes in the middle of the

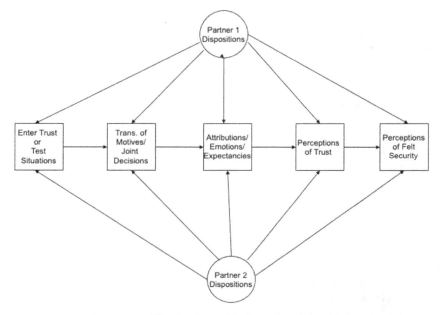

Figure 1.2   The dyadic model of trust in relationships
(Simpson, 2007).

figure) and individual difference components (represented at the top and
bottom of the figure). The individual difference components reflect the
trust-relevant dispositions of *each* relationship partner (e.g., their
attachment orientations, self-esteem, etc.) along with their associations
with each normative construct in the model. Feedback loops from the
terminal construct in the model on the far right (each partner's degree of
felt security following an interaction with their partner) to the construct
that launches the next interaction (each partner's decision about whether
or not to enter the next trust-relevant situation) are not shown, but are
presumed to exist. According to the model, each individual's perceptions
of their own *and* their partner's standing on each construct partially
explain each partner's reactions to each of the downstream constructs in
the model.

     The model also assumes that knowledge of the trust-relevant disposi-
tions of *both* partners is necessary to understand the growth of trust (or
lack of it) in a relationship over numerous interactions. The dispositional
tendencies mentioned above ought to motivate or enable individuals to
enter, transform, and occasionally create social interactions that either

increase or decrease trust over time. Two general types of situations should provide good opportunities to gauge the amount of trust warranted in a partner or relationship: (1) *trust-relevant situations* (Kelley et al., 2003) in which partners are able to repeatedly make (or fail to make) mutually beneficial A1/B1 decisions (see Figure 1.1) and (2) *strain-test* situations (Holmes, 1981), where partners are able to demonstrate (or not demonstrate) their willingness to make personal sacrifices for the good of their partner or relationship. However, before these *trust-diagnostic* situations are entered, transformed, or created, one or both partners must have enough confidence to take the interpersonal risks required to confirm or reaffirm that their partner is trustworthy. People who have positive working models (i.e., those who harbor positive attitudes and expectations about themselves and their relationship partners), such as securely attached people or those with high self-esteem, should be more likely to take these interpersonal risks.

Once they are in trust-diagnostic situations, individuals who are willing to make decisions that benefit the partner or relationship at some cost to themselves should experience greater trust and felt security. Moreover, partners with positive working models should display partner- or relationship-based transformations of motivation more regularly and extensively. As a result, they should be more able and motivated to steer trust-relevant social interactions toward mutually beneficial decisions and outcomes. After these decisions are made, working models should affect how individuals perceive the amount of transformation that they and their partner have undergone. Individuals who have positive working models may often give themselves and their partners more credit for each partner's willingness to prioritize partner and/or relationship goals and outcomes over personal goals and outcomes compared to those who have negative models (Murray et al., 2006).

This process should then generate benevolent attributions for one's own as well as the partner's relationship motives. For example, after Amanda willingly makes a major personal sacrifice to help John complete his important task, John should realize that he needs and values Amanda and their relationship, and that she truly cares for him. These attributions should stimulate constructive problem-solving, better emotion regulation, and more positive expectations about their future trust-diagnostic interactions. Patterns of attributions, emotion regulation, and situation-specific expectancies are portrayed in a single box in Figure 1.2 because the temporal order of these processes may depend on the unique features of a given interaction, the working models of each partner, and/or idiosyncratic norms or characteristics of their relationship. Collectively, these positive outcomes should sustain or increase perceptions of trust, which ought to increase felt security at least temporarily. This in turn should set up the next trust-relevant interaction, affecting whether, when, and how it is entered, transformed, or created.

On many occasions, individuals may enter trust-relevant or strain-test situations without premeditated thought or deliberately trying to do so. However, deliberate attempts to enter or create these situations should take place when important, unexpected, or suspicious events lead individuals to question whether they can continue to trust their partners. Although these interactions may be highly diagnostic, deliberate "tests" are not likely to be conducted very often given the harm they could pose to most relationships.

Across time, partners who repeatedly make and experience mutually beneficial outcomes should perceive greater "added value" due to their pro-relationship choices (see Figure 1.1), especially in trust-diagnostic situations. These repeated outcomes are likely to encourage both partners to continue to engage in relationship-sustaining or relationship-building acts (e.g., disparaging attractive alternative partners, perceiving the partner in a highly positive manner), which should sustain or facilitate mutually beneficial decisions and outcomes in the future. These effects should diminish, however, if one or both partners have negative working models, decide *not* to enter into mutually beneficial agreements, or harbor negative attributions regarding their partner's relationship-relevant goals and motives.

1.4   Recent Research on Interpersonal Trust

Trust and the underlying processes that generate, maintain, and deteriorate it are relevant to different types of relationships, ranging from brief interactions with strangers to our most intimate close relationships with family members (Simpson, 2007). These different types of relationships, however, vary on several major dimensions. They include (1) the degree to which relationships are voluntary (e.g., romantic relationships) or involuntary (e.g., family and coworker relationships), (2) the unique role expectations for each partner (e.g., parents versus their children, romantic partners, and close friends), and (3) the power dynamics involved (e.g., relatively unequal power in most parent–child dyads and most supervisor–supervisee relationships, but more equal power between romantic partners and close friends). Although the basic principles reviewed above tend to hold across different types of relationships, they have some unique features and corresponding outcomes. Thus, we now review recent research on trust, beginning with relationships that are less close (trust in strangers) and moving to closer relationships, ending with perhaps the most intimate (trust in romantic partners).

1.4.1 Trust in Strangers

Given limited information about someone, what leads people to trust and what warns them to act in a self-protective manner? Some recent work on interpersonal trust, trust in strangers, sheds light on the situations and characteristics of strangers that promote or impede the development of trust. While we do not cover a wide range of the literature on trust games (TGs) (see also Chapter 2), research utilizing TGs has also informed how trust functions at a more distal level (Johnson & Mislin, 2011).

One of the many ways in which trustworthiness can be signaled is by expressing care or concern about contentious social issues. Across a number of studies, people were more likely to trust those who care about important social issues than those who do not. This is especially true for integrity-based trust. People are also more likely to trust those who hold conflicting beliefs about social issues compared to those who do not (Zlatev, 2019). Other studies have focused on characteristics of the individual who is trusting rather than the characteristics of a stranger in calibrating trust levels. For example, people who score high on the Big 5 personality trait of openness to experience are more trusting of people who are culturally dissimilar to them (Saef et al., 2019). Furthermore, older adults are perceived as more trustworthy and they tend to be more trusting in experimental TGs (Greiner & Zednik, 2019).

According to Van Lange et al. (2014), generalized trust in both the self and others has weaker roots in genetics than is true of other constructs such as many personality traits and cognitive abilities. This is consistent with prior theories, which suggest that trust develops and is maintained primarily through interpersonal processes that reinforce or challenge working models (i.e., cognitive schemas) associated with trust. Personality traits and life circumstances, however, can also shape the development of trust. For instance, childhood socioeconomic status (SES) has been linked to trust levels in adulthood (Stamos et al., 2019). Stamos and colleagues suggest that life history theory may partially explain the connection between childhood SES and trust in adulthood. Life history theory is an evolutionary-based theory of individual differences that develop across the life span as individuals make trade-offs depending on the resources that are available to them (Del Giudice et al., 2016; Simpson & Belsky, 2016). People who grow up in lower SES environments typically encounter more threats, which usually makes them hyperaware of their surroundings and more distrustful of others in general. Income inequality and life satisfaction inequality are also associated with social trust, with the link between income inequality and social trust being mediated by life satisfaction inequality (Graafland & Lous, 2019). These studies highlight that both the environments in which individuals grow up and the ones they currently inhabit can shape the development of trust in other people, particularly strangers.

Finally, trust in strangers is also shaped by the limited interaction that people have with strangers. Such interactions may influence trust through the behavior exhibited by the stranger, which may leave the trustee feeling wary. One way in which strangers may increase their trustworthiness is by sharing information. People who receive an interesting piece of gossip, for example, tend to experience an increase in trust toward the person who confided in them. However, the accuracy of the information shared also influences how trustworthy one perceives the discloser to be. Although higher levels of inaccuracy hinder the formation of trust, misinformation, at least within limits, tends to generate higher levels of trust than sharing no information at all (Fonseca & Peters, 2018). This does not imply that people who trust strangers are more susceptible to deception; those who trust others more are often more skilled at detecting lies than those who trust others less (Carter & Weber, 2010).

1.4.2   Trust in Workplace Relationships

A substantial amount of recent work in psychology has focused on trust within work environments. Whether it be trust between coworkers or trust between an employee and their supervisor, trust is an important component of daily workplace dynamics. One important distinction to consider is that, unlike voluntary relationships, most people do not choose their coworkers yet often must trust them to some degree in order to facilitate cohesion and comradery at work. Trust in the workplace also introduces the dynamic of unique social roles and power differentials. Thus, the psychological experience of trust with coworkers may be different than other types of relationships.

Just as trust is a key social lubricant in interpersonal situations with strangers, research has confirmed that it also is important when navigating work negotiations. Although small talk may seem inconsequential in many everyday interactions, it often enhances trust between coworkers in the workplace (Mislin et al., 2011).

In addition, the impact of trust in the workplace stretches well beyond negotiations. How individuals manage team projects can differ greatly depending on how much intra-team trust exists between members on a project. For example, in a recent meta-analysis of team performance, intra-team trust significantly predicted team performance, and this effect was stronger when task interdependence was high (De Jong et al., 2016).

How accurate team members are in gauging their teammates' trust in them is another way in which intra-team trust can be affected. Greater trust meta-accuracy (i.e., how accurate people are in estimating how much team members trust them) is associated with higher levels of trust at later points in time. However, people who are less accurate in their estimations of how much their teammates trust them – specifically those who over-estimate their teammates' trust in them – report lower levels of trust over time (Brion et al., 2015). This suggests that not only is trust in coworkers important; so too is how accurate one is at perceiving coworkers' trust in them.

The degree to which coworkers trust each other is important, but what may be even more critical is how supervisors are perceived as viewing their employees. Feeling trusted versus distrusted by a supervisor can shade how employees view many experiences, which can have either positive or negative effects on numerous workplace outcomes. Indeed, being trusted by a manager and trusting in a manager generally leads to positive work outcomes, including better organizational citizenship behavior (Brower et al., 2009). Lau and colleagues (2014) clarified the mechanism through which feeling trusted yields better work outcomes. Two aspects of trust were examined: feeling relied on and being disclosed to by one's supervisor. Disclosure did not affect work performance, but employees who believed that their supervisor could rely on them had better work performance, which was mediated by having higher esteem for the organization.

Similar to how individuals gauge their teammates' level of trust in them, workplace leaders also estimate their employees' degree of trust in them. Campagna and colleagues (2020) examined what factors lead to increases in trust meta-accuracy among leaders and whether certain factors are associated with positive relational outcomes with employees. Leaders' meta-accuracy was influenced most strongly by how much they trusted specific employees, suggesting that trust tends to be reciprocal. Leaders' perceptions of who trusted them were influenced most strongly by whom they (leaders) trusted. In terms of relational outcomes, leaders who accurately detect that an employee does not trust them tend to have greater relationship conflict with that employee. In sum, people frequently gauge coworkers' trust in them and also how much they can trust their coworkers and supervisors, both of which can have a clear impact on team and workplace dynamics.

1.4.3   Trust in Family and Friends

Moving toward closer and more intimate relationships, we now focus on trust with family and friends, which has been studied less frequently than other types of relationships within the psychological literature. The role of trust within families is unique because many people are likely to expect a higher level of trust between most (but not all) family members. Furthermore, trust between parents and their children across developmental stages, between siblings, and among extended family members is likely to differ in its development and maintenance. Recent work, for example, has highlighted how parenthood can change people's levels of trust in others by making most parents less trusting of strangers (Eibach & Mock, 2011). Furthermore, greater trust in partners can make the typically stressful transition to parenthood easier. For example, new mothers and fathers who report greater trust in their partner before the birth of their first child also report smoother transitions to parenthood (Ter Kuile et al., 2017).

Within many families, a reasonably high level of trust is often assumed to exist, yet people still gauge the trustworthiness of their family members. Trustworthiness in nuclear familial relationships has been indexed by how much self-control each family member has, as perceived by other family members. In general, family members tend to trust other family members more when they are perceived to have greater self-control (i.e., the ability to refrain from undesirable behavior) (Buyukcan-Tetik et al., 2015). Unique family dynamics can also shape our trust in other family members. The number of siblings a person has, for example, can affect their generalized trust in other people, with individuals who have four or more siblings reporting lower generalized trust than those with no siblings (Yucel, 2013).

Friendship and trust have also received relatively little attention within psychology. Among the relatively few studies that have been conducted, Freitag and Bauer (2016) examined how personality traits are associated with trust in both friends and strangers. For some personality traits (e.g., openness and conscientiousness), there were no differences in perceived trust between friends and strangers. For others (e.g., agreeableness), however, there was a difference, with higher agreeableness being associated with greater trust in strangers, but less so in friends.

1.4.4   Trust in Romantic Relationships

Within the psychological literature, trust has most frequently been studied in the context of romantic relationships, with most work investigating how chronic levels of trust affect commitment, evaluations of one's partner, self-protective motives, and what occurs during discussions when partners disagree on a topic or issue. Murray and colleagues (2011), for example, have examined how different types of trust – impulsive (implicit) trust and reflective (explicit) trust – are associated with self-protection tendencies. Impulsive trust is a person's immediate, visceral evaluation of their partner's trustworthiness, presumably reflecting their automatic trust attitudes with respect to their partner. Reflective trust, by comparison, involves more conscious, deliberative evaluations of the partner's trustworthiness. In a series of studies, Murray et al. (2011) found that impulsive and reflective trust interact to affect self-protection tendencies in romantic relationships. For example, when reflective trust toward one's partner is low, higher levels of impulsive trust reduce relationship concerns and lower self-protection motivations. But when individuals are lower on impulsive trust, their level of reflective trust is more impactful and leads people to behave in a more self-protective manner. Thus, both impulsive and reflective trust are important to consider to understand when and why romantic partners take self-protective actions.

Using a behavioral observation paradigm, Shallcross and Simpson (2012) examined trust's connection to behaving in a more versus less accommodating way toward one's partner in strain-test situations (i.e., when one partner requests a major sacrifice from the other). Shallcross and Simpson had romantic couples discuss stain-test topics identified by each partner. Their discussions were video-recorded and then rated by trained observers for the amount of accommodation and compromise displayed by both partners. Greater accommodation displayed by askers (the partner requesting a sacrifice) and by responders (the partner responding to the request) predicted increases in self-reported levels of trust during the discussion. Moreover, partners who both scored higher in chronic trust entering the discussion felt closer to each other at its conclusion. Chronic levels of trust, therefore, play an important role in shaping how these difficult and taxing discussions unfold. For an example of how trust is commonly studied in interpersonal relationships within psychology, see footnote.[1]

In a study examining how romantic partners attempt to resolve major conflicts, Kim and colleagues (2015) had couples (both partners) report how close they felt to their partner both before and after a video-recorded conflict discussion. It was only during conflict discussions in which both partners were high on chronic trust that partners reported increases in feelings of closeness at the end of the discussion. Cast another way, when one partner in the relationship was less trusting, both partners reported lower levels of closeness following the conflict discussion. This highlights the trouble that just one low-trust partner can create during difficult discussions.

Campbell and colleagues (2010) examined the impact of trust during conflict on relationship evaluations across time, focusing on fluctuations in relationship evaluations in relation to each partner's level of trust. People low in trust reported greater variability in their evaluations of relationship quality gathered as part of daily diary reports over two weeks. Furthermore, low-trust partners reported more negative feelings on days when relationship conflict was high than was true of high-trust partners. Those with more trusting partners also reported more stable evaluations of the quality of their relationship. Lower levels of trust, therefore, can shape relationship processes and outcomes over time.

Duchies and colleagues (2013) demonstrated that one's degree of trust also affects memories of partners. People high in trust might benefit from positive memory biases involving their partners by remembering prior partner transgressions as being less severe, less frequent, or less damaging than is true of low-trust partners. Indeed, high-trust partners do remember relationship conflicts with a relationship-promoting bias rather than a self-protective bias. Thus, one's level of trust can slant partner perceptions and relationship evaluations in theoretically meaningful ways.

---

[1] Shallcross and Simpson (2012) provides a good example of common methods utilized to study trust in dyadic interactions among romantic partners. In this study, both partners in each relationship first completed a measure assessing their level of trust in their partner on the Trust Scale (Rempel et al., 1985). They then completed a video-recorded strain-test discussion. Strain-test discussions require each partner to choose and then discuss something they really want to do or accomplish that would require a significant sacrifice from their partner. During the study, each partner had one discussion in which they were the "asker" of a sacrifice and one in which they were the "responder" to their partner who was asking them for a sacrifice. Before and after each discussion, each partner also completed a state trust measure. Following the entire study, trained coders watched the videos of each discussion and rated both partners on their degree of accommodation to their partner when they were in the "responder" role along with several other constructs. Each partner's level of trust was then examined in relation to the degree of accommodation and other outcomes.

Not only does trust influence behaviors during conflict discussions; it also affects what follows relationship turmoil, particularly the tendency to forgive. Moulden and Finkel (2010) examined the connection between trust and forgiveness. Forgiving one's partner usually requires good self-regulation, which may depend in part on the level of trust that one has in their partner to repair the relationship and provide future benefits. In a longitudinal study of couples, Molden and Finkel found that partners who have a promotion-focus toward their relationships were more likely to have forgiven their partner for a past transgression if they were higher in trust. However, for partners who had a prevention-focus toward their relationship, commitment to the relationship was a better predictor of forgiveness than their level of trust. These findings are consistent with the notion that, amid relational transgressions, higher trust allows people to look forward to future benefits that their partner is likely to provide them, despite the risk of future betrayal.

Just as different levels of trust operate as a lens through which partners and relationships are viewed, different levels of trust may also generate reciprocal cycles that result in other relationship-promoting or -hindering behaviors. One example is self-concealment – the deliberate hiding of information. Exploring this topic, Uysal and colleagues (2012) asked romantic partners how much they perceived that their partner concealed things from them in addition to their own self-concealment efforts from their partner. Self-reports of perceived partner concealment (believing that one's partner is keeping secrets) and actual concealment (a partner's acknowledgment that they were keeping information or secrets from their partner) revealed a cyclical pattern, such that when an individual perceived that their partner was concealing something from them, their level of trust decreased, and they then engaged in greater self-concealment themselves.

On the flip side, the level of trust also appears to impact people's willingness to engage in self-disclosure with their partners. People high on self-esteem and agreeableness, for example, are more likely to self-disclose to their partners. McCarthy et al. (2017), however, revealed that this effect is mediated by each partner's degree of trusting. Thus, just as higher levels of trust allow people to see past their partner's transgressions and expect good future benefits, greater trust also permits people to have greater confidence that their partners will respond to their self-disclosures with greater understanding and care. Notably, this same pattern emerged for self-disclosure between roommates, the majority of whom were same-sex friends.

To date, most studies have focused on the distinction between low-trust and high-trust people's behaviors and evaluations in different situations. What has received less attention is how individuals involved with low-trust partners change their own behavior to adapt to the needs of their low-trust partner or attempt to buffer them so their own trust does not decline further. According to Cortes and Wood (2019), people with low-trust partners may need to be gentler in how they comfort and convey care to them. People who doubt their partner's love and report lower levels of trust tend to experience more relationship difficulties. This may force the partners of low-trust individuals to engage in more tailoring of their behavior to convey stronger, more consistent, and "genuine" care. Individuals who score lower in self-esteem and trust often have a harder time accepting such overtures (Kille et al., 2017). Thus, to identify effective, nonthreatening forms of partner care and support, Cortes and Wood (2019) examined the responses of low-trust individuals when their partners were simply told to ask them "How was your day?" This simple, subtle way of displaying care proved to be an effective way to convey care to low-trust partners without activating their relationship worries or defenses.

1.5   Summary, Future Directions, and Conclusion

Interpersonal trust poses some unique theoretical puzzles because trust in total strangers violates rational-actor models (see Dunning et al., 2019). Indeed, many people routinely underestimate how trustworthy other people actually are, yet they are willing to place a reasonable amount of initial trust in others, including total strangers. To resolve this paradox, Dunning and colleagues suggest that people trust at higher-than-expected rates because they feel strong social obligation to do so. Most people, therefore, are not really "giving" trust as much as they are "giving in" to social pressures to trust others to some degree. A large body of psychological research has documented four major findings associated with trust (Van Lange, 2015): (1) Based on prior twin studies, trusting other people stems more from culture than genetics (see also Chapter 15); (2) trust emanates mainly from social interaction experiences, including people's social networks and their exposure to media; (3) in the context of close relationships, most people place less trust in their partners than is warranted; and (4) it is adaptive to regulate, monitor, and change the level of trust placed in people.

Nevertheless, our understanding of how trust is instigated, sustained, and broken in different types of relationships remains surprisingly limited within the psychological literature. Future theory and research need to address several important issues. First, we need to understand how the dispositions and behaviors of *both* partners in a relationship shape the way in which each partner thinks, feels, and acts, especially in trust-relevant situations. Second, we need to explore how and why certain unique combinations of partner attributes facilitate or hinder the development and maintenance of trust. For example, relationships in which one partner has more power than the other might impede the development of trust if the powerful person continually takes advantage of the less powerful partner, but this combination might yield greater trust if the high-power partner consistently acts in the best interest of the low-power partner. Third, we need to determine whether the dyadic model of trust in relationships operates the same way at different stages of relationship development and across different types of relationships. Fourth, we need to examine how normative processes and individual differences *reciprocally* influence each other over time, particularly in trust-relevant situations. Fifth, we must disentangle the constructs and processes depicted in the middle part of the model (i.e., attributions/emotions/expectancies). Variables associated with the development of intimacy, such as feeling understood, validated, and cared for by one's partner, may also play a significant role in promoting trust and felt security (Reis & Shaver, 1988), especially when they occur in trust-relevant interactions. Finally, we know relatively little about how trust functions within familial relationships and friendships.

In conclusion, trust reflects the delicate juxtaposition of people's brightest hopes in relation to their worst fears. Being able to trust others is a fundamental prerequisite for establishing and maintaining various types of stable, satisfying relationships. While there has been some important theoretical and empirical work on interpersonal trust within psychology, we still do not know nearly enough about how, when, and why trust develops between two people, how it is maintained, and how and why it sometimes disintegrates. Psychological models such as the dyadic model of trust in relationships, along with the empirical findings reviewed earlier, have begun to elucidate the key variables, constructs, and interpersonal processes that lead people to trust or distrust significant others in different types of relationships. Our hope is that this overview will help future scholars interested in the neurobiology of trust gain deeper insights into the role that different areas of the brain play in the formation, maintenance, and deterioration of this critical construct.

References

Bowlby, J. (1969). *Attachment and loss: Vol. 1. Attachment.* Basic Books.

Brion, S., Lount, R. B., & Doyle, S. P. (2015). Knowing if you are trusted: Does meta-accuracy promote trust development? *Social Psychological and Personality Science,* 6(7), 823–830. https://doi.org/10.1177/1948550615590200

Brower, H. H., Lester, S. W., Korsgaard, M. A., & Dineen, B. R. (2009). A closer look at trust between managers and subordinates: Understanding the effects of both trusting and being trusted on subordinate outcomes. *Journal of Management,* 35(2), 327–347. https://doi.org/10.1177/0149206307312511

Buyukcan-Tetik, A., Finkenauer, C., Siersema, M., Vander Heyden, K., & Krabbendam, L. (2015). Social relations model analyses of perceived self-control and trust in families. *Journal of Marriage and Family,* 77(1), 209–223. https://doi.org/10.1111/jomf.12154

Campagna, R. L., Dirks, K. T., Knight, A. P., Crossley, C., & Robinson, S. L. (2020). On the relation between felt trust and actual trust: Examining pathways to and implications of leader trust meta-accuracy. *Journal of Applied Psychology,* 105(9), 994–1012. https://doi.org/10.1037/apl0000474

Campbell, L., Simpson, J. A., Boldry, J. G., & Rubin, H. (2010). Trust, variability in relationship evaluations, and relationship processes. *Journal of Personality and Social Psychology,* 99(1), 14–31. https://doi.org/10.1037/a0019714

Carter, N. L., & Weber, J. M. (2010). Not pollyannas: Higher generalized trust predicts lie detection ability. *Social Psychological and Personality Science,* 1(3), 274–279. https://doi.org/10.1177/1948550609360261

Cortes, K., & Wood, J. V. (2019). How was your day? Conveying care, but under the radar, for people lower in trust. *Journal of Experimental Social Psychology,* 83, 11–22. https://doi.org/10.1016/j.jesp.2019.03.003

De Jong, B. A., Dirks, K. T., & Gillespie, N. (2016). Trust and team performance: A meta-analysis of main effects, moderators, and covariates. *Journal of Applied Psychology,* 101(8), 1134–1150. https://doi.org/10.1037/apl0000110

Del Giudice, M., Gangestad, S. W., & Kaplan, H. S. (2016). Life history theory and evolutionary psychology. In D. M. Buss (Ed.), *The handbook of evolutionary psychology: Foundations* (pp. 88–114). John Wiley & Sons Inc.

Deutsch, M. (1973). *The resolution of conflict.* Yale University Press.

Dunning, D., Fetchenhauer, D., & Schlösser, T. (2019). Why people trust: Solved puzzles and open mysteries. *Current Directions in Psychological Science,* 28(4), 366–371. https://doi.org/10.1177/0963721419838255

Eibach, R. P., & Mock, S. E. (2011). The vigilant parent: Parental role salience affects parents' risk perceptions, risk-aversion, and trust in strangers. *Journal of Experimental Social Psychology,* 47(3), 694–697. https://doi.org/10.1016/j.jesp.2010.12.009

Erikson, E. (1963). *Childhood and society.* W. W Norton & Company.

Fonseca, M. A., & Peters, K. (2018). Will any gossip do? Gossip does not need to be perfectly accurate to promote trust. *Games and Economic Behavior*, 107, 253–281. https://doi.org/10.1016/j.geb.2017.09.015

Freitag, M., & Bauer, P. C. (2016). Personality traits and the propensity to trust friends and strangers. *The Social Science Journal*, 53(4), 467–476. https://doi.org/10.1016/j.soscij.2015.12.002

Graafland, J., & Lous, B. (2019). Income inequality, life satisfaction inequality and trust: A cross country panel analysis. *Journal of Happiness Studies*, 20(6), 1717–1737. https://doi.org/10.1007/s10902-018-0021-0

Greiner, B., & Zednik, A. (2019). Trust and age: An experiment with current and former students. *Economics Letters*, 181, 37–39. https://doi.org/10.1016/j.econlet.2019.04.004

Hardin, R. (2003). Gaming trust. In E. Ostrom & J. Walker (Eds.), *Trust and reciprocity: Interdisciplinary lessons from experimental research* (pp. 80–101). Russell Sage Foundation.

Holmes, J. G. (1981). The exchange process in close relationships: Microbehavior and macromotives. In M. J. Lerner & S. C. Lerner (Eds.), *The justice motive in social behavior* (pp. 261–284). Plenum.

Holmes, J. G., & Rempel, J. K. (1989). Trust in close relationships. In C. Hendrick (Ed.), *Close relationships* (pp. 187–220). Sage.

Johnson, N. D., & Mislin, A. A. (2011). Trust games: A meta-analysis. *Journal of Economic Psychology*, 32, 865–889. https://doi.org/10.1016/j.joep.2011.05.007

Kelley, H. H., Holmes, J. G., Kerr, N. L., Reis, H. T., Rusbult, C. E., & Van Lange, P. A. M. (2003). *An atlas of interpersonal situations*. Cambridge University Press.

Kelley, H. H., & Thibaut, J. W. (1978). *Interpersonal relations: A theory of interdependence*. Wiley.

Kille, D. R., Eibach, R. P., Wood, J. V., & Holmes, J. G. (2017). Who can't take a compliment? The role of construal level and self-esteem in accepting positive feedback from close others. *Journal of Experimental Social Psychology*, 68, 40–49. https://doi.org/10.1016/j.jesp.2016.05.003

Kim, J. S., Weisberg, Y. J., Simpson, J. A., Oriña, M. M., Farrell, A. K., & Johnson, W. F. (2015). Ruining it for both of us: The disruptive role of low-trust partners on conflict resolution in romantic relationships. *Social Cognition*, 33(5), 520–542. https://doi.org/10.1521/soco.2015.33.5.520

Kramer, R. M., & Carnevale, P. J. (2001). Trust and intergroup negotiation. In R. Brown & S. Gaertner (Eds.), *Blackwell handbook of social psychology: Intergroup processes* (pp. 431–450). Blackwell.

Lau, D. C., Lam, L. W., & Wen, S. S. (2014). Examining the effects of feeling trusted by supervisors in the workplace: A self-evaluative perspective. *Journal of Organizational Behavior*, 35(1), 112–127. https://doi.org/10.1002/job.1861

Luchies, L. B., Wieselquist, J., Rusbult, C. E., et al. (2013). Trust and biased memory of transgressions in romantic relationships. *Journal of Personality and Social Psychology*, 104(4), 673–694. https://doi.org/10.1037/a0031054

McCarthy, M. H., Wood, J. V., & Holmes, J. G. (2017). Dispositional pathways to trust: Self-esteem and agreeableness interact to predict trust and negative emotional disclosure. *Journal of Personality and Social Psychology*, 113(1), 95–116. https://doi.org/10.1037/pspi0000093

Mislin, A. A., Campagna, R. L., & Bottom, W. P. (2011). After the deal: Talk, trust building and the implementation of negotiated agreements. *Organizational Behavior and Human Decision Processes*, 115(1), 55–68. https://doi.org/10.1016/j.obhdp.2011.01.002

Molden, D. C., & Finkel, E. J. (2010). Motivations for promotion and prevention and the role of trust and commitment in interpersonal forgiveness. *Journal of Experimental Social Psychology*, 46(2), 255–268. https://doi.org/10.1016/j.jesp.2009.10.014

Murray, S. L., Holmes, J. G., & Collins, N. L. (2006). Optimizing assurance: The risk regulation system in relationships. *Psychological Bulletin*, 132(5), 641–666. https://doi.org/10.1037/0033-2909.132.5.641

Murray, S. L., Pinkus, R. T., Holmes, J. G., et al. (2011). Signaling when (and when not) to be cautious and self-protective: Impulsive and reflective trust in close relationships. *Journal of Personality and Social Psychology*, 101(3), 485–502. https://doi.org/10.1037/a0023233

Reis, H. T., & Shaver, P. R. (1988). Intimacy as an interpersonal process. In S. W. Duck (Ed.), *Handbook of personal relationships* (pp. 367–389). John Wiley & Sons.

Rempel, J. K., Holmes, J. G., & Zanna, M. P. (1985). Trust in close relationships. *Journal of Personality and Social Psychology*, 49(1), 95–112. https://doi.org/10.1037/0022-3514.49.1.95

Rotter, J. B. (1971). Generalized expectancies of interpersonal trust. *American Psychologist*, 26(5), 443–452. https://doi.org/10.1037/h0031464

Saef, R. M., Porter, C. M., Woo, S. E., & Wiese, C. (2019). Getting off on the right foot: The role of openness to experience in fostering initial trust between culturally dissimilar partners. *Journal of Research in Psychology*, 79, 176–187. https://doi.org/10.1016/j.jrp.2019.03.003

Shallcross, S. L., & Simpson, J. A. (2012). Trust and responsiveness in strain-test situations: A dyadic perspective. *Journal of Personality and Social Psychology*, 102(5), 1031–1044. https://doi.org/10.1037/a0026829

Simpson, J. A. (2007). Foundations of interpersonal trust. In A. W. Kruglanski & E. T. Higgins (Eds.), *Social psychology: Handbook of basic principles* (2nd ed., pp. 587–607). The Guilford Press.

Simpson, J. A., & Belsky, J. (2016). Attachment theory within a modern evolutionary framework. In J. Cassidy & P. R. Shaver (Eds.), *Handbook of attachment: Theory, research, and clinical applications* (3rd ed., pp. 91–116). The Guilford Press.

Stamos, A., Altsitsiadis, E., & Dewitte, S. (2019). Investigating the effect of childhood socioeconomic background on interpersonal trust: Lower childhood socioeconomic status predict lower levels of trust. *Personality and Individual Differences*, 145, 19–25. https://doi.org/10.1016/j.paid.2019.03.011

Ter Kuile, H., Kluwer, E. S., Finkenauer, C., & Van der Lippe, T. (2017). Predicting adaptation to parenthood: The role of responsiveness, gratitude, and trust. *Personal Relationship*, 24, 663–682. https://doi.org/10.1111/pere.12202

Thibaut, J. W., & Kelley, H. H. (1959). *The social psychology of groups*. Wiley.

Tooby, J., & Cosmides, L. (1996). Friendship and the banker's paradox: Other pathways to the evolution of adaptations for altruism. *Proceedings of the British Academy*, 88, 119–143.

Uysal, A., Lin, H. L., & Bush, A. L. (2012). The reciprocal cycle of self-concealment and trust in romantic relationships. *European Journal of Social Psychology*, 42(7), 844–851. https://doi.org/10.1002/ejsp.1904

Van Lange, P. A. M. (2015). Generalized trust: Four lessons from genetics and culture. *Current Directions in Psychological Science*, 24(1), 71–76. https://doi.org/10.1177/0963721414552473

Van Lange, P. A. M., Vinkhuyzen, A. A. E., & Posthuma, D. (2014). Genetic influences are virtually absent for trust. *PLoS ONE*, 9(4), e93880. https://doi.org/10.1371/journal.pone.0093880

Yucel, D. (2013). Number of siblings and generalized trust. *Social Behavior and Personality: An International Journal*, 41(8), 1399–1408. https://doi.org/10.2224/sbp.2013.41.8.1399

Zlatev, J. J. (2019). I may not agree with you, but I trust you: Caring about social issues signals integrity. *Psychological Science*, 30(6), 880–892. https://doi.org/10.1177/0956797619837948

CHAPTER 2

Trust and Behavioral Economics
Exploration of Trust Based on Game Theory

Devdeepta Bose and Colin Camerer

2.1 Introduction

This chapter is about how trust is modeled and explored in economics based on game theory. Game theory is a general mathematical language that describes the options of "players" in social interactions (called "strategies"), their interdependent consequences, and how "payoffs" (valued outcomes) are created by all the strategy choices taken together. Game theory was intended, from the start, to be applied to a wide range of settings. Games can be "one-shot" (describing how strangers might behave toward each other) or "repeated," so that the history and the shadow of the future influence interaction. Sometimes the information players have is common and complete – such as the moves and rules in chess – and sometimes there is hidden private information – such as a person's face-down cards in poker.

While it is not always obvious from public-science or even textbook introductions to game theory, there is plenty of room for human nature to influence how outcomes in games are valued. Strategy choices in games produce outcomes, and the subjective valuation of outcomes is part of the mathematical specification of a game. Therefore, numbers are needed to use game theory, but the numbers are just subjective values as judged and perceived by players. The reward medium of the outcomes can have many forms: replication of genes in biology, mating opportunities and fitness in evolutionary accounts, emotional outcomes in interpersonal encounters, status outcomes, and gains of territory in wars, etc. In game theory, these outcomes are all presumed to be reducible to numbers on an ordinal scale (that is, a ranking from worst to best) and for most cases, on a

This research was supported by the Behavioral and Neuroeconomics Discovery Fund at Caltech, and the T&C Chen Leadership Chair in Social and Decision Neuroscience. Corresponding author: Colin Camerer (camerer@hss.caltech.edu).

cardinal (or interval) scale (e.g., going from a 1 to a 2 is equally as valued as going from 2 to 3).

Even though numerical subjective values are needed, the structure is otherwise deliberately general to allow human emotions like guilt, shame, and moral obligation to enter into numerical evaluations. Although this generality was built into the mathematical possibility of outcome evaluations from the beginning, it was not put to work until several decades after the seminal contributions in the 1940s. We will next define trust in a game-theoretic sense; then will backtrack to the crucial historical steps in scholarship that got us to where we are today. Interested readers will learn even more from Alós-Ferrer and Farolfi (2019).

2.2 What Is Trust and Why Is It Important?

Our definition is that trust is defined as the expectation that another person (or entity) will repay a socially risky action by the trustor that benefited both the trustor and the trustee, in a way that makes the trustor happy that she was trusting. There are many other definitions with similar ingredients. The concept has been studied in every social science in different ways. An interdisciplinary paper on this topic in a management journal (Rousseau et al., 1998) has been cited 11,500 times (and the citation counts from year to year have steadily risen).

In theory, trust can be an important ingredient in economic analysis because it solves a problem. The problem is called "moral hazard" (an old-fashioned insurance term) or in Nobel Laureate Kenneth Arrow's rebranding, "hidden action." Hidden action means that if you agree with somebody that you will pay them $X and they will deliver Y units of quality, whether they actually deliver the promised Y units of quality cannot be specified in advance (that's the sense in which it is "hidden"). The "hazard" is that they will not actually deliver Y. It is called a "moral hazard" because they cheated you. A famous example in developing societies is simple trade. In some countries, if you buy a 20-kilo bag of rice, you may get home to find out that there are lots of heavy rocks (heavier than rice) in the bottom of the bag. Almost all "experience goods" – goods in which quality cannot be verified up front before the goods or services are experienced – have this quality.

Trust – or more precisely, trust that correctly forecasts true trustworthiness – is the solution to this problem. Trustworthiness means that even if your trading partner is not explicitly penalized for failing to deliver Y units of quality, they will choose to do so anyway, voluntarily. As Arrow (1974, p. 23) wrote, "Trust is an important lubricant of a social system.

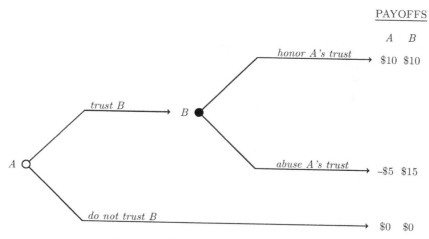

Figure 2.1   Trust game from Kreps (1990).

The trustor (A) has binary choice of whether to trust or not, and trustee (B) has binary choice of honoring or abusing that trust. If trustor (A) declines to trust, both players receive no payoff. If they do trust, trustor (B) can increase payoffs equally for both players to $10, or increase only their own payoff to $15 while harming A by costing them $5.

It is extremely efficient; it saves a lot of trouble to have a fair degree of reliance upon other people's word." The essential role of trust in lubricating market transactions is especially highlighted in the era of the Internet and digital marketplaces. While brick-and-mortar retail outlets provided a tangible process of recompensation in the case of an adverse event, the relative anonymity of the Internet forced buyers and sellers to place trust in entities that cannot see or feel. And yet the Internet provides channels for strangers to exchange goods (Facebook Marketplace, Craigslist) and services (Uber, Lyft, TaskRabbit) that have flourished largely on the basis of trust, with minimal institutional backing to help protect against opportunism (Cook & State, 2015). The "sharing" and "gig" economies of recent times are built on the foundations of trust.

2.3 Experimental Paradigms

The origin of the most widely used paradigm to study trust is in a paper by the economist David Kreps (1990), which first circulated in 1984 (see also the survey by Alós-Ferrer & Farolfi, 2019, which overlaps with many of our central points and includes more discussion of neuroscience) (Figure 2.1).

Kreps' analysis begins with the obvious fact that when two parties enter into an agreement, it is not possible (or at least prohibitively costly) to write an agreement that covers all possible contingencies in a clear way that would be enforceable by a judge or even a trusted third party (like justice in small-scale societies).

But something must be done when an unanticipated contingency occurs (such as a pandemic leading firms to lay off workers, and then accepting loans from a government to pay workers). In situations where firms are one of the partners (e.g., employer–employee contracts), there is usually some hierarchy of rights – the firm usually has more power in deciding what happens next. The principle that a firm uses to resolve outcomes in these situations is a reflection of its "corporate culture." A firm usually has decision-makers that are concentrated at the top, so the mechanisms through which these decision-makers communicate the principles being used to the workers below them in the hierarchy is one way "corporate culture" is transmitted (similar to parents, peers, teachers, and Mister Rogers "acculturating" children).

For example, a firm may use a general principle that "the customer is always right" and make every effort to resolve a dispute in the customer's favor. For example, some department stores accept returns without a receipt of original purchase, which does indeed create some fraud costs, but also earns goodwill from loyal customers who appreciate simplicity in returning goods honestly. Others might have a principle of always shortchanging contractors and forcing them to sue or accept rightful payment at a discounted rate (see Camerer & Vepsalainen, 1988 for more examples and analysis).

Even though the idea of a "firm" is intangible, the actions the management and the employees of a firm take can make or break its reputation. This attachment to maintaining a reputation allows other parties to trust a firm and enter into contracts with it, even if they know that not all outcomes are negotiable. This is because they can trust that should such an outcome occur, the firm has an incentive to act in a judicious manner, or suffer reputational harm. Thus, reputations are best preserved or destroyed if the firm acts in a manner incongruous with a contract in which the outcome is clear-cut, and easy to monitor. In Kreps' theory, the firm acts mainly as a reputation bearer – a wholly intangible object.[1]

---

[1] A literary example is the "Dread Pirate Roberts" in the film *The Princess Bride*. The original pirate built a reputation for ferocity. When he died, another pirate took on his identity and benefited from the DRP's reputation. The book's hero, Wesley, is a wonderful gentleman but is the latest incarnation of the DRP who benefits from the reputation and does not actually have to act fiercely.

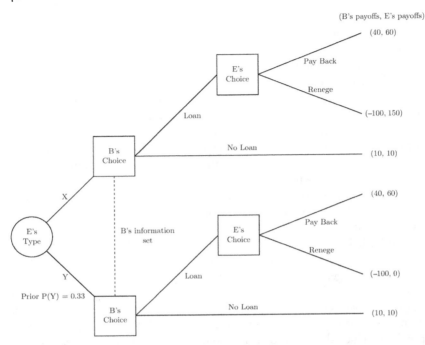

Figure 2.2   Trust game from Camerer and Weigelt (1988).
This structure highlights the fact that the trustor (B) has to make a decision without knowing if the trustee (E) is trustworthy or not. Economists refer to this as an information set where an agent can have beliefs of different levels of their partner's trustworthiness.

Kreps created the trust game (TG) shown in Figure 2.1 as a stylized example of how trust might emerge in repeated situations. If B is a long-lived entity, then players who work for B have a future incentive to honor A's trust (even though it costs a chance to earn more). The first TG experiments modeled after Kreps' investment game were done by Camerer and Weigelt (1988) (Figure 2.2). At the time, behavioral game theorists were interested not only in trust in one-shot games, but how levels of trust could unfold in a repeated "partner" interaction – because of the importance of trust being maintained over long repeated interactions, so that trust is a feature of organizational culture. Their design was heavily influenced by an important paper called the "Gang of Four" paper, referring to four prominent game theorists (Kreps et al., 1982). The paper showed something that had been a "folk theorem" for many years but never proven. Consider a prisoner's dilemma game (PDG) repeated many times between two people who keep track of their history. In the PDG players can choose to cooperate or defect. Defecting always yields a higher payoff to a player (regardless of what the other player does), but mutual defection is worse for both players than mutual cooperation. The "dilemma" is whether to choose selfishly, by defecting, or to choose for mutual group benefit by cooperating.

Suppose that most players are selfish, but a small percentage p *always* cooperate. The Gang showed that in this setting, there are equilibria in which even selfish players will cooperate repeatedly, until "close to the end." Mathematically, "close to the end" means the lowest number of periods remaining N such that $x^N < p$ (where x is a parameter less than one, that depends on payoffs). A key insight is that the breakdown in cooperation by selfish players is determined not by how many periods have been played, but by the value of N that satisfies a mathematical inequality, which depends on x and p. That is, fixing the value of the payoff parameter x, there is always a high enough number of periods N such that cooperation is supported. And oppositely, for any value of N there is a high enough value of p such that cooperation is supported. Numerical examples show that p can be very tiny, like one in a million, and still support cooperation until, say 10 or 20 trials from the end of a long-repeated game with 100 periods. The insight from this analysis is that even if essentially everybody is selfish, players will effectively *pretend* to be unselfish – and will actually cooperate – for mutual benefit (since mutual cooperation is better than mutual defection).

The analysis can be used to track the Bayesian beliefs that players should have, that their partner is selfish or purely cooperative, if their partner has cooperated thus far (that belief is thought of as the partner's "reputation"). Camerer and Weigelt (1988) showed that the relative frequencies of cooperation predicted by the Bayesian theory are quite close to what was observed in experimental data. Like other games used in strategic neuroscience, the Bayesian-Nash[2] analysis used by Camerer and Weigelt (1988) is full of interesting cognitive and neuroscientific predictions. Event-related design[3] could be used to infer the reputation values (i.e., the running value of $p(\text{selfish}|\text{history})$). After an untrustworthy move, players

---

[2] A Bayesian-Nash equilibrium is one in which players form accurate beliefs about what other players are likely to do and optimized given their beliefs (that is the Nash part). In addition, because there is hidden information Bayes' rule must be consistent with how beliefs are updated based on observable actions.

[3] An event-related fMRI design uses brain reactions at particular events, often with specific numerical values, rather than continuous activity during a block of similar activity.

in the P1 role should update p(selfish|history) and recompute the future value of expected play in more trials, which is a particular kind of computable prediction error. A general prediction is that neural activity should look similar in different game lengths for epochs that have the same number of periods remaining to the end: For example, the last 5 periods of a 20-period game should look like the last 5 periods of a 40-period game.

The next important step in experimental trust research came from an extreme simplification by Berg et al. (1995). They removed the dynamic element to focus on a single one-period TG. The game theory became less interesting but the focus on measuring sociality became sharper. One person, player 1, starts out with, say, $10. They can keep any integer amount and "invest" the rest. Denote what they invest by X. That amount grows because investment is mutually beneficial; a typical growth rate is that X triples to $3X$. Then player 2 can decide how much of the amount $3X$ to share with player 1. If we denote that repayment by Y, then player 1 ends up with $(10 - X) + Y$ and player 2 ends up with $3X - Y$. You can immediately see that since the Y payment nets out, the total win-win value for the players is $(10 - X) + 3X = 10 + 2X$. So together the players are best off if X is maximized (so $X^* = 10$). But if player 2 is maximizing just her share, which is $3X - Y$, she gets the most if $Y^* = 0$.

Berg et al. (1995)'s trimmed focus illustrates how less is often more in science. If players are selfish and both know it, player 1 will not invest because player 2 would never pay back. Nothing interesting should happen if players are selfish. But if players are *not* necessarily selfish, then many interesting empirical questions spring to life: How trusting are people? Is their trust repaid or not (i.e., are beliefs that underlie trust equal to how trustworthy player 2s are)? How do results depend on the investment multiplier? Are there stable individual differences? Can trust measured this way be associated with mental disorders, different cultural norms, personal experience, etc.?

The TG also encapsulated an essential question in organizational economics, political science, and other social sciences. Author Camerer was at the University of Chicago Business School when George Baker, an organizational economist, was visiting there in the mid-1990s. As we described earlier, there is a long history in organizational economics of trying to figure out how trust influences the nature and efficiency of contracts within and between companies (Arrow, 1974). One of the Berg et al. authors had just presented the 1995 experimental trust paper. As Camerer recalls, Prof. Baker said enthusiastically, "I never really knew what trust meant; now I know!" The point of this story is that even an organizational economist (e.g., Baker) who had thought about the nature of trust and how to model ideal contracting for many years found the experimental paradigm an insightful way to distill trust to its essence.

Pinning down how trust worked mathematically came a little later. We will give only a rough sketch here. In standard game theory with selfishness, no player 2 repays trust. This raises the question of how to model a trustworthy repayment of money. A key mathematical step is that it is natural to think of the actual trustworthiness of player 2 as being caused by two features: (1) player 2 thinks that player 1 expects to be repaid; and (2) player 2 feels some emotion, such as guilt, if she thinks player 1 expects repayment but she (player 2) does not repay.

A big mathematical step came from an innovation called "psychological game theory" (Geanakoplos et al., 1989). This paper was not properly appreciated when it was first published. The key step was to allow utilities of players for various strategic outcomes to depend on not only the series of strategies (such as the amounts X and Y that the TG players choose), but also to depend on *beliefs*.

Allowing beliefs to influence utilities makes the mathematics messy but, as a result, more psychologically interesting.[4] In TGs, the idea is that a player 2 thinks about what she can earn from choosing Y, which is $3X - Y$, and the guilt she will feel. Guilt will depend positively on $Y - E_2(E_1(Y))$. The term $E_2(E_1(Y))$ is a "second-order" expectation: It is player 2's belief about what player 1 expected her (player 2) to do. If $Y - E_2(E_1(Y)) > 0$, then player 2 exceeded player 1's expectations and may feel some pleasure from over-rewarding player 1. Choosing a higher Y then trades off the value of keeping more money (larger Y) with the moral self-satisfaction of having lived up to one's perceived obligation. If $Y - E_2(E_1(Y)) < 0$, then player 2 gave too little and feels guilty. Again, she will trade off whether it is better to have more money and more guilt, or less money and less guilt. Neuroscience has explored this structure a bit (Chang & Smith, 2015) but there is much more to do.

2.4 Advances in Trust Experiments: Betrayal Aversion and Meta-analysis

Early on, scientists began to wonder whether people were *un*trusting because of standard (in economics) aversion to risk, as captured by

---

[4] More general treatments of how reciprocity is modeled using psychological game theory are in Dufwenberg and Kirchsteiger (2004); Falk and Fischbacher (2006); and Rabin (1993).

diminishing marginal utility in a concave utility function for money. Maybe people who did not trust would also not gamble, when the social determinant of whether they get money back (determined by player 2) was replaced by a random event. This led to an important distinction between aversion to financial risk and a special "aversion to betrayal" – that is, a particular distaste for taking a risk when another person whom you trust betrays you by not repaying (see also Chapter 5).

Bohnet et al. (2008) study the prevalence of betrayal aversion in experimental samples in six countries around the world – Brazil, China, Oman, Switzerland, Turkey, and the United States. They studied the canonical one-stage Kreps TG with slightly altered payoffs. The sure outcome is (10, 10) while player 2 chooses between (15, 15) and (8, 22). Player 1 is asked for the probability p^* of player 2 choosing the (15, 15) at which they would be indifferent between choosing the sure outcome, and delegating the decision to player 2. They consider two treatments – either player 2 makes the move themselves, or their move is determined by nature (a random device). While the objective risks and likelihoods in both treatments are identical, player 1 participants state a significantly higher p^* for the treatment where player 2 is another human. The authors claim that this is driven by an aversion to the feeling of being "betrayed" by another human, something over and beyond risk aversion, which exists equally in both treatments. The authors go the extra step of collecting data from many non-WEIRD (Western, educated, industrialized, rich, and democratic) samples, and show that betrayal aversion is a broad-based phenomenon. It is found in countries that differ on many important dimensions, such as continent, political structure, economic system, culture, religion, and history.

Johnson and Mislin (2011) did an excellent meta-analysis with superb coverage. They collected 162 studies from 35 countries, mostly from North America and Europe (but also including every populated continent). Studies were found from published papers, as well as EconPapers and emailing the Economic Science Association mailing list twice. Unfortunately, their analysis does not address publication bias (e.g., do studies that report unusually high or low outlying results get underpublished?). They used a reasonable set of exclusions so that all the studies were continuous two-person TGs sticking closely to the Becker et al. (1964) structure. The strongest effects on trust (the percentage sent) are random payment, which lowers trust, and playing a real person (rather than a computer or unseen confederate), which increases trust. The size of the stakes and the investment multiplier makes no difference.

Trustworthiness varies more predictably with study features. The percentage returned (= trustworthiness) increases with the (percentage) amount trusted. The percentage returned decreases strongly with the multiplier, with student status, and when players play both player 1 and player 2 roles. There are some modest continent differences. Compared to North America, most other continents show less trust, and a little more trustworthiness. In Africa, there is less of both. Unfortunately, there are many differences across countries and continents, so only a larger meta-analysis, or studies carefully targeted to within- and between-country variation, could help us understand why the continental differences exist.

2.5   Variants of TG Experiments

The TG is a highly simplified version of when one person is unilaterally dependent on – and thus vulnerable to – another individual. Public goods games (PGGs) and PDGs are structurally similar to TGs, with a crucial difference. In the typical PDG, players choose to cooperate or defect *simultaneously*; in PGGs, there are *degrees* of cooperate/defect represented by higher or lower allocations to the shared public good.

In PDGs and PGGs, it is difficult to separate the prosocial desire to cooperate with expectations about what others will do – precisely because the game is simultaneous. A person could defect because they think others will defect, and do not want to be a sucker, or could defect because they are selfish (and they would defect no matter what they think others will do). The sequential TG is a simple way to isolate these two forces. Player 2 has a clear expectation about what the other player 1 already did. Thus, their choice is to act selfishly or to reciprocate. There is no confusion based on beliefs. Of course, it is also possible to create PDGs in which expectations are measured separately, which has led to the finding of substantial "conditional cooperation" (cooperating because others are expected to cooperate too).

The simplified TG discussed thus far, between strangers, abstracts from many real-world characteristics like communication, or promises, which are integral to the real-life situations involving trust. Papers that have included characteristics like communication, or repeated interactions in TGs include Anderhub et al. (2002), Bicchieri et al. (2011), and Ho (2012) (see Thielmann & Hilbig, 2015 for a particularly careful taxonomy).

Besides these variants of the strategic game, the simplified TG has two particularly interesting variants. Abbink et al. (2000) introduce the *moonlighting game* that adds one option to each player's strategy set: The trustor can also *take* tokens from the trustee and the trustee can also *pay* tokens to reduce the trustor's payoff. Bohnet and Meier (2012) introduced a *distrust game* where, by default, the trustor has no endowment, because all of it has been transferred to the trustee. Thus, "full trust" is the default option. These variants allow a greater exploration of the greed, competitiveness, reciprocity, and spite that can be studied through the TG. Banerjee (2018) describes some other variants of TGs that include elements of special interest to understanding corruption, such as bribery and harassment.

One way TGs, and similar economic games, can be used is in "computational psychiatry" (see also Chapters 16 and 17). This is an approach that characterizes disorders not only by symptoms and clinical evaluation, but also by their phenotypic behavior in decisions and games, often characterized by parameter values in a computational model. A good illustration using TGs is borderline personality disorder (BPD) patients. In multiround TGs, it is often the case that after a player 2 has been shown to be trustworthy, the trusting player 1 punishes the transgressor by not investing very much in the next round. That gives the player 2 a chance to "rebuild trust" by repaying an unusually high fraction after player 1's low investment (a kind of apology, which King-Casas et al. (2008) call "coaxing"). These low player 1 investments that invite coaxing normally produce insula activity in the brains of the trustee player 2's. However, BPD patients did not have the same insula signals when their partner was coaxing as neurotypicals did. They also did not show the typical phenotypical tendency to use the opportunity to rebuild trust by repaying a lot. Given that part of the name of the syndrome – "borderline" – means BPD is not well understood, the phenotypic failure to encode coaxing in the insula, if accompanied by lots of similar findings, could be one clue that will help clarify the computational phenotype and neural basis of BPD.

2.6   Social and National Trust

Besides the simplest two-person one-shot type of trust, trust can work at the organizational level (firms can engage in commerce even if every outcome cannot be contracted upon) and at the macroeconomic level (society-level trust is correlated with macroeconomic outcomes). Workers in teams trying to complete projects on a deadline rely on being able to trust that their coworkers will not shirk and will hold up their end. A firm's continued reputation, built on years of trust, can be squandered if it does not meet its financial or contractual obligations to other firms. The internal structure within companies is often affirmed by the camaraderie of the employees, enforced by gossip that plays a role in amplifying trust (Burt & Knez, 1996). Effective leadership in guiding organizational citizenship behavior is also enhanced if employees can trust that their managers have their best interests at heart (Dirks & Ferrin, 2001).

The societal-level effects of trust have also been widely studied in sociology and political science. Typically, when faced with economic hardships and loss of jobs, help often arrives from the closest social structure – family and friends. Job seeking (Granovetter, 1973) and social support (Small, 2004) are often acquired from those that are most trusted. On the other hand, sociologists and political scientists have argued that a breakdown of community and trust in communal institutions (e.g., a loss in the ability of law enforcement in treating all races equally) can lead to increases in looting, violence, and criminal activity (Hagan & McCarthy, 1998; Rose & Clear, 1998). These have obvious deleterious effects on the economic activity, particularly for small businesses.

The idea that "social capital" is important for economic development and well-being goes back a long way but was rekindled by Coleman (1988) and by Putnam et al.'s (1994) study of civic life across Italy (see Putnam, 2000). Note that social capital is typically meant to be more general than trust – it can include a community "safety net," job referrals, the ability to get help easily with expectation of repayment, etc. The idea was then taken up with vigor in development economics and related fields.

Solow (1995) argued that if social capital is to be more than a buzzword then it "should somehow be measurable, even inexactly . . . [but] measurement seems very far away" (p. 36; see also Sobel, 2002). From our perspective, a type of measurement Solow hoped for was not far away at all; Kreps laid out an approach in 1984, and it was then studied experimentally by Camerer and Weigelt (1988) several years *before* Solow wrote about his concerns.

The importance of social capital, in the specific form of trust, for economic development was noted by Arrow (1972, p. 357) who wrote, "Virtually every commercial transaction has within itself an element of trust, certainly any transaction conducted over a period of time. It can be plausibly argued that much of the economic backwardness in the world can be explained by the lack of mutual confidence."

Some striking empirical results come from using a simple survey measure of trust associated with wealth of nations. The measure most often used is an item on the World Values Survey (WVS), a large survey that has been conducted in almost 100 countries in seven waves since 1981. The WVS trust item asks: "Generally speaking, would you say that most people can be trusted or that you need to be very careful in dealing with people?"[5] The answers are binary (most can be trusted, or you need to be very careful). Higher trust levels have been associated with higher economic growth (Knack & Keefer, 1997), more financial development (Guiso et al., 2004, 2008), and greater international trade and investment (Guiso et al., 2009).

Knack and Keefer (1997)'s study shows a partial correlation (controlling for several other variables) of trust against growth in GDP from 1980 to 1992 and trust measured in 1990–1991 (the trust numbers have the cross-country average of 35.8% saying "most people can be trusted."). Trust is a substantial predictor. However, the causal pathways are complicated as trust may be both a cause of, and an effect of, other variables like "good institutions" (e.g., rule of law, democratic engagement).

A notable cross-country experiment on trust was done by Cohn et al. (2019). The measures of trust were experimental return rates, which were correlated with various measures of social institutions and demographics (though not the WVS measure). Their study was an enormous "lost-wallet" study in 355 cities in 40 different countries (mostly in Europe), which was much more careful than previous efforts. They turned in purportedly lost wallets containing a grocery list, a key, and business cards (showing an address and email). Wallets were turned in at banks, cultural institutions such as museums, post offices, hotels, and police stations or courts. Their dependent variable was whether people in those locations who got the wallet from their research assistants contacted the purported owner of the wallet. The overall return rate was 40%, and was *higher*, 51%, when the wallet also contained money ($13.45). There is large variation across countries in return rates, from 15% for China and Morocco, to 75% in Norway and Switzerland (for the no-money wallets). The cross-country variation allows a high-powered regression of many different variables that might affect this measure of "trustworthiness." The strongest predictors of more trustworthiness are geographical – higher distance from the equator, lower temperature, and lower prevalence of pathogens.[6] Unfortunately,

---

[5] Knack and Keefer (1997, p. 1257) note that return rates in a more primitive lost-wallet study done by the magazine *Reader's Digest* correlated 0.67 with WVS trust.

[6] The equator effect shows up repeatedly in analyses trying to explain differences in country wealth. It is still not thoroughly understood whether it has to do temperature, the fact that wealthier European, North American, and Asian countries are further from the equator, with pathogens from tropical climates, etc. Biology in general, and also cross-country neuroscience, could contribute to understanding this giant important effect.

they did not include the WVS trust measure. However, sociopolitical variables correlated with WVS trust – such as education, years of democracy, and political constraints on authoritarian executives – do increase wallet reporting.

Finally, modern events have proved to be a hectic kind of quasi-laboratory for changes in trust at social and national levels (even before considering the COVID-19 pandemic). While trust in institutions has been eroding steadily for a while, the Great Recession has accelerated this fall (Cook & State, 2015). This has been reflected in election outcomes around the world, with many voters clamoring for politicians who will fundamentally change the old ways of doing things. The key drivers of eroding trust appear to be rising unemployment (Stevenson & Wolfers, 2011) and sociodemographic differences (Alesina & La Ferrara, 2002). Rising suspicion of out-groups along racial and gender divisions has led to people being less likely to trust others, although religious or ethnic differences do not seem to have similar effects. A study synthesizing cross-country studies measuring trust (Bjørnskov, 2008) found that Scandinavian countries have the highest level of trust in unknown others, followed by the other Western European nations, relative to other continents.

2.7 Summary and Conclusions

This chapter reviewed how behavioral economists model trust mathematically and explore it empirically, in both highly stylized lab experiments and in field experiments (lost-wallet drops) and in field data. The standard game originated with Kreps' 1984 working paper, which was first studied experimentally by Camerer and Weigelt (1988). Berg et al. (1995) introduced a simpler two-person sequential investment game. The key feature is that the first player (trustor) invests; the investment grows large enough for both to benefit, but the second player (trustee) is not legally obligated to repay anything.

When the first experimental results emerged, economists were a bit startled how common trust was. In retrospect, the results are not **that** surprising because cooperation in one-shot prisoners' dilemma games has been well known since at least the 1980s (e.g., meta-analysis in Sally, 1995). Furthermore, Camerer and Weigelt's results are well explained by a theory in which reputation-building occurs on a foundation of expectation that a percentage of people (around 15%–20%) will always behave in a trustworthy way. The value of the TG is in its value as a tool for studying *variation* in trust, and its neural components. In TGs, player 1 is forming a belief and making a choice, waiting for player 2's decision, and reacting to player 2's decision. Player 2 waits for player 1's trust choice, faces a conflict about how much to repay, and earns a subjective reward (that may include guilt or moral satisfaction) from their trustworthiness choice (Fehr & Gächter, 2000).

There are many other interesting questions about how trust emerges in the developmental life cycle, and is acculturated locally. Another interesting question is how much an experience of rewarded or betrayed trust in one-person *P* spills over to trust in others with similar faces, accents, cultural markers, or group membership (e.g., union members, gangs, professional organizations) like *P*. The future seems bright for using social neuroscience to explore not just basic questions about trust, but different mechanistic questions that arise in the many variants of this rich game, which is a building block of so much important social activity.

References

Abbink, K., Irlenbusch, B., & Renner, E. (2000). The moonlighting game: An experimental study on reciprocity and retribution. *Journal of Economic Behavior & Organization*, 42(2), 265–277. https://doi.org/10.1016/S0167-2681(00)00089-5

Alesina, A., & La Ferrara, E. (2002). Who trusts others? *Journal of Public Economics*, 85(2), 207–234. https://doi.org/10.1016/S0047-2727(01)00084-6

Alós-Ferrer, C., & Farolfi, F. (2019). Trust games and beyond. *Frontiers in Neuroscience*, 13, 1–14. https://doi.org/10.3389/fnins.2019.00887

Anderhub, V., Engelmann, D., & Güth, W. (2002). An experimental study of the repeated trust game with incomplete information. *Journal of Economic Behavior & Organization*, 48(2), 197–216. https://doi.org/10.1016/S0167-2681(01)00216-5

Arrow, K. J. (1972). Gifts and exchanges. *Philosophy & Public Affairs*, 1(4), 343–362.

(1974). *The limits of organization*. W. W. Norton & Company. https://doi.org/10.1177/000271627541700157

Banerjee, R. (2018). On the interpretation of World Values Survey trust question: Global expectations vs. local beliefs. *European Journal of Political Economy*, 55, 491–510. https://doi.org/10.1016/j.ejpoleco.2018.04.008

Becker, G. M., DeGroot, M. H., & Marschak, J. (1964). Measuring utility by a single-response sequential method. *Behavioral Sciences*, 9(3), 226–232. https://doi.org/10.1002/bs.3830090304

Berg, J., Dickhaut, J., & McCabe, K. (1995). Trust, reciprocity, and social history. *Games and Economic Behavior*, 10(1), 122–142. https://doi.org/10.1006/game.1995.1027

Bicchieri, C., Xiao, E., & Muldoon, R. (2011). Trustworthiness is a social norm, but trusting is not. *Politics, Philosophy & Economics*, 10(2), 170–187. https://doi.org/10.1177/1470594X10387260

Bjørnskov, C. (2008). Social trust and fractionalization: A possible reinterpretation. *European Sociological Review*, 24(3), 271–283. https://doi.org/10.1093/esr/jcn004

Bohnet, I., Greig, F., Herrmann, B., & Zeckhauser, R. (2008). Betrayal aversion: Evidence from Brazil, China, Oman, Switzerland, Turkey, and the United States. *American Economic Review*, 98(1), 294–310. https://doi.org/10.1257/aer.98.1.294

Bohnet, I., & Meier, S. (2012). Trust, distrust, and bargaining. In R. Croson & G. E. Bolton (Eds.), *The Oxford handbook of economic conflict resolution* (pp. 183–198). Oxford University Press. https://doi.org/10.1093/oxfordhb/9780199730858.013.0017

Burt, R. S., & Knez, M. (1996). Trust and third-party gossip. In R. M. Kramer & T. R. Tyler (Eds.), *Trust in organizations: Frontiers of theory and research* (pp. 68–89). Sage Publications, Inc. https://doi.org/10.2307/3857331

Camerer, C., & Vepsalainen, A. (1988). The economic efficiency of corporate culture. *Strategic Management Journal*, 9(S1), 115–126. https://doi.org/10.1002/smj.4250090712

Camerer, C., & Weigelt, K. (1988). Experimental tests of a sequential equilibrium reputation model. *Econometrica: Journal of the Econometric Society*, 56(1), 1–36. https://doi.org/10.2307/1911840

Chang, L. J., & Smith, A. (2015). Social emotions and psychological games. *Current Opinion in Behavioral Sciences*, 5, 133–140. https://doi.org/10.1016/j.cobeha.2015.09.010

Cohn, A., Maréchal, M. A., Tannenbaum, D., & Zünd, C. L. (2019). Civic honesty around the globe. *Science*, 365(6448), 70–73. https://doi.org/10.1016/10.1126/science.aau8712

Coleman, J. S. (1988). Social capital in the creation of human capital. *American Journal of Sociology*, 94, S95–S120. https://doi.org/10.1086/228943

Cook, K. S., & State, B. (2015). Trust and economic organization. In R. Scott & S. Kosslyn (Eds.), *Emerging trends in the social and behavioral sciences* (pp. 1–11). Wiley.

Dirks, K. T., & Ferrin, D. L. (2001). The role of trust in organizational settings. *Organizational Science*, 12(4), 450–467. https://doi.org/10.1287/orsc.12.4.450.10640

Dufwenberg, M., & Kirchsteiger, G. (2004). A theory of sequential reciprocity. *Games and Economic Behavior*, 47(2), 268–298. https://doi.org/10.1016/j.geb.2003.06.003

Falk, A., & Fischbacher, U. (2006). A theory of reciprocity. *Games and Economic Behavior*, 54(2), 293–315. https://doi.org/10.1016/j.geb.2005.03.001

Fehr, E., & Gächter, S. (2000). Fairness and retaliation: The economics of reciprocity. *Journal of Economic Perspectives*, 14(3), 159–181. https://doi .org/10.1257/jep.14.3.159

Geanakoplos, J., Pearce, D., & Stacchetti, E. (1989). Psychological games and sequential rationality. *Games and Economic Behavior*, 1(1), 60–79. https:// doi.org/10.1016/0899-8256(89)90005-5

Granovetter, M. (1973). *Getting a job: A study of contacts and careers*. University of Chicago Press.

Guiso, L., Sapienza, P., & Zingales, L. (2004). The role of social capital in financial development. *American Economic Review*, 94(3), 526–556. https://doi.org/10.1257/0002828041464498

(2008). Trusting the stock market. *The Journal of Finance*, 63(6), 2557–2600. https://doi.org/10.1111/j.1540-6261.2008.01408.x

(2009). Cultural biases in economic exchange? *Quarterly Journal of Economics*, 124(3), 1095–1131. https://doi.org/10.1162/qjec.2009.124.3.1095

Hagan, J., & McCarthy, B. (1998). *Mean streets: Youth crime and homelessness*. Cambridge University Press. https://doi.org/10.1017/CBO9780511625497

Ho, B. (2012). Apologies as signals: With evidence from a trust game. *Management Science*, 58(1), 141–158. https://doi.org/10.1287/mnsc.1110 .1410

Johnson, N. D., & Mislin, A. A. (2011). Trust games: A meta-analysis. *Journal of Economic Psychology*, 32(5), 865–889. https://doi.org/10.1016/j.joep.2011 .05.007

King-Casas, B., Sharp, C., Lomax-Bream, L., Lohrenz, T., Fonagy, P., & Montague, P. R. (2008). The rupture and repair of cooperation in borderline personality disorder. *Science*, 321(5890), 806–810. https://doi.org/10.1126/ science.1156902

Knack, S., & Keefer, P. (1997). Does social capital have an economic payoff? A cross-country investigation. *Quarterly Journal of Economics*, 112(4), 1251–1288. https://doi.org/10.1162/003355300555475

Kreps, D. M. (1990). Corporate culture and economic theory. In J. Alt & K. Shepsle (Eds.), *Perspectives on positive political economy* (pp. 90–143). Cambridge University Press. https://doi.org/10.1017/CBO9780511571657 .006

Kreps, D. M., Milgrom, P., Roberts, J., & Wilson, R. (1982). Rational cooperation in the finitely repeated prisoners' dilemma. *Journal of Economic Theory*, 27(2), 245–252. https://doi.org/10.1016/0022-0531(82)90029-1

Putnam, R. D. (2000). *Bowling alone: The collapse and revival of American community*. Simon & Schuster. https://doi.org/10.1145/358916.361990

Putnam, R. D., Leonardi, R., & Nanetti, R. Y. (1994). *Making democracy work: Civic traditions in modern Italy*. Princeton University Press. https://doi.org/ 10.2307/2075319

Rabin, M. (1993). Incorporating fairness into game theory and economics. *American Economic Review*, 83(5), 1281–1302.

Rose, D. R., & Clear, T. R. (1998). Incarceration, social capital, and crime: Implications for social disorganization theory. *Criminology*, 36(3), 441–480. https://doi.org/10.1111/j.1745-9125.1998.tb01255.x

Rousseau, D. M., Sitkin, S. B., Burt, R. S., & Camerer, C. (1998). Not so different after all: A cross-discipline view of trust. *Academy of Management Review*, 23(3), 393–404. https://doi.org/10.5465/amr.1998.926617

Sally, D. (1995). Conversation and cooperation in social dilemmas: A meta-analysis of experiments from 1958 to 1992. *Rationality and Society*, 7(1), 58–92. https://doi.org/10.1177/1043463195007001004

Small, M. L. (2004). *Villa Victoria: The transformation of social capital in a Boston barrio*. University of Chicago Press.

Sobel, J. (2002). Can we trust social capital? *Journal of Economic Literature*, 40(1), 139–154. https://doi.org/10.1257/002205102700001

Solow, R. M. (1995). But verify. *New Republic*, 213(11), 36–39. [Review of Fukuyama, *Trust: The social virtues and the creation of prosperity*, The Free Press.]

Stevenson, B., & Wolfers, J. (2011). Trust in public institutions over the business cycle. *American Economic Review*, 101(3), 281–287. https://doi.org/10.1257/aer.101.3.281

Thielmann, I., & Hilbig, B. E. (2015). Trust: An integrative review from a person–situation perspective. *Review of General Psychology*, 19(3), 249–277. https://doi.org/10.1037/gpr0000046

CHAPTER 3

Trust and Digitalization
Review of Behavioral and Neuroscience Evidence

René Riedl

3.1 Introduction

Determining whom to trust and whom not to trust has been critical since the early days of ancient civilizations. From the time of the emergence of early hominids such as Australopithecus afarensis some million years ago until today, trust in individuals who turned out not to be trustworthy could result in significant loss, and in some cases even in death. What has characterized trust situations over the past millions of years is that human interaction typically took place in face-to-face settings. However, with the advent of digital technologies in the past decades trust situations have changed. In contrast to the former technology-free interactions, today we communicate with other people over the Internet (e.g., when we buy goods via eBay or when we use social media platforms such as Facebook), referred to as computer-mediated interaction. Moreover, we increasingly interact with technological artifacts, either directly or indirectly. Examples of direct interaction are the use of an automated airline self-check-in, autonomous vehicles, or natural language processing technologies such as Amazon's Alexa or Apple's Siri. An example of computer-mediated interaction with a technological artifact is communication with an internet chatbot that acts in the role of a virtual sales representative or a virtual doctor for diagnosis of possible diseases (e.g., https://symptomate .com/).

The International Telecommunication Union (ITU) indicated in a recent report that at the end of 2019, 4.1 billion people, or 53.6% of the global population, used the Internet; in developed countries, almost 9 out of 10 individuals used it (ITU, 2019). Further, the report shows that 97% of the entire world population lives within reach of a mobile cellular signal. Considering these numbers, the enormous impact of information

Corresponding author: René Riedl (rene.riedl@jku.at).

and communication technologies on human society is definitive. Based on recent developments in technological areas like Artificial Intelligence, Big Data, and Internet-of-Things, along with the ever-increasing use of smartphones, it is difficult to imagine that the pace and rate of digitalization will become lower in the near future. Rather, it is very likely that the opposite is the case (e.g., Yanquing et al., 2019).

This trend toward digitalization has significant implications for both the role of trust in society and for how we should conceptualize trust and trustworthiness. As will be discussed in this chapter, human perceptions of an agent's initial trustworthiness, as well as trust development processes, strongly depend on whether an interaction partner is perceived as human or technology. Such a conclusion implies that an extremist view stating that "people trust people, not technology" (Friedman et al., 2000, p. 36) has to be rejected resolutely. Rather, it is critical for research to delineate the trust differences in situations with varying levels of social and technology-related cues.

In this chapter, major insights on phenomena related to trust in a digital world are reviewed. This review integrates findings from various levels of analysis, including behavioral and neurophysiological. To structure the chapter and to organize the discussion of related work, different scenarios of trust in a digital world are developed. Next, these scenarios are introduced, followed by a discussion of both theoretical and empirical studies. Finally, a conclusion is provided to summarize the major insights of this chapter.

3.2 Scenarios of Trust in a Digital World

To better understand the nature of trust in a digital world, major trust situations, denoted as scenarios, were developed. The first scenario describes a technology-free situation of human–human interaction; see Scenario A in Figure 3.1. The remaining three scenarios refer to different trust situations that emerged inductively based on observation of social and economic interaction in today's digital world. Scenario B outlines a situation of computer-mediated human–human interaction (e.g., eBay transaction), Scenario C denotes a situation of direct human–technology interaction (e.g., ride in an autonomous vehicle), and, finally, Scenario D refers to a situation of computer-mediated human–technology interaction (e.g., communication with a chatbot on the Internet). The common denominator of all situations is that a human acts in the role of trustor, while the role of trustee can be either another human or a technological

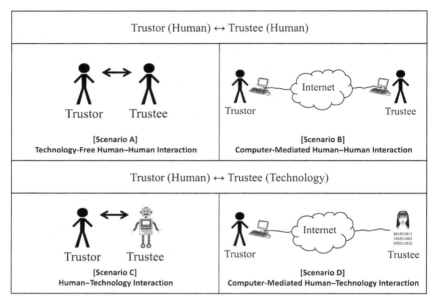

Figure 3.1   Major trust scenarios in a digital world.

artifact. The following discussion starts with a compact summary of research findings from the domain of technology-free human–human interaction. This scenario (Scenario A) is used as a conceptual basis for the three remaining scenarios B, C, and D that are directly related to trust in a digital world.

3.2.1   *Scenario A: Technology-Free Human–Human Interaction*

A vast amount of research in several scientific disciplines has investigated the nature of trust, as well as its antecedents (e.g., facial expressions in personal interactions) and consequences (e.g., cooperative behavior). Psychologists, sociologists, economists, marketers, among scholars in other academic fields, have investigated trust, both theoretically and empirically (e.g., Luhmann, 1979; Rousseau et al., 1998; Seppänen et al., 2007; Swan et al., 1999). Despite the large variety of disciplines that have studied the phenomenon, there is consensus regarding the conceptualization of trust in interpersonal relationships; note that this perspective also includes situations of interorganizational trust (e.g., firm cooperation). Most scholars describe trust as a behavior that makes one party, the trustor, vulnerable to the actions of another party, the trustee. This behavior of a trustor is affected by his or her beliefs about the trustee's trustworthiness. Further, trust behavior in a specific situation is also influenced by the trustor's general level of trust (often referred to as trust disposition), as well as by an individual's risk preferences (Riedl & Javor, 2012).

The major characteristics of a trustee are ability, benevolence, and integrity (Mayer et al., 1995). If a trustor believes in a trustee's trustworthiness, he or she believes that the trustee (a) has the competencies that are critical for the relationship (ability), (b) means well toward the trustor aside from an egocentric profit motive (benevolence), and (c) adheres to a set of principles that the trustor finds acceptable (integrity). Riedl and Javor (2012) indicate that the relevance of each characteristic may vary as a function of a trustor's inner states (e.g., high risk perceptions regarding possible betrayal may turn one's attention to benevolence rather than ability) and context factors such as the significance of the trust decision for survival (e.g., in tandem skydiving, the ability of the instructor is more important than benevolence).

Methodologically, many insights on interpersonal and interorganizational trust have been derived through survey research. Drawing upon the three trustee characteristics, items like "This person/vendor is competent and effective" (ability), "This person/vendor is interested in my well-being, not just its own" (benevolence), and "This person/vendor would keep its commitments" (integrity) have been used in combination with Likert-scales to measure trusting beliefs (e.g., McKnight et al., 2002; Nicolaou & McKnight, 2006).

In addition to surveys, researchers also used behavioral measures of trust and trustworthiness. The most prominent instrument is the trust game (TG) (Berg et al., 1995). In the mainstream version of this game, the trustor has an initial endowment of x monetary units (e.g., $10). First, the trustor decides whether to share his or her endowment (e.g., $5 for each player, then the game ends) or to send (a part of) it to the trustee. If money was sent, the trustee decides whether to keep the amount or share (some of) it with the trustor. The experimenter triples the trustor's transfer, so that both players are better off collectively if the trustor transfers money and the trustee sends back a sufficient amount. What follows is that the trustee has two possibilities: either to share the money, in which case both players are better off, or to keep all the money. If the game is played on a one-shot basis, the trustee has a strong incentive to keep all the money and repay none to the trustor. However, if the trustor anticipates this behavior, there is little reason to transfer. Therefore, if the trustor transferred no money, then a chance for higher mutual gain would be lost. In the TG, the amount sent by the trustor is used as a behavioral measure for trust, and the trustee's transfer back is used as a behavioral measure for trustworthiness.

Based on economic standard assumptions with regard to rationality and selfishness, the prediction is that a trustor passes no money to a trustee, and subsequently no money will be returned. However, in sharp contrast to this prediction, evidence of a meta-analysis with 162 studies and more than 23,000 participants indicates that trustors typically send approximately half of the initial endowment (0.502, sent fraction) and trustees frequently send a considerable amount back (0.372, proportion returned) (Johnson & Mislin, 2011). Further, this meta-analysis revealed systematic differences across geographic regions: sent fraction (trust) – Europe (0.537), North America (0.517), Asia (0.482), South America (0.458), Africa (0.456); proportion returned (trustworthiness): Europe (0.382), North America (0.340), Asia (0.460), South America (0.369), Africa (0.319).

In addition to survey results and behavioral findings, research has shown that initial trust perceptions, as well as trust and distrust development in repeated interaction, are related to activity in different brain regions. A functional magnetic resonance imaging (fMRI) study found that the amygdala and insula were significantly more activated when subjects viewed faces that they rated as most untrustworthy (Winston et al., 2002). Moreover, the study found activation in the superior temporal sulcus, a brain area relevant for mentalizing (i.e., inferring the thoughts, intentions, and feelings of other people). Based on these results, Winston et al. (2002, p. 281) concluded that "social judgments about faces reflect a combination of brain responses that are stimulus driven ... and driven by processes relating to inferences concerning the intentionality of others." After this initial study with human face stimuli, a number of further fMRI studies were conducted based on the TG. Reviews and meta-analyses (e.g., Bellucci et al., 2017; Fehr, 2009a; Hubert et al., 2018; Krueger & Meyer-Lindenberg, 2019; Riedl & Javor, 2012; Tzieropoulos, 2013) indicate that in addition to the mentioned brain areas (amygdala, insula, superior temporal sulcus), the basal ganglia (reward processing and learning), anterior cingulate cortex (conflict monitoring and regulation of social behavior), and frontal brain regions (mentalizing and regulation of social behavior) are also critical in trust situations, among some other areas.

Further, research found that trust perceptions, as well as corresponding behavior, is related to genetic and hormonal influences. Major hormones identified in trust studies and related works are oxytocin, vasopressin, testosterone, dopamine, and serotonin, among others (Krueger & Meyer-Lindenberg, 2019; Riedl & Javor, 2012). Also, research on neuro-active hormones was combined with brain imaging. One study combined intranasal administration of oxytocin and fMRI. The results of the study revealed that participants who had received oxytocin showed no change in their trust behavior after they learned that their trust had been breached several times, while participants receiving a placebo decreased their trust (Baumgartner et al., 2008) (see also Chapter 13). Regarding the genetic influences, evidence indicates that the oxytocin receptor (OXTR) gene and the arginine vasopressin 1a receptor (AVPR1a) gene (for reviews, see Riedl & Javor, 2012, and Krueger & Meyer-Lindenberg, 2019, respectively), among others, are relevant in trust situations (see also Chapter 15). Altogether, today we know that human trust perceptions and trust behavior are influenced by biological factors (genes, hormones, and the nervous system, in particular the brain) and environmental factors (e.g., socialization, culture, experience, and task demand) (Cesarini et al., 2008; Riedl & Javor, 2012).

3.2.2   *Scenario B: Computer-Mediated Human–Human Interaction*

Trust research on computer-mediated human–human interaction has dealt with a number of phenomena that characterize a digital world, such as trust in virtual teams (e.g., Gallivan, 2001; Jarvenpaa et al., 2004; Paul & McDaniel, 2004; Piccoli & Ives, 2003), trust in online social networking and virtual communities (e.g., Fogel & Nehmad, 2009; Johnson & Kaye, 2009; Junglas et al., 2007; Lankton & McKnight, 2011), and trust in e-commerce (e.g., Ba & Pavlou, 2002; Gefen et al., 2003; McKnight et al., 2002; Pavlou & Gefen, 2004). Most studies on computer-mediated human–human interaction used survey as the research method. A major finding across investigations in the different domains is that both trusting beliefs and trusting intentions are influenced by institution-based trust and a trustee's trustworthiness (ability, benevolence, integrity).

Institution-based trust describes a situation in which an individual believes that "favorable conditions are in place that are conducive to situational success in a risky endeavor" (McKnight & Chervany, 2001, p. 37). Thus, the argument is that one can rely on other individuals in computer-mediated interactions, often unknown people, because of regulations and structures that secure that things will go well. Laws and governmental enforcement bodies are an important basis for institution-based trust to develop. Thus, this kind of trust refers to beliefs about those protective institutions, not about the individual interaction partners. Evidence indicates that institution-based trust is critical to establish trustful interaction with other humans in computer-mediated environments and with online companies. Such environments include, but are not limited to, e-commerce (e.g., eBay, Amazon) and online social networking (e.g., Facebook, LinkedIn). In essence, without a minimum level of trust in the Internet in general, as well as some basic trust in a platform that constitutes the technological basis for human online interaction (e.g., eBay or Facebook), trusting beliefs and intentions toward a specific trustee, as well as subsequent behaviors (e.g., buying online, connecting with other people, information sharing), struggle to emerge (e.g., Gefen et al., 2003; McKnight et al., 2002). Seminal work on the critical role of institution-based trust in online environments has been published by Pavlou and Gefen (2004). Based on Amazon's online auction marketplace, they demonstrated that feedback mechanisms (buyers can post feedback about individual sellers), escrow services (payments are authorized only after the buyer is satisfied), and credit card guarantees (recourse is provided by financial institutions in case of fraudulent seller behavior) significantly influence both objective and self-reported transaction behavior, and that this relationship is mediated by increased trust and reduced risk perceptions.

In addition to survey research, computer-mediated interaction among humans was also investigated with fMRI. One brain imaging study used websites of eBay feedback profiles with varying levels of trustworthiness as stimuli to trigger brain activation (Dimoka, 2010). The manipulation was based on the ratio between positive, neutral, and negative feedback comments. In online environments, sellers have a strong incentive to act in a trustworthy manner because opportunistic behavior would negatively affect comments in feedback profiles and hence could erode reputation. The study found that trust is related to brain areas linked to anticipating rewards (caudate nucleus), predicting the behavior of others (anterior paracingulate cortex), and calculating uncertainty (orbitofrontal cortex). Distrust was related to brain areas linked to intense negative emotions (amygdala) and fear of loss (insular cortex). Another brain imaging study (Riedl et al., 2010) used internet offers of eBay sellers as stimuli. Toulmin's (1958) model of argumentation was applied to develop product description texts with varying degrees of trustworthiness. Findings indicate that the processing of trustworthy eBay offers activated both reward processing areas (striatum) and mentalizing areas (prefrontal regions and cingulate cortex). The processing of untrustworthy eBay offers, in contrast, activated regions associated with perception of uncertainty, in particular the insula.

Based on the same data set as used in Riedl et al. (2010), one study investigated the influence of consumer impulsiveness on trustworthiness evaluations in online settings (Hubert et al., 2018). Specifically, to investigate the differences between neural processes in the brains of shoppers with high and low impulsiveness (assessed via a survey instrument) during the trustworthiness evaluation of eBay offers, this study used a region-of-interest analysis to correlate neural activity patterns with behavioral measures. Findings show that impulsiveness can exert a significant influence on the evaluation of product offers in online environments. With respect to brain activation, both shoppers with high and low impulsiveness showed similar neural activation tendencies, but significant differences existed in the magnitude of activation patterns in brain regions that are closely related to trust and impulsiveness such as the dorsal striatum, anterior cingulate cortex, dorsolateral prefrontal cortex, and the insula.

In addition to eBay websites, Facebook was also used as stimulus in a brain imaging study. One experiment investigated trustworthiness judgments in online social networking to better understand how a picture of oneself in the Facebook profile, as well as textual information to describe oneself, influence users' initial connecting behavior (Kopton et al., 2013). Note that in such a situation the sender of a contact request acts in the role of trustor, while the recipient of the request acts in the role of trustee who can signal trustworthiness based on his or her picture and textual information. Results indicate that both pictures and textual information have strong influence on trustworthiness judgments, and these judgments are processed differently in the users' brains. Specifically, it was found that user profiles with pictures activated the fusiform area significantly more than user profiles without pictures. This result is consistent with prior evidence on the emotional processing of faces (Kanwisher et al., 1997). Moreover, the amygdala was significantly more activated for user profiles with pictures when compared to user profiles without pictures. Because the amygdala is critical for processing of emotional information, the authors hypothesize that the affective processing of trust is stronger for user profiles with pictures. Brain data analyses further revealed that perception of user profiles with textual information mainly activated brain regions responsible for cognitive processing, reading, and mentalizing, such as superior parietal lobule, frontal pole, and frontal gyrus.

When we compare the findings from trust studies in the domains of technology-free human–human interaction and computer-mediated human–human interaction it can be observed that brain activation patterns are similar. Krueger and Meyer-Lindenberg (2019) recently described the reward network (anticipation of reward as a basis for a trusting decision), salience network (incorporation of aversive feelings related to risk of treachery by another person), central-executive network (cognitively controlling immediate emotional reactions), and default-mode network (mentalizing and implementation of social cognition) as critical in trust situations. Emergence of these four brain networks, as indicated in their paper, is based on extensive investigation of studies on technology-free human–human interaction. However, the brain data presented in the studies by Dimoka (2010), Kopton et al. (2013), Hubert et al. (2018), and Riedl et al. (2010) show that trusting decisions in computer-mediated human–human interaction situation are related to activity in areas in the same four brain networks. What follows is that when human social interaction becomes computer-mediated, trust processes seem to remain relatively stable if compared to the processes observed in technology-free environments. However, further brain research studies are necessary in the domain of computer-mediated human–human interaction to replicate this conclusion.

3.2.3   Scenario C: Human–Technology Interaction

Trust between humans in computer-mediated environments resembles interpersonal trust in technology-free environments. However, there is debate over whether it is valid for technological artifacts (e.g., machines or software systems) to be considered as recipients of trust (e.g., Wang & Benbasat, 2005). Those who argue that a technology cannot be a trust target postulate that technologies lack important attributes of people, such as consciousness or experience of betrayal if trust is breached (e.g., Friedman et al., 2000; Friedman & Millett, 1997). What follows is that technological artifacts cannot be trusted, they can only be relied upon.

In sharp contrast to this view, research grounded in the Computers Are Social Actors (CASA) paradigm revealed that people follow similar social rules and heuristics when they interact with technological artifacts like computers as they do when interacting with humans (Nass et al., 1993, 1994; Reeves & Nass, 1996). For example, reciprocity is a phenomenon directly related to trust (Riedl et al., 2011). Surprisingly, people apply social reciprocity rules in their interactions with computers. What follows is that a mindless machine can be a recipient of trust, even though it lacks human attributes such as intentionality or free will (also referred to as volition). Consider the following intriguing experiment: Fogg and Nass (1997) conducted a study with two tasks: one in which the computer helped the user, and another in which the user was asked to help the computer. In the first task, subjects conducted a series of web searches with a computer and the search results were either not useful or useful. In the second task, subjects interacted with a computer that was given the task of creating a color palette to match human perceptions of color. Subjects were told that by making accurate comparisons of sets of presented colors, they could help the computer to create this palette. Importantly, subjects were free to choose the number of comparisons to make. The more comparisons a subject made, the more help was provided to the computer. In one experimental condition, subjects performed both tasks on the same computer. In another condition, subjects used one computer for the first task, and a second, though identical, computer for the second task. Results showed that subjects who worked with a helpful computer in the first task and then returned to the same computer in the second task performed significantly more work for the computer in the second task, compared to those participants who used two different computers for the two tasks. Moreover, when participants worked with a computer that was not very helpful in the first task, and then returned to the same computer in the second task, they made significantly fewer comparisons than did participants who used different computers. These results provide evidence that users apply reciprocity norms even when they interact with a mindless object like a computer that lacks agency and volition.

A fundamental question is whether humans, in their interaction with technological artifacts, do apply the same trustworthiness dimensions as in human social interaction, namely ability, benevolence, and integrity. In this context, Wang and Benbasat (2005, p. 76) write:

> [W]hile it may at first appear debatable that technological artifacts can be objects of trust, and that people assign human properties to them, evidence from a variety of relevant literature supports this argument. People respond socially to technological artifacts and perceive that they possess human characteristics (e.g. motivation, integrity, and personality). In particular, research findings have demonstrated that components of trust in humans and in technological artifacts do not differ significantly. This indicates that people not only utilize technological artifacts as tools, but also form social and trusting relationships with them.

Considering this statement and further empirical evidence from the CASA paradigm (e.g., Brave et al., 2005), it seems reasonable to assume that humans do apply the same trustworthiness dimensions, despite the fact that it is actually not rational to consider a computer with no agency and volition as benevolent or to have integrity.

However, evidence from human–computer interaction, ergonomics, and information systems research shows that the trustworthiness dimensions change, and should change, as a function of the trust target (e.g., Hancock et al., 2011; McKnight et al., 2011). Despite the fact that a huge number of possible trust targets exist in a digital world (e.g., the Internet in general, an online provider, hardware, software, or communities of internet users; Söllner et al., 2016), the major distinction to be made is inherent in the scenarios of Figure 3.1. While in scenarios A and B the trustee is human, in scenarios C and D the trustee is a technological artifact.

Referring to scenarios C and D, an early and still viable suggestion was that evaluation of a technology's trustworthiness should be based on its performance, process, and purpose rather than its ability, benevolence, and integrity (e.g., Lee & Moray, 1992; Muir, 1987; Zuboff, 1988). Performance refers to a user's expectation of consistent, stable, and reliable technology behavior. Process refers to the understanding of the underlying characteristics that govern technology behavior. Purpose refers to the technology's underlying motives and intents; the purpose of a technology reflects the developer's intention in creating the technology. One paper used this conceptualization in a mobile application context and confirmed that these three factors predict trust in a technological artifact well (Söllner et al., 2012). Moreover, this paper established eleven determinants of the three trustworthiness dimensions (three for performance, e.g., reliability; five for process, e.g., data integrity; three for purpose, e.g., designer benevolence).

During the past decade researchers directly contrasted trust in technological artifacts with computer-mediated trust in human social interaction. Table 3.1 summarizes two comparisons in which trust in technology has been contrasted with the seminal work by Mayer et al. (1995) on trusting beliefs in interpersonal and organizational relationships (ability, benevolence, integrity). The following conclusion can be highlighted: Ability of a human trustee resembles, but is different from, performance or functionality of a technology. Integrity resembles, but is different from, predictability or reliability. Finally, benevolence resembles, but is different from, helpfulness.

A fundamental question is whether the *degree of anthropomorphism* of a technological artifact alters trust perceptions and corresponding behaviors. Anthropomorphism denotes the phenomenon that humans attribute human traits, emotions, and intentions to nonhuman entities, here

Table 3.1. *Trusting beliefs in interpersonal relationships and corresponding trusting beliefs in human–technology relationships*

Trusting Beliefs in Interpersonal and Organizational Relationships	Trusting Beliefs in Human–Technology Relationships	
Mayer et al. (1995, pp. 717–719)	Paravastu et al. (2014, p. 34)	Lankton et al. (2015, p. 882)
Study context: interpersonal and organizational trust	Study context: software artifact (antiviral software)	Study context: software artifact (database management system, online social networking site)
Ability is the extent to which a trustee is believed to have the skills and competencies that are important for a relationship with the trustor.	Performance is the belief about the capability of the technology to accomplish its designated purpose.	Functionality is the belief that the technology has the capability, functions, or features to fulfill the requirements.
Benevolence is the extent to which a trustee is believed to want to do good to the trustor, aside from an egocentric profit motive.	Not applicable to technology.	Helpfulness is the belief that the specific technology provides adequate and responsive help for users.
Integrity is the extent to which a trustee is believed to adhere to a set of principles that the trustor finds acceptable.	Predictability is the belief that the technology will do what it is claimed to do without adding anything malicious on top of it.	Reliability is the belief that the technology will consistently operate properly.

Note: The definitions of the trusting beliefs have been slightly modified to be directly comparable across the three articles.

technological artifacts. Obviously, perceived anthropomorphism inherent in a technology can be manipulated based on its behavior and appearance. As an example, the reciprocity experiment by Fogg and Nass (1997) manipulated behavior. However, several studies also manipulated a technology's appearance and examined effects on trust and related processes such as mentalizing. One fMRI investigation studied whether an increase of human-likeness of interaction partners (computer, functional robot, anthropomorphic robot, human) would modulate the subjects' mentalizing brain activities (Krach et al., 2008). An iterated prisoner's dilemma game was used as a task to induce mentalizing. During the experiment subjects always played against a random sequence unknowingly to them. Irrespective of the interaction partners' responses, brain data revealed a significant linear increase of activity in mentalizing areas (medial frontal cortex, temporo-parietal junction) in correspondence with the increase of human-likeness. Consistent with this result, another experiment found that trust in an autonomous vehicle increased with rising degree of anthropomorphism (Waytz et al., 2014). Finally, a meta-analysis on trust in human–robot interaction explicitly identified anthropomorphism as a major trust determinant (Hancock et al., 2011).

3.2.4   Scenario D: Computer-Mediated Human–Technology Interaction

A detailed look at the game literature as it pertains to trust and mentalizing shows that most studies are designed so that participants play against *human* opponents, which simulates interaction in technology-free environments. However, a few game studies have also investigated participants' brain activation while playing the TG and similar games against *computer* opponents (Table 3.2). Unlike direct and hence noncomputer-mediated interaction with technological artifacts (e.g., robot, automated airline self-check-in, autonomous vehicle), the studies reviewed in this section refer to *computer-mediated* interaction with technological artifacts, including internet chatbots or software programs. Such artifacts are used on desktop PCs or mobile technologies such as the smartphone. Most notably, experiment participants playing against computer opponents are normally informed that the computer opponent "would play a fixed probabilistic strategy" (McCabe et al., 2001, p. 11832). Moreover, participants lying in the fMRI scanner are usually shown "a picture of a computer" (e.g., Rilling et al., 2004, p. 1695) or are simply informed on the screen about their interaction partner with the word "computer" (e.g., Krach et al. 2009, p. 8). Such designation of the opponent as computer creates a sharp differentiation between the technological artifact and humans, because the latter are usually shown with a picture of the face. In particular, this emphasis on the distinction between humans and technology as interaction partners in a trusting situation may explain the differences in behavior and in the underlying brain mechanisms, because technologies could be perceived as mindless, while humans are not. Table 3.2 summarizes neuroscience

Table 3.2. *Major neuroscience studies on computer-mediated human–technology interaction with a focus on trust and mentalizing*

Source	Method / Game	Major Findings
Coricelli & Nagel, (2009)	fMRI / BCG	Playing against humans versus a computer (which plays randomly) activated, among other areas, the two mentalizing regions mPFC (BA 10) and rACC (BA 32).
Gallagher et al., (2002)	PET / RPS	Bilateral anterior paracingulate cortex (BA 9 and 32), a mentalizing region, is more activated when people believed that they were playing against another human compared to playing against a computer that applied a rule-based strategy or random strategy.
Krach et al., (2009)	fMRI / PDG	Playing against putative human and computer partners resulted in activity increases in the mentalizing network. However, mPFC and ACC activity were significantly more pronounced when participants believed they were playing against the human partner rather than a mindless machine (Both the human and computer partners were programmed to play a random sequence.).
McCabe et al., (2001)	fMRI / TG	Participants with the highest cooperation scores show increases in activation in the mPFC (BA 10) during human–human interaction when compared with human–computer interaction, whereas within the group of noncooperators results did not show significant activation differences in this brain region between the human and computer condition (participants were informed that the computer would play a fixed probabilistic strategy).
Rilling et al., (2002)	fMRI / PDG	When playing the game with a computer rather than a human, cooperation was less common (although participants were actually playing against the same strategy in both conditions). The neuronal results reveal that cooperation with a computer activated regions of the vmPFC and OFC that were also activated with human playing partners. In particular, this activation could be elicited by interactive computer programs, which are programmed to be responsive to their partner's behavior. Cooperation with a computer did not activate the rACC (BA 32), which was observed for human playing partners.
Rilling et al., (2004)	fMRI / UG / PDG	For both games, activation was found in the dmPFC (BA 9) and rACC (BA 32), two mentalizing regions. Both regions responded to decisions from human

Table 3.2. (*cont.*)

Source	Method / Game	Major Findings
		and from computer partners, but showed stronger responses to human partners in both games. The stronger response to human partners is consistent with the behavioral data showing that participants distinguished between human and computer partners, rejecting unfair offers from human partners more often in the UG and cooperating more frequently with human partners in the PDG.

Notes: ACC = anterior cingulate cortex; BA = Brodmann area; BCG - beauty contest game; dmPFC = dorsomedial prefrontal cortex; fMRI = functional magnetic resonance imaging; mPFC = medial prefrontal cortex; OFC = orbitofrontal cortex; PDG = prisoner's dilemma game; PET = positron emission tomography; rACC = rostral anterior cingulate cortex; RPS = rock-paper-scissors; TG = trust game; UG = ultimatum game; vmPFC - ventromedial prefrontal cortex

studies that, by design, resemble computer-mediated human–technology interaction in reality. Note that this table only lists studies in which the technology was neither denoted nor illustrated with anthropomorphic cues. Thus, the technology was described in the most abstract way, either by simply using the label "computer" or by merely showing a picture of a computer as a mechanistic device.

What is the major insight from these brain imaging studies? It is that people typically perceive humans and technological artifacts differently. In particular, brain activation patterns differ significantly between human–human and computer-mediated human–technology interactions in mentalizing areas. A major factor that explains this difference is that people attribute consciousness to humans, but not to technological artifacts (e.g., Friedman et al., 2000; Friedman & Millett, 1997). Of note, mentalizing is a major phenomenon in a trust situation because the decision to trust implies thinking about a trustee's intentions, feelings, and thoughts (e.g., Krueger et al., 2007; Winston et al., 2002). Hence, in a trust decision situation we would definitely expect activation in mentalizing brain areas, a notion widely supported in the literature. Fehr (2009b, p. 228), for example, wrote that "[s]ince trust decisions are also likely to involve perspective-taking, they should also activate areas implicated in theory-of-mind tasks" (theory-of-mind and mentalizing are two terms that are often used interchangeably in the literature).

Anthropomorphism also plays a significant role for trust perceptions in computer-mediated human–technology interaction, not just in situations of direct interaction with a technological artifact (as described in Section 3.2.3). One study examined interaction with virtual humans (Riedl et al., 2014). These virtual humans possessed realistic, yet cartoon-like faces. Research has already determined prior to this study that communication with a virtual face may increase perceived interpersonal trust in anonymous online environments (Bente et al., 2008). Despite this trust-inducing potential of virtual faces, however, Riedl et al. (2014) hypothesized that in trust situations people would perceive human faces differently than they would perceive virtual faces. This prediction is based on evolution theory, because throughout human history the majority of interaction among people has taken place in face-to-face settings. Therefore, unlike perception of a virtual face, perception of a human face and the related trustworthiness discrimination abilities must be part of the genetic makeup of humans. Against this background, Riedl et al. (2014) conducted an experiment based on a multiround TG to gain insight into the differences and similarities of interactions between humans versus human interaction with virtual humans that lacked agency. Findings indicate that people are better able to predict the trustworthiness of humans than the trustworthiness of virtual humans. Moreover, it was found that decision making about whether or not to trust another actor activates the medial frontal cortex, a mentalizing area, significantly more during interaction with humans, if compared to interaction with virtual humans. Further, the results showed that the trustworthiness learning rate is similar, whether interacting with humans or virtual humans. Thus, this study suggests that although interaction on the Internet may have benefits, the lack of real human faces in communication may serve to reduce these benefits, in turn leading to reduced levels of collaboration effectiveness (Riedl et al., 2011, pp. 13–16).

Importantly, a follow-up study revealed that interaction with virtual faces rather than real human faces may be beneficial for specific patient populations. Specifically, this study investigated how Parkinson's disease patients would behave in a TG played with human and virtual human counterparts, and this behavior was compared to the behavior of healthy controls (HCs) (Javor et al., 2016). Based on the fact that the pathology of Parkinson's disease affects brain areas related to trust (basal ganglia, limbic structures, frontal cortex), it was predicted that trust behavior differs between Parkinson's disease patients and healthy people. In fact, what was found is intriguing. First, patients trusted human faces significantly less than HCs. Second, patients trusted virtual human faces significantly more than human faces. Third, there was no significant difference between initial trust of patients and HCs in virtual human faces. The implications of these findings are crucial. The first finding offers a plausible explanation why Parkinson's disease patients do not always follow their physician's recommendation to take their medication (Javor et al., 2015). The second and third findings suggest the solution to the problem, namely that the recommendation to take medication could be given by a virtual human (e.g., via smartphone).

In another study, subjects received advice that deteriorated gradually in reliability from a computer, a computer with a virtual face, and a human agent (De Visser et al., 2016). It is reported that anthropomorphic agents were associated with higher resistance to breakdowns in trust, referred to as trust resilience. Further, anthropomorphism decreased initial expectations, dampened impact of trust violations, and improved trust repair. Thus, endowing a technology with human characteristics can be beneficial, at least in some situations. Such characteristics may refer to both appearance and behavior (e.g., Appel et al., 2012).

3.3   Conclusion

Figure 3.1 shows major trust scenarios in a digital world. Based on this conceptual basis, the present chapter developed the following major insights. First, contrasting Scenario A versus B, it was found that trust processes in computer-mediated human–human interaction seem to resemble the processes in technology-free environments. Second, contrasting A and B versus C and D, different trustworthiness dimensions play a role. When the trustee is human, independent from whether the human interaction is computer-mediated or not, ability, benevolence, and integrity are the major dimensions. However, when the trustee is a technological artifact without agency and volition, these dimensions change, and should be changed, to functionality, performance, helpfulness, reliability, and predictability. Third, referring to scenarios C and D, when mere technological artifacts are endowed with human characteristics (e.g., appearance, behavior), trust processes resemble those that are active in situations in which the trustee is human (i.e., scenarios A and B). Intriguingly, neuroscience evidence shows that the human-likeness of an interaction partner modulates people's mentalizing and trusting brain activities. What follows is that anthropomorphism is a major "regulating screw" when trust has to be "engineered" in an increasing digitalized world. It will be rewarding to see what insight future research and engineering activities will reveal.

References

Appel, J., von der Pütten, A., Krämer, N. C., & Gratch, J. (2012). Does humanity matter? Analyzing the importance of social cues and perceived agency of a computer system for the emergence of social reactions during human-computer interaction. *Advances in Human-Computer Interaction*, 2012, Article 324694. https://doi.org/10.1155/2012/324694

Ba, S. L., & Pavlou, P. A. (2002). Evidence of the effect of trust building technology in electronic markets: Price premiums and buyer behavior. *MIS Quarterly*, 26(3), 243–268. https://doi.org/10.2307/4132332

Baumgartner, T., Heinrichs, M., Vonlanthen, A., Fischbacher, U., & Fehr, E. (2008). Oxytocin shapes the neural circuitry of trust and trust adaptation in humans. *Neuron*, 58(4), 639–650. https://doi.org/10.1016/j.neuron.2008.04.009

Bellucci, G., Chernyak, S. V., Goodyear, K., Eickhoff, S. B., & Krueger, F. (2017). Neural signatures of trust in reciprocity: A coordinate-based meta-analysis. *Human Brain Mapping*, 38(3), 1233–1248. https://doi.org/10.1002/hbm.23451

Bente, G., Rüggenberg, S., Krämer, N. C., & Eschenburg, F. (2008). Avatar-mediated networking: Increasing social presence and interpersonal trust in net-based collaborations. *Human Communication Research*, 34(2), 287–318. https://doi.org/10.1111/j.1468-2958.2008.00322.x

Berg, J., Dickhaut, J., & McCabe, K. (1995). Trust, reciprocity, and social-history. *Games and Economic Behavior*, 10(1), 122–142. https://doi.org/10.1006/game.1995.1027

Brave, S., Nass, C., & Hutchinson, K. (2005). Computers that care: Investigating the effects or orientation of emotion exhibited by an embodied computer agent. *International Journal of Human-Computer Studies*, 62(2), 161–178. https://doi.org/10.1016/j.ijhcs.2004.11.002

Cesarini, D., Dawes, C. T., Fowler, J. H., Johannesson, M., Lichtenstein, P., & Wallace, B. (2008). Heritability of cooperative behavior in the trust game. *Proceedings of the National Academy of Sciences*, 105(10), 3721–3726. https://doi.org/10.1073/pnas.0710069105

Coricelli, G., & Nagel, R. (2009). Neural correlates of depth of strategic reasoning in medial prefrontal cortex. *Proceedings of the National Academy of Sciences*, 106(23), 9163–9168. https://doi.org/10.1073/pnas.0807721106

De Visser, E. J., Monfort, S. S., McKendrick, R., et al. (2016). Almost human: Anthropomorphism increases trust resilience in cognitive agents. *Journal of Experimental Psychology: Applied*, 22(3), 331–349. https://doi.org/10.1037/xap0000092

Dimoka, A. (2010). What does the brain tell us about trust and distrust? Evidence from a functional neuroimaging study. *MIS Quarterly*, 34(2), 373–396. https://doi.org/10.2307/20721433

Fehr, E. (2009a). On the economics and biology of trust. *Journal of the European Economic Association*, 7(2–3), 235–266. https://doi.org/10.1162/JEEA.2009.7.2-3.235

(2009b). Social preferences and the brain. In P. W. Glimcher, C. F. Camerer, E. Fehr, & R. A. Poldrack (Eds.), *Neuroeconomics: Decision making and the brain* (pp. 215–232). Academic Press. https://doi.org/10.1016/B978–0-12-374176-9.00015-4

Fogel, J., & Nehmad, E. (2009). Internet social network communities: Risk taking, trust, and privacy concerns. *Computers in Human Behavior*, 25(1), 153–160. https://doi.org/10.1016/j.chb.2008.08.006

Fogg, B. J., & Nass, C. (1997). How users reciprocate to computers: An experiment that demonstrates behavior change. *Proceedings of the Conference on Human Factors in Computing Systems*, 1997, 331–332. https://doi.org/10.1145/1120212.1120419

Friedman, B., Kahn, P. H. Jr., & Howe, D. C. (2000). Trust online. *Communications of the ACM*, 43(12), 34–40. https://doi.org/10.1145/355112.355120

Friedman, B., & Millett. L. I. (1997). Reasoning about computers as moral agents: A research note. In B. Friedman (Ed.), *Human values and the design of computer technology* (pp. 201–205). CSLI Publications.

Gallagher, H. L., Jack, A. I., Roepstorff, A., & Frith, C. D. (2002). Imaging the intentional stance in a competitive game. *NeuroImage*, 16(3), 814–821. https://doi.org/10.1006/nimg.2002.1117

Gallivan, M. J. (2001). Striking a balance between trust anti control in a virtual organization: A content analysis of open source software case studies. *Information Systems Journal*, 11(4), 277–304. https://doi.org/10.1046/j.1365-2575.2001.00108.x

Gefen, D., Karahanna, E., & Straub, D. W. (2003). Trust and TAM in online shopping: An integrated model. *MIS Quarterly*, 27(1), 51–90. https://doi.org/10.2307/30036519

Hancock, P. A., Billings, D. R., Schaefer, K. E., Chen, J. Y. C., de Visser, E. J., & Parasuraman, R. (2011). A meta-analysis of factors affecting trust in human-robot interaction. *Human Factors*, 53(5), 517–527. https://doi.org/10.1177/0018720811417254

Hubert, M., Hubert, M., Linzmajer, M., Riedl, R., & Kenning, P. (2018). Trust me if you can: Neurophysiological insights on the influence of consumer impulsiveness on trustworthiness evaluations in online settings. *European Journal of Marketing*, 52(1–2), 118–146. https://doi.org/10.1108/EJM-12-2016-0870

ITU. (2019). *Measuring digital development: Facts and figures 2019*. www.itu.int/en/ITU-D/Statistics/Documents/facts/FactsFigures2019.pdf

Jarvenpaa, S. L., Shaw, T. R., & Staples, D. S. (2004). Toward contextualized theories of trust: The role of trust in global virtual teams. *Information Systems Research*, 15(3), 250–267. https://doi.org/10.1287/isre.1040.0028

Javor, A., Ransmayr, G., Struhal, W., & Riedl, R. (2016). Parkinson patients' initial trust in avatars: Theory and evidence. *PLoS ONE*, 11(11), Article e0165998. https://doi.org/10.1371/journal.pone.0165998

Javor, A., Riedl, R., Kirchmayr, M., Reichenberger, M., & Ransmayr, G. (2015). Trust behavior in Parkinson's disease: Results of a trust game experiment. *BMC Neurology*, 15(126), 1–7. https://doi.org/10.1186/s12883-015-0374-5

Johnson, N. D., & Mislin, A. A. (2011). Trust games: A meta-analysis. *Journal of Economic Psychology*, 32(5), 865–889. https://doi.org/10.1016/j.joep.2011.05.007

Johnson, T. J., & Kaye, B. K. (2009). In blog we trust? Deciphering credibility of components of the Internet among politically interested internet users. *Computers in Human Behavior*, 25(1), 175–182. https://doi.org/10.1016/j.chb.2008.08.004

Junglas, I. A., Johnson, N. A., Steel, D. J., Abraham, C., & Loughlin, P. M. (2007). Identity formation, learning styles and trust in virtual worlds. *The DATA BASE for Advances in Information Systems*, 38(4), 90–96. https://doi.org/10.1145/1314234.1314251

Kanwisher, N., McDermott, J., & Chun, M. M. (1997). The fusiform face area: A module in human extrastriate cortex specialized for face perception. *Journal of Neuroscience*, 17(11), 4302–4311. https://doi.org/10.1523/JNEUROSCI.17-11-04302.1997

Kopton, I., Sommer, J., Winkelmann, A., Riedl, R., & Kenning, P. (2013). Users' trust building processes during their initial connecting behavior in social networks: behavioral and neural evidence. *Proceedings of the International Conference on Information Systems*, 107.

Krach, S., Blümel, I., Marjoram, D., et al. (2009). Are women better mind-readers? Sex differences in neural correlates of mentalizing detected with functional MRI. *BMC Neuroscience*, 10, 1–11. https://doi.org/10.1186/1471-2202-10-9

Krach, S., Hegel, F., Wrede, B., Sagerer, G., Binkofski, F., & Kircher, T. (2008). Can machines think? Interaction and perspective taking with robots investigated via fMRI. *PLoS ONE*, 3(7), Article e2597. https://doi.org/10.1371/journal.pone.0002597

Krueger, F., McCabe, K., et al. (2007). Neural correlates of trust. *Proceedings of the National Academy of Sciences*, 104(50), 20084–20089. https://doi.org/10.1073/pnas.0710103104

Krueger, F., & Meyer-Lindenberg, A. (2019). Toward a model of interpersonal trust drawn from neuroscience, psychology, and economics. *Trends in Neurosciences*, 42(2), 92–101. https://doi.org/10.1016/j.tins.2018.10.004

Lankton, N. K., & McKnight, D. H. (2011). What does it mean to trust Facebook? Examining technology and interpersonal trust beliefs. *The DATA BASE for Advances in Information Systems*, 42(2), 32–54. https://doi.org/10.1145/1989098.1989101

Lankton, N. K., McKnight, D. H., & Tripp, J. (2015). Technology, humanness, and trust: Rethinking trust in technology. *Journal of the Association for Information Systems*, 16(10), 880–918. https://doi.org/10.17705/1jais.00411

Lee, J., & Moray, N. (1992). Trust, control strategies and allocation of function in human-machine systems. *Ergonomics*, 35(10), 1243–1270. https://doi.org/10.1080/00140139208967392

Luhmann, N. (1979). *Trust and power.* Wiley.

Mayer, R. C., Davis, J. H., & Schoorman, F. D. (1995). An integrative model of organizational trust. *Academy of Management Review,* 20(3), 709–734. https://doi.org/10.2307/258792

McCabe, K., Houser, D., Ryan, L., Smith, V., & Trouard, T. (2001). A functional imaging study of cooperation in two-person reciprocal exchange. *Proceedings of the National Academy of Sciences,* 98(20), 11832–11835. https://doi.org/10.1073/pnas.211415698

McKnight, D. H., Carter, M., Thatcher, J. B., & Clay, P. F. (2011). Trust in a specific technology: An investigation of its components and measures. *ACM Transactions on Management Information Systems,* 2(2), Article 12. https://doi.org/10.1145/1985347.1985353

McKnight, D. H., & Chervany, N. L. (2001). Trust and distrust definitions: One bite at a time. In R. Falcone, M. Singh, & Y. H. Tan (Eds.), *Trust in cybersocieties: Integrating the human and artificial perspectives* (pp. 27–54). Springer. https://doi.org/10.1007/3-540-45547-7_3

McKnight, D. H., Choudhury, V., & Kacmar, C. (2002). Developing and validating trust measures for e-commerce: An integrative typology. *Information Systems Research,* 13(3), 334–359. https://doi.org/10.1287/isre.13.3.334.81

Muir, B. M. (1987). Trust between humans and machines, and the design of decision aids. *International Journal of Man-Machine Studies,* 27(5–6), 527–539. https://doi.org/10.1016/S0020-7373(87)80013-5

Nass, C., Steuer, J. S., Henriksen, L., & Dryer, D. C. (1994). Machines, social attributions, and ethopoeia: Performance assessments of computers subsequent to "self-" or "other-" evaluations. *International Journal of Human-Computer Studies,* 40(3), 543–559. https://doi.org/10.1006/ijhc.1994.1025

Nass, C., Steuer, J. S., Tauber, E., & Reeder, H. (1993). Anthropomorphism, agency, and ethopoeia: Computers as social actors. *Proceedings of the INTERCHI '93 Conference on Human Factors in Computing Systems,* 1993, 111–112. https://doi.org/10.1145/259964.260137

Nicolaou, A. I., & McKnight, D. H. (2006). Perceived information quality in data exchanges: Effects on risk, trust, and intention to use. *Information Systems Research,* 17(4), 392–414. https://doi.org/10.1287/isre.1060.0103

Paravastu, N., Gefen, D., & Creason, S. (2014). Understanding trust in IT artifacts: An evaluation of the impact of trustworthiness and trust on satisfaction with antiviral software. *The DATA BASE for Advances in Information Systems,* 45(4), 30–50. https://doi.org/10.1145/2691517.2691520

Paul, D. L., & McDaniel, R. R. (2004). A field study of the effect of interpersonal trust on virtual collaborative relationship performance. *MIS Quarterly,* 28(2), 183–227. https://doi.org/10.2307/25148633

Pavlou, P. A., & Gefen, D. (2004). Building effective online marketplaces with institution-based trust. *Information Systems Research,* 15(1), 37–59. https://doi.org/10.1287/isre.1040.0015

Piccoli, G., & Ives, B. (2003). Trust and the unintended effects of behavior control in virtual teams. *MIS Quarterly*, 27(3), 365–395. https://doi.org/10 .2307/30036538

Reeves, B., & Nass, C. (1996). *The media equation: How people treat computers, television, and new media like real people and places.* Cambridge University Press/CSLI.

Riedl, R., Hubert, M., & Kenning, P. (2010). Are there neural gender differences in online trust? An fMRI study on the perceived trustworthiness of eBay offers. *MIS Quarterly*, 34(2), 397–428. https://doi.org/10.2307/20721434

Riedl, R., & Javor, A. (2012). The biology of trust: Integrating evidence from genetics, endocrinology and functional brain imaging. *Journal of Neuroscience, Psychology, and Economics*, 5(2), 63–91. https://doi.org/10 .1037/a0026318

Riedl, R., Mohr, P., Kenning, P., Davis, F. D., & Heekeren, H. (2011). Trusting humans and avatars: Behavioral and neural evidence. *Proceedings of the 32nd International Conference on Information Systems*, 2011, 1–23.

(2014). Trusting humans and avatars: A brain imaging study based on evolution theory. *Journal of Management Information Systems*, 30(4), 83–114. https://doi.org/10.2753/MIS0742–1222300404

Rilling, J. K, Gutman, D. A., Zeh, T. R., Pagnoni, G., Berns, G. S., & Kilts, C. D. (2002). A neural basis for social cooperation. *Neuron*, 35(2), 395–405. https://doi.org/10.1016/S0896–6273(02)00755-9

Rilling, J. K., Sanfey, A. G., Aronson, J. A., Nystrom, L. E., & Cohen, J. D. (2004). The neural correlates of theory of mind within interpersonal interactions. *NeuroImage*, 22(4), 1694–1703. https://doi.org/10.1016/j .neuroimage.2004.04.015

Rousseau, D. M., Sitkin, S. B., Burt, R. S., & Camerer, C. F. (1998). Not so different after all: A cross-discipline view of trust. *Academy of Management Review*, 23(3), 393–404. https://doi.org/10.5465/amr.1998.926617

Seppänen, R., Blomqvist, K., & Sundqvist, S. (2007). Measuring interorganizational trust: A critical review of the empirical research in 1990–2003. *Industrial Marketing Management*, 36(2), 249–265. https://doi .org/10.1016/j.indmarman.2005.09.003

Söllner, M., Hoffmann, A., Hoffmann, H., Wacker, A., & Leimeister, J. M. (2012). Understanding the formation of trust in IT artifacts. *Proceedings of the International Conference on Information Systems*, 2012.

Söllner, M., Hoffmann, A., & Leimeister, J. M. (2016). Why different trust relationships matter for information systems users. *European Journal of Information Systems*, 25(3), 274–287. https://doi.org/10.1057/ejis.2015.17

Swan, J. E., Bowers, M. R., & Richardson, L. D. (1999). Customer trust in the salesperson: An integrative review and meta-analysis of the empirical literature. *Journal of Business Research*, 44(2), 93–107. https://doi.org/10.1016/ S0148–2963(97)00244-0

Toulmin, S. (1958). *The use of argument.* Cambridge University Press.

Tzieropoulos, H. (2013). The trust game in neuroscience: A short review. *Social Neuroscience*, 8(5), 407–416. https://doi.org/10.1080/17470919.2013.832375

Wang, W., & Benbasat, I. (2005). Trust in and adoption of online recommendation agents. *Journal of the Association for Information Systems*, 6(3), 72–101. https://doi.org/10.17705/1jais.00065

Waytz, A., Heafner, J., & Epley, N. (2014). The mind in the machine: Anthropomorphism increases trust in an autonomous vehicle. *Journal of Experimental Social Psychology*, 52, 113–117. https://doi.org/10.1016/j.jesp.2014.01.005

Winston, J. S., Strange, B. A., O'Doherty, J., & Dolan, R. J. (2002). Automatic and intentional brain responses during evaluation of trustworthiness of faces. *Nature Neuroscience*, 5(3), 277–283. https://doi.org/10.1038/nn816

Yanquing, D., Edwards, J. S., & Dwivedi, Y. K. (2019). Artificial intelligence for decision making in the era of Big Data: Evolution, challenges and research agenda. *International Journal of Information Management*, 48, 63–71. https://doi.org/10.1016/j.ijinfomgt.2019.01.021

Zuboff, S. (1988). *In the age of the smart machine: The future of work and power.* Basic Books.

CHAPTER 4

Trust and Human Factors
Foundations of Trust in Automation

Tracy L. Sanders, Alexandra D. Kaplan, Keith MacArthur,
William G. Volante, and P. A. Hancock

4.1 Introduction

Human factors is a multidisciplinary field concerned with the human aspects of engineering. It aspires to optimize performance while minimizing error. In practice, this is often the study of how people use the objects, entities, and other things in their environment. In today's world the aim of human factors is generally to improve the ways in which people interact with all forms of technology, including most especially automation. The term automation covers a wide range of physical and electronic devices that conduct tasks. Automation generally promises to lower operator workload and thereby improve the quality of human life. Automated devices range in complexity and the degree of their autonomy from simple decision aids, where the automation supports users in making choices (e.g., automated lane-keeping assistance on a motor vehicle) to artificial intelligence systems that learn and change their behavior according to instructions and environmental feedback. This "intelligence" can be actualized in both physical (e.g., robot) and unembodied electronic (e.g., smart home device) systems. As such devices become ever-more integrated into all facets of human life, the quality of these interactions becomes determinative of social existence. This prospective quality of life is founded, at least to some degree, on trust.

While trust is often conceptualized as a facet of a relationship between two or more people, the rise of automation has necessitated a reconsideration and reconceptualization of trust. Now we see emerging needs for trust between humans and automated systems. Trust becomes especially important when humans and automated systems must work together toward a larger goal. However, the profile of trust is slightly different when

Approved for Public Release; Distribution Unlimited. Public Release Case Number 20-0954. The author's affiliation with The MITRE Corporation is provided for identification purposes only, and is not intended to convey or imply MITRE's concurrence with, or support for, the positions, opinions, or viewpoints expressed by the authors. Corresponding author: Tracy L. Sanders (tlsanders@mitre.org).

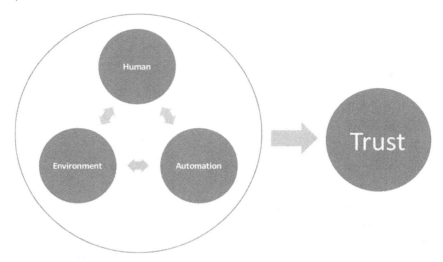

Figure 4.1   Human, environmental, and automation-specific variables interact to influence human trust in automated systems.

a person is trusting an automated system rather than another human (Hancock, Billings, & Schaefer, 2011). Specifically, trust between humans relies on the morals and motivations of the human trustee (person receiving the trust) to be coherent. However, an automated system lacks these internal motivations and currently acts only in accord with its programming or misprogramming. While there are differences between human–human and human–automation trust (Hancock et al., 2020), the overarching concept is consistent – the assumption that an entity can be relied upon to behave as expected.

Human–automation trust can be conceptualized as a three-factor model that features facets of the human trustor, the automated trustee, and the environment or context in which any such interaction occurs (Hancock, Billings, Schaefer, et al., 2011). This model, shown in Figure 4.1, presents a clear organizational schema to be able to investigate trust in all forms of technology. However, it is important that these three factors are not studied in isolation. This is because these factors necessarily interact with one another to influence how the human trustor perceives the automated trustee. Humans vary widely along many personality and performance dimensions, including variations in preexisting experience, knowledge, and cognitive capacities (i.e., individual differences). Similarly, automated systems themselves vary along comparable dimensions such as form, embodiment, behavior, capability, reliability, and level of autonomy. Further, the human and automated system interact together in a variety of ways (e.g., completing tasks on a team, business interactions) in dynamic real-world environments. The environment itself also contributes factors, including relationship and task. These experiences provide the human with the reference necessary to make trust decisions. Since each factor covaries along a number of dimensions, the interactions themselves are important because they can relatively easily and quickly change the nature of the trust relationship. For instance, a military robot may seem trustworthy if you are on a team working with that robot to rescue civilians after a disaster. However, the actions of that same robot in a daycare or shopping mall setting might induce much less trust.

Another level of complexity influencing the trust relationship between humans and automation is the passage of time. Trust represents an emergent quality that evolves, often from repeated interactions between the human trustor and the automated trustee. Each time a user interacts with a specific automated system, they bring their prior trust level to that interaction. Then, through the process of this next interaction, the human processes more information about the automated system. That, in turn, is added to their mental model, about not simply the specific automated system with which the user is interacting, but now with automated systems in general.

As our use of automation grows, so does the necessity to grant trust in automation appropriately. That is to say, it is important for humans to be able to determine correctly whether an automated system is safe and trustworthy. Here, the trust must be appropriately calibrated (Lee & Moray, 1994; Lee & See, 2004). Under-trust (i.e., too little trust) in a system can lead to its lack of use, which can be especially dangerous in situations where the automated systems' capabilities are heavily leveraged, or relied upon for safety (Parasuraman & Riley, 1997). The effects of under-trust and under-reliance often prove difficult to measure because it is difficult to demonstrate when a situation would have been safer if automation had been used. For instance, how many automobile collisions may have been avoided through more extended use of automatic emergency-breaking systems? While it is understood that this can make driving safer (National Highway Traffic Safety Administration, 2020), it proves almost impossible to quantify the number of collisions that this technology might prevent if it is not employed (Hancock, 2019). Over-trust (i.e., too much trust) in a system can lead to complacency and poor monitoring if the user overestimates the automated systems' capabilities.

For instance, a fatal 2016 car collision in Williston, Florida was attributed to a Tesla driver who failed to yield the right of way to a semitrailer. This was linked to a potential over-reliance on automation, and inattention to the status of the vehicle and roadway (National Transportation Safety Board, 2017). More egregious misuse has occurred when users try to "fool" the safety systems. For instance, a Salt Lake City man wedged an orange into the steering wheel of his Tesla Model S to put pressure on the sensors in the steering wheel so that it would appear that he had his hands on the wheel; thereby bypassing an important safety feature (Linderman, 2018).

Optimal interactions between humans and automated systems depend then upon appropriate trust calibration, and this calibration depends on all three of the identified factors of trust in automation. For the user to calibrate trust appropriately, their expectations of the automated system must be realistic. This means that they must have adequate experience with automated systems in general in order to understand their respective behaviors and limitations. It would be difficult for someone who had never seen a robot previously to properly calibrate their trust the first time they interacted with it. Features of the automated system also influence the trust calibration process through the information they provide to the human. For instance, a system that clearly indicates error to a user is more transparent than one that does not. More transparent systems may therefore better support real-time problem diagnosis, since this promotes a clear understanding of system performance. Such comprehension is key to appropriate trust calibration. The physical environment presents many factors and challenges for the human in understanding how a system is supposed to behave. The sections that follow describe the factors (human, robot, and environment) that are presently known to mediate human trust in automation. We also consider their interactions, as well as how the passage of time influences these relationships.

4.2 Human-Related Factors That Influence Trust

Many characteristics of human users (e.g., individual differences) can influence trust in human–automation interaction (HAI). These factors are generally stable, regardless of the type of entity with which the human interacts. While, to some degree they may change over time (e.g., age and experience both increase) and personality traits may fluctuate, individual differences typically remain stable across interactions with different technologies. These individual differences include everything the human brings to the encounter, including characteristics such as age, gender, and prior experience with technology or comfort with automation, as well as ability-based factors such as perceived workload.

The relationship between trust and general demographic classifications (e.g., age, gender, culture) can be difficult to analyze because humans are themselves multifaceted beings. Multiple characteristics are built up in unique configurations to create the whole person. Yet, it is undeniable that the entirety of a human being is more than the sum of measurable characteristics. Further, these characteristics interact among one another. For instance, culture can influence trust in robotics (Li et al., 2010) as can age (Erebak & Turgut, 2019; Heerink, 2011). However, the interaction between culture and age is more difficult to determine and is likely further confounded by experience with automation. With these multitudes of characteristics interacting in this fashion, it is difficult to parse the effects of specific factors and rank them in terms of which influences the trust relationship most strongly.

Time further complicates these relationships between human-related factors and trust, since the era in which a person was born (peer cohort) is likely to influence their lifetime-based experiences with automation. Research to date has indicated that age does prove to be a predictor of trust in an autonomous system; specifically, the younger the participant, the higher the level of trust in an autonomous system. This finding holds true across age groups (Scopelliti et al., 2005) including those of a largely college-aged sample (Schaefer, 2013). However, it has been difficult to parse age from experience with technology, as older people simply do not have a wealth of life-long experiences with automation from which to draw. This can be compared to younger people who have been raised in environments where automated systems have been commonplace. As these younger people, who have been steeped in technology since their birth get older, the influence of age on the human–autonomous system trust relationship will itself most probably change.

Various types of prior experience can serve to influence an individual's trust in an automated system. More experience with a robot, for example, is typically correlated with higher trust levels (Heerink, 2011). This is true whether people's experience is measured in hands-on activities like experience building and/or controlling robots, or in indirect encounters such as the number of feature movies about robots they have watched (Schaefer, 2013). Popular media radically influences public perceptions, including perceptions of automation. Hancock and colleagues discussed the fundamental attribution error in perceiving robots as operating and behaving like humans (Hancock, Billings, & Schaefer, 2011). Nevertheless, science fiction has frequently portrayed this situation and influenced public perception across the years. These authors indicated that this propensity proves concerning, since the intention of automation (more specifically, the human's perception of this intention) is critical to trust development.

An individual's preconceived notions concerning robots (derived from various sources) can have adverse effects on trust. One way to measure pre-existing attitudes toward automation empirically is through use of the Negative Attitudes toward Robots Scale (NARS; Nomura et al., 2006) The NARS measures individuals' negative attitudes surrounding interactions with robots, their perceptions of the social influence of robots, and their emotions regarding robots. It is unsurprising that studies have demonstrated that the higher ratings of negative attitudes toward robots are related to lower trust in robots in general (Wang et al., 2010).

Though examinations of how individual difference factors influence trust in automation vary, there remain some consistent findings related to human expectations. One such finding is the effect of the human user's understanding of their role in shared work with an automated system. Specifically, the more clarity an individual is provided concerning their own role, the higher their level of trust. For example, a study of home health aid workers found that when people believed their interactions with a robot would be simple to understand, they exhibited higher levels of trust than those who believed there would be some confusion about how to interact (Alaiad & Zhou, 2014). Similarly, in another study, those who had received a clear written explanation of a robot's role in an interaction showed higher trust in that robot as compared to those who had not been told about the robot's role (Groom et al., 2011). Users' perceived control over the interaction also influences trust level. Users who have contribution to the decision-making process of an autonomous entity proceed to report higher levels of trust (Phillips et al., 2017) than those who had less perceived control. Further, users with lower levels of expertise are more likely to blindly trust an automated system than those with high levels of expertise (McBride & Morgan, 2010). This implies a relationship between the users' perception and use of automation. These studies demonstrate that the way in which a human user perceives an automated system is influenced by their expectations of their own role and their ability to control the situation while performing the tasks in question.

Expectations and prospects of cognitive workload also serve to influence trust. Most automation, particularly if it is properly calibrated, can be used to reduce operator workload (Endsley & Kaber, 1999). Often, users do expect an automated system to decrease their workload, but may worry that the difficulty of using a nonintuitive interface, while interacting with technology that is unfamiliar to them, will increase that workload. Thus, the effect of expectancy on trust promises to be an effect of perceived workload. While increased workload can correlate with higher trust in autonomous systems (Biros et al., 2004), it is likely that this is only because the automation has the potential to decrease the operator workload by taking on some responsibilities for overall performance.

Personality factors have been found to influence trust in automated systems. Specifically, both extroversion (Haring et al., 2013; Szalma & Taylor, 2011) and agreeableness (Chien et al., 2016) have been demonstrated to influence trust respective of HAI. However, Block warned that personality in general is difficult to define (Block, 2001) and even more difficult to successfully measure in a consistent and reliable way. One issue is that the personality dimensions (e.g., extraversion, agreeableness, openness) are measured differently based on the type that is tested (e.g., Meyers-Briggs Type Indicator, the Revised NEO Personality Inventory). These tests are not necessarily consistent one with another. The complication of multiple uncorrelated tests is worsened in analysis and reporting, whereby results of these respective tests are often modeled to fit data.

While the performance characteristics of the robot are often considered, those of the human (both real and perceived) involved in the HAI are also relevant. Indeed, a certain level of familiarity in many diverse domains (e.g., basic technology knowledge, eyesight, manual dexterity) is often required to operate any given automated system. In addition, the human users' perceptions of those abilities, their expectations, and understanding of the situation persistently serve to shape the nature of HAI.

4.3 Automated System-Related Factors That Influence Trust

Implementing automation in any context requires consideration of its human operator, and good design practices encourage its intended and continuing use. As discussed before, trust in autonomation increases the likelihood of its appropriate use and discourages misuse, disuse, and abuse. Therefore, it is vital to consider the specific facets of automation that engender greater levels of trust.

Multiple meta-analyses have served as foundations for models of trust in HAI. These have found two categories of trust antecedents that are related to the automated system itself. That is, its physical and behavioral aspects and its performance (Hancock, Billings, Schaefer, et al., 2011; Hancock et al., 2020; Kessler et al., 2017). Performance refers to such characteristics as reliability and dependability. Physical and social aspects of the automated system, such as personality and proximity to the human user, are comprised of identified traits that relate to the capability of the autonomous entity and have the strongest influence on trust in automation (Hancock, Billings, Schaefer, et al., 2011).

4.3.1   *Physical and Behavior-Based Factors*

Physical system attributes, or the "look and feel" of a system, provide the initial basis for trust assessment in most HAI. Similar to the case with humans themselves, the more attractive an automated system is, the more likely it is to be accepted and trusted. However, the influence of these attributes does not cease after the first glance. Humans tend to make far-reaching attributions based solely on attractiveness (Ellis et al., 2005; Goetz et al., 2003). While this is obviously important for understanding trust in HAI, it is also difficult to tease apart the individual components that make up attractiveness. For this reason, it may be helpful to envision an automated system in a Gestalt fashion, that is, as a single cohesive unit (Koffka, 1935). Gestalt, which means a whole of something is different than the sum of its parts, is often used to describe something's overall aesthetic value. In reality, it applies to every factor that influences human perception in the interaction. That is to say, how a person perceives an automated system and judges it to be trustworthy or not is based on one integrated model of that system during any real-world interaction. A user does not mentally disassemble a system into its various aesthetic and functional features, then consciously consider past information and interactions they've had with similar systems. In actuality, the person perceives the automated system as the sum of all its parts.

In addition to physical attributes, certain behavioral qualities are desirable in order for autonomous systems to be accepted. This is especially the case if they have a social component or they work as part of a team. Generally, autonomous entities should behave in the same way humans are expected to in a given circumstance. Robots maintaining social conventions, such as social cues, emotive expression, and empathy, improve trust in such autonomous systems (Evers et al., 2008; Looije et al., 2010). Similarly, autonomous entities that have enhanced socialization aspects, including verbal communication, alongside extroverted personalities are more approachable (Joosse et al., 2013), just as politeness, etiquette, and dependability support trust, especially when the system malfunctions or behaves unexpectedly (Biros et al., 2004; Tsui et al., 2010). However, to design the desired behavioral qualities into a robot, it is necessary to first understand the intended users and their particular needs. Through a detailed understanding of an intended human user in a given role, the expectations governing the trust relationship in HAI can guide the behavioral characteristics of the system.

One important automation characteristic influencing trust in HAI is anthropomorphism, or the magnitude of human likeness of any given automated system. Some findings have shown that the level of anthropomorphism that a robot presents is correlated to the level of trust humans place in it (Erebak & Turgut, 2019; Evers et al., 2008). However, when robots become too anthropomorphic (i.e., mimic human appearance and behavior too closely), they are perceived as "creepy." This phenomenon is known as the uncanny valley (Mori, 2012). These findings are not necessarily disparate – anthropomorphism is a combination of physical and behavioral attributes.

Embodiment itself (or lack thereof) can also influence trust ratings. For instance, embodied systems (e.g., robots) have received greater trust ratings than virtual autonomous entities (e.g., software programs; Looije et al., 2010). However, this may be mediated by a user's perceived control over the automated system or situation. This is also likely changing as everyday interaction with unembodied robots (e.g., Amazon's Alexa and Apple's Siri) continues to increase.

4.3.2 *Performance-Based Factors*

Reliability has, to date, been treated as the single-most important factor in the level of human–automation trust. This assertion is so well accepted that many experiments manipulate reliability in order to measure trust. The assumption is that low reliability leads to low trust and vice versa. However, performance is perceived by the human trustor, who, depending on their knowledge, may or may not even know that a given system is not behaving reliably. While reliability is certainly important for HAI, trust can recover after automation failure (Desai et al., 2013).

The components and characteristics of the automated system work together to provide an integrated automated system. Ideally, autonomous systems need to be competent and capable in the context of their purpose, concede to humans with which they interact, adapt to changes in humans and the environment, actively attempt to forge relationships of trust, and be effective in communication with humans. These are all qualities they convey through their overall appearance and behavior.

4.4   Environment-Related Factors Influencing Trust

While both the human and the automated system present elements that influence trust, a third major category from which influencing variables emerge is the environment. This is illustrated in two recent meta-analyses of antecedents of trust in human–robot interaction and HAI respectively (Hancock, Billings, Schaefer, et al., 2011; Schaefer et al., 2016). Environmental factors (also referred to as contextual factors) cover nearly every facet of the interaction that is not directly related to the human- or automation-related factors. These environmental factors fall generally into two major categories: team collaboration and task-based factors. Team collaboration factors include in-group membership, cultural dynamics, communication, and shared mental models. Task-based factors include task type, task complexity, and other aspects of the physical environment. Each of these components plays a role in the development, facilitation, and maintenance of trust between humans and automated systems.

4.4.1   Team Collaboration Factors

Similarities are evident between trust that is shared by two humans, and the trust between people and automation. Many argue that trust stems from social interaction (Blau, 1964), present in both interactions with other humans and interaction with automated systems. Further, trust is often contingent on an attribution process, events based on the personality or disposition of the person (Reeder & Brewer, 1979; Rempel et al., 1985). These types of influences have been shown to be present not only in human–human trust, but in human–computer trust as well (Earley, 1988). This social aspect of trust plays a role when making judgments based on advice from an outside source. Dijkstra examined the effect of trust on a decision-making task, when advice was given either by a human or an automated advisor (Dijkstra, 1995). Participants rated the automated advisor as more objective and rational and then followed its advice more often than that of the human advisor. A follow-up study found similar results, even when the information provided by the system was objectively less accurate than that of the human (Dijkstra, 1999). This finding suggests that humans may be aware, either explicitly or implicitly, how social factors play a role in trust. In turn, this relates to how such factors can affect the degree of trust given to an entity. Importantly, it also demonstrates that social bias can lead individuals to miscalibrate trust toward certain entities or teammates.

The pattern of trusting inaccurate systems has also been observed more recently in the area of conformity. Early work on the topic of social conformity, conducted by Asch (1951, 1955), observed the occurrence of individuals conforming to seemingly incorrect answers, their reactions being based on the majority of their group's responses. Recently, the power of conformity has been investigated in the context of human–robot interaction (HRI). Work performed by Hertz and Weise (2018) has demonstrated robust findings that conformity is observed between a human and a group of robotic devices. Further, Volante and colleagues (2019) showed the importance of communication on conforming to decisions made about a group of robots. In this latter work, attitudes expressed about a robot performing a task influenced the trust ratings made by other observers toward that robot. Along with communication, these social aspects are critical environmental factors that influence the trust relationship.

Team-based factors such as coordination and collaboration certainly impact trust levels. Gauging the power of these factors is built upon understanding from human teaming research. Trust in teams is developed through task performance perception, team satisfaction, and organizational commitment. The development of trust in teams is important in determining the overall effectiveness of such teams (Costa, 2003). Models of human team-based trust incorporate both aspects of the people involved as well as the environment they act within. This is similar to the HRI trust models (e.g., Hancock, Billings, Schaefer, et al., 2011; Hancock et al., 2020; Kessler et al., 2017). Individual difference measures, such as propensity to trust, perceived trustworthiness, and cooperative behavior help to predict the effective levels of trust present in working teams. In human–robot teams, these human characteristics are still present; however, they only account for a portion of the overall team composition. While it is important to study, model, and design robotic systems to promote trust, it is also important to feature the human role in this dynamic. The models of human–robot and human–automation trust both incorporate these aspects of the human into a larger picture of overall trust, enabling researchers to appropriately ascribe the weight of each of these components in the overall model of trust.

Overall, trust is a complex facet of relationships, be it between two people or a larger group consisting of humans and nonhuman machines. However, these factors must be weighed accordingly. Both the aspects of the automation and the environment play critical roles in the overall trust relationship. Understanding team-based effects is critical in designing automation that works to promote accurately calibrated trust.

4.5   Interactions Between the Factors That Influence Trust

While it is useful for research purposes to isolate these individual factors, the real-world situations that researchers typically want to generalize findings to are dynamic, emergent, and messy. This makes the process of quantifying trust in automation or extracting specific trust measures for the purpose of predicting automation use difficult. While it may be desirable from a research standpoint to evaluate these individual factors of trust in automation singly, real-world interactions cannot so easily be parsed – the description provided in earlier sections of the human, robot, and environmental factors influencing trust in automation demonstrates the extent to which the trust relationships are actually built upon the interactions between the three factors, at least as much as their individual effects.

As discussed, trust calibration is key to effective and productive interactions between humans and automated systems. Both under- and over-trust can prove problematic. For instance, under-trust can occur even with perfectly competent automation. Imagine an operator who is required to monitor a mixed team to find and disable incendiary explosive devices. This soldier is somewhat wary of robots in general. The task and environment are dangerous, adding to the overall level of stress. The robot's processes may not be totally transparent, so, while it maybe performs correctly, it does not provide the soldier with sufficient information to know that it is totally reliable. This leads to a situation where the soldier does not know why the robot is doing what it does. This results in excessive monitoring of the robot and perhaps missing their own tasks in the process. In this case, the robot functioned exactly as it should. However, lacking transparency, its human user was not able to understand its underlying logic and decision making. The interaction between the information the robot was providing about its behavior, the human user's understanding of that information, and a high-stress environment may often lead to poor trust calibration (the human trusted the robot less than they should have). Such under-trust can have potentially disastrous consequences if, as is often the case, the team was structured to depend on the robot for a specific task.

In contrast, interactions between trust antecedents can result in over-trust, which also proves problematic. For instance, imagine a person has just purchased an expensive vehicle with automation capabilities such as advanced cruise control. They have bought into the idea of a "self-driving" car, and they believe that this vehicle is capable of autonomously navigating the environment. They have so much faith in this vehicle that they ignore the operational guidance mandates requiring that they actively engage in monitoring the vehicle and environment. Here they fail to maintain vigilance and stop paying attention to the road. It is then that a collision occurs, caused by under-monitoring related to excessive trust in the system. In this case the user trusted the system to perform beyond its capabilities, an example of over-trust. While automated vehicles ought to provide clear guidance to their drivers through a number of communication cues (e.g., the vehicle's manual, driver education, instructions at the dealership, interface components such as alerts), drivers can neglect this information in favor of an incorrect preconception based on their previous observations and experiences, which can include even fictional interpretations of automation and artificial intelligence. The interaction between the information that the automated vehicle is providing and what the driver is perceiving can result in suboptimal trust calibration and outright over-reliance. Equally important is the environmental context. The vehicle interacts with its surroundings to influence trust. In a perfectly safe environment such as a protected closed course, driver inattention might be, to a degree, tolerable. However, in a busy urban environment replete with unexpected events, maintaining vigilance is crucial to safety (and see Hancock, 2013). The human user also interacts with the environment to impact trust. If they are less familiar with the roadway, they may be more likely to maintain such vigilance and attend to the automated system.

Another dimension that complicates this dynamic relationship between trust antecedents is time (Kaplan et al., 2020). While initial trust is based on both prior experiences on behalf of the user and the immediately observable characteristics of the automated system, each subsequent interaction provides sequentially more information upon which the human user can base their trust judgments. Trust is constantly recalibrating. The user considers trust, as well as other criteria (e.g., how important the task is; whether it is possible for a human to perform the task; the risk to human welfare) to make choices as to whether to use the automation. Predictable performance by that system is one critical key to fostering human trust over time (Lee & Moray, 1992).

4.6 Trust Measurement

Latent, or unobservable, variables are by nature unmeasurable. They require "proxy" variables in order to be employed as indicators. While it is possible to simply ask a person questions regarding their trust level in a given automated system, people are notoriously poor reporters of their own prospective behavior (Hancock, 1996; Natsoulas, 1967). Although a user may report high trust in an automated system, that does not necessarily mean they will then subsequently use it (Chen & Terrence, 2009). A number of factors are likely responsible for this dissociation. For instance, people are often unaware of their own internal biases, as demonstrated by work concerning implicit associations (Greenwald et al., 1998). The environment can also influence trust ratings. If a participant in a research study thinks that the researcher has a vested interest in positive results, they may provide trust ratings that they believe will please that researcher (i.e., experimenter bias). While it is challenging, fostering an appropriate trust relationship is crucial to quality HAI, and proper measurement is necessary to understand trust relationships.

Many methods have been proposed to measure trust, by both subjective and objective means. Trust is measured subjectively by asking people how much they trust someone or something using surveys or verbal measures. Subjective trust measures are the most common way of assessing trust in experimental settings. One widely used survey is the Trust in Automation Scale (Jian et al., 2000), with other trust scales including Merritt's (2011) Trust Scale, and Yagoda and Gillan's (2012) Human–Robot Interaction Scale and, as mentioned previously, a user's preexisting attitude toward trust in robots can be measured using the Negative Attitude toward Robots Scale (Nomura et al., 2006). Similarly, propensity to trust automation has been measured (see Lee & See, 2004) using the Automation-Induced Complacency Potential Rating Scale (Singh et al., 1993).

While subjective trust measures may be useful in some circumstances, they do not lend themselves to clear comparisons across time. One scale has addressed this using a prepost comparison (e.g., Schaefer, 2013). Here trust is measured before and after a participant interacts with a robot. While this begins to address the time issue in trust measurement, it can introduce test fatigue. Another solution employed by Desai and colleagues (2013) is to ask participants only the direction of change in trust, not the magnitude of the change. While this would tend to reduce the likelihood of test fatigue, it remains difficult to quantify the degree of change in trust participants experienced.

Measures that are not based on self-reporting are considered more objective, and therefore thought to be free of some of the issues plaguing subjective measures. However, construct validity (i.e., the degree to which the test measures what it claims to), is difficult to demonstrate using direct measures because it is the measures' correlations with the aforementioned trust scales (or some other less-than-perfect measure) that demonstrate their validity. Some objective measures that have been explored for trust measurement include eye tracking (Djamasbi et al., 2010; Jenkins & Jiang, 2010), skin response (Akash et al., 2018; Khawaji et al., 2015), and other neurobiological measurements.

Evidence suggests functional neuroimaging may be instrumental in understanding and quantifying trust behaviors by measuring biological changes in the trustor. A recent meta-analysis of 30 articles that leveraged the "trust game" (TG) to explore brain activation reported activation in the anterior insula was associated with trust behaviors (Bellucci et al., 2017). In the TG (also referred to as the investment game; Berg et al., 1995), participants are given money and instructed to choose some amount from the money they received and send it to the other player (see also Chapter 2). Participants are told that the amount they send will be tripled by the experimenter. The other player may be another participant, but could also be an experimenter or an automated system. Next, the other player sends some amount of money back to the participant. Since the experimenter triples the initial sum sent by the participant, sending more money to the other player during the first turn increases the overall amount of money in the game, and thereby increases the amount of money the participant could potentially receive. However, the amount the participant actually receives is determined by the amount the other player returns. Thus, the participant can potentially increase the amount of money they receive by trusting the other player, but there is the risk of loss as well. This game is often used to elicit trust behaviors during experimentation.

One experiment leveraging the TG to observe measurable behaviors involved comparing participants' interactions with humans to their interactions with avatars during the TG using functional magnetic resonance imaging (fMRI) (see also Chapter 3). In this experiment, Riedl and colleagues (2014) reported that decision making about whether or not to trust another actor activated the medial frontal cortex (an area thought to be important for predicting others' thoughts and intentions) significantly more during interaction with humans than with interaction with avatars. In another type of experiment, Hubert and colleagues (2018) classified participants based on their impulsiveness levels and compared them during shopping scenarios. These authors found differences between more impulsive (i.e., hedonistic) and less impulsive (i.e., prudent) shoppers in terms of the magnitude of activations patterns in brain regions related to trust and impulsiveness (dorsal striatum, anterior cingulate, dorsolateral prefrontal cortex, and insula cortex) using fMRI.

The electroencephalogram has also been hypothesized as a measure of universal trust. In an experiment involving monitoring algorithms and identifying errors, De Visser and colleagues (2018) manipulated the credibility and reliability of algorithms provided to participants. These authors reported that neural markers of action monitoring (observational error-related negativity and observed error positivity) were significantly different based on algorithm reliability, and correlated with the subjective measures of trust.

One issue plaguing trust measurement is that it does not necessarily lead to use. As demonstrated by Sanders and colleagues (2019), other factors, such as concern over human welfare, may use decisions more than trust. Similarly, Drnec and colleagues (2016) posit that while it is generally understood that trust influences use, there is not necessarily a direct relationship between any trust measure and use behavior. For this reason, the latter authors recommend measuring interactional behaviors such as reliance and compliance instead, indicating these are "a more fruitful and immediate route" (Drnec et al. 2016, p. 2) to dealing with real-world problems arising from poorly calibrated trust in automation.

Riedl and Javor (2012) point out that trust can be conceptualized in different ways, and measurement needs to be based on the type of trust being measured. For instance, by conceptualizing trust as a belief, the characteristics of the trustee become the object of investigations. In such cases, self-report measures are appropriate. However, conceptualizing trust as a behavioral intention necessitates measuring actual behavior. Functional neuroimaging can offer an objective measure of biological processes when participants are making use-choice decisions, thereby supporting investigations into the relationship between trust and use behavior.

4.7 Conclusion

Defining and measuring trust in automation is indeed a challenging task. Interactive factors across human, automated system, and the environment further complicate the issue. However, definition and measurement are key to fostering appropriately calibrated trust and reliance on automated systems. Such calibration has important and far-reaching implications. While these measures may be imperfect, there is still a need to understand and quantify trust in automation in both laboratory and real-world settings. Examining each individual situation for the best combination of measurements to deploy currently represents best practice.

References

Akash, K., Hu, W. L., Jain, N., & Reid, T. (2018). A classification model for sensing human trust in machines using EEG and GSR. *ACM Transactions on Interactive Intelligent Systems*, 8(4), Article 27. https://doi.org/10.1145/3132743

Alaiad, A., & Zhou, L. (2014). The determinants of home healthcare robots adoption: An empirical investigation. *International Journal of Medical Informatics*, 83(11), 825–840. https://doi.org/10.1016/j.ijmedinf.2014.07.003

Asch, S. E. (1951). Effects of group pressure on the modification and distortion of judgments. In H. Guetzkow (Ed.), *Groups, leadership and men: Research in human relations* (pp. 177–190). Carnegie Press.

(1955). Opinions and social pressure. *Scientific American*, 193(5), 31–35.

Bellucci, G., Chernyak, S. V., Goodyear, K., Eickhoff, S. B., & Krueger, F. (2017). Neural signatures of trust in reciprocity: A coordinate-based meta-analysis. *Human Brain Mapping*, 38(3), 1233–1248. https://doi.org/10.1002/hbm.23451

Berg, J., Dickhaut, J., & McCabe, K. (1995). Trust, reciprocity, and social-history. *Games and Economic Behavior*, 10(1), 122–142. https://doi.org/10.1006/game.1995.1027

Biros, D. P., Daly, M., & Gunsch, G. (2004). The influence of task load and automation trust on deception detection. *Group Decision and Negotiation*, 13(2), 173–189. https://doi.org/10.1023/B:GRUP.0000021840.85686.57

Blau, P. M. (1964). *Exchange and power in social life*. Wiley.

Block, J. (2001). Millennial contrarianism: The five-factor approach to personality description 5 years later. *Journal of Research in Personality*, 35(1), 98–107. https://doi.org/10.1006/jrpe.2000.2293

Chen, J. Y. C., & Terrence, P. I. (2009). Effects of imperfect automation and individual differences on concurrent performance of military and robotics tasks in a simulated multitasking environment. *Ergonomics*, 52(8), 907–920. https://doi.org/10.1080/00140130802680773

Chien, S. Y., Lewis, M., Sycara, K., Liu, J. S., & Kumru, A. (2016). Relation between trust attitudes toward automation, Hofstede's cultural dimensions, and big five personality traits. *Proceedings of the Human Factors and Ergonomics Society*, 840–844. https://doi.org/10.1177/1541931213601192

Costa, A. C. (2003). Work team trust and effectiveness. *Personnel Review*, 32(5), 605–622. https://doi.org/10.1108/00483480310488360

De Visser, E. J., Beatty, P. J., Estepp, J. R., et al. (2018). Learning from the slips of others: Neural correlates of trust in automated agents. *Frontiers in Human Neuroscience*, 12(309), 1–15. https://doi.org/10.3389/fnhum.2018.00309

Desai, M., Kaniarasu, P., Medvedev, M., Steinfeld, A., & Yanco, H. (2013). Impact of robot failures and feedback on real-time trust. *8th ACM/IEEE International Conference on Human-Robot Interaction, HRI '13*, 251–258. https://doi.org/10.1109/HRI.2013.6483596

Dijkstra, J. (1995). The influence of an expert system on the user's view: How to fool a lawyer. *New Review of Applied Expert Systems*, 1, 123–138.

———. (1999). User agreement with incorrect expert system advice. *Behaviour & Information Technology*, 18(6), 399–411. https://doi.org/10.1080/01449299118832

Djamasbi, S., Siegel, M., Tullis, T., & Dai, R. (2010). Efficiency, trust, and visual appeal: Usability testing through eye tracking. *Proceedings of the Annual Hawaii International Conference on System Sciences*, 1–10. https://doi.org/10.1109/HICSS.2010.171

Drnec, K., Marathe, A. R., Lukos, J. R., & Metcalfe, J. S. (2016). From trust in automation to decision neuroscience: Applying cognitive neuroscience methods to understand and improve interaction decisions involved in human automation interaction. *Frontiers in Human Neuroscience*, 10(290), 1–14. https://doi.org/10.3389/fnhum.2016.00290

Earley, P. C. (1988). Computer-generated performance feedback in the magazine-subscription industry. *Organizational Behavior and Human Decision Processes*, 41(1), 50–64. https://doi.org/10.1016/0749-5978(88)90046-5

Ellis, L. U., Sims, V. K., Chin, M. G., et al. (2005). Those a-maze-ing robots: Attributions of ability are based on form, not behavior. *Proceedings of the Human Factors and Ergonomics Society Annual Meeting*, 49(3), 598–601. https://doi.org/10.1177/154193120504900382

Endsley, M. R., & Kaber, D. B. (1999). Level of automation effects on performance, situation awareness and workload in a dynamic control task. *Ergonomics*, 42(3), 462–492. https://doi.org/10.1080/001401399185595

Erebak, S., & Turgut, T. (2019). Caregivers' attitudes toward potential robot coworkers in elder care. *Cognition, Technology and Work*, 21(2), 327–336. https://doi.org/10.1007/s10111-018-0512-0

Evers, V., Maldonado, H. C., Brodecki, T. L., & Hinds, P. J. (2008). Relational vs. group self-construal. *3rd ACM/IEEE International Conference on Human-Robot Interaction, HRI '08*, 255–262. https://doi.org/10.1145/1349822.1349856

Goetz, J., Kiesler, S., & Powers, A. (2003). Matching robot appearance and behavior to tasks to improve human-robot cooperation. *IEEE International Workshop on Robot and Human Interactive Communication*, 55–60. https://doi.org/10.1109/ROMAN.2003.1251796

Greenwald, A. G., McGhee, D. E., & Schwartz, J. L. K. (1998). Measuring individual differences in implicit cognition: The implicit association test. *Journal of Personality and Social Psychology*, 74(6), 1464–1480. https://doi.org/10.1037/0022-3514.74.6.1464

Groom, V., Srinivasan, V., Bethel, C. L., Murphy, R., Dole, L., & Nass, C. (2011). Responses to robot social roles and social role framing. *International Conference on Collaboration Technologies and Systems*, 194–203. https://doi.org/10.1109/CTS.2011.5928687

Hancock, P. A. (1996). Effects of control order, augmented feedback, input device and practice on tracking performance and perceived workload. *Ergonomics*, 39(9), 1146–1162. https://doi.org/10.1080/00140139608964535

(2013). In search of vigilance: The problem of iatrogenically created psychological phenomena. *The American Psychologist*, 68(2), 97–109. https://doi.org/10.1037/a0030214

(2019). Some pitfalls in the promises of automated and autonomous vehicles. *Ergonomics*, 62(4), 479–495. https://doi.org/10.1080/00140139.2018.1498136

Hancock, P. A., Billings, D. R., & Schaefer, K. E. (2011). Can you trust your robot? *Ergonomics in Design*, 19(3), 24–29. https://doi.org/10.1177/1064804611415045

Hancock, P. A., Billings, D. R., Schaefer, K. E., Chen, J. Y. C., De Visser, E. J., & Parasuraman, R. (2011). A meta-analysis of factors affecting trust in human-robot interaction. *Human Factors*, 53(5), 517–527. https://doi.org/10.1177/0018720811417254

Hancock, P. A., Kessler, T. T., Kaplan, A. D., Brill, J. C., & Szalma, J. L. (2020). Evolving trust in robots: Specification through sequential and comparative meta-analyses. *Human Factors*, 62(4). https://doi.org/https://doi.org/10.1177/0018720820922080

Haring, K. S., Matsumoto, Y., & Watanabe, K. (2013). How do people perceive and trust a lifelike robot. *Lecture Notes in Engineering and Computer Science*, 1, 425–430.

Heerink, M. (2011). Exploring the influence of age, gender, education and computer experience on robot acceptance by older adults. *6th ACM/IEEE International Conference on Human-Robot Interaction, HRI '11*, 147–148. https://doi.org/10.1145/1957656.1957704

Hertz, N., & Wiese, E. (2018). Under pressure: Examining social conformity with computer and robot groups. *Human Factors*, 60(8), 1207–1218. https://doi.org/10.1177/0018720818788473

Hubert, M., Hubert, M., Linzmajer, M., Riedl, R., & Kenning, P. (2018). Trust me if you can: Neurophysiological insights on the influence of consumer impulsiveness on trustworthiness evaluations in online settings. *European Journal of Marketing*, 52(1–2), 118–146. https://doi.org/10.1108/EJM-12-2016-0870

Jenkins, Q., & Jiang, X. (2010). Measuring trust and application of eye tracking in human robotic interaction. *IIE Annual Conference Proceedings*, 1.

Jian, J.-Y., Bisantz, A. M., & Drury, C. G. (2000). Foundations for an empirically determined scale of trust in automated systems. *International Journal of Cognitive Ergonomics*, 4(1), 53–71. https://doi.org/10.1207/S15327566IJCE0401_04

Joosse, M., Lohse, M., Perez, J. G., & Evers, V. (2013). What you do is who you are: The role of task context in perceived social robot personality. *Proceedings of the IEEE International Conference on Robotics and Automation*, 2134–2139. https://doi.org/10.1109/ICRA.2013.6630863

Kaplan, A. D., Kessler, T. T., Sanders, T. L., Cruit, J., Brill, J. C., & Hancock, P. A. (2020). Time to trust: Trust as a function of time in human-robot interaction. In C. Nam & J. Lyons (Eds.), *Trust in human-robot interaction* (pp. 143–159). Academic Press.

Kessler, T., Stowers, K., Brill, J. C., & Hancock, P. A. (2017). Comparisons of human-human trust with other forms of human-technology trust. *Proceedings of the Human Factors and Ergonomics Society Annual Meeting*, 61(1), 1303–1307. https://doi.org/10.1177/1541931213601808

Khawaji, A., Zhou, J., Chen, F., & Marcus, N. (2015). Using galvanic skin response (GSR) to measure trust and cognitive load in the text-chat environment. *Proceedings of the 33rd Annual ACM Conference Extended Abstracts on Human Factors in Computing Systems, CHI EA'15*, 1989–1994. https://doi.org/10.1145/2702613.2732766

Koffka, K. (1935). *Principles of gestalt psychology*. Routledge.

Lee, J. D., & Moray, N. (1992). Trust, control strategies and allocation of function in human-machine systems. *Ergonomics*, 35(10), 1243–1270. https://doi.org/10.1080/00140139208967392

     (1994). Trust, self-confidence, and operators' adaptation to automation. *International Journal of Human-Computer Studies*, 40(1), 153–184. https://doi.org/10.1006/ijhc.1994.1007

Lee, J. D., & See, K. A. (2004). Trust in automation: Designing for appropriate reliance. *Human Factors*, 46(1), 50–80. https://doi.org/10.1518/hfes.46.1.50_30392

Li, D., Rau, P. L. P., & Li, Y. (2010). A cross-cultural study: Effect of robot appearance and task. *International Journal of Social Robotics*, 2(2), 175–186. https://doi.org/10.1007/s12369-010-0056-9

Linderman, T. (2018). *Using an orange to fool Tesla's autopilot is probably a really bad ideas*. Motherboard: Tech by Vice. www.vice.com/en_us/article/a3na9p/tesla-autosteer-orange-hack

Looije, R., Neerincx, M. A., & Cnossen, F. (2010). Persuasive robotic assistant for health self-management of older adults: Design and evaluation of social behaviors. *International Journal of Human-Computer Studies*, 68(6), 386–397. https://doi.org/10.1016/j.ijhcs.2009.08.007

McBride, M., & Morgan, S. (2010). Trust calibration for automated decision aids. *Research Brief*, 9, 1–11.

Merritt, S. M. (2011). Affective processes in human-automation interactions. *Human Factors*, 53(4), 356–370. https://doi.org/10.1177/0018720811411912

Mori, M. (2012). The uncanny valley. *IEEE Robotics and Automation Magazine*, 19(2), 98–100. https://doi.org/10.1109/MRA.2012.2192811

National Highway Traffic Safety Administration. (2020). *Driver assistance technologies*. United States Department of Transportation. www.nhtsa.gov/equipment/driver-assistance-technologies

National Transportation Safety Board. (2017). Collision between a car operating with automated vehicle control systems and a tractor-semitrailer truck. *Highway Accident Report*.

Natsoulas, T. (1967). What are perceptual reports about? *Psychological Bulletin*, 67(4), 249–272. https://doi.org/10.1037/h0024320

Nomura, T., Suzuki, T., Kanda, T., & Kato, K. (2006). Measurement of negative attitudes toward robots. *Interaction Studies*, 7(3), 437–454. https://doi.org/10.1075/is.7.3.14nom

Parasuraman, R., & Riley, V. (1997). Humans and automation: Use, misuse, disuse, abuse. *Human Factors*, 39(2), 230–253. https://doi.org/10.1518/001872097778543886

Phillips, E., Ullman, D., De Graaf, M. M. A., & Malle, B. F. (2017). What does a robot look like?: A multi-site examination of user expectations about robot appearance. *Proceedings of the Human Factors and Ergonomics Society Annual Meeting*, 61(1), 1215–1219. https://doi.org/10.1177/1541931213601786

Reeder, G. D., & Brewer, M. B. (1979). A schematic model of dispositional attribution in interpersonal perception. *Psychological Review*, 86(1), 61–79. https://doi.org/10.1037/0033-295X.86.1.61

Rempel, J. K., Holmes, J. G., & Zanna, M. P. (1985). Trust in close relationships. *Journal of Personality and Social Psychology*, 49(1), 95–112. https://doi.org/10.1037/0022-3514.49.1.95

Riedl, R., & Javor, A. (2012). The biology of trust: Integrating evidence from genetics, endocrinology, and functional brain imaging. *Journal of Neuroscience, Psychology, and Economics*, 5(2), 63–91. https://doi.org/10.1037/a0026318

Riedl, R., Mohr, P., Kenning, P., Davis, F., & Heekeren, H. (2014). Trusting humans and avatars: A brain imaging study based on evolution theory. *Journal of Management Information Systems*, 30(4), 83–114. https://doi.org/10.2753/MIS0742-1222300404

Sanders, T. L., Kaplan, A. P., Koch, R., Schwartz, M., & Hancock, P. A. (2019). The relationship between trust and use choice in human-robot interaction. *Human Factors*, 61(4), 614–626. https://doi.org/10.1177/0018720818816838

Schaefer, K. E. (2013). *The perception and measurement of human-robot trust* [Doctoral dissertation]. University of Central Florida.

Schaefer, K. E., Chen, J. Y. C., Szalma, J. L., & Hancock, P. A. (2016). A meta-analysis of factors influencing the development of trust in automation: Implications for understanding autonomy in future systems. *Human Factors*, 58(3), 377–400. https://doi.org/10.1177/0018720816634228

Scopelliti, M., Giuliani, M. V., & Fornara, F. (2005). Robots in a domestic setting: A psychological approach. *Universal Access in the Information Society*, 4(2), 146–155. https://doi.org/10.1007/s10209-005-0118-1

Singh, I. L., Molloy, R., & Parasuraman, R. (1993). Automation-induced "complacency": Development of the complacency-potential rating scale. *The International Journal of Aviation Psychology*, 3(2), 111–122. https://doi.org/10.1207/s15327108ijap0302_2

Szalma, J. L., & Taylor, G. S. (2011). Individual differences in response to automation: The five-factor model of personality. *Journal of Experimental Psychology: Applied*, 17(2), 71–96. https://doi.org/10.1037/a0024170

Tsui, K. M., Desai, M., & Yanco, H. A. (2010). Considering the bystander's perspective for indirect human-robot interaction. *5th ACM/IEEE International Conference on Human-Robot Interaction, HRI '10*, 129–130. https://doi.org/10.1145/1734454.1734506

Volante, W. G., Sosna, J., Kessler, T., Sanders, T. L., & Hancock, P. A. (2019). Social conformity effects on trust in simulation-based human-robot interaction. *Human Factors*, 61(5), 805–815. https://doi.org/10.1177/00187208 18811190

Wang, L., Rau, P. L. P., Evers, V., Robinson, B. K., & Hinds, P. (2010). When in Rome: The role of culture and context in adherence to robot recommendations. *5th ACM/IEEE International Conference on Human-Robot Interaction, HRI '10*, 359–366. https://doi.org/10.1145/1734454.1734578

Yagoda, R. E., & Gillan, D. J. (2012). You want me to trust a ROBOT? The development of a human-robot interaction trust scale. *International Journal of Social Robotics*, 4(3), 235–248. https://doi.org/10.1007/s12369-012-0144-0

PART II

Neuropsychological Level of Trust

CHAPTER 5

Trust and Risk

Neuroeconomic Foundations of Trust Based on Social Risk

Nina Lauharatanahirun and Jason A. Aimone

5.1 Introduction

Trust decisions permeate the daily lives of individuals. Sometimes those decisions do not involve other people, like when a hiker decides whether to trust an old rope bridge to cross a ravine. At other times individuals are faced with decisions that involve trusting another person. At the individual level, such social trust decisions range from relatively small transactions, such as deciding whether to trust your Uber driver to get you home safely, to much larger ones, such as trusting your spouse to reciprocate your affections, loyalty, and fidelity. These interpersonal trust decisions are important for shaping our social lives and can have cascading positive and negative consequences. While nonsocial trust decisions are important to understand in their own right, in the last few decades, researchers from many fields of study (psychology, economics, neuroscience, computer science) have focused on understanding social trust behavior using experimental paradigms (perhaps most notably in economics the Berg et al., 1995 investment game; see also Chapter 2). From these empirical efforts, it is clear that trust is a multidimensional construct shaped by many neuroeconomic features at the biological, psychological, and behavioral levels. We begin by first defining trust as we use the concept in this chapter. We then describe our conceptualization of how interpersonal trust behavior can ultimately be thought of as a *decision based on social risk*. Next, we discuss potential psychological aspects of trust behavior such as risk preferences and betrayal aversion. We then review the current state of the literature on the neurobiological mechanisms of such psychological features. Finally, we turn to open questions and future directions for research in this area.

We would like to thank the reviewers for their insightful and constructive feedback. We also thank Derek Spangler and Mary Zhuo Ke for reviewing previous versions of this chapter prior to submission. Corresponding author: Nina Lauharatanahirun (nina.lauhara@psu.edu).

5.2   Trust as a Behavior

While being the focus of many empirical studies over the last few decades across many disciplines, there is no clear cross-disciplinary consensus on the definition of "trust." The disagreement in definitions often rests in the fundamental question of whether trust is characterized as a belief (Hardin, 2001, 2002, 2006; Sapienza et al., 2013) or a behavior (Coleman, 1990; Elster, 2007; Fehr, 2009). The different approaches vary in whether trust is based on the trustor's knowledge (Hardin, 2006) and/or expectations (Rousseau et al., 1998) about their trustee counterpart or whether trust is defined off of the action of the trustor toward the trustee (Coleman, 1990; Fehr, 2009).

Ultimately, how we define trust in different situations is important because it forms the scientific bedrock of how we understand social behavior and, just as importantly, informs the particular methods by which we probe trust and refine existing theories on the topic. In this chapter, we take the *trust as a behavior* approach. The *act* of trusting can be thought of as an investment of resources in another that may (with some degree of uncertainty) provide future benefits (Coleman, 1990; Fehr 2009). These investments may vary in type such as money, time, effort, and emotional engagement. By characterizing trust as a behavior, we are able to measure the willingness of a trustor to make themselves vulnerable to a trustee's actions, which includes the possibility of betrayal. This vulnerability to place resources at the disposal of another, without any guarantee that these resources will be returned, is what some may argue is the key feature of trust (Coleman, 1990; Fairley et al., 2016; Fehr, 2009; Hong & Bohnet, 2007). In this chapter, we adopt Thielmann and Hilbig's (2015, p. 251) definition of interpersonal trust as "a risky choice of making oneself dependent on the actions of another in a situation of uncertainty, based upon some expectation of whether the other will act in a benevolent fashion despite an opportunity to betray." Our adopted definition implicitly acknowledges that individual differences in beliefs are likely to influence trust behaviors. We assume that these beliefs exist and have a critical role in trust behavior, likely forming the priors of the probability of beneficial or costly outcomes resulting from trust. These beliefs, however, are not the focus of the current chapter.

Figure 5.1 lays out a diagram of our conceptualization of interpersonal trust behavior as a microeconomic system. This conceptualization provides us with a framework for understanding the various features that may affect trust behavior. We will elaborate on important elements of this figure as

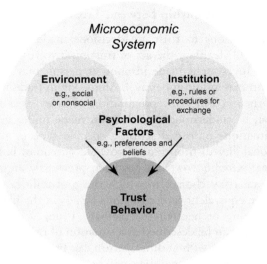

Figure 5.1 Conceptualization of trust behavior.
Trust is not a unitary construct and fundamentally can be characterized as a decision made under uncertainty. Trust can be described as a risk environment (a type of uncertain situation) where the likelihood that another person will reciprocate or betray one's trust is based on expectations formed over time. Furthermore, trust can be understood as a function of the components of an economic system (along the lines of Smith, 1982) in which the decision environment (e.g., source generating potential outcomes), institutional rules and procedures of the interaction (e.g., one interaction or repeated interactions), and psychological factors (e.g., preferences and/or beliefs) all contribute to trust behavior.

we proceed. The darkest circle represents trust as an outcome behavior that is dependent upon both the institutional and environmental elements of the economic system. The environment of a microeconomic system can be characterized as a "set of initial circumstances that cannot be altered by the agents or the institutions within which they interact" (Smith, 1982, p. 924). The institution within this system refers to the rules and procedures of the trust exchange (Smith, 1982). There are also psychological factors that may depend on the type of environment or institution in which trust occurs, ultimately influencing trust behavior. All of these components within this microeconomic system have the potential to influence trust behavior. This system allows us to identify or focus on a particular component of the system to assess its impact or influence on trust behavior.

5.3   The Relationship between Trust and Social Risk

At their root, decisions to trust are decisions made under uncertainty (Gambetta, 1988). Meaning, the act of trusting involves accepting a level of *risk* that the investment made in another person may or may not be reciprocated and may result in betrayal. Aligned with traditional economic and decision theory, our conceptualization of trust as a behavior (see Figure 5.1) can be understood as a decision made under uncertainty. In economics, situations of *risk* describe a specific type of uncertainty in which the probability distribution of possible outcomes is known (Holt & Laury, 2002; Knight, 1921). It has been previously argued that decisions to trust are risky choices in which the probabilities of betrayal or reciprocation are equivalent to the trustor's beliefs in the likelihood of the trustee reciprocating or betraying (Coleman, 1990; Williamson, 1993). Alternatively, trust can be described as a situation of risk where beliefs and a history of experiences with another person can build over time akin to a probability distribution of how others will behave in a given environment. When someone chooses to expose themselves to risk, the uncertainty of reciprocation and betrayal is situated within this expected probability distribution. This does not mean, however, that all trust is social risk or vice versa. Trust stems from uncertainty that may or may not be social in nature (and there may be social risk situations that do not involve trust). For instance, trust behavior can be present during interpersonal interactions as well as within exchanges involving technology or other nonsocial environments. Within this chapter, we will focus on trust behavior within social environments.

In most of the influential research examining the relationship between trust and risk (e.g., Bohnet et al., 2008, 2010; Bohnet & Zeckhauser, 2004; Eckel & Wilson, 2004; Fairley et al., 2016; Houser et al., 2010; Kosfeld et al., 2005), the experimental environments were manipulated such that probability distributions were able to be estimated or known in order for formal comparisons to be tested between decisions made in trust versus risk conditions. If trust decisions can be thought of as simple decisions under risk, then theoretically trust behavior should be able to be predicted from an individual's risk preferences, when outcome probabilities are clearly defined and known (Coleman, 1990). There is mixed evidence about this connection. Based on some studies (e.g., Fairley et al., 2016; Schecter, 2007), trust behavior can be explained well by individual risk attitudes, while a separate set of studies (Ashraf et al., 2006; Eckel & Grossman, 1996; Eckel & Wilson, 2004; Houser et al., 2010) show no evidence of a substantial relationship between trust and risk decisions. These inconsistent findings can be partially reconciled by taking into account that the relationship between risk and trust may be different depending on the environment and institution in which risk and trust decisions are assessed.

There are several studies that exemplify evidence against an association between risk preferences elicited from standard nonsocial risk elicitation paradigms (e.g., Eckel & Grossman, 1996; Holt & Laury, 2002) and trust behavior. For instance, Eckel and Wilson (2004) used two behavioral measures of risk preferences (Holt & Laury, 2002; Zuckerman et al., 1964) and found that neither of the behavioral measures of risk were associated with trust game (TG) behavior (Berg et al., 1995). Similarly, Houser and colleagues (2010) found that risk preferences predicted individual investment decisions in risk games but not in corresponding TGs after accounting for individual differences in risk preferences. These findings initially suggest that trust behaviors cannot be fully captured by risk attitudes assessed using standard risk elicitation paradigms. While these studies were well designed and used standard ways of measuring risk and trust, the risk, environments, and institutions in these studies differ in subtle but potentially important ways as compared to TGs. For instance, the lottery task used to measure risk in both Eckel and Wilson (2004) and Houser et al. (2010) uses nonstrategic (state uncertainty)-generated probabilities from a nonsocial source (computer), while the TG uses strategically generated probabilities (strategic uncertainty) from a social source (humans in same or previous session).

Indeed, a recent study by Fairley and colleagues (2016) showed that individual socially sourced risk attitudes can explain decisions to trust when they are measured in a more similar environment and institution. In this study, researchers used a standard TG (Berg et al., 1995) and a novel risky TG to measure risk preferences. As opposed to a lottery choice mechanism, participants were asked to make risky decisions in a similarly constructed environment as the TG with the exception that trustors are able to condition their decisions on all possible trustees' decisions. Trustors are told that four trustees have been randomly assigned to them and that after all trustees' decisions are made, one of these four trustees will be randomly assigned to them. This leaves the trustor with five potential outcomes: Either none, one, two, three, or all four of the trustees may choose to return half of the invested amount, and it is unknown which of these outcomes will come to fruition. Thus, the risky TG transforms the standard TG into a decision under risk with a known probability distribution of the potential outcomes trustees may provide. Using the same environment (i.e., source of risk) and institution (context of exchange), Fairley and colleagues (2016) demonstrate that risk preferences are strongly associated with investment decisions in the standard TG. Support for these findings is also seen in experiments done outside the laboratory within diverse samples (Schecter, 2007).

As a caveat, it is worth noting that all these studies involved making trust decisions within a specific institution (i.e., one-shot interactions) and environment (i.e., economic social risk). There may be other institutions (such as repeated interactions) under which trust behaviors occur as well (or other environments). Just as nonsocial risk decisions may be domain-specific (Blais & Weber, 2006), decisions to trust may also be domain-specific. For instance, decisions under similar economic social risk may differ whether the risk stems from a recreational or health domain. Future studies may find research along these lines beneficial.

5.4   An Exemplar of Social Risk: Betrayal Aversion

Among the many environmental factors that differentiate trust decisions from other monetary risk decisions is the source generating the uncertainty. In many (if not the majority of) trust environments, the source of risk that determines possible outcomes is another person or people (i.e., social), which is inherently different from a nonsocial environment where the source of risk is a random process mechanism (e.g., dice or a computer). Decision makers face social risk when another individual is the primary source of uncertainty and, as Yamagashi (2011, p. 11) says, "it is in situations in which social uncertainty is large that trust is needed." From a mathematical perspective it is perhaps odd that identical monetary risk situations would be treated differently by decision makers based upon the source of objective risk outcome probabilities. "Traditional" outcome-centered economic theory would predict that rational decision makers, when given the same outcomes and probabilities, should make the same decision, even if taking into account social preferences (inequity aversion [Fehr & Schmidt, 1999], altruism [Andreoni & Miller, 2002]), etc. that have preferences concerned with end division of earnings). However, in many studies over the last decade, researchers have found that social versus nonsocial sources of uncertainty produce varying effects on behavior despite having identical outcomes and probabilities (Abdellaoui et al., 2011; Aimone & Houser, 2012; Bohnet et al., 2008, 2010; Bohnet & Zeckhauser, 2004; Fairley et al, 2016; Lauharatanahirun et al., 2012).

While there are many neurobiological and psychological reasons why social and nonsocial risk environments result in disparate behaviors, we will focus initially upon betrayal aversion as an illustration. In their seminal study, Bohnet and Zeckhauser (2004) show that people make different decisions in environments that involve trusting a stranger in a one-shot interaction compared with taking a risky bet with an identical payoff structure. Using binary choice TGs, risky dictator games (DGs), and lottery choice games as treatments, they ask participants to choose between a certain outcome and a lottery, where the lottery could produce either positive or negative outcomes for themselves and, in some treatments, differential payments for a partner as well. If a participant chose the lottery in the TG, a human trustee partner determines the outcomes for both players. If a participant chose the lottery in the risky DG, a random mechanism, not another human, determines the outcomes for both the participant and a human partner. The same process is followed for the lottery choice game, but there were no payoffs to another human partner. A risk environment was ensured using a minimum acceptable probability (MAP) elicitation mechanism (similar to a Becker DeGroot Marshack mechanism; Becker et al., 1964) for choosing the risky option over the safe choice in each treatment. We would expect to observe the same behavior in all conditions under standard risk preference models. However, their results show that trustors report lower MAPs in the lottery when a nonsocial mechanism generates the outcomes relative to when outcomes are decided by another person in the TG. The authors attributed this finding being due to aversion to betrayal. In other words, people may demand a higher likelihood of gaining a larger payoff for taking the risky option when outcomes are determined by another person rather than a nonsocial mechanism. Ultimately, this study speaks to the importance of the decision environment in shaping trust decisions and has led to a number of studies examining decision-making behavior within social and nonsocial contexts.

It is perhaps strange to imagine why a phenomenon like betrayal aversion would persist in an evolutionary sense considering it leads individuals to require higher probabilities of high outcomes to trust, all else equal, compared to otherwise equivalent monetary environments. This is akin to leaving money on the table. Aimone and Houser (2011, 2013) examined whether betrayal aversion brings an advantage, in an evolutionary sense, to groups of betrayal-averse agents compared to nonbetrayal-averse agents. In their study, the authors hold the social risk source constant in each of their treatments. In one condition, participants played a standard binary choice TG with a randomly matched human trustee. In another, some trustor participants (not all, in order to avoid deception) were told that while they were randomly matched with a specific human trustee (who was paid based upon their own decision to betray or reciprocate), a computer would randomly match the trustor to the decision of the anonymous trustee, not necessarily with the decision of their partner trustee (computer-mediated trust). The main difference between these conditions rests on the information that subjects have regarding whether a betrayal outcome comes from their own counterpart's decision or someone else's counterpart's decision. The authors find that participants made significantly more risky decisions to trust in the computer condition relative to the standard TG, suggesting support for betrayal-averse behavior.

Some of the benefits of betrayal aversion are made clear in the Aimone and Houser (2011, 2013) studies when considering how trustees perceive the environment. In a different treatment, both trustors and trustees were informed that trustors would be shielded from personal betrayal via the computer-mediation procedure. When this procedure was commonly known, betrayal rates from trustees increased significantly. In other words, trustees appear to be implicitly aware of the added social risk component of betrayal aversion in the trustors' decision-making process (e.g., they are betraying averse). This knowledge of extra disutility from betrayal appears to deter betrayal actions, thus making the social exchange environment more cooperative and mutually beneficial. When betrayal aversion was removed, not only did trustees become more willing to betray, but trustors appear to have foreseen that change in trustee behavior revealed by a drop in trust rates. This benefit of betrayal aversion was recovered and an increase of trust was generated, when the trust institution in the Aimone and Houser (2011, 2013) studies provided trustors the option to avoid the knowledge of betrayal but did not force it. Even though trustees knew of this option, the potential for their partner to be exposed to the disutility of betrayal was sufficient to maintain relatively lower rates of betrayal. Aimone and Houser (2011 and 2013) demonstrate how knowledge of the source generating uncertainty (i.e., environment) shapes decision-making behavior. These findings are also supported by other studies showing more socially risk-adverse decisions in environments where the source of uncertainty is another person relative to a nonsocial one (Aimone & Houser, 2012; Aimone et al., 2014; Butler & Miller, 2018; Quercia, 2016). Additionally, these results have also been replicated in diverse samples from across six different countries (Bohnet et al., 2008).

It is worth noting that these studies use social and nonsocial conditions within a binary choice TG. Upon examining other studies that use nonbinary-choice TG institutions, we find evidence that trustors' decisions in nonsocial and social environments do not necessarily differ. For instance, in Kosfeld et al. (2005), participants engage in a TG where they are presented with options to invest nothing, 4, 8, or 12 units in a trustee. As a control, a separate sample of participants completed the same TG with the exception that people were asked to invest in a project rather than in another person, and the distribution of payoffs determining risk was equivalent in each game. Kosfeld and colleagues (2005) did not observe any differences between the two groups who completed the nonbinary-choice TG and the nonsocial control condition. The combination of results across different institutions demonstrates how subtle differences across experimental designs can lead to largely disparate results, speaking to what some may claim are discrepancies across research studies.

5.5 Psychological Determinants of Trust as a Social Risk

Arriving at the decision to trust often involves multiple psychological processes that occur at the cognitive, emotional, and social levels. These psychological processes are not mutually exclusive, but each contributes distinct features that ultimately shape trust behaviors. At the cognitive level, trust may require that individuals weigh information about themselves and others in the pursuit of their goals. For instance, the "intentions" of the source of risk have little to no relevance in nonsocial sourced risk situations; however, social risk attitudes may heavily depend on another's intentions and thus may vary as these intentions change. Butler and Miller (2018) conducted a study to test whether three key features of human intentionality could potentially be determinants of socially risk-adverse behavior. Using Bohnet and Zeckhauser's (2004) binary TG, they constructed three treatments in which they manipulated whether the trustor thinks the trustee (i) can voluntarily act, (ii) foresees consequences of their actions, and (iii) desires these consequences. While they could replicate Bohnet and Zeckhauser (2004) when all three features were provided to the participant, they found that when removing the ability for the trustee to foresee their actions, trustors had smaller on average MAPs relative to the treatment when all information was provided. This suggests that the transparency of a counterparty's intentions is a key determinant of trust and/or socially risky behavior rather than simply the mere presence of interacting with another human. Broadly, these findings demonstrate that people consider not only the consequences of trusting another person, but also the psychological motives of that person.

At the emotional level (see also Chapter 6), the anticipation of trust violations may bring on "feelings of being a sucker" (Vohs et al., 2007) a phenomenon also known as the sucker effect (Kerr, 1983). The sucker effect describes situations in which an individual exhibits aversive emotional response as the result of perceiving that one has been taken advantage of during an interpersonal interaction with the shared understanding of a fair exchange (Vohs et al., 2007). Based on this fear invoked by this phenomenon, people may be more likely to avoid taking social risks or express a decreased willingness to trust. Support for this effect was demonstrated by Effron and Miller (2011) who found that anticipated self-blame or feeling foolish like one should have known better mediated the effect of conditions (nonsocial or social) on participants' trust decisions. This result suggests that people exhibit more negative emotional responses when feeling betrayed or exploited by another person compared with a nonsocial mechanism. In a recent multidisciplinary and integrative review on trust (Thielmann & Hilbig, 2015), betrayal sensitivity was identified as one of the three central features of trust behavior.

In Section 5.4 we discussed how betrayal aversion might be beneficial in generating a more cooperative economic system. Negative emotions associated with betrayal aversion may also arise as a protective mechanism that prevents oneself from being hurt or taken advantage of by another person, leading people to avoid situations in which they are vulnerable to another's trustworthiness. Deviating from studies using economic paradigms, Koehler and Gershoff (2003) showed support for betrayal-averse behavior in several studies that examined how people respond to various crimes involving betrayal, betrayal of safety products, and the risk of future betrayal by such products. They found that people reported experiencing greater levels of negative emotions in all betrayal conditions as compared to nonbetrayal conditions, indicating that betrayal aversion elicits aversive emotional responses. Perhaps their most interesting finding, however, was that people were willing to select products (air bag, alarm, vaccine) that substantially increased their risk for dying to avoid a small chance of dying due to betrayal rather than choosing products that lowered their overall risk of dying but exposed them to betrayal. In a more recent study also involving consumer behavior of safety products, they found that the effects of betrayal aversion could be reduced when interventions were introduced to attenuate negative emotional responses such as introducing positive imagery (Gershoff & Koehler, 2011). These findings on consumer behavior lend insights into the potential negative health outcomes that can arise from betrayal aversion and suggest ways to curb such effects. The strong emotional and betrayal aversion responses seen with these inanimate products suggests that we may grow close or develop a type of "social" relationship with our trusted safety products, expecting from them what we expect from trusted human counterparts.

Social norms (i.e., implicit expectations, rules, and procedures that are widely accepted by groups and societies) can also influence social behavior, like trust, at the individual level (Lapinski & Rimal, 2005; Sherif, 1936). From this normative perspective, people may engage in trust behavior to reap the "downstream benefits as much as they follow an injunction (i.e., a normative obligation) to do so" (Dunning et al., 2019, p. 367; Dunning et al., 2014). In other words, people may trust because they perceive that this is the appropriate action approved by others in their social group. Interestingly this mental framework of trust would lead one to engage in social trust more often than an equivalent nonsocial risk environment (opposite the direction of betrayal aversion). For instance, Dunning and colleagues (2014) endowed participants with $5 and were presented with two options: (i) keep the money for themselves or (ii) give it to another person in the room that they were matched with by the experimenter. The participant's identity was not revealed to the other person and vice versa. If people chose to give it to the other person, the $5 was increased to $20. The other person was then faced with a decision to either keep the $20 or give $10 back to the participant. Dunning et al. (2014) find that a majority of people decide to entrust their $5 to another person. Consistent with these findings, Fetchenhauer and Dunning (2012) asked people to play a TG and found that 54% of people were willing to choose the risky option to trust compared to 29% who opted to choose the risky option determined by a lottery with the same payoff structure. Taken altogether, these findings support the normative perspective proposed by Dunning et al. (2019) and provide evidence for a phenomenon called principled trustfulness (Fetchenhauer & Dunning, 2012; Fetchenhauer et al., 2020). Principled trustfulness is the idea that people trust to avoid sending a negative social signal that the trustor thinks their counterpart is not trustworthy (Fetchenhauer et al., 2020), which is driven by injunctive norms in which individuals believe that they should trust others (Dunning et al., 2014). Within our conceptualization, a concern for principled trustfulness is a psychological factor that arises from social risk environments. Intriguingly, Fetchenhauer et al. (2020) conducted a study in which they compared betrayal-aversion treatments alongside principled trustfulness treatments and find evidence suggesting that principled trust-fulness may be a stronger phenomenon.

While the literature has primarily focused on studying how each of these psychological processes (and others) at the cognitive, emotional, and social levels *separately* contribute to risky decisions to trust, these processes often do not occur in isolation in the real world. It is likely that trust behavior involves an interaction of these psychological processes. On the one hand, strong experimental designs enabling identification of phenomenon of interest such as betrayal aversion or principled trustfulness often attempt to hold all other factors constant. On the other hand, these designs may be telling only part of a story such that betrayal aversion or principled trustfulness may be moderated by other psychological factors. These interactions of psychological processes may be difficult to disentangle from behavioral data alone. Given that certain neural structures may be associated with distinct psychological functions, functional neuroimaging studies may help disambiguate the contribution of these separate psychological factors to trust behavior.

5.6   Neural Mechanisms of Social Risk and Trust

Research in the area of neuroeconomics broadly seeks to identify connections between behavioral economic parameters, decision-making processes, and brain function (Rangel et al., 2008). Neuroeconomics is an interdisciplinary research area that integrates theories and methods from economics (economic decision-making paradigms and formal models), psychology (psychological theory of cognition and human behavior), and neuroscience (methods and knowledge for understanding brain function). In the proceeding sections of this chapter, we have discussed the economic and psychological processes affecting economic social-risk-based trust behavior. In this section, we focus our attention on decision neuroscience studies of social risk and trust. Specifically, we review functional neuroimaging studies that use either functional magnetic resonance imaging (fMRI) or electroencephalography (EEG).

Functional neuroimaging is a unique and critically valuable tool for uncovering the neural processes and events associated with economic decision making. Behavioral studies provide a means to explore revealed preferences of participants under a variety of treatments and conditions to identify robust causal influences on decision making. However, in many circumstances neurobiological mechanism or process differences may exist but be hidden, since the ultimate behavior may be similar between experimental treatments. Neuroimaging studies, as discussed throughout this book, help shed light on the underlying processes or neurobiological mechanisms that may give rise to behavioral differences.

With respect to trust and social risk, the majority of functional neuro-imaging work is particularly focused on elucidating the role of specific brain regions in encoding economic variables from traditional expected utility and value-based decision-making models (Rangel et al., 2008). Within the area of decision making under uncertainty, the coding of objective risk information in nonsocial contexts has been linked to a specific network of regions: the bilateral insular cortex, medial prefrontal cortex including the dorsal anterior cingulate cortex (dACC) (Christopoulos et al., 2009), and thalamus (see meta-analysis, Mohr et al., 2010). Greater hemodynamic responses in these brain areas have been associated with the encoding of higher levels of risk (Mohr et al., 2010). There are also several studies that show that adolescents process risk in a similar network of brain regions (e.g., bilateral insular cortex and dACC) showing that risk processing in this set of brain regions is not specific to adults (Kim-Spoon et al., 2017; Lauharatanahirun et al., 2018). The activation of these brain areas within a risky decision-making context is consistent with the broader functional roles of these brain regions (especially the anterior insular cortex and anterior cingulate cortex) within the salience system to detect salient stimuli and recruit other relevant functional systems (Menon & Uddin, 2010). Neural responses in this network of regions have also been shown to be modulated by nonsocial economic risk preferences, indicating those who are risk adverse exhibit greater hemodynamic responses in the lateral orbiotfrontal cortex (Tobler et al., 2007), inferior frontal gyrus (Christopoulos et al., 2009), and caudate (Engelmann & Tamir, 2009). It is thought that these regions may function as an inhibitory response that also signals salient risky options within nonsocial environments (Christopoulos et al., 2009; Lauharatanahirun et al., 2018). Risk-seeking attitudes, however, have been linked to greater hemodynamic responses in the posterior parietal cortex (Huettel et al., 2006), medial orbitofrontal cortex (Engelmann & Tamir, 2009; Tobler et al., 2007), and superior and inferior frontal gyri (Engelmann & Tamir, 2009).

The neuroeconomics literature has primarily studied risky decision making within nonsocial contexts and little work has focused on the neurobiological differences between social and nonsocially sourced risk. Some work exists though and suggests greater exploration of the topic may be fruitful. Researchers have started to build upon existing work to examine whether similar neural correlates of nonsocial risk are also involved in social risk decisions. For example, one study examined both distinct and separable features of decision making under risk in social and nonsocial contexts (Lauharatanahirun et al., 2012). In this study, Lauharatanahirun and colleagues (2012) asked people to play an investment game while their hemodynamic responses were monitored using fMRI. In the investment game, participants were faced with two decision options: (i) keep an endowment ranging between $5 and $15 dollars or (ii) invest their endowment in a risky option where possible outcomes were either determined by a random process (nonsocial risk) or another person (social risk). While on the surface this task may appear to be the same as standard TGs, the investment game used in this study differs from prior work in that the possibility of betrayal in the social risk condition is removed. Specifically, the distribution of potential outcomes in the social risk condition was determined from a sample of previous participants' decisions and, thus, the other person in the social risk condition did not have a stake in the current game. As such, the risk (known probabilities over known outcomes) in the social and nonsocial conditions was identical.

From this task, the authors calculated economic risk preferences using a standard expected utility function for each participant within the social and nonsocial risk conditions. Within their sample, they found that there were two social risk-sensitivity groups: people that displayed higher levels of risk aversion in the nonsocial (relative to social) risk condition and another group that displayed higher levels of risk aversion in the social (relative to nonsocial) risk condition. Importantly, these social risk sensitivities appeared to be distinguished by neural sensitivities to risk information in the amygdala prior to making a decision. Specifically, individuals showing less risk aversion to nonsocial (relative to social) sources also exhibited reduced amygdala activation prior to choosing risky options in the nonsocial (relative to social) condition. Conversely, those showing less risk aversion to social (relative to nonsocial) sources also displayed reduced amygdala activation prior to choosing risky options in the social (relative to nonsocial) condition. This pattern of results suggests that the amygdala may be an important information-processing mechanism by which individuals are guided to engage (or not) in socially risky behavior. These results are also in line with recent work linking economic risk tolerance to greater functional connectivity between the amygdala and the medial prefrontal cortex (Jung et al., 2018).

In their review chapter on neuroeconomics and trust, Aimone and Houser (2016) drew a connection between the role of the amygdala in social and nonsocial risk and the literature on the amygdala and trust. The results of lesion studies (Adolphs et al.,1998; Koscik & Tranel, 2011) on the amygdala can be interpreted to suggest that the default for humans is to trust and that the amygdala acts to rein in trust by signaling fear to an initial trust decision (see also Chapter 18). Likewise, oxytocin/placebo studies (Kirsch et al., 2005; Kosfeld et al. 2005) suggest that the neuro-peptide oxytocin causally acts to increase trust and may be due to a reduced fear response in the amygdala when presented with a trust decision under increased levels of oxytocin (see also Chapter 13). Although Kosfeld et al. (2005) suggested that oxytocin might be acting upon betrayal aversion, oxytocin's relationship with amygdala function (Kirsch et al., 2005) suggests that oxytocin may actually be affecting individual responses to social relative to nonsocial sources of uncertainty via the amygdala (Aimone & Houser, 2016; Lauharatanahirun et al., 2012).

While the amygdala appears to respond to differences in the source generating uncertainty, and thus is important for shaping risky decisions, behavioral evidence suggests that how this uncertainty is resolved also contributes to risky decisions. To expand on their line of work in this area, Aimone et al. (2014) sought to explore the neural correlates of betrayal aversion. Participants in this study were asked to play a binary TG as the investor while undergoing an fMRI scan. Similar to the Aimone and Houser (2011, 2012, and 2013) designs, half of the games were standard TGs where a decision to trust resulted in a payment based on their own counterpart trustee's decision (exposure to possible personal betrayal). The other half were TGs in which decisions to trust were computer-mediated games based on a computer's random draw from the pool of that session's trustee decisions, shielding investors from betrayal knowledge in those games (i.e., no exposure to personal betrayal knowl-edge). Replicating their previous findings, Aimone and Houser find that there were more decisions to trust when payments were determined by a computer mediator rather than their counterpart. When participants decided to trust, participants on average showed higher activation in the right insular cortex as compared to when they decided to not trust their counterpart. This result supports previous assertions that anticipated aver-sive emotions may be present when investors are exposed to the possibility of betrayal, as recruitment of the insular cortex is associated with the subjective experience of anticipating potentially emotionally aversive stim-uli (Simmons et al., 2004). The insular cortex has been implicated in the processing of emotional responses (Craig, 2002; Damasio et al., 2000) and is a key region in the salience (Menon & Uddin, 2010) and risk processing

(Mohr et al., 2010) networks. Aimone and Houser also found significant differences in medial frontal cortex and right dorsolateral prefrontal cortex response difference which they attributed to emotion regulation.

The absence of amygdala activation differences observed between Aimone et al. (2014)'s TG and computer-mediated TGs may reflect that the perception of a social risk source was consistent across conditions, leaving no room for the Lauharatanahirun et al., (2012) social/nonsocial amygdala differences to arise. Likewise, the absence of amygdala activation differences in Aimone et al. (2014) also calls into question the role of oxytocin and betrayal aversion. Subsequent to the Kirsch et al. (2005) and Kosfeld et al. (2005) oxytocin studies, there have been mixed results regarding the replication of oxytocin's role in increasing trust behavior. For instance, Mikolajczak et al. (2010) were able to replicate previous work showing that oxytocin increases trust, but a recent review by Nave et al. (2015) demonstrates that in large-sample studies researchers have "failed to find consistent associations of specific OXT-related genetic polymorphisms and trust" and they "conclude that the cumulative evidence does not provide robust convergent evidence that human trust is reliably associated with OXT" (p. 772; see also Chapter 13).

While the first two studies reviewed above use fMRI that has high spatial resolution, other neuroimaging modalities such as EEG may provide additional information regarding the dynamic mechanisms of social risk-based trust decisions that unfold over time. EEG, unlike fMRI, has greater temporal resolution and may be more sensitive to understanding the time course of neural activity. To investigate how individual differences in social risk seeking affect trust behavior, Wang et al. (2017) examined differences in EEG activity during a standard TG between low and high social risk seekers. The social risk-seeking groups were determined using the social domain from the Domain-Specific Risk-Taking Scale (DOSPERT; Blais & Weber, 2006). They found that high social risk seekers display a larger N2 event-related potential (200–330 ms) and increased ß frequency band activity (12–30 Hz) when deciding to distrust as compared to trusting their counterparts, whereas no such effects were observed for low social risk seekers. Specifically, N2 is thought to be generated from the anterior cingulate cortex (Wang et al., 2017; Yeung et al., 2004). Both N2 and increased ß frequency band activity are implicated in response inhibition or effortful cognitive control (Huster et al., 2013), suggesting that high social risk seekers may require greater cognitive control to trust a nonsocial mechanism rather than a social one. This result complements the finding in Lauharatanahirun et al. (2012), which shows that those exhibiting less risk aversion to social (relative to nonsocial) sources of uncertainty (i.e., more socially risk seeking) show greater deactivation of fear-related responses in the amygdala. In other words, high social risk seekers require more cognitive effort that may be due to a low fear or inhibitory signals to social sources of uncertainty.

5.7 Discussion and Future Directions

As evidenced by past research, using both behavioral and functional neuroimaging methods, the source of risk is of critical importance in economic decisions. Some risk derives from a social source, such as other people's decisions, while other risk derives from a nonsocial source, such as a coin flip. Interestingly, the population appears divided with some individuals preferring social risk and others preferring nonsocial risk. While some initial research has been done, as we discussed in this chapter, this work is sparse and there appears to be fertile ground for other neuroscience, psychology, and economics research to be conducted.

It is puzzling why individuals would adopt a preference for one type of risk over the other, especially considering these preferences were identified (in studies like Lauharatanahirun et al., 2012) in environments where the social or nonsocial source of risk carried no strategic importance. Studies attempting to identify the evolutionary benefit of these preferences could be valuable. Similarly, it is unknown currently how deep a preference for "nonsocial" risk runs in an individual. For most nonsocial sources of risk (with the exception of a few known probability uncertain events like half-lives of elements) an ultimate social source could be argued to underpin the nonsocial source. For instance, a coin flip must be flipped by a person (social) or a machine or computer that was somehow manufactured or programmed by a person to generate the risky outcome. Are these social/nonsocial risk studies picking up social/nonsocial source differences, or something different like k-level reasoning or a preference for computer mediation?

While we focus on the social risk dimension in this chapter, various institutional features and preferences can be active under either of these risk source environments, features, and preferences that research show lead to different behavioral and neural differences. Betrayal aversion is one such phenomenon that we discuss in this chapter. As we mentioned briefly, a smaller amount of research (e.g., Koehler & Gershoff, 2003 and related studies) exists that shows betrayal aversion exists even in the nonsocial domain as well. How connected social and nonsocial betrayal aversion are to each other is not currently well understood; nor do we know whether there are similar neural mechanisms underpinning these behavioral phenomena. Likewise, risk uncertainty (known probabilities) is also intuitively closely connected to ambiguity uncertainty (unknown probabilities). All the environmental and institutional components of trust we discussed under risk intuitively exist in trust environments characterized as ambiguity and may reflect similar or different neural processes.

As for trust as a social risk, as we discuss in this chapter, very few functional neuroimaging studies have been conducted. The ability to distinguish between different mechanisms when behavior is similar may be very profitable for research. Take, for instance, the puzzle Fetchenhauer et al. (2020) tackle in their study trying to disentangle betrayal aversion from principled trustfulness. They draw conclusions based upon a relatively large sample of participants in a within-subjects design study, that 19.3% of participants make decisions consistent with principled trustfulness and only 6.7% consistent with betrayal aversion. However, as is common in many within-subject behavioral studies, many participants make the same decisions in both treatments and thus cannot be "typed." Over 70% of individuals in Fetchenhauer et al. (2020) make the same decisions in both of the within-subjects treatments. A neuroimaging study, while expensive, can help in such a situation since even though the behavior of subjects has no differences, the neural mechanisms may. Researchers interested in such questions would benefit from future work in this area.

Overall, research has begun to examine social risk-based trust and has shown promising and informative results. Socially sourced nonstrategic risk environments have been shown to be processed differently by individuals and lead to diverse behaviors and revealed preferences. These influences of sources of risk appear to also spill over into richer strategic risk environments, such as trust, and play an important role in factors like betrayal aversion. However, the current number of imaging studies in this area remain limited and are predominately correlational. There are a number of other neuroimaging methods such as transcranial magnetic stimulation and transcranial direct current stimulation, which may help researchers understand causal relationships in this area of trust research.

References

Abdellaoui, M., Baillon, A., Placido, L., & Wakker, P. P. (2011). The rich domain of uncertainty: Source functions and their experimental implementation. *American Economic Review*, 101(2), 695–723. https://doi.org/10.1257/aer.101.2.695

Adolphs, R., Tranel, D., & Damasio, A. R. (1998). The human amygdala in social judgment. *Nature*, 393(6684), 470–474. https://doi.org/10.1038/30982

Aimone, J. A., & Houser, D. (2011). Beneficial betrayal aversion. *PLoS ONE*, 6 (3), Article e17725. https://doi.org/10.1371/journal.pone.0017725

(2012). What you don't know won't hurt you: A laboratory analysis of betrayal aversion. *Experimental Economics*, 15(4), 571–588. https://doi.org/10.1007/s10683–012-9314-z

(2013). Harnessing the benefits of betrayal aversion. *Journal of Economic Behavior & Organization*, 89, 1–8. https://doi.org/10.1016/j.jebo.2013.02.001

(2016). Neuroeconomics: A flourishing field. In J. Komlos & I. R. Kelly (Eds.), *The Oxford handbook of economics and human biology*. (pp. 649–666). Oxford University Press. https://doi.org/10.1093/oxfordhb/9780199389292.013.1

Aimone, J. A., Houser, D., & Weber, B. (2014). Neural signatures of betrayal aversion: An fMRI study of trust. *Proceedings of the Royal Society B: Biological Sciences*, 281(1782), Article 20132127. https://doi.org/10.1098/rspb.2013.2127

Andreoni, J., & Miller, J. (2002). Giving according to GARP: An experimental test of the consistency of preferences for altruism. *Econometrica*, 70, 737–753. https://doi.org/10.1111/1468-0262.00302

Ashraf, N., Bohnet, I., & Piankov, N. (2006). Decomposing trust and trustworthiness. *Experimental Economics*, 9(3), 193–208. https://doi.org/10.1007/s10683–006-9122-4

Becker, G. M., DeGroot, M. H., & Marschak, J. (1964). Measuring utility by a single-response sequential method. *Behavioral Science*, 9(3), 226–232. https://doi.org/10.1002/bs.3830090304

Berg, J., Dickhaut, J., & McCabe, K. (1995). Trust, reciprocity, and social history. *Games and Economic Behavior*, 10(1), 122–142. https://doi.org/10.1006/game.1995.1027

Blais, A. R., & Weber, E. U. (2006). A domain-specific risk-taking (DOSPERT) scale for adult populations. *Judgment and Decision Making*, 1(1), 33–47. https://doi.org/10.1037/t13084-000

Bohnet, I., Greig, F., Herrmann, B., & Zeckhauser, R. (2008). Betrayal aversion: Evidence from Brazil, China, Oman, Switzerland, Turkey, and the United States. *American Economic Review*, 98(1), 294–310. https://doi.org/10.1257/aer.98.1.294

Bohnet, I., Herrmann, B., & Zeckhauser, R. (2010). Trust and the reference points for trustworthiness in Gulf and Western countries. *The Quarterly Journal of Economics*, 125(2), 811–828. https://doi.org/10.1162/qjec.2010.125.2.811

Bohnet, I., & Zeckhauser, R. (2004). Trust, risk and betrayal. *Journal of Economic Behavior & Organization*, 55(4), 467–484. https://doi.org/10.1016/j.jebo.2003.11.004

Butler, J. V., & Miller, J. B. (2018). Social risk and the dimensionality of intentions. *Management Science*, 64(6), 2787–2796. https://doi.org/10.1287/mnsc.2016.2694

Christopoulos, G. I., Tobler, P. N., Bossaerts, P., Dolan, R. J., & Schultz, W. (2009). Neural correlates of value, risk, and risk aversion contributing to decision making under risk. *Journal of Neuroscience*, 29(40), 12574–12583. https://doi.org/10.1523/JNEUROSCI.2614-09.2009

Coleman, J. (1990) *Foundation of social theory*. The Belknap Press of Harvard University Press.

Craig, A. D. (2002). How do you feel? Interoception: The sense of the physiological condition of the body. *Nature Reviews Neuroscience*, 3(8), 655–666. https://doi.org/10.1038/nrn894

Damasio, A. R., Grabowski, T. J., Bechara, A., et al. (2000). Subcortical and cortical brain activity during the feeling of self-generated emotions. *Nature Neuroscience*, 3(10), 1049–1056. https://doi.org/10.1038/79871

Dunning, D., Anderson, J. E., Schlösser, T., Ehlebracht, D., & Fetchenhauer, D. (2014). Trust at zero acquaintance: More a matter of respect than expectation of reward. *Journal of Personality and Social Psychology*, 107(1), 122–141. https://doi.org/10.1037/a0036673

Dunning, D., Fetchenhauer, D., & Schlösser, T. (2019). Why people trust: Solved puzzles and open mysteries. *Current Directions in Psychological Science*, 28(4), 366–371. https://doi.org/10.1177/0963721419838255

Eckel, C. C., & Grossman, P. J. (1996). Altruism in anonymous dictator games. *Games and Economic Behavior*, 16(2), 181–191. https://doi.org/10.1006/game.1996.0081

Eckel, C. C., & Wilson, R. K. (2004). Is trust a risky decision? *Journal of Economic Behavior & Organization*, 55(4), 447–465. https://doi.org/10.1016/j.jebo.2003.11.003

Effron, D. A., & Miller, D. T. (2011). Reducing exposure to trust-related risks to avoid self-blame. *Personality and Social Psychology Bulletin*, 37(2), 181–192. https://doi.org/10.1177/0146167210393532

Elster, J. (2007) *Explaining social behavior*. Cambridge University Press. https://doi.org/10.1017/CBO9780511806421

Engelmann, J. B., & Tamir, D. (2009). Individual differences in risk preference predict neural responses during financial decision making. *Brain Research*, 1290, 28–51. https://doi.org/10.1016/j.brainres.2009.06.078

Fairley, K., Sanfey, A., Vyrastekova, J., & Weitzel, U. (2016). Trust and risk revisited. *Journal of Economic Psychology*, 57, 74–85. https://doi.org/10.1016/j.joep.2016.10.001

Fehr, E. (2009). On the economics and biology of trust. *Journal of the European Economic Association*, 7(2–3), 235–266. https://doi.org/10.1162/JEEA.2009.7.2-3.235

Fehr, E., & Schmidt, K. M. (1999) A theory of fairness, competition, and cooperation. *The Quarterly Journal of Economics*, 114(3), 817–868. https://doi.org/10.2139/ssrn.106228

Fetchenhauer, D., & Dunning, D. (2012). Betrayal aversion versus principled trustfulness: How to explain risk avoidance and risky choices in trust games. *Journal of Economic Behavior & Organization*, 81(2), 534–541. https://doi .org/10.1016/j.jebo.2011.07.017

Fetchenhauer, D., Lang, A. S., Ehlebracht, D., Schlösser, T., & Dunning, D. (2020). Does betrayal aversion really guide trust decisions towards strangers? *Journal of Behavioral Decision Making*, 33(4), 556–566. https://doi.org/10 .1002/bdm.2166

Gambetta, D. (1988). *Trust: Making and breaking cooperative relations.* Blackwell.

Gershoff, A. D., & Koehler, J. J. (2011). Safety first? The role of emotion in safety product betrayal aversion. *Journal of Consumer Research*, 38(1), 140–150. https://doi.org/10.1086/658883

Hardin, R. (2001) Conceptions and explanations of trust. In K. S. Cook (Ed.), *Trust in society* (pp. 3–39). Russell Sage Foundation. http://www.jstor.org/ stable/10.7758/9781610441322.5

(2002). *Trust and trustworthiness.* Russell Sage Foundation.

(2006). *Trust.* Polity Press.

Holt, C. A., & Laury, S. K. (2002). Risk aversion and incentive effects. *American Economic Review*, 92(5), 1644–1655. https://doi.org/10.1257/ 000282802762024700

Hong, K., & Bohnet, I. (2007). Status and distrust: The relevance of inequality and betrayal aversion. *Journal of Economic Psychology*, 28(2), 197–213. https://doi.org/10.1016/j.joep.2006.06.003

Houser, D., Schunk, D., & Winter, J. (2010). Distinguishing trust from risk: An anatomy of the investment game. *Journal of Economic Behavior & Organization*, 74(1–2), 72–81. https://doi.org/10.1016/j.jebo.2010.01.002

Huettel, S. A., Stowe, C. J., Gordon, E. M., Warner, B. T., & Platt, M. L. (2006). Neural signatures of economic preferences for risk and ambiguity. *Neuron*, 49(5), 765–775. https://doi.org/10.1016/j.neuron.2006.01.024

Huster, R. J., Enriquez-Geppert, S., Lavallee, C. F., Falkenstein, M., & Herrmann, C. S. (2013). Electroencephalography of response inhibition tasks: Functional networks and cognitive contributions. *International Journal of Psychophysiology*, 87(3), 217–233. https://doi.org/10.1016/j .ijpsycho.2012.08.001

Jung, W. H., Lee, S., Lerman, C., & Kable, J. W. (2018). Amygdala functional and structural connectivity predicts individual risk tolerance. *Neuron*, 98(2), 394–404. https://doi.org/10.1016/j.neuron.2018.03.019

Kerr, N. L. (1983). Motivation losses in small groups: A social dilemma analysis. *Journal of Personality and Social Psychology*, 45(4), 819–828. https://doi.org/ 10.1037/0022-3514.45.4.819

Kim-Spoon, J., Deater-Deckard, K., Lauharatanahirun, N., et al. (2017). Neural interaction between risk sensitivity and cognitive control predicting health risk behaviors among late adolescents. *Journal of Research on Adolescence*, 27 (3), 674–682. https://doi.org/10.1111/jora.12295

Kirsch, P., Esslinger, C., Chen, Q., et al. (2005). Oxytocin modulates neural circuitry for social cognition and fear in humans. *Journal of Neuroscience*, 25 (49), 11489–11493. https://doi.org/10.1523/JNEUROSCI.3984-05.2005

Knight, F. H. (1921). *Risk, uncertainty and profit*. Houghton Mifflin.

Koehler, J. J., & Gershoff, A. D. (2003). Betrayal aversion: When agents of protection become agents of harm. *Organizational Behavior and Human Decision Processes*, 90(2), 244–261. https://doi.org/10.1016/S0749-5978(02)00518-6

Koscik, T. R., & Tranel, D. (2011). The human amygdala is necessary for developing and expressing normal interpersonal trust. *Neuropsychologia*, 49 (4), 602–611. https://doi.org/10.1016/j.neuropsychologia.2010.09.023

Kosfeld, M., Heinrichs, M., Zak, P. J., Fischbacher, U., & Fehr, E. (2005). Oxytocin increases trust in humans. *Nature*, 435(7042), 673–676. https:// doi.org/10.1038/nature03701

Lapinski, M. K., & Rimal, R. N. (2005). An explication of social norms. *Communication Theory*, 15(2), 127–147. https://doi.org/10.1111/j.1468-2885.2005.tb00329.x

Lauharatanahirun, N., Christopoulos, G. I., & King-Casas, B. (2012). Neural computations underlying social risk sensitivity. *Frontiers in Human Neuroscience*, 6, Article 213. https://doi.org/10.3389/fnhum.2012.00213

Lauharatanahirun, N., Maciejewski, D., Holmes, C., Deater-Deckard, K., Kim-Spoon, J., & King-Casas, B. (2018). Neural correlates of risk processing among adolescents: Influences of parental monitoring and household chaos. *Child Development*, 89(3), 784–796. https://doi.org/10.1111/cdev.13036

Menon, V., & Uddin, L. Q. (2010). Saliency, switching, attention and control: A network model of insula function. *Brain Structure and Function*, 214(5–6), 655–667. https://doi.org/10.1007/s00429-010-0262-0

Mikolajczak, M., Gross, J. J., Lane, A., Corneille, O., de Timary, P., & Luminet, O. (2010). Oxytocin makes people trusting, not gullible. *Psychological Science*, 21(8), 1072–1074. https://doi.org/10.1177/0956797610377343

Mohr, P. N., Biele, G., & Heekeren, H. R. (2010). Neural processing of risk. *Journal of Neuroscience*, 30(19), 6613–6619. https://doi.org/10.1523/ JNEUROSCI.0003-10.2010

Nave, G., Camerer, C., & McCullough, M. (2015). Does oxytocin increase trust in humans? A critical review of research. *Perspectives on Psychological Science*, 10(6), 772–789. https://doi.org/10.1177/1745691615600138

Quercia, S. (2016). Eliciting and measuring betrayal aversion using the BDM mechanism. *Journal of the Economic Science Association*, 2(1), 48–59. https:// doi.org/10.1007/s40881-015-0021-3

Rangel, A., Camerer, C., & Montague, P. R. (2008). A framework for studying the neurobiology of value-based decision making. *Nature Reviews Neuroscience*, 9(7), 545–556. https://doi.org/10.1038/nrn2357

Rousseau, D., Sitkin, S. B., Burt, R., & Camerer, C. (1998). Not so different after all: A cross-discipline view of trust. *Academy of Management Review*, 23(3), 393–404. https://doi.org/10.5465/AMR.1998.926617

Sapienza, P., Toldra-Simats, A., & Zingales, L. (2013). Understanding trust. *The Economic Journal*, 123(573), 1313–1332. https://doi.org/10.1111/ecoj.12036

Schechter, L. (2007). Traditional trust measurement and the risk confound: An experiment in rural Paraguay. *Journal of Economic Behavior & Organization*, 62(2), 272–292. https://doi.org/10.1016/j.jebo.2005.03.006

Sherif, M. (1936). *The psychology of social norms*. Harper & Brothers.

Simmons, A., Matthews, S. C., Stein, M. B., & Paulus, M. P. (2004). Anticipation of emotionally aversive visual stimuli activates right insula. *Neuroreport*, 15(14), 2261–2265. https://doi.org/10.1097/00001756-200410050-00024

Smith, V. L. (1982). Microeconomic systems as an experimental science. *The American Economic Review*, 72(5), 923–955. http://www.jstor.org/stable/1812014

Thielmann, I., & Hilbig, B. E. (2015). Trust: An integrative review from a person–situation perspective. *Review of General Psychology*, 19(3), 249–277. https://doi.org/10.1037/gpr0000046

Tobler, P. N., O'Doherty, J. P., Dolan, R. J., & Schultz, W. (2007). Reward value coding distinct from risk attitude-related uncertainty coding in human reward systems. *Journal of Neurophysiology*, 97(2), 1621–1632. https://doi.org/10.1152/jn.00745.2006

Vohs, K. D., Baumeister, R. F., & Chin, J. (2007). Feeling duped: Emotional, motivational, and cognitive aspects of being exploited by others. *Review of General Psychology*, 11(2), 127–141. https://doi.org/10.1037/1089-2680.11.2.127

Wang, Y., Jing, Y., Zhang, Z., Lin, C., & Valadez, E. A. (2017). How dispositional social risk-seeking promotes trusting strangers: Evidence based on brain potentials and neural oscillations. *Journal of Experimental Psychology: General*, 146(8), 1150–1163. https://doi.org/10.1037/xge0000328

Williamson, O. E. (1993). Calculativeness, trust, and economic organization. *The Journal of Law and Economics*, 36(1, Part 2), 453–486. https://doi.org/10.1086/467284

Yamagishi, T. (2011). *Trust: The evolutionary game of mind and society*. Springer. https://doi.org/10.1007/978-4-431-53936-0

Yeung, N., Botvinick, M. M., & Cohen, J. D. (2004). The neural basis of error detection: Conflict monitoring and the error-related negativity. *Psychological Review*, 111(4), 931–959. https://doi.org/10.1037/0033-295X.111.4.931

Zuckerman, M., Kolin, E. A., Price, L., & Zoob, I. (1964). Development of a sensation-seeking scale. *Journal of Consulting Psychology*, 28(6), 477–482. https://doi.org/10.1037/h0040995

CHAPTER 6

Trust and Emotion
The Effects of Incidental and Integral Affect

Federica Farolfi, Li-Ang Chang, and Jan B. Engelmann

6.1 Introduction

Decisions whether to trust someone are complex and require the support of a multitude of cognitive, affective, and motivational processes. A common conceptualization of the neurocognitive processes involved in social decisions, including trust decisions, posits the following steps that the decision-maker is required to undergo at minimum (see for instance Engelmann & Hare, 2018; Rangel et al., 2008): (1) forming a perceptual representation of the choice space, including what the choice options are and who is affected by the decision outcomes; (2) evaluating the different outcomes in terms of their costs and benefits to self and others; (3) planning and executing an action that reflects the choice; and (4) consuming the outcome of the choice, which involves comparing the observed with the expected value of the outcome (which gives rise to the prediction error) to update the subjective value of the chosen option for future decisions. Multiple cognitive processes support the above decision steps, including attention (e.g., Hare et al., 2011; Lim et al., 2011; Rangel & Hare, 2010), memory (e.g., Bechara & Martin, 2004; Hinson et al., 2003), theory of mind (e.g., Cutler & Campbell-Meiklejohn, 2019; Rilling et al., 2004; Schurz et al., 2014), and learning (e.g., Niv et al., 2012; Schönberg et al., 2007; Schultz, 2002). A plethora of research in cognitive and affective neuroscience on emotion–cognition interactions has shown that many of these cognitive processes are readily influenced by affective processes (e.g., Pessoa, 2008). Attention, for instance, is commonly captured by emotional stimuli (Mulckhuyse et al., 2013, 2017; Yiend, 2010), leading to preferential processing of emotional stimuli over others. Given the tight integration between emotional and choice-relevant cognitive processes (Pessoa, 2008), as well as significant overlap in the

Corresponding author: Jan B. Engelmann (j.b.engelmann@uva.nl).

neural circuitry of cognitive and affective processes (Engelmann & Hare, 2018), emotions can be expected to influence cognitive mechanisms that support trust decisions at all stages outlined above.

In the current chapter, we review research from multiple fields, including behavioral economics and neuroeconomics, that investigates the influences of affect on trust. We focus on the relationship between emotional states and trusting behavior by looking at behavioral and neural evidence that examined moods and emotions[1] experienced at the moment of the choice (Loewenstein et al., 2001). This type of emotions, known as *immediate emotions* (Dunning et al., 2017; Lerner et al., 2015; Loewenstein & Lerner, 2003; Rick & Loewenstein, 2008; Schlösser et al., 2016), falls into two categories: *incidental emotions,* as those whose source is unrelated to the target decision; and *integral emotions,* which arise from directly contemplating features of the decision, such as thinking about the consequences of a choice (Lerner & Keltner, 2000; Pham, 2007).

The majority of the experiments we review here employ the trust game (TG), a game-theoretic approach developed in experimental economics to model the decision to trust (for a detailed review of the TG see Alós-Ferrer & Farolfi, 2019; Engelmann, 2010) (see also Chapter 2). In the TG, two agents are facing a social dilemma in a strategic incentivized scenario. In its continuous version, as proposed by Berg et al. (1995), two agents, a trustor and a trustee, engage in a sequential one-shot interaction. The trustor acts as a first mover and decides how much of her endowment to allocate to the second agent, the trustee, where zero is an option (effectively ending the game). The amount sent is then tripled by the experimenter and given to the trustee, who decides how much of this magnified amount to return to the trustor, where again, zero is an option. The portion of endowment sent to the trustee is considered to be a measure of trust, while the amount returned to the trustor represents a measure of trustworthiness or reciprocity. The rules of the game (i.e., monetary payoffs) are common knowledge to both agents, and the theoretical prediction for a rational self-interested trustor would be not to make any transfer to the trustee by anticipating

---

[1] From a theoretical standpoint, there is a generally accepted distinction between emotions and moods. Emotions are characterized as affect that arises from a clear specific event, they occur at high intensity, and they are short-lived. Moods are described as states without a clear point of formation, which present low intensity but a long duration such as hours or days (Capra, 2004; Forgas, 1995; Lench et al., 2011; Schwarz, 1990). While it would be meaningful to investigate the different impact of emotions and moods on trusting behavior, in this chapter the term emotion refers to both emotions and moods (Pham, 2007).

that a selfish opponent would return nothing (subgame perfect equilibrium). As might be expected, actual human behavior significantly differs from the economically rational choice to act selfishly as indicated by the positive levels of both trust and reciprocity commonly observed in laboratory settings (Berg et al., 1995; Camerer, 2003; Johnson & Mislin, 2011).

Initially seen as an emotionless cognitive task, the literature on the TG did not immediately include affective states as factors that could potentially affect or explain the observed "irrational" behavior in the laboratory. Subsequently, social preferences such as altruism and other-regarding preferences (e.g., inequity aversion) and possible cognitive limits entered into the equation (Camerer, 2003; Fehr et al., 2005). Nowadays, the tendency is to perceive emotions as an integral part of the decision-making process (e.g., as factors producing biases) and a valuable, albeit not always behaviorally transparent, source of information (Engelmann & Fehr, 2017; Engelmann & Hare, 2018; Lerner et al., 2015; Loewenstein et al., 2001).

6.2 Behavioral Effects of Incidental Emotions on Trust Behavior

Because real-world decisions are rarely made within an emotional vacuum, incidental emotions are ubiquitous in real life and understanding their influence on decision processes is therefore important. From the perspective of economic rationality, incidental emotions should not affect the decision at hand, since the origin of these emotional states is unrelated to the targets of the decision. Psychological intuition, on the other hand, supports the view that our current affective states may influence our decisions. A large body of empirical evidence agrees with our psychological intuition and has already established that these emotional states can affect how people interpret the possible outcomes of their decisions (Andrade & Ho, 2007; Capra, 2004; Dunn & Schweitzer, 2005; Schwarz, 1990). Incidental emotions are therefore increasingly accepted as a core part of judgment and decision making in different domains such as risk (Cohn et al., 2015; Engelmann & Fehr, 2017; Engelmann & Hare, 2018; Engelmann et al., 2015; Lerner et al., 2015; Loewenstein et al., 2001; Mellers et al., 1997; Phelps et al., 2014) and interpersonal trust (Dunn & Schweitzer, 2005; Engelmann, Meyer, et al., 2019).

To observe how emotions and moods affect behavior, experimentalists rely on a gamut of emotion-induction techniques in the laboratory (also known as mood induction procedures, MIPs) that temporarily place the participants in a particular mood state (e.g., anger, sadness, happiness) immediately before performing an unrelated task. Examples are the autobiographical emotional memory task (AEMT) that asks participants to reactivate past memories; the Velten method (Velten, 1968), where subjects read emotionally loaded sentences to endogenously generate the suggested mood; hypnosis (Maccallum et al. 2000); or by using emotion-inducing material such as movie clips (Kirchsteiger et al., 2006) and music (Kenealy, 1988). The effectiveness of such emotion manipulations is typically assessed by measuring neurophysiological responses that reflect autonomic nervous system arousal and include heart rate (Roelofs, 2017), galvanic skin conductance levels (Eimontaite et al., 2013), and salivary cortisol levels (Hellhammer et al., 2009), self-report measures such as the Positive And Negative Affect Schedule (PANAS; Saadaoui et al., 2019), correlation with the observed behavior, or by using face-reading technology that assesses moment-to-moment changes in facial expressions of emotion (Kugler et al., 2020). While all these procedures have been corroborated along the years, but less effectively by using an internet-based setting (Ferrer et al., 2015; Göritz & Moser, 2006), they present limitations in terms of timing of the effect, contamination of other nontarget affects (Myers & Tingley, 2016), and ethical admissibility in some settings (Ferrer et al., 2015; Gerrards-Hesse et al., 1994). More recently, studies have addressed some shortcomings of MIPs and induced negative affect via the threat of shock procedure (ToS; Schmitz & Grillon, 2012) in which participants receive unpredictable and mildly painful electrical shocks in a threatening condition, and no or nonpainful shocks in a safe condition (Cohn et al., 2015; Engelmann, Meyer, et al., 2019). Importantly, converging evidence from different methods provides relatively strong support for the role of particular emotions in trust decisions.

6.2.1 *Positive Incidental Emotions*

Capra (2004) has conducted one of the first studies that tested the impact of positive (and negative) induced mood on behavior in a one-shot TG. This initial study found no evidence that emotions influence trust behavior. As a mood-inducer, the author used both an AEMT, where subjects had to write an autobiographical essay, and experienced success or failure throughout the experiment (by receiving hard or easy sets of MENSA questions). In the same study, she found that subjects in a positive mood were more altruistic in the dictator game (DG)[2] (suggesting that positive

---

[2] In the dictator game (Kahneman et al., 1986) the investors are facing a similar choice as in the trust game, but the recipients are passive (they have no chance to counteract) thus putting the investors in

affect makes people more aware of the other player's payoffs). In line with the latter result, Mellers et al. (2010) found that a positive mood (induced by giving subjects a candy bag and a movie clip to watch) generally increased the level of cooperation in both the DG and ultimatum game (UG).[3] Saadaoui et al. (2019) explore the effects of positive (and negative) emotions on trust and risk attitude. In their study, emotion induction was performed by showing subjects a slideshow of pictures (International Affective Picture System) followed by the assessment of participants' emotional state using the Self-Assessment Manikin scale. Subjects performed a TG, a DG, and, ultimately, a risk and ambiguity game. The authors implemented two treatments, a *safe* treatment (TG/DG) and a *risky* treatment (RTG/RDG) with the main difference that the amount sent by the investor was multiplied by three with a probability of 50% and multiplied by one with the remaining probability in the risky conditions (RTG/RDG). Their results indicate that in the risky treatment, both positive and negative emotions decrease pro-social behavior in the DG, whereas emotions do not affect trusting behavior in the TG. In the safe treatment, however, trustors showed higher levels of trust after negative compared to positive mood induction. Finally, individuals in the positive mood condition were more likely to be risk takers compared to the negative mood condition.

A more specific and discrete positive emotion that has been addressed in the literature is happiness. Mislin et al. (2015) asked subjects to recall and write about a happy and joyful memory and watch commercial film clips before engaging in a TG. Results indicate that happy people are more likely to trust, particularly in the condition that offered a relatively lower overall gain from the initial trust (Figure 6.1A). These results are in line with a study of emotions on interpersonal trust by Dunn and Schweitzer (2005). Myers and Tingley (2016) used a similar procedure to induce happiness (together with anger, anxiety, guilt, and self-assurance) by means

complete control and not exposed to financial risk (loss of the investment) and social risk (possibility of being betrayed by the opponent). See Alós-Ferrer and Farolfi (2019) for a critical survey of the use of the game in comparison with the trust game.

[3] In the ultimatum game (Güth et al., 1982) the first mover (the proposer) makes an offer on how to split her endowment between her and the second mover (the receiver). The latter observes the proposed offer and decides between rejecting the offer (where both players get a null payoff) or accepting the offer (where the suggested split of the amount occurs). Experimental evidence indicates that proposers usually offer between 40% and 50% of their endowment (which is usually accepted), while rejections are observed when proposers offer below their 20% of the endowment (Camerer, 2003). Although inefficient from an economic point of view (i.e., the receivers would be better off by accepting any positive amount) the rejection of the offer signals to the proposer the unfairness of the implied division.

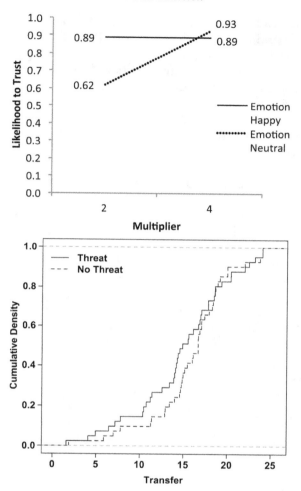

Figure 6.1   Effects of the induction of specific incidental emotions on trust.
Figure 6.1A shows that the positive emotion of happiness increases trust decisions under
specific conditions in the trust game. Figure 6.1B shows the effect of the specific emotion of
anxiety, induced via threat of shock, on trust. In particular, fewer subjects transfer low
amounts (below 15 MU) in the no-threat condition (ca. one-half in the threat condition vs.
ca. one-third in the no threat condition), while more subjects transferred relatively large
amounts in the no-threat condition. Note that Figure 6.1A is reproduced with permission
from Mislin et al. (2015). Figure 6.1B was created using publicly available data from
Engelmann, Schmid, et al. (2019).

of the AEMT and subsequently asked subjects to complete the expanded form Positive And Negative Affect Schedule (PANAS-X) questionnaire to measure general positive and negative affect. The autobiographical memory task failed to manipulate positive emotions.[4] An interesting aspect that has been explored within the realm of incidental emotions and cooperative behavior is whether emotion manipulation has an impact on the cognitive processing style. In this strand of research, Hertel et al. (2000) used a modified version of a public goods game[5] and induced happiness and sadness by asking subjects to watch two film excerpts. The authors found that happy people were more likely to use a heuristics processing strategy, whereas sad people favored a more careful, gathering-information approach.

In sum, the results reviewed in Section 6.2.1 suggest that positive mood states have relatively little influence on trust decisions, with two studies showing a null effect of induced positive mood on trust, while positive effects were observed on cooperation and altruism. On the other hand, the specific emotion of happiness has been shown to lead to an increase in trust across multiple studies, likely by increasing participants' optimism and therefore their expectations of a positive back-transfer (Fredrickson et al., 2003). This agrees with previous findings demonstrating a consistent association between happiness and enhanced risk seeking across a number of studies (Engelmann & Hare, 2018). The results reviewed in Section 6.2.1 suggest that this effect of positive emotions on decision making extends also to the domain of social decision making, including decisions to trust. A likely mechanism for the specific effects of happiness on trust is by enhancing cognitive mechanisms that support approach behaviors, such as reward seeking, as well as inducing optimistic beliefs.

---

[4] Note that one reason for the relative sparsity of studies investigating the causal role of positive affect is that it remains relatively difficult to induce positive emotional states, especially for longer periods of time.

[5] In the public goods game (Andreoni, 1995; Fehr & Gächter, 2000; Isaac & Walker, 1988) a group of individuals must decide independently how to allocate their initial endowment between a private and a group account. While the resources allocated to the private account exclusively benefit the individual, the total contributions donated to the group account are multiplied by an efficiency factor by the experimenter and equally redistributed among all the individuals of the group. The game mimics common social dilemmas, and in its standard form the optimum would require for the individuals to give full contribution to the group account while the prescription for a rational individual would be to defect and contribute nothing to the group account. Empirically, it has been shown that the average contribution to the group account is about 60% of the endowment, showing that individuals are not entirely free-riders, but fall short from the social optimum.

6.2.2 *Negative Incidental Emotions*

The study done by Capra (2004) found no impact of negative induced mood on trusting behavior. An emotion-specific analysis conducted by Myers and Tingley (2016) revealed that anxiety (an emotion with low certainty about the negative consequences of the event) has a negative influence on trust, contrary to guilt or anger. Similar behavioral results were obtained in a recent neuroimaging study that induced incidental anxiety via ToS and found significant decreases in trust as a consequence (Figure 6.1B, Engelmann, Meyer, et al., 2019). Two other important negative emotions that have been tested within a TG environment are incidental regret and disappointment. Martinez and Zeelenberg (2015) induced these emotions via both a scrambled sentence task and a standard recall memory procedure. The authors showed that the feeling of regret decreased trusting behavior whereas disappointment increased it. The authors suggest that the positive effect of disappointment on trust levels might reflect the willingness to avoid future disappointments and the attempt to gain a better final outcome. The decreasing levels of trust observed by participants feeling regret might be seen as a correcting maneuver with the intent of avoiding reexperiencing the same feeling in the future.

Nelissen et al. (2007) induced guilt and fear by using an autobiographical recall procedure and asked participants to play a social dilemma game (give-some dilemma) that is similar to the TG in the respect that highly cooperative subjects can be taken advantage of by the interaction partner. Additionally, participants' social value orientation was assessed to account for possible individual differences in terms of pro-social or pro-self preferences. Their findings reveal that incidental fear reduced cooperation, but only for those subjects with a pro-social value orientation, while incidental guilt increased cooperation, but only for those individuals showing a pro-self orientation. In line with this result, De Hooge et al. (2011) showed that incidental guilt promotes pro-social behavior toward the "victim" of a multiplayer DG, even if it is done at the expenses of the others. Regarding interpersonal trust, Dunn and Schweitzer (2005) showed that incidental anger decreased levels of trust, but with emotional cognitive appraisal the effects on trust disappeared.

Affective dispositions in the form of character traits can be considered another form of incidental affect, as they are unrelated to the decision outcomes. A recent study assessing such affective character traits and investigating individual differences in trust behavior showed that trait anger significantly reduced trust (Engelmann, Schmid, et al., 2019). Moreover, people with high levels of dispositional anger also had more pessimistic beliefs about the back-transfers of trustees, and changed their behavior significantly in the context of a punishment opportunity. These results generally agree with a recent meta-analysis of personality traits and behavior in social dilemmas (see figure 4 in Thielmann et al., 2020), showing that two related dispositional negative emotions (aggression and anger) reduce pro-social decisions in the context of multiple games. Interestingly, positive dispositional affect showed no influence on pro-social decisions, while the personality traits of honesty-humility and its negatively correlated construct of antisociality (including Machiavellianism and psychopathy) significantly enhanced (honesty-humility) and reduced (antisocial traits) pro-social behaviors, such as trusting and reciprocating (Engelmann, Schmid, et al., 2019; Thielmann et al., 2020).

In sum, induced negative mood seems to have little to no effect on trust decisions. Specific negative emotions, on the other hand, have varying effects. Reduced trust was observed in response to induced anxiety and fear, which is consistent with the action tendencies of these emotions that enhance avoidant and withdrawal-related behavior (Chen & Bargh, 1999; Roelofs et al., 2010). Anger, both as incidental and dispositional affect, has been shown to reduce trust, which at first glance is inconsistent with the approach motivation associated with this emotion. However, in the setting of the TG, it is likely that anger reduces the participants' willingness to be placed in a situation that renders participants vulnerable to the betrayal of another. In agreement with this hypothesis, Engelmann, Schmid, et al. (2019) find that under conditions in which the trustor is able to punish the trustee, and therefore is no longer powerless and can respond to potential betrayal, trust in dispositionally angry participants significantly increased. In addition to these basic emotions, more complex social emotions, such as guilt, shame, disappointment, and regret have also been successfully induced in previous work. Disappointment and guilt both consistently increased cooperation, while regret decreased trust.

While incidental emotions have been shown to have an important effect on trust behavior, further research will be necessary to identify whether and how emotions influence not just trust, but also belief formation and whether their effects on behavior and beliefs occur consciously or not. In tackling these questions, future research will need to circumvent methodological limitations related to the MIPs, including subjects' different susceptibility to the techniques and avoiding potential demand effects (for instance, by possibly avoiding self-report questions that might cause subjects to reflect on their emotional state). Recent approaches relying on the ToS procedure tackle many of the limitations of mood inductions (e.g., Engelmann et al., 2015; Engelmann, Meyer, et al., 2019), but are currently limited to negative affect only.

6.3 Behavioral Effects of Integral Emotions

Unlike incidental emotions, integral emotions are directly related to the decision outcomes. Within this category, a meaningful distinction concerns those emotions that are experienced before making the actual decision, known as *anticipatory emotions* (Engelmann & Hare, 2018; Loewenstein & Lerner, 2003); and those emerging as a consequence of the revealed outcome. Examples of the latter are disappointment in case of losses (Loomes & Sugden, 1986), regret about a nonchosen and better option (Loomes & Sugden, 1982), pleasure and gratitude if decisions are rewarded (Rabin, 1993), negative emotional reactions due to unfair offers (Sanfey, 2009; Tabibnia et al., 2008), or forgiveness after a transgression (Desmet et al., 2011). These types of emotions are experienced once the outcome is known (postdecisional phase) and therefore are integral to the decision process. They are particularly important for the computation of prediction errors, as well as updating future expectations and decisions based on the experienced outcomes. Because here we are interested mainly in how emotions influence trust at the time the decision is made, we focus on the more impactful role of anticipatory emotions, as the affective responses triggered by thinking about the future consequences of one's behavior (predecisional phase) (Loewenstein & Lerner, 2003).[6]

Although the decision to trust could be rewarding in itself (Engelmann & Fehr, 2017), from a strictly monetary point of view, trust decisions are favorable only if the trustee is in fact trustworthy and reciprocates the initial investment of the trustor. There are two important sources that can influence the decision to trust: (1) the perceived trustworthiness of the interaction partner during the decision, which is commonly measured in experiments as an expectation or belief about how much the interaction partner will return; and (2) the participant's willingness to take a social risk that, in the context of the TG, is related to the perceived likelihood of

---

[6] Dunning et al. (2012) and Schlösser et al. (2016) advocate the importance of emotions that are not attached to the outcome of the decision, but rather to the specific action a person is contemplating to take. In this less consequentialist vision, the authors argue that a person may feel anxiety just about the thought of engaging in a trust decision, and feel guilty about the thought or distrust the human counterpart (without cogitating on the possible consequences).

betrayal by the trustee. Both sources can influence decision-relevant cognitive processes, such as the perceived social risk involved in trusting another person, and affective processes, such as the emotion involved in anticipating betrayal (betrayal aversion). In this respect, the trustor forms a belief about her opponent's level of trustworthiness and subsequently relies on her expectations when forming a decision (Thielmann & Hilbig, 2015).

To form a belief the trustor could integrate information (if available) from cues that are directly related to her opponent's reciprocity such as history and reputational mechanism (Charness et al., 2011; Delgado et al., 2005); or unrelated and normatively uninformative cues such as (fictional) opponents' handwritten essays (Eimontaite et al., 2013), resemblance (DeBruine, 2002), and pupil mimicry (Prochazkova et al., 2018; Wehebrink et al., 2018) (see also Chapter 7). Research in social neuroscience suggests that in the absence of such cues, trustors likely form reciprocity expectations based on how they would behave if placed in the shoes of the trustee, an approach based on self-projection (e.g., Engelmann, Meyer, et al., 2019; Waytz & Mitchell, 2011). A downside of self-projection is that it can lead to decision biases in overly pro- and antisocial individuals (Engelmann, Schmid, et al., 2019). Opponents' facial expressions are also very influential for decisions to trust or distrust (Alguacil et al., 2015; Ekman & Friesen, 2003), whether the visual clue is provided by means of photographs (Franzen et al., 2011; Jaeger et al., 2019; Scharlemann et al., 2001), line drawings (Eckel & Wilson, 2003), video clips of facial dynamics (Krumhuber et al., 2007), or virtual reality (Kugler et al., 2020).

Numerous studies have used facial stimuli to inspect the role of trustworthiness judgments in decisions to trust, because trustworthiness judgments are made spontaneously (Klapper et al., 2016) and quickly (Willis & Todorov, 2006) from others' faces and have a clear neural representation in the amygdala (Engell et al., 2007; Winston et al., 2002). Capnellane and Kring (2013) found that facial expressions of anger reduced trust, while facial expressions of happiness, contrary to the authors' expectations, had no influence on decisions to trust. Similarly, Tortosa et al. (2013) found that trustors were more willing to trust happy partners compared to angry partners in a repeated TG environment. On a more subtle level, Krumhuber et al. (2007) investigated the dual nature of a smile (fake vs. genuine) showing video clips (fewer than 6 s) of opponent players where only the mouth region was animated. Subjects chose more often a counterpart with an authentic smile and engaged more often in trusting behavior in the TG. Interestingly, participants perceived opponents showing a neutral expression (used as a control) as less trustworthy than either a genuine or fake smile. Informing trustors about their opponents' incidental emotional state could also affect behavior. Kausel and Connolly (2014) found that trustors associated their opponent's anger with untrustworthiness and acted accordingly.

In the TG, the trustor needs to overcome two different sources of risk: a financial one, which represents the risk of not receiving a return on the investment; and a social one, which is the risk of being betrayed (Aimone et al., 2014, 2015; Bohnet et al., 2008; Bohnet & Zeckhauser, 2004; Fehr, 2009; Fetchenhauer & Dunning, 2012; Quercia, 2016). The argument has been made that betrayal aversion has important emotional consequences that can affect trust decisions (Engelmann & Fehr, 2017). One way to measure betrayal aversion has been developed by Bohnet and Zeckhauser (2004). In their paradigm, participants complete an equivalently framed binary TG, a risk game, and a risky DG, but unlike the standard TG, participants do not indicate how much they would invest in each scenario. Instead, participants are asked to indicate their minimum acceptable probabilities (MAP), that is, the probability of positive and fair repayment of the investment that they require to make the (socially) risky investment (Bohnet & Zeckhauser, 2004; for a global replication, see Bohnet et al., 2008). The risky DG provides the most interesting comparison to trust behavior, as the risky DG includes a passive recipient who has no opportunity to betray the trustor. Both the trustor and this recipient receive the equivalent payment to the one in the TG, but how much is determined by a random mechanism (instead of the trustee who decides in the standard TG). Social preferences therefore should be (almost) equal across the two games. Results from multiple experiments employing this method (Bohnet et al., 2008; Bohnet & Zeckhauser, 2004) indicate that there is an additional cost when taking social compared to nonsocial risk, as reflected by a higher MAP in the TG, compared to all other games. Additional behavioral paradigms have been developed to measure betrayal aversion (Aimone & Houser, 2012), which have shown that the decision to trust can be affected by the possibility of finding out whether betrayal occurred. Interestingly, Aimone and Houser (2012) report that levels of trust are higher when investors are forced to stay in the dark about the trustee's betrayal. There is an ongoing debate regarding how different methods of elicitation of betrayal aversion (i.e., the tendency to avoid social risk) could lead to mixed results in literature (e.g., use of minimum accepted probability vs. choice lists; see Engelmann & Fehr, 2017 for a discussion; see Alós-Ferrer & Farolfi, 2019 for the analysis of the two sources of risk).

In sum, integral emotions have been shown to significantly affect trust decisions. Specifically, facial emotional expressions communicated by the interaction partner during the trust decision can have significant influences on trust, with facial expressions of negative affect, such as anger, reducing and positive facial expressions, such as happiness, enhancing trust. It is noteworthy that while participants readily use facial expressions of emotions and the facial appearance of counterparts to infer their trustworthiness, only conflicting evidence exists about whether such inferences can in fact be made accurately. While initial reports showed that trustworthiness can be detected at levels slightly above chance from neutral photographs (Bonnefon et al., 2017; De Neys et al., 2017; Tognetti et al., 2013; Verplaetse et al., 2007), more recent work suggests that participants are in fact unable to do so (Efferson & Vogt, 2013; Jaeger et al., 2020). One important reason for this inaccuracy is that, when making trustworthiness inferences, participants seem to be easily swayed by the emotional features of faces that are in fact unpredictable of a counterpart's trait pro-sociality (Jaeger et al., 2020; Scharlemann et al., 2001). Moreover, betrayal aversion (not an emotional state in itself, but a dispositional attitude favoring specific emotions) and its affective consequences during the time of choice can significantly reduce trust decisions. Future research is needed to further understand the specific emotional consequences of betrayal aversion and their influence on trust decisions. One promising route to take may be to investigate individual differences in betrayal aversion and its relationship with dispositional character traits, emotions, and theory of mind abilities.

6.4   The Neural Basis of Emotional Influences on Trust Decisions

The neural basis of trust has received significant attention in the field of neuroeconomics. It is generally acknowledged that two processes interact during trust decisions (Figure 6.2), which are: (1) a social cognitive component that assesses the trustworthiness and intentions of interaction partners and is processed in a social cognition network consisting of the temporoparietal junction (TPJ), superior temporal sulcus (STS), and dorsomedial prefrontal cortex (dmPFC); and (2) an evaluative component that assesses the subjective value of the decision and is processed in the ventral striatum (vSTR) and ventromedial prefrontal cortex (vmPFC) (e.g., Engelmann & Fehr, 2017; Ruff & Fehr, 2014). Multiple neuroimaging studies employing the TG have shown activation in social cognition areas when participants were actively making trust decisions (e.g., Engelmann,

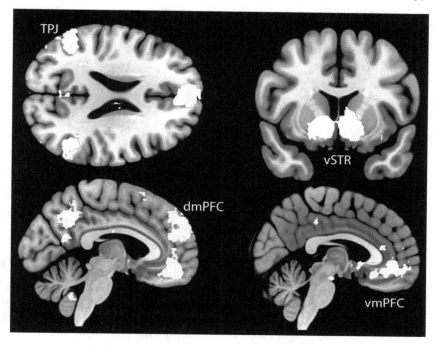

Figure 6.2   Brain networks involved in trust decisions.

Meyer, et al., 2019; Gromann et al., 2013; Krueger et al., 2008; McCabe et al., 2001; Sripada et al., 2009; Stanley et al., 2012). Such activations of social cognition regions during trust decisions likely reflect mentalizing, as the agent needs to take the perspective of the trustee and simulate how she will react to given transfers. This is because of the presence of a strong incentive to avoid being betrayed, which is unique to decisions to trust as opposed to matched risky decisions. Moreover, a recent meta-analysis of the neuroimaging literature around the TG also implicated the anterior insula in one-shot trust decisions (Bellucci, Feng, Camilleri, Eickhoff, & Krueger, 2018), likely reflecting this region's involvement in assessing social norm deviations (Krueger, Bellucci, Xu, & Feng, 2020).

The mentalizing, or "theory of mind" network that includes the TPJ and dmPFC is shown in the left of Figure 6.2. The regions depicted are thought to be involved in social cognitive functions that include taking the perspective of another person to understand their intentions and beliefs. The right side shows the valuation network that includes the vSTR and vmPFC. This network has been implicated in subjective value computations and reward processing. The figure shows meta-analyses (association tests) obtained from https://neurosynth.org using the search terms "mentalizing" and "value."

6.4.1   Incidental Affect: Anxiety Suppresses Social Cognitive Neural Circuitry

While converging evidence points to the involvement of social cognitive and valuation processes during trust decisions, relatively little is known about the effects of emotions on the neural networks supporting trust decisions. The effects of anxiety on the neural circuitry involved in trust decisions was recently investigated in a functional magnetic resonance imaging (fMRI) study by Engelmann, Meyer, et al. (2019). The authors employed a one-shot TG in which participants made decisions in either a trust or matched nonsocial control game. Importantly, participants made these decisions in the context of incidental anxiety, which was induced using the ToS paradigm. At the behavioral level, the presence of ToS-induced anxiety led to a reduction in trust (Figure 6.1B), an observation that agrees with the behavioral results reviewed in Section 6.2.2 (Myers & Tingley, 2016).

Moreover, neuroimaging results showed that the left TPJ is specifically engaged during trust decisions, and this activation is suppressed by the presence of incidental anxiety. In addition, the researchers identified a "trust network" in which functional connectivity (FC) with the left TPJ correlated with transfers in the TG, but not in an equivalent nonsocial control game. This brain–behavior relationship reflects increased FC between the left TPJ and dmPFC, as well as the ventrolateral prefrontal cortex (vlPFC, extending into the anterior insula) with increasing trust levels. Importantly, the aversive emotion induced by the threat of shock significantly reduced the connectivity between the left TPJ and posterior STS, and this neural breakdown was associated with reduced trust at the behavioral level. The neural effects of anxiety therefore reflect a suppression of the activity and connectivity of social cognition regions, particularly the left TPJ, while participants were making trust decisions. Similar suppressions of choice-relevant brain regions have also been observed in the context of risky decision making, specifically in the vSTR and vmPFC (Engelmann et al., 2015). Moreover, social cognition regions have also been shown to be suppressed under conditions of stress, which is a natural consequence of anxiety (Nolte et al., 2013). Jointly, these results support the notion that the effects of anxiety play out at the neural level by suppressing specific neural circuitry that importantly supports decision-relevant cognitive processes (Engelmann & Hare, 2018).

A study by Kang et al. (2011) used temperature priming, that is, exposure to cold and warm packs, to induce feelings of (un)pleasantness immediately before participants played a TG. Behavioral results show that cold priming reduced investments in the TG relative to warm primes. A follow-up fMRI study by the same authors showed increased activity in the anterior insula during trust decisions in the cold (compared to warm) condition. The results suggest that enhanced insular activity after an unpleasant prime may be associated with reduced behavioral trust. The anterior insula is an interesting region that is relevant for trust decisions, as it has been implicated in multiple processes that support trust decisions, including negative affect and withdrawal motivation (Caria et al., 2010; Craig, 2009; Harlé et al., 2012; Wager & Barrett, 2017). It commonly activates during trust decisions as indicated by recent meta-analysis (Bellucci et al., 2017), potentially reflecting negative affect in anticipation and response to unfair offers (Sanfey et al., 2003; Tabibnia et al., 2008), which are likely triggered by deviations from expectations or social norms (Krueger et al., 2020). An additional possibility of anterior insula activation at the time of choice is that it might be involved in the anticipatory affective component of betrayal aversion (as opposed to the social cognitive component of mentalizing).

6.4.2 *Integral Affect: Betrayal Aversion Is Computed in the Anterior Insula*

As discussed above, betrayal aversion is associated with negative integral emotions at the time of choice (Engelmann & Fehr, 2017). Betrayal aversion has been directly investigated in an imaging context. Aimone et al. (2014) adopted their approach used in behavioral studies of betrayal aversion (Aimone & Houser, 2011, 2012; Bohnet et al., 2008; Houser et al., 2010), for use in the context of an fMRI experiment to investigate the neural correlates of betrayal aversion. Specifically, subjects made decisions about whether to trust or not to trust in the context of two binary TGs: (1) in the standard version, the trustor makes a binary decision between a fair option, in which each agent receives an equal payout, and an option that leads to clear advantages for the trustee, but losses for the trustor; (2) in the computer-mediated condition, which is similar to the risky DG of Bohnet and Zeckhauser (2004), a random mechanism (not the trustee) decides how much the trustor and trustee receive. Therefore, while payouts are matched across both conditions, the trustee can actively betray the trust of the trustor in the standard TG, but not in the computer-mediated condition. Behavioral results showed increased trust in the computer-mediated condition, mirroring the results of Bohnet and Zeckhauser (2004) and supporting the presence of betrayal aversion. Importantly, the anterior insula showed increased activation when participants made the decision to trust during the standard TG, but not when they made the same decision during the computer-mediated game, nor when they decided to play it safe by not trusting. Since betrayal is only possible when subjects decided to trust in the TG, but none of the other conditions, the increased insula signal during this condition supports the view that this region is involved in betrayal aversion.

In sum, while neuroimaging results on the affective processes of trust decisions are relatively sparse at the moment, there is a clear picture emerging from these studies. Both incidental and anticipatory negative affect are associated with trust-suppressive consequences at the time of choice, and this behavioral effect is paralleled by the suppression of social cognition regions at the neural level. Specifically, incidental anxiety was shown to suppress activity and connectivity within the social cognition network, consisting of the TPJ, STS, and dmPFC (Figure 6.2). Additionally, experiencing an unpleasant (relative to a pleasant) stimulation immediately before making trust decisions suppresses trust and enhances activity in the anterior insula during trust decisions. Given the involvement of the anterior insula in aversive affective processes related to social decisions (Lamm & Singer, 2010), it is likely that contextual and anticipatory affective signals from the anterior insula, and the amygdala (see Engelmann, Meyer, et al., 2019) are communicated to social cognition regions such as the TPJ, STS, and dmPFC. That the effect of negative affect on these regions is one of suppression makes much sense at the neural level: As the need to focus on immediate biological needs and safety increases under conditions of threat, the need to consider others in one's decision decreases and thereby the need to recruit social cognitive regions involved in mentalizing. In fact, participants should be more selfish when threatened (by external circumstances or the likelihood of betrayal) and perform safer actions to protect their interests. In the context of the TG this should be reflected by decreased social risk taking and reduced considerations of the benefit of one's actions for others. This conjecture, however, needs to be confirmed by future studies investigating how affective and cognitive components are integrated via the activity and connectivity patterns of affective and social cognitive neural circuits.

6.5   Conclusions, Future Directions, and Open Questions

The evidence we reviewed strongly suggests that both incidental and integral emotions can influence decisions to trust and, at the same time, decision-relevant neural circuitry. Importantly, this largely occurs in a manner that is consistent with the action tendencies associated with specific emotions (Engelmann & Hare, 2018). On the one hand, anxiety (and the related emotion of fear) serves the function of initiating behaviors that protect the organism and in many cases are related to defensive behaviors such as withdrawal from threatening situations (Mulckhuyse et al., 2017). Situations that trigger withdrawal, such as ToS, therefore lead to reductions in trust. On the other hand, happiness is an approach-related emotion that can promote optimism (e.g., Lyubomirsky et al., 2005) and generally leads to increased trust in game-theoretical settings. Interestingly, the effects of negative incidental and integral affect have recently been investigated at the neural level, with anxiety suppressing social cognitive neural circuitry that supports trust decisions, such as the TPJ, STS, and dmPFC, while unpleasant experiences preceding decisions, as well as the possibility of betrayal, enhanced activity in a region associated with negative affect, the anterior insula.

An open avenue of research on trust and emotions concerns the role played by past negative and positive experiences with other people. How we learn in social contexts, how our experiences are generalized to novel contexts, and what role emotions play in social learning are important aspects of trust behavior that need to be investigated by future studies. Real-life interactions with other people are typically repeated and differ from the one-shot, anonymous interactions commonly used in laboratory experiments (Engelmann, 2010). Despite its importance for the generalizability of the research on trust and emotions, this aspect of trust behavior remains to be assessed in depth. Promising first steps in this direction have been taken in a study conducted by FeldmanHall et al. (2018), in which subjects played an iterative TG against three partners exhibiting a high, neutral, or low level of trustworthiness. Once they learned who can and can't be trusted in part 1 of the study, subjects faced new players that had a certain resemblance with the previous players in part 2. In this second part of the game, participants picked their new interaction partners from a list of new players that had different levels of similarity with the players from part 1 that subjects had interacted with. The goal of this study was to investigate how perceptual similarity between known individuals and unfamiliar strangers shapes social learning. In part 2 of the study, subjects preferred to play with strangers that resembled the highly trustworthy players from the first part and refused to play with strangers that resembled the untrustworthy known players. Additionally, these behavioral tuning profiles were asymmetrically applied, in the sense that individuals were distrusted more when they presented a minimal resemblance with the untrustworthy players from the first game. At the neural level, during the second part of the game, amygdala activation was found to track the levels of resemblance with the untrustworthy types. Given that the amygdala is commonly associated with negative affect (Lindquist et al., 2012) and, at the same time, trustworthiness judgments (Winston et al., 2002), such results suggest that affective processes might play a role in learning about the trustworthiness of interaction partners.

While negative experiences with interaction partners and their generalization are reflected in the amygdala, positive experiences have been shown to be tracked by the vmPFC (Bellucci et al., 2019). This recent experiment commenced in two stages: While in the scanner, participants played the take advice game (TAG), in which they chose one of two cards that faced upside down. Importantly, participants had no information about the cards, but were paid for selecting the card with a higher numeric value, providing a 50% chance of winning. Advisers were able to improve those odds by providing information about one of the two cards that could either be correct (honest advice), or incorrect (dishonest advice). Importantly, participants could identify the intentions of the advisors when given feedback about their choices. After scanning, participants played a TG with the honest and dishonest advisors. Results indicate that advisors that proved to be trustworthy during the TAG game were trusted more in the subsequent TG. Multivariate analyses of the fMRI responses during the TAG game identified that honesty was represented in a network consisting of the vmPFC, dorsolateral PFC, intraparietal sulcus, and posterior cingulate cortex. Moreover, FC strength between the vmPFC and TPJ was positively and significantly associated with trust in the subsequent TG. Jointly, results from Bellucci et al. (2019) and FeldmanHall et al. (2018) implicate both affective (learning from betrayal) and cognitive (e.g., learning and generalization to novel contexts) processes in learning about the trustworthiness of others. Future research is needed to more clearly identify the interactions between affective and cognitive processes during trust decisions and learning whom to trust.

Finally, recent research in the field of psychiatry has begun investigating social interactions in chronic mood disorders such as depression, anxiety, and borderline personality disorder (see also Chapters 16 and 17). Such investigations enable observation of the effects of chronic changes of affective states on social decision making and related neural circuitry. Indeed, perturbed social decision making and difficulties maintaining functioning social relationships is frequently reported in mood disorders (Hirschfeld et al., 2000) and can be particularly distressing to patients. Investigating how subjects affected by mood disorders that experience chronic and relatively intense distortions of specific emotions and how these disturbances affect trusting behavior could provide a better understanding of the neural basis of the role of emotions in complex social interactions. Borderline personality disorder (BPD) patients, for instance, have been shown to report lower trustworthiness in faces of interaction partners than normal controls (Fertuck et al., 2018). Interestingly, rejection sensitivity mediates the relationship between mistrust and increased BPD symptoms, which agrees with core symptoms of BPD, including mistrustful, negative representations of the self and others (Hallquist & Pilkonis, 2012).

At the neural level, BPD patients have been shown to exhibit abnormal anterior insula activity during repeated TGs in which they were not able to maintain trust (King-Casas et al., 2008). Abnormal responses in the anterior insula were observed in BPD patients: While the anterior insula in healthy control subjects clearly tracked level of cooperation (with greater responses seen when norms were violated), this was not the case in BPD patients. Mood disorders have also been associated with abnormal neural responses during social interactions including the TG and UG. In an earlier study (Sripada et al., 2009), patients with social anxiety disorder showed decreased activation in the medial PFC during trust decisions compared to healthy controls. A study by Gradin et al. (2015) showed that, while healthy control participants showed increased responses in the vSTR as the fairness of proposers' offers increased, such fairness tracking was absent in depressed patients. Jointly, these results indicate that important choice-relevant and social cognitive brain regions show abnormal activation patterns in patients experiencing chronic distortions of emotions. This lends further support to the above conclusions that core neural circuitry involved in trust decisions, including valuation regions in the vSTR and vmPFC, as well as social cognition regions such as the dmPFC, and affective regions such as the anterior insula, are intimately involved in integrating emotion and cognition during trust decisions.

References

Aimone, J., Ball, S., & King-Casas, B. (2015). The betrayal aversion elicitation task: An individual level betrayal aversion measure. *PLoS ONE*, 10(9), Article e0137491. https://doi.org/10.1371/journal.pone.0137491

Aimone, J. A., & Houser, D. (2011). Beneficial betrayal aversion. *PLoS ONE*, 6 (3), Article e17725. https://doi.org/10.1371/journal.pone.0017725

(2012). What you don't know won't hurt you: A laboratory analysis of betrayal aversion. *Experimental Economics*, 15(4), 571–588. https://doi.org/10.2139/ssrn.1589146

Aimone, J. A., Houser, D., & Weber, B. (2014). Neural signatures of betrayal aversion: An fMRI study of trust. *Proceedings of the Royal Society B: Biological Sciences*, 281(1782), 20132127. https://doi.org/10.1098/rspb.2013.2127

Alguacil, S., Tudela, P., & Ruz, M. (2015). Ignoring facial emotion expressions does not eliminate their influence on cooperation decisions. *Psicológica*, 36 (2), 309–335. www.redalyc.org/articulo.oa?id=16941182006

Alós-Ferrer, C., & Farolfi, F. (2019). Trust games and beyond. *Frontiers in Neuroscience*, 13(887), 1–14. https://doi.org/10.3389/fnins.2019.00887

Andrade, E. B., & Ho, T.-H. (2007). How is the boss's mood today? I want a raise. *Psychological Science*, 18(8), 668–671. https://doi.org/10.1111/j.1467-9280.2007.01956.x

Andreoni, J. (1995). Warm-glow versus cold-prickle: The effects of positive and negative framing on cooperation in experiments. *The Quarterly Journal of Economics*, 110(1), 1–21. https://doi.org/10.2307/2118508

Bechara, A., & Martin, E. M. (2004). Impaired decision making related to working memory deficits in individuals with substance addictions. *Neuropsychology*, 18(1), 152–162. https://doi.org/10.1037/0894-4105.18.1.152

Bellucci, G., Chernyak, S. V., Goodyear, K., Eickhoff, S. B., & Krueger, F. (2017). Neural signatures of trust in reciprocity: A coordinate-based meta-analysis. *Human Brain Mapping*, 38(3), 1233–1248. https://doi.org/10.1002/hbm.23451

Bellucci, G., Feng, C., Camilleri, J., Eickhoff, S. B., & Krueger, F. (2018). The role of the anterior insula in social norm compliance and enforcement: Evidence from coordinate-based and functional connectivity meta-analyses. *Neuroscience & Biobehavioral Reviews*, 92, 378–389. https://doi.org/10.1016/j.neubiorev.2018.06.024

Bellucci, G., Molter, F., & Park, S. Q. (2019). Neural representations of honesty predict future trust behavior. *Nature Communications*, 10(1), 1–12. https://doi.org/10.1038/s41467-019-13261-8

Berg, J., Dickhaut, J., & McCabe, K. (1995). Trust, reciprocity, and social history. *Games and Economic Behavior*, 10(1), 122–142. https://doi.org/10.1006/game.1995.1027

Bohnet, I., Greig, F., Herrmann, B., & Zeckhauser, R. (2008). Betrayal aversion: Evidence from Brazil, China, Oman, Switzerland, Turkey, and the United States. *American Economic Review*, 98(1), 294–310. https://doi.org/10.1257/aer.98.1.294

Bohnet, I., & Zeckhauser, R. (2004). Trust, risk and betrayal. *Journal of Economic Behavior & Organization*, 55(4), 467–484. https://doi.org/10.2139/ssrn.478424

Bonnefon, J.-F., Hopfensitz, A., & De Neys, W. (2017). Can we detect cooperators by looking at their face? *Current Directions in Psychological Science*, 26 (3), 276–281. https://doi.org/10.1177/0963721417693352

Camerer, C. F. (2003). *Behavioral game theory: Experiments in strategic interaction*. Princeton University Press.

Campellone, T. R., & Kring, A. M. (2013). Who do you trust? The impact of facial emotion and behaviour on decision making. *Cognition & Emotion*, 27 (4), 603–620. https://doi.org/10.1080/02699931.2012.726608

Capra, M. C. (2004). Mood-driven behavior in strategic interactions. *American Economic Review*, 94(2), 367–372. https://doi.org/10.1257/0002828041301885

Caria, A., Sitaram, R., Veit, R., Begliomini, C., & Birbaumer, N. (2010). Volitional control of anterior insula activity modulates the response to aversive stimuli: A real-time functional magnetic resonance imaging study. *Biological Psychiatry*, 68(5), 425–432. https://doi.org/10.1016/j.biopsych.2010.04.020

Charness, G., Du, N., & Yang, C.-L. (2011). Trust and trustworthiness reputations in an investment game. *Games and Economic Behavior*, 72(2), 361–375. https://doi.org/10.1016/j.geb.2010.09.002

Chen, M., & Bargh, J. A. (1999). Consequences of automatic evaluation: Immediate behavioral predispositions to approach or avoid the stimulus. *Personality and Social Psychology Bulletin*, 25(2), 215–224. https://doi.org/10.1177/0146167299025002007

Cohn, A., Engelmann, J., Fehr, E., & Maréchal, M. A. (2015). Evidence for countercyclical risk aversion: An experiment with financial professionals. *American Economic Review*, 105(2), 860–885. https://doi.org/10.1257/aer.20131314

Craig, A. (2009). Emotional moments across time: A possible neural basis for time perception in the anterior insula. *Philosophical Transactions of the Royal Society B: Biological Sciences*, 364(1525), 1933–1942. https://doi.org/10.1098/rstb.2009.0008

Cutler, J., & Campbell-Meiklejohn, D. (2019). A comparative fMRI meta-analysis of altruistic and strategic decisions to give. *NeuroImage*, 184, 227–241. https://doi.org/10.1016/j.neuroimage.2018.09.009

De Hooge, I. E., Nelissen, R., Breugelmans, S. M., & Zeelenberg, M. (2011). What is moral about guilt? Acting "prosocially" at the disadvantage of others. *Journal of Personality and Social Psychology*, 100(3), 462–473. https://doi.org/10.1037/a0021459

De Neys, W., Hopfensitz, A., & Bonnefon, J.-F. (2017). Split-second trustworthiness detection from faces in an economic game. *Experimental Psychology*, 64(4), 231–239. https://doi.org/10.1027/1618-3169/a000367

DeBruine, L. M. (2002). Facial resemblance enhances trust. *Proceedings of the Royal Society B: Biological Sciences*, 269(1498), 1307–1312. https://doi.org/10.1098/rspb.2002.2034

Delgado, M. R., Frank, R. H., & Phelps, E. A. (2005). Perceptions of moral character modulate the neural systems of reward during the trust game. *Nature Neuroscience*, 8(11), 1611–1618. https://doi.org/10.1038/nn1575

Desmet, P. T., De Cremer, D., & Van Dijk, E. (2011). In money we trust? The use of financial compensations to repair trust in the aftermath of distributive harm. *Organizational Behavior and Human Decision Processes*, 114(2), 75–86. https://doi.org/10.1016/j.obhdp.2010.10.006

Dunn, J. R., & Schweitzer, M. E. (2005). Feeling and believing: The influence of emotion on trust. *Journal of Personality and Social Psychology*, 88(5), 736–748. https://doi.org/10.1037/0022-3514.88.5.736

Dunning, D., Fetchenhauer, D., & Schlösser, T. (2012). Trust as a social and emotional act: Noneconomic considerations in trust behavior. *Journal of Economic Psychology*, 33(3), 686–694. https://doi.org/10.1016/j.joep.2011.09.005

(2017). The varying roles played by emotion in economic decision making. *Current Opinion in Behavioral Sciences*, 15, 33–38. https://doi.org/10.1016/j.cobeha.2017.05.006

Eckel, C. C., & Wilson, R. K. (2003). The human face of game theory. In E. Ostrom & J. M. Walker (Eds.), *Trust and reciprocity: Interdisciplinary lessons from experimental research* (pp. 245–274). Russell Sage Foundation.

Efferson, C., & Vogt, S. (2013). Viewing men's faces does not lead to accurate predictions of trustworthiness. *Scientific Reports*, 3, Article 1047. https://doi.org/10.1038/srep01047

Eimontaite, I., Nicolle, A., Schindler, I. C., & Goel, V. (2013). The effect of partner-directed emotion in social exchange decision making. *Frontiers in Psychology*, 4(469), 1–11. https://doi.org/10.3389/fpsyg.2013.00469

Ekman, P., & Friesen, W. V. (2003). *Unmasking the face: A guide to recognizing emotions from facial clues*. Malor Books.

Engell, A. D., Haxby, J. V., & Todorov, A. (2007). Implicit trustworthiness decisions: Automatic coding of face properties in the human amygdala. *Journal of Cognitive Neuroscience*, 19(9), 1508–1519. https://doi.org/10.1162/jocn.2007.19.9.1508

Engelmann, J. B. (2010). Measuring trust in social neuroeconomics: A tutorial. *Hermeneutische Blätter*, 1(2), 225–242.

Engelmann, J. B., & Fehr, E. (2017). The neurobiology of trust and social decision: The important role of emotions. In P. A. M. Van Lange, B. Rockenbach, & T. Yamagishi (Eds.), *Trust in social dilemmas* (pp. 33–56). Oxford University Press.

Engelmann, J. B., & Hare, T. A. (2018). Emotions can bias decision making processes by promoting specific behavior. In A. S. Fox, R. C. Lapate, A. J. Shackman, & R. J. Davidson (Eds.), *The nature of emotion: Fundamental questions* (2nd ed., pp. 355–370). Oxford University Press.

Engelmann, J. B., Meyer, F., Fehr, E., & Ruff, C. C. (2015). Anticipatory anxiety disrupts neural valuation during risky choice. *Journal of Neuroscience*, 35(7), 3085–3099. https://doi.org/10.1523/jneurosci.2880-14.2015

Engelmann, J. B., Meyer, F., Ruff, C. C., & Fehr, E. (2019). The neural circuitry of affect-induced distortions of trust. *Science Advances*, 5(3), Article eaau3413. https://doi.org/10.1126/sciadv.aau3413

Engelmann, J. B., Schmid, B., De Dreu, C. K., Chumbley, J., & Fehr, E. (2019). On the psychology and economics of antisocial personality. *Proceedings of the National Academy of Sciences*, 116(26), 12781–12786. https://doi.org/10.1073/pnas.1820133116

Fehr, E. (2009). On the economics and biology of trust. *Journal of the European Economic Association*, 7(2–3), 235–266. https://doi.org/10.1162/JEEA.2009.7.2-3.235

Fehr, E., Fischbacher, U., & Kosfeld, M. (2005). Neuroeconomic foundations of trust and social preferences: Initial evidence. *American Economic Review*, 95(2), 346–351. https://doi.org/10.1257/000282805774669736

Fehr, E., & Gächter, S. (2000). Cooperation and punishment in public goods experiments. *American Economic Review*, 90(4), 980–994. http://doi.org/10.1257/aer.90.4.980

FeldmanHall, O., Dunsmoor, J. E., Tompary, A., Hunter, L. E., Todorov, A., & Phelps, E. A. (2018). Stimulus generalization as a mechanism for learning to trust. *Proceedings of the National Academy of Sciences*, 115(7), E1690–E1697. https://doi.org/10.1073/pnas.1715227115

Ferrer, R. A., Grenen, E. G., & Taber, J. M. (2015). Effectiveness of internet-based affect induction procedures: A systematic review and meta-analysis. *Emotion*, 15(6), 752–762. https://doi.org/10.1037/emo0000035

Fertuck, E. A., Fischer, S., & Beeney, J. (2018). Social cognition and borderline personality disorder: Splitting and trust impairment findings. *Psychiatric Clinics*, 41(4), 613–632. https://doi.org/10.1016/j.psc.2018.07.003

Fetchenhauer, D., & Dunning, D. (2012). Betrayal aversion versus principled trustfulness: How to explain risk avoidance and risky choices in trust games. *Journal of Economic Behavior & Organization*, 81(2), 534–541. https://doi.org/10.1016/j.jebo.2011.07.017

Forgas, J. P. (1995). Mood and judgment: The affect infusion model (AIM). *Psychological Bulletin*, 117(1), 39–66. https://doi.org/10.1037/0033-2909.117.1.39

Franzen, N., Hagenhoff, M., Baer, N., et al. (2011). Superior "theory of mind" in borderline personality disorder: An analysis of interaction behavior in a virtual trust game. *Psychiatry Research*, 187(1–2), 224–233. https://doi.org/10.1016/j.psychres.2010.11.012

Fredrickson, B. L., Tugade, M. M., Waugh, C. E., & Larkin, G. R. (2003). What good are positive emotions in crisis? A prospective study of resilience and emotions following the terrorist attacks on the United States on September 11th, 2001. *Journal of Personality and Social Psychology*, 84(2), 365–376. https://doi.org/10.1037/0022-3514.84.2.365

Gerrards-Hesse, A., Spies, K., & Hesse, F. W. (1994). Experimental inductions of emotional states and their effectiveness: A review. *British Journal of Psychology*, 85(1), 55–78. https://doi.org/10.1111/j.2044-8295.1994.tb02508.x

Göritz, A. S., & Moser, K. (2006). Web-based mood induction. *Cognition and Emotion*, 20(6), 887–896. https://doi.org/10.1080/02699930500405386

Gradin, V., Pérez, A., MacFarlane, J., et al. (2015). Abnormal brain responses to social fairness in depression: An fMRI study using the Ultimatum Game. *Psychological Medicine*, 45(6), 1241–1251. https://doi.org/10.1017/s0033291714002347

Gromann, P. M., Heslenfeld, D. J., Fett, A.-K., Joyce, D. W., Shergill, S. S., & Krabbendam, L. (2013). Trust versus paranoia: Abnormal response to social reward in psychotic illness. *Brain*, 136(6), 1968–1975. https://doi.org/10.1093/brain/awt076

Güth, W., Schmittberger, R., & Schwarze, B. (1982). An experimental analysis of ultimatum bargaining. *Journal of Economic Behavior & Organization*, 3(4), 367–388. https://doi.org/10.1016/0167-2681(82)90011-7

Hallquist, M. N., & Pilkonis, P. A. (2012). Refining the phenotype of borderline personality disorder: Diagnostic criteria and beyond. *Personality Disorders: Theory, Research, and Treatment*, 3(3), 228–246. https://doi.org/10.1037/a0027953

Hare, T. A., Malmaud, J., & Rangel, A. (2011). Focusing attention on the health aspects of foods changes value signals in vmPFC and improves dietary choice. *Journal of Neuroscience*, 31(30), 11077–11087. https://doi.org/10.1523/jneurosci.6383-10.2011

Harlé, K. M., Chang, L. J., van't Wout, M., & Sanfey, A. G. (2012). The neural mechanisms of affect infusion in social economic decision making: A mediating role of the anterior insula. *NeuroImage*, 61(1), 32–40. https://doi.org/10.1016/j.neuroimage.2012.02.027

Hellhammer, D. H., Wüst, S., & Kudielka, B. M. (2009). Salivary cortisol as a biomarker in stress research. *Psychoneuroendocrinology*, 34(2), 163–171. https://doi.org/10.1016/j.psyneuen.2008.10.026

Hertel, G., Neuhof, J., Theuer, T., & Kerr, N. L. (2000). Mood effects on cooperation in small groups: Does positive mood simply lead to more cooperation? *Cognition & Emotion*, 14(4), 441–472. https://doi.org/10.1080/026999300402754

Hinson, J. M., Jameson, T. L., & Whitney, P. (2003). Impulsive decision making and working memory. *Journal of Experimental Psychology: Learning, Memory, and Cognition*, 29(2), 298–306. https://doi.org/10.1037/0278-7393.29.2.298

Hirschfeld, R., Montgomery, S. A., Keller, M. B., et al. (2000). Social functioning in depression: A review. *The Journal of Clinical Psychiatry*, 61(4), 268–275. https://doi.org/10.4088/JCP.v61n0405

Houser, D., Schunk, D., & Winter, J. (2010). Distinguishing trust from risk: An anatomy of the investment game. *Journal of Economic Behavior & Organization*, 74(1–2), 72–81. https://doi.org/10.1016/j.jebo.2010.01.002

Isaac, R. M., & Walker, J. M. (1988). Group size effects in public goods provision: The voluntary contributions mechanism. *The Quarterly Journal of Economics*, 103(1), 179–199. https://doi.org/10.2307/1882648

Jaeger, B., Evans, A. M., Stel, M., & Van Beest, I. (2019). Explaining the persistent influence of facial cues in social decision making. *Journal of Experimental Psychology: General*, 148(6), 1008–1021. https://doi.org/10.1037/xge0000591

Jaeger, B., Oud, B., Williams, T., Krumhuber, E. G., Fehr, E., & Engelmann, J. B. (2020). Trustworthiness detection from faces: Does reliance on facial impressions pay off? *PsyArXiv preprint*. https://doi.org/10.31234/osf.io/ayqeh

Johnson, N. D., & Mislin, A. A. (2011). Trust games: A meta-analysis. *Journal of Economic Psychology*, 32(5), 865–889. https://doi.org/10.1016/j.joep.2011.05.007

Kahneman, D., Knetsch, J. L., & Thaler, R. H. (1986). Fairness and the assumptions of economics. *Journal of Business*, 59(4), S285–S300. https://doi.org/10.1086/296367

Kang, Y., Williams, L. E., Clark, M. S., Gray, J. R., & Bargh, J. A. (2011). Physical temperature effects on trust behavior: The role of insula. *Social Cognitive and Affective Neuroscience*, 6(4), 507–515. https://doi.org/10.1093/scan/nsq077

Kausel, E. E., & Connolly, T. (2014). Do people have accurate beliefs about the behavioral consequences of incidental emotions? Evidence from trust games. *Journal of Economic Psychology*, 42, 96–111. https://doi.org/10.1016/j.joep.2014.02.002

Kenealy, P. (1988). Validation of a music mood induction procedure: Some preliminary findings. *Cognition & Emotion*, 2(1), 41–48. https://doi.org/10.1080/02699938808415228

King-Casas, B., Sharp, C., Lomax-Bream, L., Lohrenz, T., Fonagy, P., & Montague, P. R. (2008). The rupture and repair of cooperation in borderline personality disorder. *Science*, 321(5890), 806–810. https://doi.org/10.1126/science.1156902

Kirchsteiger, G., Rigotti, L., & Rustichini, A. (2006). Your morals might be your moods. *Journal of Economic Behavior & Organization*, 59(2), 155–172. https://doi.org/10.1016/j.jebo.2004.07.004

Klapper, A., Dotsch, R., Van Rooij, I., & Wigboldus, D. H. (2016). Do we spontaneously form stable trustworthiness impressions from facial appearance? *Journal of Personality and Social Psychology*, 111(5), 655–664. https://doi.org/10.1037/pspa0000062

Krueger, F., Bellucci, G., Xu, P., & Feng, C. (2020). The critical role of the right dorsal and ventral anterior insula in reciprocity: Evidence from the trust and ultimatum games. *Frontiers in Human Neuroscience*, 14(176), 1–6. https://doi.org/10.3389/fnhum.2020.00176

Krueger, F., Grafman, J., & McCabe, K. (2008). Neural correlates of economic game playing. *Philosophical Transactions of the Royal Society B: Biological Sciences*, 363(1511), 3859–3874. https://doi.org/10.1098/rstb.2008.0165

Krumhuber, E., Manstead, A. S., Cosker, D., Marshall, D., Rosin, P. L., & Kappas, A. (2007). Facial dynamics as indicators of trustworthiness and

cooperative behavior. *Emotion*, 7(4), 730–735. https://doi.org/10.1037/
1528-3542.7.4.730

Kugler, T., Ye, B., Motro, D., & Noussair, C. N. (2020). On trust and disgust:
Evidence from face reading and virtual reality. *Social Psychological and
Personality Science*, 11(3), 317–325. https://doi.org/10.1177/
1948550619856302

Lamm, C., & Singer, T. (2010). The role of anterior insular cortex in social
emotions. *Brain Structure and Function*, 214(5–6), 579–591. https://doi.org/
10.1007/s00429–010-0251-3

Lench, H. C., Flores, S. A., & Bench, S. W. (2011). Discrete emotions predict
changes in cognition, judgment, experience, behavior, and physiology:
A meta-analysis of experimental emotion elicitations. *Psychological Bulletin*,
137(5), 834–855. https://doi.org/10.1037/a0024244

Lerner, J. S., & Keltner, D. (2000). Beyond valence: Toward a model of emotion-
specific influences on judgement and choice. *Cognition & Emotion*, 14(4),
473–493. https://doi.org/10.1080/026999300402763

Lerner, J. S., Li, Y., Valdesolo, P., & Kassam, K. S. (2015). Emotion and decision
making. *Annual Review of Psychology*, 66(1), 799–823. https://doi.org/10
.1146/annurev-psych-010213-115043

Lim, S.-L., O'Doherty, J. P., & Rangel, A. (2011). The decision value computations in the vmPFC and striatum use a relative value code that is guided by
visual attention. *Journal of Neuroscience*, 31(37), 13214–13223. https://doi
.org/10.1523/jneurosci.1246-11.2011

Lindquist, K. A., Wager, T. D., Kober, H., Bliss-Moreau, E., & Barrett, L. F.
(2012). The brain basis of emotion: A meta-analytic review. *The Behavioral
and Brain Sciences*, 35(3), 121–143. https://doi.org/10.1017/
s0140525x11000446

Loewenstein, G., & Lerner, J. S. (2003). The role of affect in decision making. In
R. J. Davidson, K. R. Scherer, & H. H. Goldsmith (Eds.), *Handbook of
affective science* (pp. 619–642). Oxford University Press.

Loewenstein, G. F., Weber, E. U., Hsee, C. K., & Welch, N. (2001). Risk as
feelings. *Psychological Bulletin*, 127(2), 267–286. https://doi.org/10.1037/
0033-2909.127.2.267

Loomes, G., & Sugden, R. (1982). Regret theory: An alternative theory of
rational choice under uncertainty. *The Economic Journal*, 92(368),
805–824. https://doi.org/10.2307/2232669

(1986). Disappointment and dynamic consistency in choice under uncertainty. *The
Review of Economic Studies*, 53(2), 271–282. https://doi.org/10.2307/2297651

Lyubomirsky, S., King, L., & Diener, E. (2005). The benefits of frequent positive
affect: Does happiness lead to success? *Psychological Bulletin*, 131(6),
803–855. https://doi.org/10.1037/0033-2909.131.6.803

Maccallum, F., McConkey, K. M., Bryant, R. A., & Barnier, A. J. (2000).
Specific autobiographical memory following hypnotically induced mood
state. *International Journal of Clinical and Experimental Hypnosis*, 48(4),
361–373. https://doi.org/10.1080/00207140008410366

Martinez, L. F., & Zeelenberg, M. (2015). Trust me (or not): Regret and disappointment in experimental economic games. *Decision*, 2(2), 118–126. https://doi.org/10.1037/dec0000025

McCabe, K., Houser, D., Ryan, L., Smith, V., & Trouard, T. (2001). A functional imaging study of cooperation in two-person reciprocal exchange. *Proceedings of the National Academy of Sciences*, 98(20), 11832–11835. https://doi.org/10.1073/pnas.211415698

Mellers, B. A., Haselhuhn, M. P., Tetlock, P. E., Silva, J. C., & Isen, A. M. (2010). Predicting behavior in economic games by looking through the eyes of the players. *Journal of Experimental Psychology: General*, 139(4), 743–755. https://doi.org/10.1037/a0020280

Mellers, B. A., Schwartz, A., Ho, K., & Ritov, I. (1997). Decision affect theory: Emotional reactions to the outcomes of risky options. *Psychological Science*, 8(6), 423–429. https://doi.org/10.1111/j.1467-9280.1997.tb00455.x

Mislin, A., Williams, L. V., & Shaughnessy, B. A. (2015). Motivating trust: Can mood and incentives increase interpersonal trust? *Journal of Behavioral and Experimental Economics*, 58, 11–19. https://doi.org/10.1016/j.socec.2015.06.001

Mulckhuyse, M., Crombez, G., & Van der Stigchel, S. (2013). Conditioned fear modulates visual selection. *Emotion*, 13(3), 529–536. https://doi.org/10.1037/a0031076

Mulckhuyse, M., Engelmann, J. B., Schutter, D. J., & Roelofs, K. (2017). Right posterior parietal cortex is involved in disengaging from threat: A 1-Hz rTMS study. *Social Cognitive and Affective Neuroscience*, 12(11), 1814–1822. https://doi.org/10.1093/scan/nsx111

Myers, C. D., & Tingley, D. (2016). The influence of emotion on trust. *Political Analysis*, 24(4), 492–500. https://doi.org/10.1093/pan/mpw026

Nelissen, R. M., Dijker, A. J., & deVries, N. K. (2007). How to turn a hawk into a dove and vice versa: Interactions between emotions and goals in a give-some dilemma game. *Journal of Experimental Social Psychology*, 43(2), 280–286. https://doi.org/10.1016/j.jesp.2006.01.009

Niv, Y., Edlund, J. A., Dayan, P., & O'Doherty, J. P. (2012). Neural prediction errors reveal a risk-sensitive reinforcement-learning process in the human brain. *Journal of Neuroscience*, 32(2), 551–562. https://doi.org/10.1523/jneurosci.5498-10.2012

Nolte, T., Bolling, D. Z., Hudac, C., Fonagy, P., Mayes, L. C., & Pelphrey, K. A. (2013). Brain mechanisms underlying the impact of attachment-related stress on social cognition. *Frontiers in Human Neuroscience*, 7(816), 1–12. https://doi.org/10.3389/fnhum.2013.00816

Pessoa, L. (2008). On the relationship between emotion and cognition. *Nature Reviews Neuroscience*, 9(2), 148–158. https://doi.org/10.1038/nrn2317

Pham, M. T. (2007). Emotion and rationality: A critical review and interpretation of empirical evidence. *Review of General Psychology*, 11(2), 155–178. https://doi.org/10.1037/1089-2680.11.2.155

Phelps, E. A., Lempert, K. M., & Sokol-Hessner, P. (2014). Emotion and decision making: Multiple modulatory neural circuits. *Annual Review of Neuroscience*, 37(1), 263–287. https://doi.org/10.1146/annurev-neuro-071013-014119

Prochazkova, E., Prochazkova, L., Giffin, M. R., Scholte, H. S., De Dreu, C. K., & Kret, M. E. (2018). Pupil mimicry promotes trust through the theory-of-mind network. *Proceedings of the National Academy of Sciences*, 115(31), E7265–E7274. https://doi.org/10.1073/pnas.1803916115

Quercia, S. (2016). Eliciting and measuring betrayal aversion using the BDM mechanism. *Journal of the Economic Science Association*, 2(1), 48–59. https://doi.org/10.1007/s40881-015-0021-3

Rabin, M. (1993). Incorporating fairness into game theory and economics. *The American Economic Review*, 83(5), 1281–1302. www.jstor.org/stable/2117561?seq=1#metadata_info_tab_contents

Rangel, A., Camerer, C., & Montague, P. R. (2008). A framework for studying the neurobiology of value-based decision making. *Nature Reviews Neuroscience*, 9(7), 545–556. https://doi.org/10.1038/nrn2357

Rangel, A., & Hare, T. (2010). Neural computations associated with goal-directed choice. *Current Opinion in Neurobiology*, 20(2), 262–270. https://doi.org/10.1016/j.conb.2010.03.001

Rick, S., & Loewenstein, G. (2008). The role of emotion in economic behavior. In M. Lewis, J. M. Haviland-Jones, & L. F. Barrett (Eds.), *Handbook of emotions* (3rd ed.; pp. 138–158). The Guilford Press.

Rilling, J. K., Sanfey, A. G., Aronson, J. A., Nystrom, L. E., & Cohen, J. D. (2004). The neural correlates of theory of mind within interpersonal interactions. *NeuroImage*, 22(4), 1694–1703. https://doi.org/10.1016/j.neuroimage.2004.04.015

Roelofs, K. (2017). Freeze for action: Neurobiological mechanisms in animal and human freezing. *Philosophical Transactions of the Royal Society B: Biological Sciences*, 372(1718), 20160206. https://doi.org/10.1098/rstb.2016.0206

Roelofs, K., Putman, P., Schouten, S., Lange, W.-G., Volman, I., & Rinck, M. (2010). Gaze direction differentially affects avoidance tendencies to happy and angry faces in socially anxious individuals. *Behaviour Research and Therapy*, 48(4), 290–294. https://doi.org/10.1016/j.brat.2009.11.008

Ruff, C. C., & Fehr, E. (2014). The neurobiology of rewards and values in social decision making. *Nature Reviews Neuroscience*, 15(8), 549–562. https://doi.org/10.1038/nrn3776

Saadaoui, H., El Harbi, S., & Ibanez, L. (2019). Do people trust more when they are happy or when they are sad? Evidence from an experiment. *Managerial and Decision Economics*, 40(4), 374–383. https://doi.org/10.1002/mde.3008

Sanfey, A. G. (2009). Expectations and social decision making: Biasing effects of prior knowledge on Ultimatum responses. *Mind & Society*, 8(1), 93–107. https://doi.org/10.1007/s11299-009-0053-6

Sanfey, A. G., Rilling, J. K., Aronson, J. A., Nystrom, L. E., & Cohen, J. D. (2003). The neural basis of economic decision making in the Ultimatum

Game. *Science*, 300(5626), 1755–1758. https://doi.org/10.1126/science
.1082976

Scharlemann, J. P., Eckel, C. C., Kacelnik, A., & Wilson, R. K. (2001). The value
of a smile: Game theory with a human face. *Journal of Economic Psychology*,
22(5), 617–640. https://doi.org/10.1016/s0167-4870(01)00059-9

Schlösser, T., Fetchenhauer, D., & Dunning, D. (2016). Trust against all odds?
Emotional dynamics in trust behavior. *Decision*, 3(3), 216–230. https://doi
.org/10.1037/dec0000048

Schmitz, A., & Grillon, C. (2012). Assessing fear and anxiety in humans using the
threat of predictable and unpredictable aversive events (the NPU-threat test).
Nature Protocols, 7(3), 527–532. https://doi.org/10.1038/nprot.2012.001

Schönberg, T., Daw, N. D., Joel, D., & O'Doherty, J. P. (2007). Reinforcement
learning signals in the human striatum distinguish learners from nonlearners
during reward-based decision making. *Journal of Neuroscience*, 27(47),
12860–12867. https://doi.org/10.1523/jneurosci.2496-07.2007

Schultz, W. (2002). Getting formal with dopamine and reward. *Neuron*, 36(2),
241–263. https://doi.org/10.1016/s0896-6273(02)00967-4

Schurz, M., Radua, J., Aichhorn, M., Richlan, F., & Perner, J. (2014).
Fractionating theory of mind: A meta-analysis of functional brain imaging
studies. *Neuroscience & Biobehavioral Reviews*, 42, 9–34. https://doi.org/10
.1016/j.neubiorev.2014.01.009

Schwarz, N. (1990). Feelings as information: Informational and motivational
functions of affective states. In T. E. Higgins & R. M. Sorrentino (Eds.),
Handbook of motivation and cognition: Foundations of social behavior (Vol. 1;
pp. 527–561). The Guilford Press.

Sripada, C. S., Angstadt, M., Banks, S., Nathan, P. J., Liberzon, I., & Phan, K. L.
(2009). Functional neuroimaging of mentalizing during the trust game in
social anxiety disorder. *Neuroreport*, 20(11), 984–989. https://doi.org/10
.1097/wnr.0b013e32832d0a67

Stanley, D. A., Sokol-Hessner, P., Fareri, D. S., et al. (2012). Race and reputation: Perceived racial group trustworthiness influences the neural correlates
of trust decisions. *Philosophical Transactions of the Royal Society B: Biological
Sciences*, 367(1589), 744–753. https://doi.org/10.1098/rstb.2011.0300

Tabibnia, G., Satpute, A. B., & Lieberman, M. D. (2008). The sunny side of
fairness: Preference for fairness activates reward circuitry (and disregarding
unfairness activates self-control circuitry). *Psychological Science*, 19(4),
339–347. https://doi.org/10.1111/j.1467-9280.2008.02091.x

Thielmann, I., & Hilbig, B. E. (2015). Trust: An integrative review from a
person–situation perspective. *Review of General Psychology*, 19(3), 249–277.
https://doi.org/10.1037/gpr0000046

Thielmann, I., Spadaro, G., & Balliet, D. (2020). Personality and prosocial
behavior: A theoretical framework and meta-analysis. *Psychological Bulletin*,
146(1), 30–39. https://doi.org/10.1037/bul0000217

Tognetti, A., Berticat, C., Raymond, M., & Faurie, C. (2013). Is cooperativeness
readable in static facial features? An inter-cultural approach. *Evolution and*

Human Behavior, 34(6), 427–432. https://doi.org/10.1016/j.evolhumbehav
.2013.08.002

Tortosa, M. I., Strizhko, T., Capizzi, M., & Ruz, M. (2013). Interpersonal effects
of emotion in a multi-round trust game. *Psicologica: International Journal of
Methodology and Experimental Psychology*, 34(2), 179–198.

Velten, J. E. (1968). A laboratory task for induction of mood states. *Behaviour
Research and Therapy*, 6(4), 473–482. https://doi.org/10.1016/0005-7967(
68)90028-4

Verplaetse, J., Vanneste, S., & Braeckman, J. (2007). You can judge a book by its
cover: The sequel. A kernel of truth in predictive cheating detection.
Evolution and Human Behavior, 28(4), 260–271. https://doi.org/10.1016/j
.evolhumbehav.2007.04.006

Wager, T. D., & Barrett, L. F. (2017). From affect to control: Functional
specialization of the insula in motivation and regulation. *BioRxiv*, Article
102368. https://doi.org/10.1101/102368

Waytz, A., & Mitchell, J. P. (2011). Two mechanisms for simulating other
minds: Dissociations between mirroring and self-projection. *Current
Directions in Psychological Science*, 20(3), 197–200. https://doi.org/10
.1177/0963721411409007

Wehebrink, K. S., Koelkebeck, K., Piest, S., de Dreu, C. K., & Kret, M. E.
(2018). Pupil mimicry and trust—implication for depression. *Journal of
Psychiatric Research*, 97, 70–76. https://doi.org/10.1016/j.jpsychires.2017
.11.007

Willis, J., & Todorov, A. (2006). First impressions: Making up your mind after a
100-ms exposure to a face. *Psychological Science*, 17(7), 592–598. https://doi
.org/10.1111/j.1467-9280.2006.01750.x

Winston, J. S., Strange, B. A., O'Doherty, J., & Dolan, R. J. (2002). Automatic
and intentional brain responses during evaluation of trustworthiness of faces.
Nature Neuroscience, 5(3), 277–283. https://doi.org/10.1038/nn816

Yiend, J. (2010). The effects of emotion on attention: A review of attentional
processing of emotional information. *Cognition and Emotion*, 24(1), 3–47.
https://doi.org/10.1080/02699930903205698

Trust and Reputation
How Knowledge about Others Shapes Our Decisions

*Emily G. Brudner, Alec J. Karousatos, Dominic S. Fareri,
and Mauricio R. Delgado*

7.1 Introduction

The ability to make adaptive trust decisions in a novel or familiar social environment is critical to avoiding harm, cooperating with others, and maintaining healthy social bonds. The reputation of a social partner – that is, the belief about or notoriety of a person's trait characteristics or general behavioral tendencies – is an important indicator that can be used to predict whether that social partner can be trusted in a given interaction. For example, when choosing a new physician, a patient may seek out information about the physician's reputation by simply looking at their photo online and making a snap judgment about how friendly or competent they seem. Or perhaps the patient may form an opinion based on a richer set of information by, for instance, examining the physician's credentials or reading reviews from other patients. If perceived as trustworthy from these initial impressions, the patient may learn more about the doctor's trustworthiness through direct interactions at her first visit and continue updating her beliefs about them as the relationship progresses, building a reputation and foundation of trust through this repeated social exchange.

In this chapter, we review fundamental and contemporary research on the neurobiological underpinnings of how trustworthiness reputations are developed and how they guide social decision making and behavior. We start by describing the basic neural processes involved in forming rapid, perceptual-based trustworthiness impressions when more comprehensive social information is unavailable. Next, we delve into the computational mechanisms that guide moment-to-moment reputation learning through direct experience and explore how reputational information from indirect

This work was supported by funding from the McKnight Foundation. Corresponding author: Mauricio R. Delgado (delgado@psychology.rutgers.edu).

sources interacts with these direct experiences to drive trust behavior. We then shift from reputations formed in novel social environments to those shaped by a wide array of social experiences and long-standing, established relationships. Finally, we discuss the broader implications of reputation-based trust behavior in real-world social settings and put forth avenues for future research to investigate how adverse environments impact reputation formation and trust decisions.

7.2   Forming Initial Trust Reputations through Perceptual Judgments and Contextual Cues

We often rely on prior information about others and past experiences with them to guide trust decisions. However, novel or unfamiliar social environments present a unique challenge where we have little to no prior information off of which to base trust reputations. In these situations, we may be susceptible to snap judgments, in which the brain relies on available perceptual and contextual information from the environment to form an initial impression of perceived trustworthiness. In this section, we review the extensive literature on how the brain forms rapid impressions of an individual's trustworthiness based on perceptual social cues and discuss how the context in which these cues are presented may or may not update initial impressions to guide trust behavior.

7.2.1   Forming Impressions of Trustworthiness from Facial Features

One of the most accessible sources of social information is the human face. Humans, like other social animals, are especially sensitive to and value social stimuli (Bhanji & Delgado, 2014; Gluckman & Johnson, 2013; Theeuwes & Van der Stigchel, 2006) and facial cues in particular provide a wealth of information that is used to establish initial impressions and guide trust decisions (Rezlescu et al., 2012; Todorov et al., 2015). For example, faces that are perceived as less trustworthy are interpreted as being angrier than perceived trustworthy faces (Oosterhof & Todorov, 2009) and are less likely to receive investments in a classic trust game (TG) paradigm (Krumhuber et al., 2007; Van't Wout & Sanfey, 2008). The tendency to form an impression of perceived trustworthiness from facial cues occurs as early as 33 milliseconds after initial face presentation (De Neys et al., 2017; Marzi et al., 2014; Todorov et al., 2009), is present early in childhood (Ewing et al., 2015), and parallels developmental trajectories of other socio-emotional processes through adolescence (Fett et al., 2014; Tashjian et al., 2019). Furthermore, perceptions of trustworthiness seem to be especially unique to human faces, as artificial (computer-generated) faces elicit lower and less consistent perceived trustworthiness judgments and are less memorable than human faces (Balas & Pacella, 2017). Thus, initial impressions formed from perceptual features of the human face can be thought of as one of the most powerful drivers of trust behavior in otherwise novel or impoverished social settings.

The amygdala, a subcortical structure in the medial temporal lobe, is highly sensitive to social and emotional cues from facial features (Adolphs & Spezio, 2006; Benuzzi et al., 2007; Todorov et al., 2008). In addition to being involved in a host of other social and emotional functions (see Adolphs, 2010 for review), it is thought to play an integral role in forming initial perceptions of trustworthiness and other face-based impressions, such as attractiveness (Bzdok et al., 2011; Freeman et al., 2014; Mende-Siedlecki, Said, & Todorov, 2013; Mende-Siedlecki, Verosky, et al., 2013; Santos et al., 2016; Todorov, 2012; Todorov et al., 2013). Functional neuroimaging paradigms presenting novel, decontextualized faces (i.e., without hair, clothing, information about the surrounding environment, etc.) have found that amygdala activity is strongest in response to faces that are subjectively rated as less trustworthy (Baron et al., 2011; Engell et al., 2007; Tashjian et al., 2019; Todorov et al., 2008; Winston et al., 2002) even when faces are presented subliminally (Freeman et al., 2014). Amygdala activation also seems to be nonlinearly related to group consensus of perceived trustworthiness, where faces that have high group consensus as being perceived as either trustworthy or untrustworthy elicit greater amygdala activity than faces that have low group consensus on perceived trustworthiness (Rule et al., 2013; Said et al., 2009). A meta-analysis of face-based impressions of perceived trustworthiness suggests that this dissociation between linear and nonlinear representations of perceived trustworthiness may reflect nuanced anatomical distinctions within amygdala function, where more ventral portions track the negative linear relationship with individual differences in perceived trustworthiness impressions and dorsal portions track more nonlinear group consensus information (Mende-Siedlecki, Verosky, et al., 2013). However, it should be noted that the spatial resolution of functional magnetic resonance imaging (fMRI) may not be sufficient to fully capture this functional distinction, and future studies are needed to confirm these findings.

7.2.2   *Contextual Influences on Facial Trustworthiness Judgments*

Though decontextualized designs can provide controlled environments in which to study facial evaluations of perceived trustworthiness, first impressions in daily life are rarely formed on the basis of a single piece of information or without broader context. Indeed, initial impressions from facial features can be influenced by other social cues (e.g., hair, clothing; Bonnefon et al., 2013; Oh et al., 2020) and emotional information in the surrounding environment (Keres & Chartier, 2016). For example, a study using computer mouse-tracking technology revealed that threatening (vs. negative or neutral) backdrops facilitated more direct untrustworthy judgments and more indirect trustworthy judgments of faces, highlighting the impact of emotional context on face-based impression formation (Brambilla et al., 2018). Furthermore, implicit perceptions of trustworthiness from faces can also be updated over the course of social interactions when met with salient or new social information (Ames & Fiske, 2013; Campellone & Kring, 2013; D. Li et al., 2017). Indeed, trust behavior can be guided initially by perceptions of the trustworthiness of a face, but can be shaped by experiences via trial-by-trial learning (Chang et al., 2010; see Section 7.3; see Chapter 8).

Updating initial face-based impressions with contextual or social information is thought to recruit a host of neural systems involved in social cognition, expectancy violation and conflict, and cognitive control (for review, see Mende-Siedlecki, Said, & Todorov, 2013). In the context of initial trustworthiness evaluations specifically, the dorsomedial prefrontal cortex (dmPFC), a region generally associated with inferring the mental states of others (Amodio & Frith, 2006), is thought to integrate social and contextual information to update perceived trustworthiness impressions initially formed through face perception. For example, in a study using noninvasive transcranial magnetic stimulation, stimulation applied over the dmPFC reduced the speed at which participants were able to confirm whether a face–adjective combination was congruent with their initial impressions about that face (Ferrari et al., 2014). Importantly, this effect did not occur when the adjective or face were presented separately, providing evidence that the dmPFC integrates social information from multiple sources to update initial impressions. Interactions between the dmPFC and the amygdala are also thought to determine whether initial trustworthiness impressions are swayed by new contextual information. Specifically, stronger amygdala activation during initial impression formation is related to weaker dmPFC activity during updating

(Baron et al., 2011). These findings highlight that, despite some influence from contextual information, strong initial impressions formed through facial features can be inflexible to updating from outside sources, and that this process occurs through coordination between multiple neural systems involved in impression formation and social cognition.

7.2.3 *Trustworthiness Impressions Based on Group Membership*

Perceptual and contextual cues in novel social environments can also signal group membership and lead to biased impressions of trustworthiness. In line with theories of social identity (Tajfel & Turner, 1986) and motivated cognition (Hughes & Zaki, 2015; Kunda, 1990), people tend to form rapid and effortless reputational biases and learn more from trust outcomes when interacting with ingroup relative to outgroup members (Olcaysoy Okten et al., 2020; Sofer et al., 2017). Furthermore, overcoming these biases may require effortful and explicit cognitive control (Hughes, Ambady, & Zaki, 2017). For example, students who trust peers from their same university (ingroup) over peers from a different university (outgroup) tend to recruit brain regions associated with value-based decision making (Hughes, Zaki, & Ambady, 2017), such as the ventromedial prefrontal cortex (vmPFC; e.g., Bartra et al., 2013). In contrast, trusting outgroup members or individuals with poor reputations tends to be associated with activation in regions generally linked with cognitive control and conflict, including the dorsal anterior cingulate cortex (dACC); regions that are perhaps necessary to assess conflict in the decision process and inhibit prepotent responses driven by prior knowledge (Delgado et al., 2005; Hughes, Zaki, & Ambady, 2017). Group-based trustworthiness biases are also thought to be driven by both a strong ingroup identity and an expectation that ingroup members will reciprocate more than outgroup members. Wu et al. (2018), for example, found that trustworthiness biases based on political affiliation were unique to members of a political party that had stronger overall partisanship and group identity. When trust was violated by ingroup members, people affiliated with this political party showed greater activation in regions involved in cognitive control (e.g., dorsolateral prefrontal cortex, dlPFC) and mentalizing (e.g., temporoparietal junction, TPJ), but showed greater reward prediction error activity in the caudate nucleus (a subcomponent of the striatum, STR) when the violations came from outgroup members. These findings are consistent with other recent work demonstrating the role of social cognitive mechanisms in ingroup biases and trust decisions based on reciprocity (Bellucci et al., 2018; Fujino et al., 2020).

It is important to note that biases in trustworthiness impressions are not always unilaterally directed toward ingroup members. In many cases, implicit attitudes toward specific social groups, regardless of one's own group membership, can also influence trust decisions in novel social settings. Implicit racial biases are a powerful example of this, as they can predict perceived trustworthiness judgments independent of one's own race or explicit racial attitudes. Implicit bias can be measured via the Implicit Association Test (Greenwald et al., 1998) and has been found to predict perceived trustworthiness ratings and actual trust decisions, such that participants with more pro-white or pro-Black implicit biases were more trusting of white or Black partners, respectively (Stanley et al., 2011). These findings were replicated in perceptions of fairness in an ultimatum game, where implicit racial biases predicted fewer accepted offers from Black versus white partners (Kubota et al., 2013). Furthermore, activation in reward-related regions such as the STR during investment decisions in a one-shot TG positively predicted individual investment biases toward one race or another, while amygdala activation may have reflected greater perceived risk in trusting Black versus white partners overall (Stanley et al., 2012). Together, these findings are suggestive of how implicit biases about different social groups can have a powerful and potentially prejudiced impact on reputation formation and trust decisions in novel social environments.

In sum, the ability to form initial trustworthiness impressions based on perceptual facial cues provides a means of navigating novel or unfamiliar social environments where more comprehensive reputation information is unavailable. Neural systems that are sensitive to social information from facial cues form rapid and robust perceptual biases that guide trust decisions, even if these biases do not accurately predict actual trustworthiness of real-world partners. These biases are often strong enough to govern trust decisions even in the face of conflicting information, but they can also be influenced by the surrounding emotional environment and updated over time with new social information.

7.3   Learning about Trust Reputations from Direct and Indirect Sources

Although initial trustworthiness impressions in novel social environments can be formed through the rapid detection of perceptual and contextual cues, in the real world we often become privy to more detailed information about a social partner by interacting with them directly, by observing their behavior, or by receiving information about them from others. In this section, we review the computational mechanisms that facilitate learning about others' trustworthiness through direct experience, and then discuss how the reputational information we receive from outside sources can interact with direct learning experiences to drive trust behavior (see Chapters 8 and 10).

7.3.1 Reinforcement Learning Mechanisms Guide Reputation Formation

The brain is constantly forming and updating predictive models about the environment on the basis of new information and prior experiences. In some cases, our brains are attuned to the consequences of our own actions and the actions of others, and update internal working models of these actions through a computational process known as reinforcement learning (RL; O'Doherty et al., 2015; Rescorla & Wagner, 1972; Shteingart & Loewenstein, 2014; Sutton & Barto, 1998). When prior information is unavailable, such as in a novel social environment, the brain relies on direct experiences with others to form a model about a social partner and to maximize the outcomes of future interactions. Updating such models via RL is thought to recruit circuitry involved in reward valuation, such as the caudate and the nucleus accumbens (Daw et al., 2006; Fareri et al., 2012; O'Doherty et al., 2004; Phan et al., 2010; Zaki et al., 2016).

The caudate is thought to play a key role in forming trust reputations through RL mechanisms during repeated experiences with novel social partners (Bellucci et al., 2017; King-Casas, 2005; Lambert et al., 2017; Wardle et al., 2013). In their landmark study, for example, King-Casas et al. (2005) used hyperscanning (simultaneous fMRI scanning of multiple people; Montague et al., 2002) to study real-time reputation formation during an iterative TG between strangers. They found that trust reputations are formed through updating processes in the caudate that are akin to dopaminergic reward prediction-error mechanisms observed in classic animal studies (e.g., Schultz et al., 1997). At the beginning of the task, the caudate was sensitive to whether one's partner reciprocated or violated trust investments. However, as the task progressed, caudate responses shifted from the outcome phase to the decision phase, signaling that participants had learned to predict their partner's reciprocation patterns and made investment decisions accordingly.

Neural systems involved in social cognition may also be important for forming models of novel social partners based on their trustworthiness and reputation (e.g., Hackel et al., 2015). For example, Bault et al. (2015) fit an RL model to cooperative decisions in a public goods game with parameters that not only accounted for behavioral updates based on trial-by-trial feedback, but also for a more cumulative "social tie" signal that represented the formation of a social bond. This model outperformed other RL models to predict cooperation decisions and revealed activity in the posterior superior temporal sulcus and the TPJ, which tracked the integration of trial-by-trial outcomes with cumulative social tie signals. Interestingly this activity decreased over the course of the task, potentially reflecting a reduced need for social cognitive processes as participants grew closer to their partners. Related findings suggest that computational signals reflective of social learning recruit other regions implicated in social cognition (i.e., precuneus; Stanley, 2016). Taken together, these findings demonstrate that both subcortical computations of value and learning and higher-order social cognitive mechanisms help to shape trustworthiness reputations over the course of repeated social interactions.

7.3.2   Reputations from Indirect Sources Bias Learning and Trust Decisions

In some cases, we may become privileged to initial reputational information about a novel social partner prior to interacting with them. For example, before interviewing a candidate for graduate school, an admissions committee may form an initial reputation about the candidate through their curriculum vitae, examples of their prior work, and letters of recommendation from their past advisors. Indirect information such as this helps to form a reputational "prior" from which one can make trust decisions during subsequent interactions. One common way that this is studied in the literature is by measuring trust and cooperation decisions as a function of prior knowledge about a partner's moral character (Charness et al., 2011; Everett et al., 2016; Falvello et al., 2015; Hackel et al., 2020; Radell et al., 2016; Suzuki et al., 2016; Zarolia et al., 2017). For example, in a study by Delgado et al. (2005), participants were introduced to three fictional partners with unique biographies about their moral character: One partner was depicted as good (philanthropic and altruistic), one as bad (deceptive and criminal), and one as neutral (no moral information provided). After reading these biographies, participants played an iterative TG with each of the three partners. At the beginning of the task, participants perceived the good partner as more trustworthy than the bad or neutral partners, and this translated to more investment decisions with the good partner throughout the task. This bias is especially telling given that reciprocation rates across all three partners were set at 50%, meaning that despite equal patterns of reciprocation and defection, participants biased trust decisions according to prior reputational information. Furthermore, this trust bias was reflected in the caudate nucleus, which exhibited differential responses to reciprocation or defection in the neutral condition (and in a nonsocial lottery condition), but not in response to outcomes from the good or bad partners. This study provided further evidence that the caudate plays an important role in forming trust reputations through RL mechanisms, but additionally revealed that prior information can circumvent this learning process and bias trust decisions by making outcomes less informative.

One potential explanation for why it is difficult to overcome initial reputational biases when new information is available is the influence of oxytocin on trust behavior (Ide et al., 2018; Kosfeld et al., 2005; Van IJzendoorn & Bakermans-Kranenburg, 2012; Yan et al., 2018; see Chapter 13). For example, participants who were administered intranasal oxytocin before playing a TG with anonymous partners did not show typical behavioral modification following negative feedback, while participants who were administered a placebo reduced their overall subsequent investments, as expected (Baumgartner et al., 2008). The placebo group also demonstrated enhanced amygdala and caudate activity during investment decisions after receiving negative feedback (suggestive of typically functioning RL mechanisms), while the oxytocin group did not. Importantly, these effects occurred only during the TG, and did not replicate during a comparable nonsocial lottery task. These findings highlight that oxytocin regulation in neural circuits that are responsible for social valuation and learning may guide trust reputation formation during social interactions; however, further studies are still needed to confirm the replicability of these effects (Declerck et al., 2020).

In recent years, a number of studies have emerged using advanced neuroimaging analysis techniques and computational RL models to further evince how direct and indirect reputational information interact to guide trust decisions. For example, when prior reputations are available, stronger effective connectivity (i.e., psychophysiological interaction; Friston, 2011) between the caudate and the ventrolateral prefrontal cortex (vlPFC) in response to violations of trust has been associated with continued investment decisions on subsequent trials (Fouragnan et al., 2013), suggesting that cortical regions may disrupt RL or updating in the STR in certain situations, leading to continued trust decisions that favor existing reputations (see also J. Li et al., 2011 for an example of this disruption in a probabilistic learning setting). Furthermore, computational RL models that take into account prior beliefs (expectations about how a partner will respond) better predict trust and cooperation decisions than standard RL models when reputational information is available (Fouragnan et al., 2013; Hackel et al., 2020; Vanyukov et al., 2019). Taken together, these findings demonstrate corticostriatal sensitivity to trust outcomes that are biased by reputational priors.

In sum, several processes and their respective neural correlates – from action–outcome learning and value-based decision making to social cognition –work in tandem to build trust reputations through both direct experiences and prior information from indirect sources. Such information is integrated through reinforcement learning mechanisms that guide moment-to-moment trust decisions and form cumulative social ties, but can be biased or circumvented altogether when strong prior information is available. The reviewed studies provide insights into the neurological underpinnings of trust reputation formation in novel social environments, and shed light on how social bonds are formed and maintained over the course of a repeated social interaction.

7.4 Trust Reputations in Established Social Relationships

The focus of this chapter thus far has been on reputations and trust decisions in novel social environments. However, some of our most important social interactions occur with those with whom we have strengthened and maintained relationships through a variety of social settings or over the course of many years. These recurring social interactions provide opportunities to form deeper and more complex representations of a partner's trustworthiness and ultimately foster healthy (or harmful) social bonds. In this section, we discuss how trust reputations are generalized from prior nontrust-related social interactions, as well as how reputations formed over extended periods of time can bias trust behavior in established interpersonal relationships.

7.4.1 Generalizing Trust Reputations from Prior Social Interactions

Observing a partner's behavior over the course of repeated social experiences may contribute to a more generalized reputation of their character and inform subsequent trust decisions. For example, perceptions of moral character gleaned through honest or dishonest advice in a card-guessing task informed investments in a subsequent TG (Bellucci et al., 2019).

Furthermore, multivoxel pattern analysis revealed neural representations of social character during an advice-taking task in brain regions including the posterior cingulate cortex and dlPFC that were separate from the representation of outcome valence in the STR and ACC. Critically, regions decoding reputation based on honesty significantly predicted later trust decisions in interactions with the same partners. These findings provide evidence that perceptions of moral character formed through past experiences can subsequently be integrated into trust decisions. In some cases, reputations formed through past experiences with one person may also generalize to a similar looking, but novel social partner (FeldmanHall et al., 2018). After learning a set of partners' trust reputations through an iterative TG, participants played a new game with new partners whose faces were perceptually similar morphs of those of the original partners. New partners received comparable investments to their perceptually similar counterparts and showed similar activation patterns in the vmPFC and amygdala, revealing how past experiences can even influence future trust decisions with novel, but similar-looking individuals.

Other, nontrust-related past experiences can also contribute to perceptions of social character and influence later trust behavior. For example, Fareri et al. (2012) found that while ventral striatal activation correlated with social prediction error signals during an iterative TG, initial reputations formed during a preceding Cyberball game (a ball-tossing game in which partners can be exclusionary or inclusive; Williams et al., 2000) biased feedback learning, such that participants learned more from defection when interacting with exclusionary partners and learned more from reciprocation when interacting with inclusive partners. These differential learning signals further correlated with activation of regions associated with salience and executive control (e.g., dACC, anterior insula; Seeley et al., 2007). Learning about reputations from nontrust-related experiences may also extend to interactions on social media. In a recent study by Brudner et al. (2019), participants decided whether to share their own Instagram photos with three (fictitious) peers who then provided variable amounts of positive ("likes") and negative ("dislikes") feedback. In a subsequent TG, participants disproportionately trusted peers that provided more positive feedback than peers who provided more negative feedback. Together, these findings highlight the ways in which reputations formed through past experiences can bias trust decisions to strengthen or weaken social bonds, even when these past experiences do not provide any information about trustworthiness directly.

7.4.2 Trust Based on Close Interpersonal Relationships

Our strongest and arguably most important social bonds, those of close interpersonal relationships, are deeply rooted in trust reputations that have been formed and strengthened over extended periods of time. Indeed, the mere presence of a close social partner can shape perception of rewards (Fareri et al., 2012), influence prosociality (Morelli et al., 2018), and even shift risky decisions (Chein et al., 2011). Thus, it is perhaps unsurprising that close relationships have a profound impact on trust, as trust requires a relationship of reliance. When an individual relies on their social partner, they potentially expose their own vulnerabilities while taking the calculated risk that their partner will behave in a predictable and supportive manner.

In the neuroscience literature, the formation and maintenance of trust in interpersonal relationships has often been studied in the context of friendships. In a study by Fareri et al. (2015), for example, participants played an iterative TG with a same-sex close friend, a same-sex stranger, and a computer. Despite partners' responses being surreptitiously preprogrammed to equate rates of reciprocity at 50%, participants were more likely to invest in a close friend than in a stranger or computer, suggesting that social closeness can actively bias trust decisions (Figure 7.1A). Furthermore, a social value RL model that integrated parameters of subjective closeness with the value of experienced reciprocity revealed that participants assigned greater social value to reciprocation from their close friend compared with that from the stranger or computer. This social value "bonus" was also reflected in the bilateral ventral striatum (vSTR) and medial prefrontal cortex (mPFC), such that reciprocation from the close friend showed increased activation when compared to reciprocation from the stranger, tracking with the learning signal from the social value model (Figure 7.1B). Thus, even when partners defect and reciprocate at similar rates, the heightened social value of an established relationship enhances the experience of reciprocity and biases subsequent decisions to trust close friends more often than strangers.

To further understand the neural underpinnings of reputational bias in trust decisions, Fareri et al. (2020) conducted a secondary analysis of their 2015 data to examine network connectivity during trust-based interactions with close others and strangers. A network psychophysiological interaction analysis (Utevsky et al., 2017) probing connectivity of the default mode network (DMN) revealed an enhanced positive coupling with areas of the frontoparietal control network during reciprocity from friends relative to strangers that scaled with social closeness. These findings suggest that the

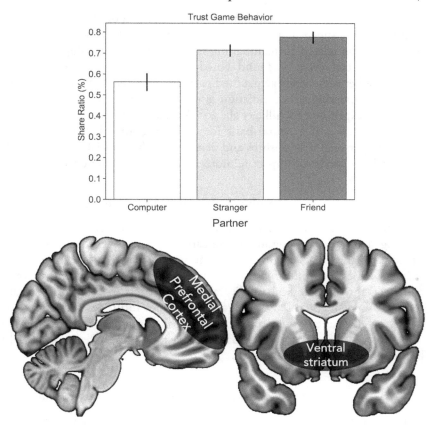

Figure 7.1   Iterative trust game with partners varying in terms of closeness
(computer, stranger, and close friend).
(A) Participants demonstrate trust based on reputation by investing money with different
partners at increased rates as a function of social closeness, despite equal rates of reciprocation
across partners. (B) Activity of corticostriatal circuits (vSTR, mPFC) was observed during the
outcome phase when participants learned whether their decision to trust was reciprocated or
not. The magnitude of the reward response predicted a model-derived parameter of the social
value of reciprocity that accounted for partners' reputations
(adapted from Fareri et al. 2015).

heightened salience or importance of positive interactions with close others
may be encoded by interactions between these neural networks, which
could facilitate our ability to adapt and predict others' future behavior.
Relatedly, reduced activity in the right TPJ, a key node within the DMN,
has been associated with both resistance to updating impressions for close

friends (Park et al., 2020) and self-reports of having more friends (Park & Young, 2020), suggesting that discounting negative behavior from close others may be related to maintaining interpersonal relationships. Similar trust biases can even be found based on the amount of relationship experience between newly acquainted partners, such that participants resist reputation updating after a violation of trust for partners with whom they have more experience (Schilke et al., 2013). Taken together, these findings provide evidence of a neural basis for the reputational bias observed in close interpersonal relationships and demonstrate how social closeness and relationship experience impact reinforcement-based reputation updating.

7.5   Broader Implications and Future Directions

Grounded in the foundational evidence described in this chapter, new and exciting steps are emerging in trust research and social neuroscience more broadly. In this final section, we outline some ways in which innovative methodologies and more naturalistic paradigms are contributing to the enhancement of ecological validity and connections to real-world social settings. We will also discuss potential avenues for future research into the effects of adverse environments on reputation formation and trust decisions, as well as discuss the broader impact of these effects on social bonding and psychological health.

7.5.1   Real-World Consequences of Reputation-Based Trust Decisions

In the past, trust paradigms used in neuroscience research have primarily been simplified to be conducive to the fMRI scanning environment. However, recent work has sought to link the neural mechanisms of trust reputation formation to trust behavior in real-life social settings. For example, split-second perceived trustworthiness impressions formed from facial features have been linked to legal sentencing in criminal cases, even in the face of contrasting knowledge or if such impressions do not accurately predict real-world behavior (Rule et al., 2013; Wilson & Rule, 2015). Jaeger et al. (2020), for instance, found that faces that were perceived as less trustworthy were more likely to be given a guilty verdict in a legal sentencing paradigm than faces that were perceived as more trustworthy. Interestingly, systematically providing participants with knowledge about the effects of facial stereotypes on sentencing decisions did not reduce this perceptual bias, and participants even revised their verdicts when perceived facial trustworthiness did not align with their initial face-blind decisions. Knowledge about a person's prior record may also shape reputational biases in these circumstances and may impact whether a person is considered guilty of alleged wrongdoing. Specifically, social partners who proved to be untrustworthy in a TG were subsequently judged to be more blameworthy in a vignette of negative behaviors than partners who were previously more trustworthy (Kliemann et al., 2008). The effects of these prior records were also reflected in greater right TPJ activity in response to negative vignettes about untrustworthy versus trustworthy partners, suggesting that social cognitive mechanisms may contribute to biased verdicts for people with untrustworthy prior records.

Beyond the legal domain, understanding how reputations bias trust behavior also informs what we know about how people choose to trust others in a variety of social settings and emotional contexts (see also Chapter 6). For example, perceived trustworthiness impressions and amygdala activation in response to facial features predict political preferences and hypothetical (but perhaps not actual) voting behavior (Hetherington, 1999; Rule et al., 2010; Todorov et al., 2005; see Olivola & Todorov, 2010 for review). Furthermore, perceived trustworthiness impressions based on racial group membership is related to discrimination on share economy services such as Airbnb; however, this effect is diminished when other reputational cues are available, such as perceived social similarity or recommendations from other consumers (Abrahao et al., 2017; Berg Nødtvedt et al., 2020). As a final example, trustworthiness reputations can have an important impact on public opinion of science (Fiske & Dupree, 2014), where people perceive a scientist's research to be more interesting and competent when the scientist is perceived as having a more trustworthy-looking face (Gheorghiu et al., 2017). Together, these findings highlight the importance of connecting basic insights about reputation formation in the brain with real-world trust behaviors and social outcomes.

7.5.2 How Do Adverse Environments Influence Reputation-Based Trust Decisions?

An emerging avenue of research in social neuroscience is the investigation into how environmental adversity (e.g., acute and chronic stress, resource scarcity, exposure to threat) shapes decision making and social interactions that inform reputation building. Although the effects of adverse environments have been heavily studied in nonsocial contexts, such as anticipating and receiving personal rewards or making independent economic decisions

(Bogdan & Pizzagalli, 2006; Corral-Frías et al., 2015; Dillon et al., 2009; Huijsmans et al., 2019; Mather & Lighthall, 2012; Porcelli & Delgado, 2017; Porcelli et al., 2012), less is known about how such environments affect decisions when social partners are involved.

One possibility is that people cope with adversity by seeking out positive social resources. Indeed, the tend-and-befriend hypothesis posits that adverse environments motivate people to form and strengthen social bonds in order to share critical resources, ensure personal safety, and receive emotional support (Taylor, 2006; Taylor & Master, 2011). When successful, positive social relationships and a sense of community can safeguard against the harmful physical and psychological consequences resulting from adverse experiences (Ditzen & Heinrichs, 2014; Eisenberger et al., 2007; Jachimowicz et al., 2017; Raposa et al., 2015). In the context of trust and other prosocial behaviors, it is plausible that coping with adversity involves forming more positive reputations about others as a means of strengthening and maintaining these crucial social bonds. However, research in this domain is still nascent and the results thus far are mixed. On the one hand, acute psychosocial stressors have indeed been shown to enhance trust and prosocial behavior (Vieira et al., 2020; von Dawans et al., 2012, 2019) and strengthen feelings of interpersonal closeness (Berger et al., 2016). Yet other similar paradigms examining both acute and chronic stress have shown the opposite effect (Engelmann et al., 2019; FeldmanHall et al., 2015; Jirsaraie et al., 2019) or no effect at all (Buchanan & Passarelli, 2020). There are a number of potential methodological explanations for these discrepancies, including variability in the type of adverse events being measured (e.g., threat of shock vs. psychosocial stressor), individual differences in physiological responses to adversity (e.g., rise in cortisol levels), and disparities across the parameters of the paradigms themselves (e.g., one-shot vs. iterative TG). Thus, future work in this domain should seek to clarify these effects through more refined methodological approaches.

Another potential reason for these inconsistent findings may be that adversity differentially affects trust and other prosocial behaviors depending on the perceived trustworthiness reputation of the social partner, which could be driven by factors such as interpersonal closeness or group membership. Indeed, acute psychosocial stress manipulations have led to greater monetary allocation to close versus distant social partners (Margittai et al., 2015) and greater subjective ratings of trustworthiness for members of one's racial ingroup versus outgroup (Salam et al., 2017). Furthermore, acute economic resource scarcity has been shown to alter perceptual judgments and neural responses to faces of different races, leading to a reduction in allocation of monetary resources to minoritized groups (Krosch & Amodio, 2014, 2019). This bias toward perceived social reputation may occur because adverse events consume and deplete cognitive resources (Alexander et al., 2007; Arnsten et al., 2012; Duncko et al., 2009; Elzinga & Roelofs, 2005; Luethi et al., 2009; Raio et al., 2013; Roozendaal et al., 2009; Schoofs et al., 2009), reducing one's capacity to engage in explicit, goal-directed behavior and instead defaulting to more habitual (though often biased or inaccurate) choices (Heatherton, 2011; Plessow et al., 2011, 2012; Porcelli & Delgado, 2017). Finally, trust and other prosocial behaviors in the face of adversity may also be influenced by individual differences in factors such as biological sex (Berger et al., 2016; Schweda et al., 2019; Steinbeis et al., 2015) or chronic exposure to adverse environments (Chang & Baskin-Sommers, 2020; H. Li et al., 2019). Taken together, we are just now beginning to understand how environmental adversity impacts trust and other prosocial behaviors. There remain many open questions about how adverse events shape how we form initial perceived trustworthiness impressions, learn from repeated trust interactions, and make decisions based on prior trust reputations, and future research in this domain should apply extra consideration to how social factors and individual differences bias such processes.

7.6 Conclusion

The act of trust can be thought of as a prediction of the reliability of a social partner based on our knowledge about them. While trust is often based on established interpersonal relationships, where a prior history of predictable behaviors helps to direct our decisions to trust, at times in the absence of personal experience or in a novel social setting, we rely on incomplete reputations to predict reciprocity. Indeed, the ability to form generalized beliefs about others is critical to predicting social outcomes and driving trust decisions. The brain is well equipped to form impressions about others, either by rapidly detecting perceptual social cues via regions such as the amygdala, learning from repeated action–outcome contingencies and integrating indirect information via corticostriatal circuits, or by drawing on years' worth of past experiences through social cognitive mechanisms. Although reputation formation processes have clear benefits for adapting to one's environment and forming healthy social bonds, they can also bias trust decisions in ways that are inaccurate, maladaptive to a given situation, or even harmful to marginalized social groups. This wealth of research on how reputation shapes decisions to trust has identified key neurobiological and computational mechanisms that support impression formation, reputation updating, and decision making in a variety of social contexts. This work sets the stage upon which future research can expand to translate basic findings to more real-world settings and to understand how these processes are impacted by adverse environments.

References

Abrahao, B., Parigi, P., Gupta, A., & Cook, K. S. (2017). Reputation offsets trust judgments based on social biases among Airbnb users. *Proceedings of the National Academy of Sciences*, 114(37), 9848–9853. https://doi.org/10.1073/pnas.1604234114

Adolphs, R. (2010). What does the amygdala contribute to social cognition?. *Annals of the New York Academy of Sciences*, 1191(1), 42–61. https://doi.org/10.1111/j.1749-6632.2010.05445.x

Adolphs, R., & Spezio, M. (2006). Role of the amygdala in processing visual social stimuli. In *Progress in brain research* (Vol. 156, pp. 363–378). Elsevier. https://doi.org/10.1016/S0079-6123(06)56020-0

Alexander, J. K., Hillier, A., Smith, R. M., Tivarus, M. E., & Beversdorf, D. Q. (2007). Beta-adrenergic modulation of cognitive flexibility during stress. *Journal of Cognitive Neuroscience*, 19(3), 468–478. https://doi.org/10.1162/jocn.2007.19.3.468

Ames, D. L., & Fiske, S. T. (2013). Outcome dependency alters the neural substrates of impression formation. *NeuroImage*, 83, 599–608. https://doi.org/10.1016/j.neuroimage.2013.07.001

Amodio, D. M., & Frith, C. D. (2006). Meeting of minds: The medial frontal cortex and social cognition. *Nature Reviews Neuroscience*, 7(4), 268–277. https://doi.org/10.1038/nrn1884

Arnsten, A. F. T., Wang, M. J., & Paspalas, C. D. (2012). Neuromodulation of thought: Flexibilities and vulnerabilities in prefrontal cortical network synapses. *Neuron*, 76(1), 223–239. https://doi.org/10.1016/j.neuron.2012.08.038

Balas, B., & Pacella, J. (2017). Trustworthiness perception is disrupted in artificial faces. *Computers in Human Behavior*, 77, 240–248. https://doi.org/10.1016/j.chb.2017.08.045

Baron, S. G., Gobbini, M. I., Engell, A. D., & Todorov, A. (2011). Amygdala and dorsomedial prefrontal cortex responses to appearance-based and behavior-based person impressions. *Social Cognitive and Affective Neuroscience*, 6(5), 572–581. https://doi.org/10.1093/scan/nsq086

Bartra, O., McGuire, J. T., & Kable, J. W. (2013). The valuation system: A coordinate-based meta-analysis of BOLD fMRI experiments examining neural correlates of subjective value. *NeuroImage*, 76, 412–427. https://doi.org/10.1016/j.neuroimage.2013.02.063

Bault, N., Pelloux, B., Fahrenfort, J. J., Ridderinkhof, K. R., & Van Winden, F. (2015). Neural dynamics of social tie formation in economic decision making. *Social Cognitive and Affective Neuroscience*, 10(6), 877–884. https://doi.org/10.1093/scan/nsu138

Baumgartner, T., Heinrichs, M., Vonlanthen, A., Fischbacher, U., & Fehr, E. (2008). Oxytocin shapes the neural circuitry of trust and trust adaptation in humans. *Neuron*, 58(4), 639–650. https://doi.org/10.1016/j.neuron.2008.04.009

Bellucci, G., Chernyak, S. V., Goodyear, K., Eickhoff, S. B., & Krueger, F. (2017). Neural signatures of trust in reciprocity: A coordinate-based meta-analysis. *Human Brain Mapping*, 38(3), 1233–1248. https://doi.org/10.1002/hbm.23451

Bellucci, G., Hahn, T., Deshpande, G., & Krueger, F. (2018). Functional connectivity of specific resting-state networks predicts trust and reciprocity in the trust game. *Cognitive, Affective, & Behavioral Neuroscience*, 19(1), 165–176. https://doi.org/10.3758/s13415-018-00654-3

Bellucci, G., Molter, F., & Park, S. Q. (2019). Neural representations of honesty predict future trust behavior. *Nature Communications*, 10(1), Article 5184. https://doi.org/10.1038/s41467-019-13261-8

Benuzzi, F., Pugnaghi, M., Meletti, S., et al. (2007). Processing the socially relevant parts of faces. *Brain Research Bulletin*, 74(5), 344–356. https://doi.org/10.1016/j.brainresbull.2007.07.010

Berg Nødtvedt, K., Sjåstad, H., Skard, S., Thorbjørnsen, H., & Van Bavel, J. (2020). Racial bias in the sharing economy and the role of trust and self-congruence. *Social Science Research Network*. https://dx.doi.org/10.2139/ssrn.3434463

Berger, J., Heinrichs, M., von Dawans, B., Way, B. M., & Chen, F. S. (2016). Cortisol modulates men's affiliative responses to acute social stress. *Psychoneuroendocrinology*, 63, 1–9. https://doi.org/10.1016/j.psyneuen.2015.09.004

Bhanji, J. P., & Delgado, M. R. (2014). Perceived control influences neural responses to setbacks and promotes persistence. *Neuron*, 83(6), 1369–1375. https://doi.org/10.1016/j.neuron.2014.08.012

Bogdan, R., & Pizzagalli, D. A. (2006). Acute stress reduces reward responsiveness: Implications for depression. *Biological Psychiatry*, 60(10), 1147–1154. https://doi.org/10.1016/j.biopsych.2006.03.037

Bonnefon, J.-F., Hopfensitz, A., & De Neys, W. (2013). The modular nature of trustworthiness detection. *Journal of Experimental Psychology: General*, 142(1), 143–150. https://doi.org/10.1037/a0028930

Brambilla, M., Biella, M., & Freeman, J. B. (2018). The influence of visual context on the evaluation of facial trustworthiness. *Journal of Experimental Social Psychology*, 78, 34–42. https://doi.org/10.1016/j.jesp.2018.04.011

Brudner, E. G., Khalil, A., & Delgado, M. R. (2019, August). *The upside of social media: The influence of peer 'likes' on adaptive social behavior.* Flux Congress, New York, NY.

Buchanan, T. W., & Passarelli, T. O. (2020). How do stress and social closeness impact prosocial behavior? *Experimental Psychology*, 67(2), 123–131. https://doi.org/10.1027/1618-3169/a000482

Bzdok, D., Langner, R., Caspers, S., et al. (2011). ALE meta-analysis on facial judgments of trustworthiness and attractiveness. *Brain Structure and Function*, 215(3–4), 209–223. https://doi.org/10.1007/s00429-010-0287-4

Campellone, T. R., & Kring, A. M. (2013). Who do you trust? The impact of facial emotion and behaviour on decision making. *Cognition & Emotion*, 27(4), 603–620. https://doi.org/10.1080/02699931.2012.726608

Chang, L. J., Doll, B. B., van't Wout, M., Frank, M. J., & Sanfey, A. G. (2010). Seeing is believing: Trustworthiness as a dynamic belief. *Cognitive Psychology*, 61(2), 87–105. https://doi.org/10.1016/j.cogpsych.2010.03.001

Chang, S.-A. A., & Baskin-Sommers, A. (2020). Living in a disadvantaged neighborhood affects neural processing of facial trustworthiness. *Frontiers in Psychology*, 11, Article 409. https://doi.org/10.3389/fpsyg.2020.00409

Charness, G., Du, N., & Yang, C.-L. (2011). Trust and trustworthiness reputations in an investment game. *Games and Economic Behavior*, 72(2), 361–375. https://doi.org/10.1016/j.geb.2010.09.002

Chein, J., Albert, D., O'Brien, L., Uckert, K., & Steinberg, L. (2011). Peers increase adolescent risk taking by enhancing activity in the brain's reward circuitry. *Developmental Science*, 14(2), F1–F10. https://doi.org/10.1111/j.1467-7687.2010.01035.x

Corral-Frías, N. S., Nikolova, Y. S., Michalski, L. J., Baranger, D. A. A., Hariri, A. R., & Bogdan, R. (2015). Stress-related anhedonia is associated with ventral striatum reactivity to reward and transdiagnostic psychiatric symptomatology. *Psychological Medicine*, 45(12), 2605–2617. https://doi.org/10.1017/S0033291715000525

Daw, N. D., O'Doherty, J. P., Dayan, P., Seymour, B., & Dolan, R. J. (2006). Cortical substrates for exploratory decisions in humans. *Nature*, 441(7095), 876–879. https://doi.org/10.1038/nature04766

Declerck, C. H., Boone, C., Pauwels, L., Vogt, B., & Fehr, E. (2020). A registered replication study on oxytocin and trust. *Nature Human Behaviour*, 4(6), 646–655. https://doi.org/10.1038/s41562-020-0878-x

Delgado, M. R., Frank, R. H., & Phelps, E. A. (2005). Perceptions of moral character modulate the neural systems of reward during the trust game. *Nature Neuroscience*, 8(11), 1611–1618. https://doi.org/10.1038/nn1575

De Neys, W., Hopfensitz, A., & Bonnefon, J. F. (2017). Split-second trustworthiness detection from faces in an economic game. *Experimental Psychology*, 64(4), 231–239. https://doi.org/10.1027/1618-3169/a000367

Dillon, D. G., Holmes, A. J., Birk, J. L., Brooks, N., Lyons-Ruth, K., & Pizzagalli, D. A. (2009). Childhood adversity is associated with left basal ganglia dysfunction during reward anticipation in adulthood. *Biological Psychiatry*, 66(3), 206–213. https://doi.org/10.1016/j.biopsych.2009.02.019

Ditzen, B., & Heinrichs, M. (2014). Psychobiology of social support: The social dimension of stress buffering. *Restorative Neurology and Neuroscience*, 32(1), 149–162. https://doi.org/10.3233/RNN-139008

Duncko, R., Johnson, L., Merikangas, K., & Grillon, C. (2009). Working memory performance after acute exposure to the cold pressor stress in healthy volunteers. *Neurobiology of Learning and Memory*, 91(4), 377–381. https://doi.org/10.1016/j.nlm.2009.01.006

Eisenberger, N. I., Taylor, S. E., Gable, S. L., Hilmert, C. J., & Lieberman, M. D. (2007). Neural pathways link social support to attenuated neuroendocrine stress responses. *NeuroImage*, 35(4), 1601–1612. https://doi.org/10.1016/j.neuroimage.2007.01.038

Elzinga, B. M., & Roelofs, K. (2005). Cortisol-induced impairments of working memory require acute sympathetic activation. *Behavioral Neuroscience*, 119(1), 98–103. https://doi.org/10.1037/0735-7044.119.1.98

Engell, A. D., Haxby, J. V., & Todorov, A. (2007). Implicit trustworthiness decisions: Automatic coding of face properties in the human amygdala. *Journal of Cognitive Neuroscience*, 19(9), 1508–1519. https://doi.org/10.1162/jocn.2007.19.9.1508

Engelmann, J. B., Meyer, F., Ruff, C. C., & Fehr, E. (2019). The neural circuitry of affect-induced distortions of trust. *Science Advances*, 5(3), Article eaau3413. https://doi.org/10.1126/sciadv.aau3413

Everett, J. A. C., Pizarro, D. A., & Crockett, M. J. (2016). Inference of trustworthiness from intuitive moral judgments. *Journal of Experimental Psychology: General*, 145(6), 772–787. https://doi.org/10.1037/xge0000165

Ewing, L., Caulfield, F., Read, A., & Rhodes, G. (2015). Perceived trustworthiness of faces drives trust behaviour in children. *Developmental Science*, 18(2), 327–334. https://doi.org/10.1111/desc.12218

Falvello, V., Vinson, M., Ferrari, C., & Todorov, A. (2015). The robustness of learning about the trustworthiness of other people. *Social Cognition*, 33(5), 368–386. https://doi.org/10.1521/soco.2015.33.5.368

Fareri, D. S., Chang, L. J., & Delgado, M. R. (2012). Effects of direct social experience on trust decisions and neural reward circuitry. *Frontiers in Neuroscience*, 6(148), 1–17. https://doi.org/10.3389/fnins.2012.00148

(2015). Computational substrates of social value in interpersonal collaboration. *Journal of Neuroscience*, 35(21), 8170–8180. https://doi.org/10.1523/jneurosci.4775-14.2015

Fareri, D. S., Smith, D. V., & Delgado, M. R. (2020). The influence of relationship closeness on default-mode network connectivity during social interactions. *Social Cognitive and Affective Neuroscience*, 15(3), 261–271. https://doi.org/10.1093/scan/nsaa031

FeldmanHall, O., Dunsmoor, J. E., Tompary, A., Hunter, L. E., Todorov, A., & Phelps, E. A. (2018). Stimulus generalization as a mechanism for learning to trust. *Proceedings of the National Academy of Sciences*, 115(7), E1690–E1697. https://doi.org/10.1073/pnas.1715227115

FeldmanHall, O., Raio, C. M., Kubota, J. T., Seiler, M. G., & Phelps, E. A. (2015). The effects of social context and acute stress on decision making under uncertainty. *Psychological Science*, 26(12), 1918–1926. https://doi.org/10.1177/0956797615605807

Ferrari, C., Lega, C., Vernice, M., et al. (2014). The dorsomedial prefrontal cortex plays a causal role in integrating social impressions from faces and verbal descriptions. *Cerebral Cortex*, 26(1), 156–165. https://doi.org/10.1093/cercor/bhu186

Fett, A. K. J., Gromann, P. M., Giampietro, V., Shergill, S. S., & Krabbendam, L. (2014). Default distrust? An fMRI investigation of the neural development of trust and cooperation. *Social Cognitive and Affective Neuroscience*, 9 (4), 395–402. https://doi.org/10.1093/scan/nss144

Fiske, S. T., & Dupree, C. (2014). Gaining trust as well as respect in communicating to motivated audiences about science topics. *Proceedings of the National Academy of Sciences*, 111(Suppl. 4), 13593–13597. https://doi.org/10.1073/pnas.1317505111

Fouragnan, E., Chierchia, G., Greiner, S., Neveu, R., Avesani, P., & Coricelli, G. (2013). Reputational priors magnify striatal responses to violations of trust. *Journal of Neuroscience*, 33(8), 3602–3611. https://doi.org/10.1523/jneurosci.3086-12.2013

Freeman, J. B., Stolier, R. M., Ingbretsen, Z. A., & Hehman, E. A. (2014). Amygdala responsivity to high-level social information from unseen faces. *Journal of Neuroscience*, 34(32), 10573–10581. https://doi.org/10.1523/jneurosci.5063-13.2014

Friston, K. J. (2011). Functional and effective connectivity: A review. *Brain Connectivity*, 1(1), 13–36. https://doi.org/10.1089/brain.2011.0008

Fujino, J., Tei, S., Itahashi, T., et al. (2020). Role of the right temporoparietal junction in intergroup bias in trust decisions. *Human Brain Mapping*, 41(6), 1677–1688. https://doi.org/10.1002/hbm.24903

Gheorghiu, A. I., Callan, M. J., & Skylark, W. J. (2017). Facial appearance affects science communication. *Proceedings of the National Academy of Sciences*, 114 (23), 5970–5975. https://doi.org/10.1073/pnas.1620542114

Gluckman, M., & Johnson, S. P. (2013). Attentional capture by social stimuli in young infants. *Frontiers in Psychology*, 4, Article 527. https://doi.org/10.3389/fpsyg.2013.00527

Greenwald, A. G., McGhee, D. E., & Schwartz, J. L. K. (1998). Measuring individual differences in implicit cognition: The implicit association test. *Journal of Personality and Social Psychology*, 74(6), 1464–1480. https://doi.org/10.1037/0022-3514.74.6.1464

Hackel, L. M., Doll, B. B., & Amodio, D. M. (2015). Instrumental learning of traits versus rewards: Dissociable neural correlates and effects on choice. *Nature Neuroscience*, 18(9), 1233–1235. https://doi.org/10.1038/nn.4080

Hackel, L. M., Wills, J. A., & Van Bavel, J. J. (2020). Shifting prosocial intuitions: Neurocognitive evidence for a value-based account of group-based cooperation. *Social Cognitive and Affective Neuroscience*, 15(4), 371–381. https://doi.org/10.1093/scan/nsaa055

Heatherton, T. F. (2011). Neuroscience of self and self-regulation. *Annual Review of Psychology*, 62(1), 363–390. https://doi.org/10.1146/annurev.psych.121208.131616

Hetherington, M. J. (1999). The effect of political trust on the presidential vote, 1968–96. *American Political Science Review*, 93(2), 311–326. https://doi.org/10.2307/2585398

Hughes, B. L., Ambady, N., & Zaki, J. (2017). Trusting outgroup, but not ingroup members, requires control: Neural and behavioral evidence. *Social Cognitive and Affective Neuroscience*, 12(3), 372–381. https://doi.org/10.1093/scan/nsw139

Hughes, B. L., & Zaki, J. (2015). The neuroscience of motivated cognition. *Trends in Cognitive Sciences*, 19(2), 62–64. https://doi.org/10.1016/j.tics.2014.12.006

Hughes, B. L., Zaki, J., & Ambady, N. (2017). Motivation alters impression formation and related neural systems. *Social Cognitive and Affective Neuroscience*, 12(1), 49–60. https://doi.org/10.1093/scan/nsw147

Huijsmans, I., Ma, I., Micheli, L., Civai, C., Stallen, M., & Sanfey, A. G. (2019). A scarcity mindset alters neural processing underlying consumer decision making. *Proceedings of the National Academy of Sciences*, 116(24), 11699–11704. https://doi.org/10.1073/pnas.1818572116

Ide, J. S., Nedic, S., Wong, K. F., et al. (2018). Oxytocin attenuates trust as a subset of more general reinforcement learning, with altered reward circuit functional connectivity in males. *NeuroImage*, 174, 35–43. https://doi.org/10.1016/j.neuroimage.2018.02.035

Jachimowicz, J. M., Chafik, S., Munrat, S., Prabhu, J. C., & Weber, E. U. (2017). Community trust reduces myopic decisions of low-income individuals. *Proceedings of the National Academy of Sciences*, 114(21), 5401–5406. https://doi.org/10.1073/pnas.1617395114

Jaeger, B., Todorov, A. T., Evans, A. M., & Van Beest, I. (2020). Can we reduce facial biases? Persistent effects of facial trustworthiness on sentencing decisions. *Journal of Experimental Social Psychology*, 90, Article 104004. https://doi.org/10.1016/j.jesp.2020.104004

Jirsaraie, R. J., Ranby, K. W., & Albeck, D. S. (2019). Early life stress moderates the relationship between age and prosocial behaviors. *Child Abuse & Neglect*, 94, Article 104029. https://doi.org/10.1016/j.chiabu.2019.104029

Keres, A., & Chartier, C. R. (2016). The biasing effects of visual background on perceived facial trustworthiness. *Psi Chi Journal of Psychological Research*, 21(3), 170–175.

King-Casas, B. (2005). Getting to know you: Reputation and trust in a two-person economic exchange. *Science*, 308(5718), 78–83. https://doi.org/10.1126/science.1108062

King-Casas, B., Tomlin, D., Anen, C., Camerer, C. F., Quartz, S. R., & Montague, P. R. (2005). Getting to know you: Reputation and trust in a two-person economic exchange. *Science*, 308(5718), 78–83. https://doi.org/10.1126/science.1108062

Kliemann, D., Young, L., Scholz, J., & Saxe, R. (2008). The influence of prior record on moral judgment. *Neuropsychologia*, 46(12), 2949–2957. https://doi.org/10.1016/j.neuropsychologia.2008.06.010

Kosfeld, M., Heinrichs, M., Zak, P. J., Fischbacher, U., & Fehr, E. (2005). Oxytocin increases trust in humans. *Nature*, 435(7042), 673–676. https://doi.org/10.1038/nature03701

Krosch, A. R., & Amodio, D. M. (2014). Economic scarcity alters the perception of race. *Proceedings of the National Academy of Sciences*, 111(25), 9079–9084. https://doi.org/10.1073/pnas.1404448111

(2019). Scarcity disrupts the neural encoding of Black faces: A socioperceptual pathway to discrimination. *Journal of Personality and Social Psychology*, 117(5), 859–875. https://doi.org/10.1037/pspa0000168

Krumhuber, E., Manstead, A. S. R., Cosker, D., Marshall, D., Rosin, P. L., & Kappas, A. (2007). Facial dynamics as indicators of trustworthiness and cooperative behavior. *Emotion*, 7(4), 730–735. https://doi.org/10.1037/1528-3542.7.4.730

Kubota, J. T., Li, J., Bar-David, E., Banaji, M. R., & Phelps, E. A. (2013). The price of racial bias: Intergroup negotiations in the ultimatum game. *Psychological Science*, 24(12), 2498–2504. https://doi.org/10.1177/0956797613496435

Kunda, Z. (1990). The case for motivated reasoning. *Psychological Bulletin*, 108(3), 480–498. https://doi.org/10.1037/0033-2909.108.3.480

Lambert, B., Declerck, C. H., Emonds, G., & Boone, C. (2017). Trust as commodity: Social value orientation affects the neural substrates of learning to cooperate. *Social Cognitive and Affective Neuroscience*, 12(4), 609–617. https://doi.org/10.1093/scan/nsw170

Li, D., Meng, L., & Ma, Q. (2017). Who deserves my trust? Cue-elicited feedback negativity tracks reputation learning in repeated social interactions. *Frontiers in Human Neuroscience*, 11, Article 307. https://doi.org/10.3389/fnhum.2017.00307

Li, H., Song, Y., & Xie, X. (2019). Altruistic or selfish? Responses when safety is threatened depend on childhood socioeconomic status. *European Journal of Social Psychology*, 50(5), 1001–1016. https://doi.org/10.1002/ejsp.2651

Li, J., Delgado, M. R., & Phelps, E. A. (2011). How instructed knowledge modulates the neural systems of reward learning. *Proceedings of the National Academy of Sciences*, 108(1), 55–60. https://doi.org/10.1073/pnas.1014938108

Luethi, M., Meier, B., & Sandi, C. (2009). Stress effects on working memory, explicit memory, and implicit memory for neutral and emotional stimuli in healthy men. *Frontiers in Behavioral Neuroscience*, 2(5). https://doi.org/10.3389/neuro.08.005.2008

Margittai, Z., Strombach, T., Van Wingerden, M., Joëls, M., Schwabe, L., & Kalenscher, T. (2015). A friend in need: Time-dependent effects of stress on social discounting in men. *Hormones and Behavior*, 73, 75–82. https://doi.org/10.1016/j.yhbeh.2015.05.019

Marzi, T., Righi, S., Ottonello, S., Cincotta, M., & Viggiano, M. P. (2014). Trust at first sight: Evidence from ERPs. *Social Cognitive and Affective Neuroscience*, 9(1), 63–72. https://doi.org/10.1093/scan/nss102

Mather, M., & Lighthall, N. R. (2012). Risk and reward are processed differently in decisions made under stress. *Current Directions in Psychological Science*, 21 (1), 36–41. https://doi.org/10.1177/0963721411429452

Mende-Siedlecki, P., Said, C. P., & Todorov, A. (2013). The social evaluation of faces: A meta-analysis of functional neuroimaging studies. *Social Cognitive and Affective Neuroscience*, 8(3), 285–299. https://doi.org/10.1093/scan/nsr090

Mende-Siedlecki, P., Verosky, S. C., Turk-Browne, N. B., & Todorov, A. (2013). Robust selectivity for faces in the human amygdala in the absence of expressions. *Journal of Cognitive Neuroscience*, 25(12), 2086–2106. https://doi.org/10.1162/jocn_a_00469

Morelli, S. A., Leong, Y. C., Carlson, R. W., Kullar, M., & Zaki, J. (2018). Neural detection of socially valued community members. *Proceedings of the National Academy of Sciences*, 115(32), 8149–8154. https://doi.org/10.1073/pnas.1712811115

Montague, P. R., Berns, G. S., Cohen, J. D., et al. (2002). Hyperscanning: Simultaneous fMRI during linked social interactions. *NeuroImage*, 16(4), 1159–1164. https://doi.org/10.1006/nimg.2002.1150

O'Doherty, J., Dayan, P., Schultz, J., Deichmann, R., Friston, K., & Dolan, R. J. (2004). Dissociable roles of ventral and dorsal striatum in instrumental conditioning. *Science*, 304(5669), 452–454. https://doi.org/10.1126/science.1094285

O'Doherty, J. P., Lee, S. W., & McNamee, D. (2015). The structure of reinforcement-learning mechanisms in the human brain. *Current Opinion in Behavioral Sciences*, 1, 94–100. https://doi.org/10.1016/j.cobeha.2014.10.004

Oh, D., Shafir, E., & Todorov, A. (2020). Economic status cues from clothes affect perceived competence from faces. *Nature Human Behaviour*, 4(3), 287–293. https://doi.org/10.1038/s41562-019-0782-4

Olcaysoy Okten, I., Magerman, A., & Forbes, C. E. (2020). Behavioral and neural indices of trust formation in cross-race and same-race interactions. *Journal of Neuroscience, Psychology, and Economics*, 13(2), 100–125. https://doi.org/10.1037/npe0000127

Olivola, C. Y., & Todorov, A. (2010). Elected in 100 milliseconds: Appearance-based trait inferences and voting. *Journal of Nonverbal Behavior*, 34(2), 83–110. https://doi.org/10.1007/s10919-009-0082-1

Oosterhof, N. N., & Todorov, A. (2009). Shared perceptual basis of emotional expressions and trustworthiness impressions from faces. *Emotion*, 9(1), 128–133. https://doi.org/10.1037/a0014520

Park, B., Fareri, D., Delgado, M., & Young, L. (2020). The role of right temporoparietal junction in processing social prediction error across relationship contexts. *Social Cognitive and Affective Neuroscience*. https://doi.org/10.1093/scan/nsaa072

Park, B., & Young, L. (2020). An association between biased impression updating and relationship facilitation: A behavioral and fMRI investigation. *Journal of

Experimental Social Psychology, 87, Article 103916. https://doi.org/10.1016/j .jesp.2019.103916

Phan, K. L., Sripada, C. S., Angstadt, M., & McCabe, K. (2010). Reputation for reciprocity engages the brain reward center. *Proceedings of the National Academy of Sciences*, 107(29), 13099–13104. https://doi.org/10.1073/pnas .1008137107

Plessow, F., Fischer, R., Kirschbaum, C., & Goschke, T. (2011). Inflexibly focused under stress: Acute psychosocial stress increases shielding of action goals at the expense of reduced cognitive flexibility with increasing time lag to the stressor. *Journal of Cognitive Neuroscience*, 23(11), 3218–3227. https://doi.org/10.1162/jocn_a_00024

Plessow, F., Kiesel, A., & Kirschbaum, C. (2012). The stressed prefrontal cortex and goal-directed behaviour: Acute psychosocial stress impairs the flexible implementation of task goals. *Experimental Brain Research*, 216(3), 397–408. https://doi.org/10.1007/s00221-011-2943-1

Porcelli, A. J., & Delgado, M. R. (2017). Stress and decision making: Effects on valuation, learning, and risk-taking. *Current Opinion in Behavioral Sciences*, 14, 33–39. https://doi.org/10.1016/j.cobeha.2016.11.015

Porcelli, A. J., Lewis, A. H., & Delgado, M. R. (2012). Acute stress influences neural circuits of reward processing. *Frontiers in Neuroscience*, 6(157). https://doi.org/10.3389/fnins.2012.00157

Radell, M. L., Sanchez, R., Weinflash, N., & Myers, C. E. (2016). The personality trait of behavioral inhibition modulates perceptions of moral character and performance during the trust game: Behavioral results and computational modeling. *PeerJ*, 4, Article e1631. https://doi.org/10.7717/peerj.1631

Raio, C. M., Orederu, T. A., Palazzolo, L., Shurick, A. A., & Phelps, E. A. (2013). Cognitive emotion regulation fails the stress test. *Proceedings of the National Academy of Sciences*, 110(37), 15139–15144. https://doi.org/10 .1073/pnas.1305706110

Raposa, E. B., Laws, H. B., & Ansell, E. B. (2015). Prosocial behavior mitigates the negative effects of stress in everyday life. *Clinical Psychological Science*, 4 (4), 691–698. https://doi.org/10.1177/2167702615611073

Rescorla, R., & Wagner, A. (1972). A theory of Pavlovian conditioning: Variations in the effectiveness of reinforcement and nonreinforcement. In A. H. Black & W. F. Prokasy (Eds.), *Classical conditioning II: Current research and theory* (Vol. 2, pp. 64–99). Appleton-Century-Crofts.

Rezlescu, C., Duchaine, B., Olivola, C. Y., & Chater, N. (2012). Unfakeable facial configurations affect strategic choices in trust games with or without information about past behavior. *PLoS ONE*, 7(3), Article e34293. https:// doi.org/10.1371/journal.pone.0034293

Roozendaal, B., McReynolds, J. R., Van der Zee, E. A., Lee, S., McGaugh, J. L., & McIntyre, C. K. (2009). Glucocorticoid effects on memory consolidation depend on functional interactions between the medial prefrontal cortex and basolateral amygdala. *Journal of Neuroscience*, 29(45), 14299–14308. https:// doi.org/10.1523/JNEUROSCI.3626-09.2009

Rule, N. O., Freeman, J. B., Moran, J. M., Gabrieli, J. D. E., Adams, R. B., & Ambady, N. (2010). Voting behavior is reflected in amygdala response across cultures. *Social Cognitive and Affective Neuroscience*, 5(2–3), 349–355. https://doi.org/10.1093/scan/nsp046

Rule, N. O., Krendl, A. C., Ivcevic, Z., & Ambady, N. (2013). Accuracy and consensus in judgments of trustworthiness from faces: Behavioral and neural correlates. *Journal of Personality and Social Psychology*, 104(3), 409–426. https://doi.org/10.1037/a0031050

Said, C. P., Baron, S. G., & Todorov, A. (2009). Nonlinear amygdala response to face trustworthiness: Contributions of high and low spatial frequency information. *Journal of Cognitive Neuroscience*, 21(3), 519–528. https://doi.org/10.1162/jocn.2009.21041

Salam, A. P., Rainford, E., Van Vugt, M., & Ronay, R. (2017). Acute stress reduces perceived trustworthiness of male racial outgroup faces. *Adaptive Human Behavior and Physiology*, 3(4), 282–292. https://doi.org/10.1007/s40750-017-0065-0

Santos, S., Almeida, I., Oliveiros, B., & Castelo-Branco, M. (2016). The role of the amygdala in facial trustworthiness processing: A systematic review and meta-analyses of fMRI Studies. *PLoS ONE*, 11(11), Article e0167276. https://doi.org/10.1371/journal.pone.0167276

Schilke, O., Reimann, M., & Cook, K. S. (2013). Effect of relationship experience on trust recovery following a breach. *Proceedings of the National Academy of Sciences*, 110(38), 15236–15241. https://doi.org/10.1073/pnas.1314857110

Schoofs, D., Wolf, O. T., & Smeets, T. (2009). Cold pressor stress impairs performance on working memory tasks requiring executive functions in healthy young men. *Behavioral Neuroscience*, 123(5), 1066–1075. https://doi.org/10.1037/a0016980

Schultz, W., Dayan, P., & Montague, P. R. (1997). A neural substrate of prediction and reward. *Science*, 275(5306), 1593–1599. https://doi.org/10.1126/science.275.5306.1593

Schweda, A., Faber, N. S., Crockett, M. J., & Kalenscher, T. (2019). The effects of psychosocial stress on intergroup resource allocation. *Scientific Reports*, 9(1), Article 18620. https://doi.org/10.1038/s41598-019-54954-w

Seeley, W. W., Menon, V., Schatzberg, A. F., et al. (2007). Dissociable intrinsic connectivity networks for salience processing and executive control. *Journal of Neuroscience*, 27(9), 2349–2356. https://doi.org/10.1523/jneurosci.5587-06.2007

Shteingart, H., & Loewenstein, Y. (2014). Reinforcement learning and human behavior. *Current Opinion in Neurobiology*, 25, 93–98. https://doi.org/10.1016/j.conb.2013.12.004

Sofer, C., Dotsch, R., Oikawa, M., Oikawa, H., Wigboldus, D. H. J., & Todorov, A. (2017). For your local eyes only: Culture-specific face typicality influences perceptions of trustworthiness. *Perception*, 46(8), 914–928. https://doi.org/10.1177/0301006617691786

Stanley, D. A. (2016). Getting to know you: General and specific neural computations for learning about people. *Social Cognitive and Affective Neuroscience*, 11(4), 525–536. https://doi.org/10.1093/scan/nsv145

Stanley, D. A., Sokol-Hessner, P., Banaji, M. R., & Phelps, E. A. (2011). Implicit race attitudes predict trustworthiness judgments and economic trust decisions. *Proceedings of the National Academy of Sciences*, 108(19), 7710–7715. https://doi.org/10.1073/pnas.1014345108

Stanley, D. A., Sokol-Hessner, P., Fareri, D. S., et al. (2012). Race and reputation: Perceived racial group trustworthiness influences the neural correlates of trust decisions. *Philosophical Transactions of the Royal Society B: Biological Sciences*, 367(1589), 744–753. https://doi.org/10.1098/rstb.2011.0300

Steinbeis, N., Engert, V., Linz, R., & Singer, T. (2015). The effects of stress and affiliation on social decision making: Investigating the tend-and-befriend pattern. *Psychoneuroendocrinology*, 62, 138–148. https://doi.org/10.1016/j.psyneuen.2015.08.003

Sutton, R. S., & Barto, A. G. (1998). *Reinforcement learning: An introduction*. The MIT Press. https://muse.jhu.edu/book/60836

Suzuki, A., Ito, Y., Kiyama, S., et al. (2016). Involvement of the ventrolateral prefrontal cortex in learning others' bad reputations and indelible distrust. *Frontiers in Human Neuroscience*, 10, Article 28. https://doi.org/10.3389/fnhum.2016.00028

Tajfel, H., & Turner, J. C. (1986). The social identity theory of intergroup behavior. In S. Worchel and W. G. Austin (Eds.), *Psychology of intergroup relations* (pp. 7–24). Hall Publishers.

Tashjian, S. M., Guassi Moreira, J. F., & Galván, A. (2019). Multivoxel pattern analysis reveals a neural phenotype for trust bias in adolescents. *Journal of Cognitive Neuroscience*, 31(11), 1726–1741. https://doi.org/10.1162/jocn_a_01448

Taylor, S. E. (2006). Tend and befriend: Biobehavioral bases of affiliation under stress. *Current Directions in Psychological Science*, 15(6), 273–277. https://doi.org/10.1111/j.1467-8721.2006.00451.x

Taylor, S. E., & Master, S. L. (2011). Social responses to stress: The tend-and-befriend model. In R. J. Contrada & A. Baum (Eds.), *The handbook of stress science: Biology, psychology, and health* (pp. 101–109). Springer.

Theeuwes, J., & Van der Stigchel, S. (2006). Faces capture attention: Evidence from inhibition of return. *Visual Cognition*, 13(6), 657–665. https://doi.org/10.1080/13506280500410949

Todorov, A. (2012). The role of the amygdala in face perception and evaluation. *Motivation and Emotion*, 36(1), 16–26. https://doi.org/10.1007/s11031-011-9238-5

Todorov, A., Baron, S. G., & Oosterhof, N. N. (2008). Evaluating face trustworthiness: A model based approach. *Social Cognitive and Affective Neuroscience*, 3(2), 119–127. https://doi.org/10.1093/scan/nsn009

Todorov, A., Mandisodza, A. N., Goren, A., & Hall, C. C. (2005). Inferences of competence from faces predict election outcomes. *Science*, 308(5728), 1623–1626. https://doi.org/10.1126/science.1110589

Todorov, A., Mende-Siedlecki, P., & Dotsch, R. (2013). Social judgments from faces. *Current Opinion in Neurobiology*, 23(3), 373–380. https://doi.org/10 .1016/j.conb.2012.12.010

Todorov, A., Olivola, C. Y., Dotsch, R., & Mende-Siedlecki, P. (2015). Social attributions from faces: Determinants, consequences, accuracy, and functional significance. *Annual Review of Psychology*, 66, 519–545. https://doi .org/10.1146/annurev-psych-113011-143831

Todorov, A., Pakrashi, M., & Oosterhof, N. N. (2009). Evaluating faces on trustworthiness after minimal time exposure. *Social Cognition*, 27(6), 813–833. https://doi.org/10.1521/soco.2009.27.6.813

Utevsky, A. V., Smith, D. V., Young, J. S., & Huettel, S. A. (2017). Large-scale network coupling with the fusiform cortex facilitates future social motivation. *ENeuro*, 4(5). https://doi.org/10.1523/ENEURO.0084-17.2017

Van IJzendoorn, M. H., & Bakermans-Kranenburg, M. J. (2012). Differential susceptibility experiments: Going beyond correlational evidence: Comment on beyond mental health, differential susceptibility articles. *Developmental Psychology*, 48(3), 769–774. https://doi.org/10.1037/a0027536

Van't Wout, M., & Sanfey, A. G. (2008). Friend or foe: The effect of implicit trustworthiness judgments in social decision making. *Cognition*, 108(3), 796–803. https://doi.org/10.1016/j.cognition.2008.07.002

Vanyukov, P. M., Hallquist, M. N., Delgado, M., Szanto, K., & Dombrovski, A. Y. (2019). Neurocomputational mechanisms of adaptive learning in social exchanges. *Cognitive, Affective, & Behavioral Neuroscience*, 19(4), 985–997. https://doi.org/10.3758/s13415-019-00697-0

Vieira, J., Schellhaas, S., Enström, E., & Olsson, A. (2020). Help or flight? Increased threat imminence promotes defensive helping in humans. https://doi.org/10.31234/osf.io/bckn3

von Dawans, B., Ditzen, B., Trueg, A., Fischbacher, U., & Heinrichs, M. (2019). Effects of acute stress on social behavior in women. *Psychoneuroendocrinology*, 99, 137–144. https://doi.org/10.1016/j.psyneuen.2018.08.031

von Dawans, B., Fischbacher, U., Kirschbaum, C., Fehr, E., & Heinrichs, M. (2012). The social dimension of stress reactivity: Acute stress increases prosocial behavior in humans. *Psychological Science*, 23(6), 651–660. https://doi.org/10.1177/0956797611431576

Wardle, M. C., Fitzgerald, D. A., Angstadt, M., Sripada, C. S., McCabe, K., & Luan Phan, K. (2013). The caudate signals bad reputation during trust decisions. *PLoS ONE*, 8(6), Article e68884. https://doi.org/10.1371/ journal.pone.0068884

Williams, K. D., Cheung, C. K. T., & Choi, W. (2000). Cyberostracism: Effects of being ignored over the Internet. *Journal of Personality and Social Psychology*, 79(5), 748–762. https://doi.org/10.1037/0022-3514.79.5.748

Wilson, J. P., & Rule, N. O. (2015). Facial trustworthiness predicts extreme criminal-sentencing outcomes. *Psychological Science*, 26(8), 1325–1331. https://doi.org/10.1177/0956797615590992

Winston, J. S., Strange, B. A., O'Doherty, J., & Dolan, R. J. (2002). Automatic and intentional brain responses during evaluation of trustworthiness of faces. *Nature Neuroscience*, 5(3), 277–283. https://doi.org/10.1038/nn816

Wu, C.-T., Fan, Y.-T., Du, Y.-R., et al. (2018). How do acquired political identities influence our neural processing toward others within the context of a trust game? *Frontiers in Human Neuroscience*, 12, Article 23. https://doi.org/10.3389/fnhum.2018.00023

Yan, X., Yong, X., Huang, W., & Ma, Y. (2018). Placebo treatment facilitates social trust and approach behavior. *Proceedings of the National Academy of Sciences*, 115(22), 5732–5737. https://doi.org/10.1073/pnas.1800779115

Zaki, J., Kallman, S., Wimmer, G. E., Ochsner, K., & Shohamy, D. (2016). Social cognition as reinforcement learning: Feedback modulates emotion inference. *Journal of Cognitive Neuroscience*, 28(9), 1270–1282. https://doi.org/10.1162/jocn_a_00978

Zarolia, P., Weisbuch, M., & McRae, K. (2017). Influence of indirect information on interpersonal trust despite direct information. *Journal of Personality and Social Psychology*, 112(1), 39–57. https://doi.org/10.1037/pspi0000074

CHAPTER 8

Trust and Learning
Neurocomputational Signatures of Learning to Trust

Gabriele Bellucci and Jean-Claude Dreher

8.1 Introduction

Learning whom to trust or distrust is an important skill in building social relationships. This chapter focuses on learning dynamics underlying decisions whether to trust or distrust other partners in social interactions. Two main experimental paradigms have been employed to investigate how people learn whom to trust. One experimental setting refers to advice-taking paradigms (Yaniv & Kleinberger, 2000). In this type of paradigm, two partners interact with each other as adviser and advisee, respectively. Participants take in general the role of advisee and need to decide whether to trust the information provided by the advisers. Advice utilization operationalizes trusting and reciprocal behaviors in these paradigms. In general, two estimates are required from participants, before and after seeing the advice of an adviser, and the degree to which participants revise their opinion after receiving advice measures their willingness to trust the received information and hence, by proxy, its source. Participants' trust and reciprocity are further modulated in these paradigms by manipulating social characteristics of the advisers, such as their competence, confidence, and kindness (Biele et al., 2009, 2011; Hertz et al., 2017; Mahmoodi et al., 2018; Meshi et al., 2012; Toelch et al., 2014).

Another experimental setting is the economic game known as the investment (or trust) game (Berg et al., 1995) (see also Chapter 2). In a standard investment game, a player in the role of investor receives an initial endowment and needs to decide whether to share some of it with a partner

Gabriele Bellucci is supported by the Max Planck Society. Jean-Claude Dreher was funded by the IDEX-LYON from the University of Lyon (project INDEPTH) within the program Investissements d'Avenir (ANR-16-IDEX-0005) and by the LABEX CORTEX (ANR-11-LABX-0042) of the University of Lyon, within the program Investissements d'Avenir (ANR-11-IDEX-007) operated by the French National Research Agency (ANR), and grants from the ANR and the National Science Foundation, within the Collaborative Research in Computational Neuroscience program (ANR-16-NEUC-0003-01). Corresponding author: Gabriele Bellucci (gbellucc@gmail.com).

in the role of trustee. If any money is shared, the amount is multiplied (usually tripled) and passed on to the trustee. The trustee needs now to decide whether to share any portion of the multiplied amount back to the investor or keep the entire amount. The investor's decision is regarded as a trust decision, while the trustee's decision is regarded as reciprocity (Chaudhuri & Gangadharan, 2007; Csukás et al., 2008). Such a version of the investment game has mainly been used to study trust in reciprocity and cooperation, but lends itself to also investigate more strategic forms of behaviors (Camerer, 2003; Chaudhuri et al., 2002; Krueger et al., 2007, 2008).

In Section 8.2, we review evidence about the type of social information about others (i.e., their social characteristics and psychological traits) that functions as central determinant and predictor of trustworthiness impressions and trusting behaviors. In Section 8.3, we turn to examine the learning dynamics and computational mechanisms that unravel how people integrate these different pieces of social information about others to update their trustworthiness beliefs and revise their trusting behaviors. In Section 8.4, we review neuroimaging evidence on the neural underpinnings of these learning processes. Finally, in Section 8.5, we draw conclusions on the neurocomputational processes underlying learning to trust, draft possible insights for clinical research, and propose future directions for forthcoming investigations.

8.2   Shades of Trust

8.2.1   The Traits One Can Trust

Across disciplines, trust is defined as the willingness to be vulnerable to another on the basis of positive expectations of the other's intentions and behaviors (Rousseau et al., 1998). A similar multidisciplinary definition of trust underlines that trust occurs when no control over the other's behavior is possible (Mayer et al., 1995). The absence of control refers to cases in which an agent's decision outcomes depend on someone else's decisions that the agent cannot (or does not want to) monitor or regulate. Interactions where rules and monitoring activities are in place, such as contracts that regulate the expected behavior of another person and define deterrents for deviant behaviors, do not require trust. Importantly, when an agent eschews the imposition of regulatory frames, the ultimate decision to trust lies in the positive expectations of the other person's intentions. Information that drives an individual to focus on the possible bad

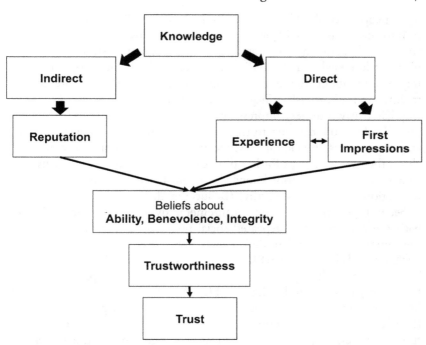

Figure 8.1 Schematic formation of trustworthiness impressions guiding trust behavior. Information leading to the formation of trustworthiness judgments is based on either direct or indirect information about the partner's character and behaviors. Indirect information refers mostly to the other's reputation. On the contrary, direct knowledge might vary in nature depending on how well the other person is known. Literature on trust can be roughly divided into studies on first impressions about others and repeated interactions (establishing a history of experiences with the other person). This information helps build beliefs about three main characteristics of the other person: her ability, benevolence, and integrity. Judgments about others' trustworthiness are formed on the basis of these beliefs and ultimately guide trust decisions in social interactions.

intentions of another, for instance, by simply calling the other person an "opponent," evokes negative expectations that corrupt trust (Burnham et al., 2000). Similarly, showing distrustful behavior toward another person elicits the expectation that the target of such distrustful behavior is herself untrustworthy and need to be avoided, or ostracized (Hillebrandt et al., 2011). However, how do people form such expectations?

Expectations might arise from indirect or direct knowledge (Figure 8.1). Individuals might form trustworthiness judgments based on a person's reputation, which mainly originates in indirect information received from other people (see also Chapter 7). On the contrary, direct knowledge refers to information gathered from a more or less shallow, personal interaction with the other person. The literature on trust has mainly studied two forms of direct knowledge. First, individuals might rely on subjective (implicit) impressions about the other person's trustworthiness that are formed rapidly and effortlessly (Siegel et al., 2019; Todorov et al., 2009). Implicit trustworthiness impressions have reliably been shown to play a pivotal role in the decision to trust unknown others or strangers in single and anonymous interactions, where individuals do not know anything about the partner except for her physical appearance (e.g., facial trustworthiness) and/or some prior knowledge about her reputation (e.g., indirect reputation of being trustworthy) (Bellucci et al., 2020).

Second, positive expectations can emerge dynamically from experience with the partner during repeated social interactions that give individuals the opportunity to update their beliefs about the partner's character and behaviors (Hula et al., 2018). For instance, an individual can learn the benevolence of her partner over the course of multiple interactions from the partner's kind behavior (Ho & Weigelt, 2005), and be more likely to reciprocate if she learns that the partner has previously trusted (McCabe et al., 2003). Importantly, also in repeated interactions, implicit trustworthiness impressions formed at the beginning of the interaction with the partner are not completely discarded but slowly integrated into the learning dynamics underlying trusting interactions, influencing the final trustworthiness judgments resulting from the social interaction (Chang et al., 2010).

Now, the question arises as to what kind of information individuals seek, gather, and integrate in these different contexts to make inferences about the other person's trustworthiness. A classic model posits that at least three characteristics (or traits) are central to the formation of trustworthiness impressions and the final trust decision (Figure 8.1). These characteristics hence constitute factors of perceived trustworthiness or antecedents of trust, and include the following: ability, benevolence, and integrity (Mayer et al., 1995).

Ability refers to skills and competencies of the trustee that are taken into consideration before a trust decision is made. The trustee might want to use her skills to help the trustor reach his goals. In general, the trustor might be more or less dependent on the trustee's skills for his actions. This interdependency creates the conditions for trust, as the trustor needs to believe that the trustee's skills can ultimately benefit him and that he cannot easily and inexpensively do well without them. These skills and abilities might be domain- or situation-specific, as individuals would rely on a doctor for a medical problem and ask a lawyer for a legal counseling and not vice versa. However, this restriction does not need to be valid in general, as competent individuals are perceived as domain-general authorities and might be asked for advice in other domains than the one they are known to be expert in. One reason for this is that individuals turn to experts not only because of their technical expertise in a specific field but also for their general, analytic skills that made them the experts they are in the first place. Hence, individuals might reach out to other-field experts to sample a different type of information from them, for instance, a methodological approach to make a specific decision, instead of requiring a specific solution to the problem at hand. Finally, individuals might also turn to experts just to receive a boost in their confidence.

Benevolence refers to the positive intentions and attitudes of the trustee. A trustee is benevolent to the extent to which she is willing to engage in actions that benefit the trustor despite their cognitive, physical, or monetary costs and beyond a strictly egocentric motivation for self-profit. With this respect, being altruistic and inclusive induces trustworthiness impressions in others that make the altruistic individual more likely to be trusted in social interactions, whereas excluding others for no ostensive reasons evokes impressions of a malevolent character that promote distrustful behaviors (Delgado et al., 2005; Frost et al., 1978). Benevolence is central to one's decision to trust (King-Casas et al., 2005). Signs that the other might have bad intentions or might not be well minded decrease one's willingness to trust, even when other information is available that would otherwise evoke trustworthiness impressions. For instance, individuals are more likely to be influenced by the advice of nonexperts with good intentions than by the advice of experts with likely bad intentions (McGinnies & Ward, 1980), suggesting that benevolence outweighs expertise when these types of information compete. Furthermore, unconditional kindness, but neither positive nor negative reciprocity, has strongly been associated with trusting behaviors (Thielmann & Hilbig, 2015). However, further studies are needed to better understand how individuals weight different trustworthiness sources for a decision to trust, as an expert is likely to be trusted despite a reputation of being untrustworthy if one's personal experience is inconsistent with the expert's reputation.

Finally, integrity refers to the extent to which the trustee adheres to a set of principles that the trustor finds acceptable. This factor closely relates to the moral dimension or the moral character of the trustee, and highlights the trustee's behavioral consistency that reflects the trustee's congruence to a determined set of values. For example, individuals with strong moral characteristics are perceived as more trustworthy, trusted more, preferred as social partner, and are believed to be more likely to reciprocate trust (Everett et al., 2016). However, simple behavioral consistency is not sufficient, as a trustee might consistently act in a self-serving manner (see also the relationship between trust and behavioral predictability). Recently, it has been proposed that integrity is not only an important characteristic of the trustee but also a relevant characteristic of the trustor, although for different reasons. While in the trustee integrity signals trustworthiness, in the trustor it impels to trust. Previous studies found, for example, that the sense of compliance with a trust norm and the sense of respect for the other person predict individual trust (Dunning et al., 2014), suggesting a normative (moral) component inherent to trust decisions (Dunning et al., 2019).

It has been shown that these factors of trust and trustworthiness are partly captured by three personality traits. In particular, a model of personality, namely the HEXACO Personality Inventory, has been operationalized in a self- and observer-report instrument consisting of six dimensions – Honesty-Humility (H), Emotionality (E), Extraversion (X), Agreeableness (A), Conscientiousness (C), and Openness to Experience (O) (Ashton & Lee, 2007; Ashton et al., 2004; Lee & Ashton, 2004). Studies using this inventory show that propensity to trust relies on positive expectations of social partners held by individuals who do not perceive others as exploitative (i.e., higher agreeableness), who feel optimistic in general (i.e., higher extraversion), and who are not themselves inclined to exploit others (i.e., higher honesty-humility) (Ashton et al., 2014).

8.2.2   *The Distrusting Side of Control*

In Section 8.2.1, we described factors that play a role in an individual's willingness to trust others. However, we have not yet touched on a related topic. In fact, it is not enough to identify which information is important for a trust decision. Most of the time, information is noisy or comes from individuals who are themselves untrustworthy or might have reasons to hide relevant information. To decrease decisional uncertainty originating from noisy sources, individuals might engage in different control strategies to check the other person's trustworthiness and boost one's confidence before trusting. But how much information is necessary to trust someone?

Is not seeking out more information to prove a source's reliability as such already a sign of distrust? The trade-off between exerting control (increasing one's confidence about the other person's trustworthiness) and giving up on control (blind trust) is extremely fragile.

Previous evidence has consistently shown that attempts to exert control signal untrustworthiness impressions and decrease others' trust. For example, requiring a partner to give up on control decreases the partner's willingness to trust, likely because it signals to the partner that she is not trusted (Das & Teng, 1998, 2001; Malhotra, 2004). That control behavior reflects untrustworthiness impressions was first investigated in a seminal work by Strickland (1958), where participants as supervisors needed to decide whether to monitor other participants playing the role of workers. Supervisors were incentivized to keep the workers' performance high over the course of the task but, at first, could only monitor in predetermined trials (monitored trials). However, after having received feedback about the history of the workers' performance in both monitored and nonmonitored trials at the end of the first part of the experiment, supervisors were allowed to freely choose whom to monitor in the second part. Results showed that workers who performed poorly in nonmonitored trials were judged as less trustworthy and monitored more often by supervisors.

Complementarily, individuals refrain from control behaviors to avoid inducing untrustworthiness impressions that might have a negative impact on a partner's decisions. For instance, in a recent study, participants had the opportunity to sample information about the history of their partners' reciprocal behavior before a decision to trust (Ma et al., 2020). In one condition, participants were told that the partner would be informed about how much they sampled (overt sampling condition), while in the other condition they were told that the partner would not know about their information-sampling behavior (covert sampling condition). Behavioral results showed that participants sampled less when sampling was overt and reported that they believed overt sampling information would make the partner's reciprocation less likely, suggesting that participants refrained from sampling to avoid inducing negative impressions.

Attempts to impose binding contracts have similar effects on trustworthiness impressions and trusting behaviors. Malhotra and Murnighan (2002) propose that trust and binding contrasts represent two mutually exclusive mechanisms of social behavior control and regulation. Trust is an informal mechanism of risk management for uncertainty reduction in social interactions, whereas binding contracts represent more a formal mechanism thereof. Importantly, while binding contracts facilitate exchanges and allow for successful negotiations, their enforcement erodes the development of interpersonal bonds and the establishment of interpersonal trust, which emerges only in situations where the partner's good intentions can be put at test (e.g., when there are incentives not to cooperate). Importantly, enforcing binding contracts are detrimental to trust, while trust increases in situations regulated by nonbinding contracts. This is because nonbinding contracts allow for attributions of positive, dispositional attitudes, as the partner's behavior is not dictated by exogenous, contextual factors (like in binding contracts) but by her personal choices and personality. As nonbinding contracts enable inferences on personal attributions for cooperation, they provide a better basis for building interpersonal trust and control uncertainty in several social interactions (Malhotra, 2004; Pillutla et al., 2003).

This raises the question as to whether efforts to detect trustworthiness can be seen as attempts to predict a partner's behavior for uncertainty reduction, given that trustworthiness hints at an individual's behavioral consistency (Lewis & Weigert, 1985). For instance, if I know that my decisions' outcomes hinge on your well-minded behavior, information about your trustworthiness will decrease the outcome uncertainty associated with my decisions. All things being equal, if you are trustworthy, the outcome I expect is the one that will realize. Similarly, if I have reasons to believe that you are not to be trusted, I will probably gauge the chances to be pretty low that a particular outcome contingent on our joint decisions will realize. Hence, trust might be compared to a probability distribution over outcome occurrences, giving the idea that trust is a form of risk (Coleman, 1990; Deutsch, 1958; Luhmann, 1979). However, recent empirical results refute this equation between trust and risk.

For example, previous studies have found no relationships between risk preferences and trust (Ashraf et al., 2006; Berg et al., 1995) (see also Chapter 5). Moreover, risk-averse behaviors in trusting interactions are very different from risk-averse behaviors in gambling contexts, as they yield different individual aversion parameters that do not map onto each other (Fairley et al., 2016). Several studies have provided evidence on the differences between trust and risk decisions. For example, individuals have been shown to be more reluctant to take a chance on another individual than on a lottery that randomly determines decision outcomes (Bohnet & Zeckhauser, 2004). Other studies have suggested a similar difference but in the opposite direction. In particular, a reduced willingness to trust a partner in Bohnet and Zeckhauser (2004) might be due to the fact that the partners had incentives to be untrustworthy (Snijders & Keren, 2001) and participants might have underestimated the proportion of those who would reciprocate (Dunning et al., 2019; Fetchenhauer & Dunning, 2009). In a recent study, individuals were found to be more likely to play a gamble when its outcomes depended on a partner with no incentives to be malevolent as opposed to chance (Bellucci et al., in press). These results accord with previous evidence that individuals are more likely to trust a partner who reciprocates frequently than playing with a slot machine that rewards with the same probability (Chang et al., 2010). Interestingly, the opposite effect was observed for untrustworthy partners. Specifically, participants are less willing to trust a partner who reciprocates infrequently than playing with a slot machine that rewards with the same probability (Chang et al., 2010). Overall, these results suggest that a partner's intentions are central to trust decisions in social interactions, which do not simply reduce to risk behaviors in nonsocial interactions.

A recent study extended these results. By eliminating incentives to be untrustworthy, participants were observed to have similar trust levels toward partners whose reputation was unknown and partners with a reputation of being trustworthy (Bellucci & Park, 2020). On the contrary, all untrustworthy partners were distrusted to a similar extent despite different degrees of untrustworthiness. These results suggest that people discriminate degrees of trustworthiness in a coarser way than risk probabilities – being more extreme in their trustworthiness perceptions. In this sense, trustworthiness impressions might be more discrete or even categorical, likely because another agent's behavior is traced back to a stable personality that is believed to bear a higher degree of consistency and coherence than agency-independent events. These behavioral observations have important implications for learning dynamics in social contexts.

These studies suggest that behavioral consistency, as a feature of an individual's trustworthiness, is pivotal for trust. Yet, trust cannot be reduced to a form of control behavior nor trustworthiness to predictability. This is because trust signals giving up on exerting control over other individuals. Indeed, people with low need to control others are perceived as more trustworthy, while attempts of control signal distrust (Frost et al., 1978). And finally, predictable peers are not necessarily trusted and the learning processes underlying the formation of trustworthiness beliefs about social partners manifest themselves as fundamentally different from learning patterns linked to the learning of outcome probabilities and event contingencies in nonsocial contexts (such as the risk domain).

8.3   Learning to Trust

8.3.1   Computational Models of Learning

The studies discussed so far provide evidence on behavioral differences across social and nonsocial contexts that hint at different underlying learning dynamics. Now, we turn to studies that analyze and formalize these learning dynamics (Cheong et al., 2017; Park et al., 2019). As previously mentioned, trustworthiness beliefs rely on indirect knowledge originating from another person's reputation, and from direct knowledge based on subjective first impressions or dynamic learning of the other's behavior through repeated experiences (Figure 8.2). This dynamic learning has been linked to reinforcement learning processes. Reinforcement learning describes how organisms learn by trial and error to predict and acquire rewards (Gershman & Daw, 2017). Reinforcement learning relies on prediction error (PE, or surprise), which signals the discrepancy between actual and expected rewards (Rudebeck et al., 2013; Tsuchida et al., 2010). The Rescorla–Wagner model formalizes learning as trial-by-trial updates of expectations according to the current prediction error (Rescorla & Wagner, 1972). Expectations (or predictions) of the obtainable reward

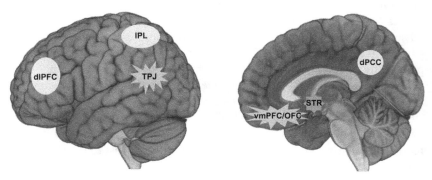

Figure 8.2   Brain regions involved in trust learning.
The STR underlies action–outcome associative learning allowing the identification of discrepancies in another person's behavior. Activity in the ventromedial prefrontal cortex/orbitofrontal cortex (vmPFC/OFC) encodes character trait information about the other. The temporoparietal junction (TPJ) represents current beliefs about the other's likely behavior. The inferior parietal lobule (IPL), dorsolateral prefrontal cortex (dlPFC), and dorsal posterior cingulate cortex (dPCC) integrate current feedback about others' trustworthiness with knowledge about their reputation to guide present and future decisions.

associated with a stimulus *s* are encapsulated by $V_t(s_t)$, that is, the value associated with a particular stimulus at trial *t*. Given that R_t describes the received reward at trial *t*, updates of reward expectations are formalized as follows:

$$PE_t = R_t - V_t(s_t), \tag{1}$$

where PE_t is the prediction error at trial *t*. PEs are smaller when the received reward is close to what is expected and larger when the received reward is far from what is expected. The PE can be thought of as the quantity that determines how much update is needed. The more we learn about the associative strength between a particular stimulus and its reward, the less learning occurs, as the expected reward approximates the actual reward. This implies that our expectation (prediction) of a reward *R* given a stimulus *s* will increase in accuracy over time with a concomitant reduction of discrepancy (error). Importantly, this learning process is not linear but hinges on individual learning parameters that determine the size of the update step and so affect the magnitude of the changes involved. Hence, the predicted value of a stimulus *s* on the next trial *t* is updated as follows:

$$V_{t+1}(s_t) = V_t(s_t) + \alpha * PE_t, \tag{2}$$

where α is the individual learning rate (usually between 0 and 1) updating the reward expectation. The value of a stimulus updated with large learning rates reflects the more recent history of received rewards, as reward expectations are updated by more heavily weighting the current reward. On the contrary, the value of a stimulus updated with small learning rates reflects the more remote history of rewards, as reward expectations are updated by more strongly weighting the expectations.

On the neural level, PEs are carried by dopaminergic neurons (Montague et al., 1996; Schultz et al., 1997). In particular, phasic dopaminergic responses in the midbrain, striatum (STR), and orbitofrontal cortex (OFC) show properties similar to reward PEs as described by the Rescorla–Wagner model (Hollerman & Schultz, 1998; Schultz, 2000; Schultz et al., 1997). Combining reinforcement learning models with neuroimaging, correlations between neural signals and model-based PEs have been observed in humans as well, such as in the ventral striatum (vSTR) (Dreher et al., 2006; O'Doherty et al., 2004), anterior insula (Preuschoff et al., 2006), hippocampus (Vanni-Mercier et al., 2009), OFC (Li et al., 2016; Metereau & Dreher, 2015), and midbrain (Howard & Kahnt, 2018). While reinforcement learning models were initially employed to describe instrumental learning (i.e., Pavlovian conditioning), they have recently been used to characterize other forms of learning (Joiner et al., 2017), like learning another person's character traits (Biele et al., 2009; Chang et al., 2010; Delgado et al., 2005; Fouragnan et al., 2013).

In social interactions, learning is complicated by the intentional stance of the interacting partner. Hence, an agent does not only need to learn the associations between events to identify actions for reward maximization and loss avoidance, but it also needs to consider the intentions of the interacting partner to correctly weight the outcomes of the social interaction. Indeed, positive outcomes can hide bad intentions and negative outcomes can be the by-product of a well-minded action. Hence, in social contexts, events bear information about the partners' action utilities, which allow estimations of their interests, inferences on their intentions, and predictions of their future behavior. A well-known formalization of action utilities for social behaviors in simple two-person interactions is provided by the Fehr–Schmidt model (Fehr & Schmidt, 1999).

Within the Fehr–Schmidt framework, kind and unkind intentions are reflected by fair and unfair behaviors, which can be described as self- and other-centered inequity aversion. Individuals are inequity averse if they dislike outcomes that are perceived as inequitable (Fehr & Schmidt, 1999). Inequity aversion is self-centered when individuals care about their own material payoff relative to the payoff of others and increases with increasing disadvantageous inequity (the less the individual has relative to others). Inequity aversion is other-centered when individuals care about the payoff of others relative to their own material payoff and increases with increasing advantageous inequity (the more the individual has relative to others). Given this definition of fairness, which is exclusively based on the importance (or weighting) people ascribe to outcomes of joint behaviors in social interactions, fair and unfair behaviors can be formalized with a utility function. Let $x = x_1, \ldots, x_n$ denote the vector of outcomes (e.g., monetary payoffs) for specific actions of a set of n players indexed by $i \in \{1, \ldots, n\}$. The utility function of player $i \in \{1, \ldots, n\}$ is given by:

$$U_i(x) = x_i - \alpha_i \, max \left\{ x_j - x_i, 0 \right\} - \beta_i \, max \left\{ x_i - x_j, 0 \right\}, \qquad i \neq j. \quad (3)$$

As can be seen in Equation (3), the utility U_i of player i is a weighted sum of the utility gain from player i's outcome (i.e., x_i) and the utility losses from disadvantageous (i.e., $\alpha_i \, max \left\{ x_j - x_i, 0 \right\}$) and advantageous (i.e., $\beta_i \, max \left\{ x_i - x_j, 0 \right\}$) inequities. That is, when player i has much less than player j (i.e., $x_j > x_i$), the utility of player i's outcome is reduced by disadvantageous inequity aversion (or envy), as individuals dislike having less than others. Similarly, when player i has much more than player j (i.e., $x_j < x_i$), the utility of player i's outcome is reduced by advantageous inequity aversion (or guilt), as individuals feel guilty for having more than others. In Equation (3), α_i and β_i are subject-specific parameters that capture individual differences in how much people value the disutilities from disadvantageous and advantageous inequities.

Despite this model neatly capturing mentalizing processes (e.g., how people think about others' fairness) in trusting interactions (Hula et al., 2015, 2018; Khalvati et al., 2019; Xiang et al., 2012), it still has important limitations. For instance, it does not take into consideration that the costs of mentalizing are cognitively nonnegligible (e.g., limited working memory), especially when mentalizing involves prospection (Na et al., 2019). To reduce such costs, individuals use trustworthiness as a safety signal that allows them to engage in costly inferences on a partner's behavior only when the partner's trustworthiness is low or unknown (Sperber et al., 2010; Wu et al., 2020). Hence, computational models attempting to formalize social learning and mentalizing dynamics need to reliably address such a trade-off.

8.3.2   The Endurance of a Good Reputation

In social interactions, individuals are mainly tasked with the challenge of learning another person's character. The character of another points to generally stable traits that allow reliable inferences on the other person's intentions and actions, and on the quality of the information she has and communicates (e.g., her credibility). Reliable group members are believed to be a source of accurate information (Gordon & Spears, 2012) and information sharing is associated with trust (Burt & Knez, 1995). In contrast, a bad reputation has a deleterious effect on beliefs about others' trustworthiness and credibility (McGinnies & Ward, 1980; Reichelt, Sievert, & Jacob, 2013; Weiner & Mowen, 1986). Similarly, lying, both in the forms of concealment of information and sharing of inaccurate information, calls for norm-enforcing behaviors such as punishment (Fehr & Fischbacher, 2003; Sánchez-Pagés & Vorsatz, 2007).

Because reliable, trustworthy, and credible individuals are likely to benefit the group as a whole by sharing accurate information, engaging in prosocial behaviors, or holding their word in task assignments and promises (Becker et al., 2017; Galton, 1907; Mellers et al., 2014; Sjöberg, 2009), societies have a strong interest of promoting and reinforcing good, prosocial qualities. Reputation functions as a proxy for credit assignment based on a person's past behavior in a social group and represents an important mechanism for cooperation in heterogeneous, large-scale societies (Fehr & Fischbacher, 2004). Reputation works like a social tag to easily distinguish good cooperators from bad ones, especially when no prior information about the partners is provided. In this sense, it can be used as a prior for first interactions with other people that is subsequently updated based on new incoming information about the partner's behavior. Hence, with new information about a partner's character traits, individuals should be able to successfully update their trustworthiness beliefs about the partner. However, we will see that reputation strongly biases people's initial impressions and learning, even impacting neural responses to rewards.

In particular, individuals believe that positive traits are more frequent than negative traits and that positive traits are more easily lost than negative ones (Rothbart & Park, 1986). Consequently, the theory of trust asymmetry posits that a good reputation is more easily lost than gained and hence individuals are faster at adapting their behavior after feedback about another person's untrustworthiness than after feedback about another person's trustworthiness. This prediction is based on early evidence that trust is decreased more by negative events than increased by positive ones (Slovic, 1993). These results chime well with a general pattern of evaluations of good and positive feedbacks in humans, which suggests that negative information (e.g., negative events and monetary losses) loom greater than positive ones (e.g., positive events and monetary gains) (Kahneman & Tversky, 1979; Platt & Huettel, 2008; Tversky & Kahneman, 1992).

The theory of trust asymmetry relies on evidence that impressions about favorable traits (such as one's ability and integrity) require more instances to form than impressions about unfavorable traits and unfavorable traits are harder to lose. For example, a previous study has found that individuals more strongly distrust nonexpert advisers with a reputation of being expert than trust expert advisers with a reputation of being nonexpert (Yaniv & Kleinberger, 2000). Hence, individuals seem to more readily distrust those with a good reputation when current disconfirming information is provided. On the contrary, a bad reputation hampers attempts to regain trust, confirming that negative experiences with a social partner have greater influence than positive ones (Yaniv, 2006). Despite this apparently confirming evidence, another important phenomenon that generally goes overlooked is that impressions about others' traits that are more easily formed are also harder to lose irrespective of the favorability of the trait (Rothbart & Park, 1986). Consequently, if it is easier to form a positive impression (maybe because of some prior beliefs or the particular situation and context), that impression will be also more enduring and harder to lose.

In the previous study by Yaniv and Kleinberger (2000), participants had to learn advisers' expertise from feedback about complicated factual knowledge and the advisers were deprived of intentionality, as participants believed the advisers were always communicating their best guess. A recent study tried to overcome this limitation by allowing advisers to deliberately decide whether to be honest or dishonest in advice giving (Bellucci & Park, 2020). Being honest was a reasonable behavioral strategy for advisers to build a good reputation that could have paid off in a subsequent interaction, where participants could repay the advisers for their advice-giving behavior. This established a social context that facilitated the formation of positive trustworthiness impressions. However, being dishonest was not disincentivized and represented a cognitively, less costly strategy. Results show that initial levels of trust were very high for all advisers, confirming that the experimental situation induced positive priors about the interacting partners. However, after a couple of trials (during the reputation-building phase) participants realized that some advisers were not honest and quickly adjusted their behavioral strategy accordingly. At the end of the reputation-building phase, participants could clearly distinguish advisers with a reputation of being dishonest from advisers with a reputation of being honest.

Now, later on in the experiment, advisers with a bad reputation began to show signs of honesty, while advisers with a good reputation turned dishonest. Notably, participants successfully revised their first impressions of the advisers with a bad reputation and trusted them increasingly more, but did not change their behavior toward the advisers with a good reputation, suggesting a learning impairment for the latter. A reinforcement learning model indicated a reputation-dependent asymmetry in the valuation of the advisers' honesty and dishonesty. Contrary to the theory of trust asymmetry, participants did not weight dishonesty more than honesty, and the dishonesty of the advisers with a good reputation was not weighted more than the dishonesty of the advisers with a bad reputation. On the contrary, a good reputation strengthened the valuation of honest behavior, whereas a bad reputation corroborated valuation of dishonest behavior (Bellucci & Park, 2020).

Virtually the same results were found by Siegel et al. (2018) in a moral decision-making task, where participants observed the moral decisions of other co-players and rated their moral impressions of them. Participants learnt the reputation of the co-players who initially were either bad or good but then began to make decisions that were more or less moral than previously. Results showed that participants updated their moral impressions more for bad than for good co-players, suggesting that good impressions of a moral co-player did not optimally change when that co-player was less moral than previously, while bad impressions of an immoral co-player did not impair the accurate tracking of the co-player's morality (Siegel et al., 2018). Comparable results were found in a study by Fareri et al. (2012), where participants learnt the moral (first interaction) and trustworthy character (second interaction) of their partners in two consequential interactions. Despite similar trustworthy behaviors of the partners in the second interaction, participants were more likely to trust those partners who established a reputation of being moral in the first interaction. A reinforcement learning model indicated a reputation-dependent asymmetry in belief updating with trustworthiness beliefs being more likely updated after positive feedbacks for the partner with a good reputation but after negative feedbacks for the partner with a bad reputation. Finally, a recent study extended these results showing that such reputational bias can be observed only in social interactions with trustworthy partners but not in nonsocial contexts when playing with rewarding slot machines (Lamba et al., 2020).

These results suggest that the three antecedents of trust discussed in the previous paragraph contribute to trustworthiness impressions differently depending on the context. Moreover, traits closely related to the intentionality dimension are learnt faster and impact learning and trusting behavior more profoundly than traits associated with individual ability and expertise. However, to our knowledge, no study has directly compared how different antecedents of trust impact people's trustworthiness impressions in the same experiment. Future studies are thus necessary to understand whether and how different sources of information about others' traits are sampled and integrated for a decision to trust. In particular, computational research on how intentions of others are inferred and integrated into outcome valuations is still at an embryonic stage. Recent investigations implementing the Fehr–Schmidt model have revealed different levels of mentalizing sophistication. For example, a study by Xiang et al. (2012) estimated individual depth-of-thoughts (cognitive levels of sophistication of one's model of a partner's intentions) from trusting behavior in response to a partner's reciprocity. Results indicated at least three levels of depth-of-thought and showed that participants with the least sophisticated model of the partner's intentions were less successful at learning the partner's reciprocity for efficient cooperation. By highlighting the importance of mentalizing processes for accurate learning and adequate behavior revision in social interactions, these findings call for more investigations on the intentionality aspect inherent to social learning dynamics and the interactions with the types of situations where they occur.

8.4 Brain Trust

8.4.1 Identifying Signs of Distrust

Different neuroimaging studies have addressed the question as to which brain areas are involved in learning a partner's trustworthiness during social interactions (see also Chapter 7). An early study by Delgado et al. (2005) investigated neural responses to feedback about behaviors of partners of different moral character traits. Results demonstrated striatal responses underlying both a decision to trust a partner and learning that the partner reciprocated. Further, higher activations in the vSTR (Figure 8.2) were observed for trust in the partner with a bad reputation and in the caudate for reciprocal behavior of the same partner. On the contrary, no differences in neural responses in these regions were observed for the partner with a good reputation. These differences in neural responses in the STR might underlie the behavioral patterns discussed in the previous paragraph. In particular, as individuals seem to optimally revise their impressions of partners with a bad but not a good reputation, recruitment of the STR might support such behavioral updating for more efficient learning by integrating the relevant information. The caudate nucleus might specifically underlie updating of behaviorally relevant information about others, as this region is recruited particularly during interactions with individuals with a bad reputation (Wardle et al., 2013), and is consistently engaged in information processing about another person's behavior in trusting interactions (Bellucci et al., 2017).

Similarly, a study by King-Casas et al. (2005) found the caudate to be involved in learning from a partner's reciprocal behavior. In particular, activations in the caudate peaked during the feedback phase at the beginning of the trusting interaction but shifted over time from the period of the revelation of the other person's behavior to the period prior to it. These findings seem to suggest that striatal activity tracks the partner's reciprocity over time and its temporal shift might represent a signature of learning dynamics, according to which the STR integrates information about the other's reputation for belief updating in early states but signals predictions or inferences on the other's likely reciprocal behavior in later stages. Another study has provided first evidence for the selective role of the STR in learning others' reciprocity. In particular, neural responses to cooperative partners with a reputation for reciprocity were observed both in the STR and OFC, another important region for learning (Gottfried & Dolan, 2004; Phan et al., 2010; Rudebeck & Murray, 2014). However, greater striatal activations for the cooperative than the uncooperative or neutral partners were observed only in the STR. Moreover, these striatal activations were specifically driven by stronger neural responses to feedbacks on the reciprocity of the cooperative partner (Phan et al., 2010), suggesting that striatal neural responses were selective to information received about the behavior of partners with a reputation for reciprocity.

If striatal activity plays a role in belief updating about others' trustworthiness for behavioral adaptation, activity in the STR should specifically track value updating over time. In particular, within the framework of reinforcement learning models, striatal activity should reflect PE trustworthiness signals in response to the partner's trustworthy behavior. The temporal shift of striatal activity in King-Casas et al. (2005) points to a role for the STR in PEs about others' traits (e.g., social PEs). Another neuroimaging study provided first model-based evidence to this hypothesis (Fareri et al., 2012). Model-based PEs correlated with neural signal in the STR during the revelation of the other person's behavior, suggesting that the STR was integrating information about the partner's trustworthiness based on feedback about the partner's reciprocal behavior. Importantly, however, no differences in neural signals were observed for partners with different reputations. Hence, despite this evidence on the involvement of striatal activity in trustworthiness belief updating for behavior adaptation to others' reputation, it is unclear whether the STR specifically reflects an individual's expectations of the partner (e.g., her reputation) or rather more general computational processes, such as information integration processes related to action–outcome associative learning.

8.4.2   Tracking Trustworthiness

The evidence discussed so far suggests a role of striatal regions in learning dynamics during trusting interactions, which are also involved in learning of other characteristics of social partners such as their prosocial tendencies (Lockwood et al., 2016). Further, recent pharmacological evidence has provided converging evidence for a role of the dopaminergic system in trusting behaviors (Bellucci et al., 2020). Given the high shared variance between trustworthiness and attractiveness – a primary reward (Bellucci et al., 2020; Stirrat & Perrett, 2010; Wilson & Eckel, 2006), it is not surprising that trustworthiness recruits brain areas known to encode several rewards (Aharon et al., 2001; O'Doherty et al., 2003; Pegors et al., 2015; Winston et al., 2007). Further, given the role of the STR in learning, the involvement of striatal structures during social learning seems to confirm investigations in the nonsocial domain. However, at least two limitations can be highlighted. First, most of this evidence comes from experimental paradigms, such as economic games, where "trust decisions" are inextricably intertwined with monetary rewards. Thus, paradigms and computational models that investigate belief updating in these experiments need to control for neural signatures associated with reward PEs, especially because those striatal activations were consistently observed during feedback phases where participants not only learn about the partner's behavior but also get to know how much they earned in the trial. Second, neural patterns in these brain structures are mostly associated with associative learning but not with other forms of learning such as language learning (Ekerdt et al., 2020; Finkl et al., 2020; Price, 2012; Zatorre, 2013) and might hence only represent forms of associative learning involved in social learning. Hence, it is unclear whether they are specific to social learning or rather reflect other processes woven into the social behaviors in those experimental paradigms, such as associative learning to track changes in the environment that might be caused by the other person's behavior.

If striatal neural patterns reflect learning dynamics related to understanding whether the partner is trustworthy, those same neural patterns should generalize to other experimental paradigms. Neuroimaging studies investigating trustworthiness learning in advice-taking paradigms, however, seem to provide a negative answer. For example, a recent neuroimaging study was able to isolate social evaluation signals related to another person's trustworthiness (learnt through the other's honesty and dishonesty) from nonsocial value signals related to rewards (i.e., winnings and losses) received during the feedback phase (Bellucci, Molter, & Park, 2019). Disentangling these two signals further allowed the investigation of neural signatures specifically related to trustworthiness representations and their modulatory effects on reward processing. Results showed that the STR and anterior cingulate cortex specifically encoded reward information, while feedbacks about the other person's trustworthiness were represented in the dlPFC, dorsal posterior cingulate cortex, and parietal cortex (e.g., inferior parietal lobule, IPL) (Figure 8.2). Importantly, neural signal from these regions was able to predict reputation-dependent trust in the partner during a subsequent interaction, whereas neural signal from the STR was not informative of an individual's future trust (Bellucci, Molter, & Park, 2019). These findings represent the first evidence that other brain regions than striatal structures represent social information relevant to reputation-dependent trustworthiness beliefs.

Another work using a reinforcement learning model further indicates that social PEs about a partner's trustworthiness correlates with activity in the medial prefrontal cortex, TPJ, and posterior superior temporal cortex (Behrens et al., 2008) – important mentalizing brain regions (Grèzes et al., 2001; Koster-Hale et al., 2017; Saxe & Kanwisher, 2003). On the contrary, reward PEs correlated with neural activity in the STR and anterior cingulate cortex, suggesting a dissociation between trustworthiness updating signals and reward PE signals. Similar results were found in a similar paradigm by Diaconescu et al. (2017), despite the use of a different reinforcement learning model. A recent neuroimaging study extends these findings showing that social PEs correlate with neural activity in the medial prefrontal cortex (i.e., OFC) and TPJ (Figure 8.2). Importantly, OFC activity preferentially encoded information about another person's trustworthiness but not subjective trustworthiness impressions of the other person (Bellucci & Park, in press). On the contrary, stronger functional connectivity between the OFC and TPJ was associated with more favorable trustworthiness impressions, suggesting that the OFC entails positive character trait information that supports belief updating about another person's behavior in the TPJ for trustworthiness impressions formation.

Further evidence on these dissociable signals comes from results observed in a different paradigm investigating the neural correlates of strategic behavior in an inspection game (Hampton et al., 2008). In this study, pairs of participants played in a two-player strategic game in which opponents have competing goals. One participant played as employer and could either inspect (distrust) or not inspect (trust), while the other played as employee and could either work (be trustworthy) or shirk (be untrustworthy). Computational modeling results showed that participants were not only using representations of the opponents' future choices to guide their own choice, but were also incorporating knowledge of how one's own actions influenced the partner's strategy, that is, how much the partner was showing reciprocal cooperation, which is a central feature of trustworthiness signals (Mahmoodi et al., 2018). Moreover, at the time of outcome revelation, influence updates of the partner's inferred trustworthiness and reward PEs were correlated with different neural signatures. In particular, trustworthiness update signals were found in the posterior superior temporal sulcus, while reward PEs were found in the vSTR. Importantly, also in this study, parameter values for trustworthiness updating and reward PEs were estimated from the same model, suggesting that they reliably captured independent and dissociable signals.

Finally, evidence on the role of mentalizing brain regions in trusting behaviors comes from brain network analyses of resting-state functional brain connectivity. Those brain regions that have been found to be consistently engaged by mentalizing tasks also cluster into an interconnected network at rest, known as the default-mode network (DMN; Alves et al., 2019; Ingvar, 1974; Raichle et al., 2001). Previous evidence has shown that resting-state functional connectivity bears predictive information about individuals' behavior (Rosenberg et al., 2016), personality traits (Adelstein et al., 2011; Kunisato et al., 2011), and social preferences (Hahn, Notebaert, Anderl, Reicherts, et al., 2015) (see also Chapter 12). Two studies provided evidence that whole-brain resting-state connectivity also predicts propensity to trust (Hahn, Notebaert, Anderl, Teckentrup, et al., 2015; Lu et al., 2019) but left open the question whether there is any specificity in the brain networks that preferentially represent information underlying trusting behavior. A recent study filled this gap by testing five classic resting-state networks, namely the default-mode, frontoparietal, sensorimotor, cinguloopercular, and occipital networks (Bellucci, Hahn, et al., 2019; Dosenbach et al., 2007, 2010). These networks have been associated with different functions, such as central-executive functions for the frontoparietal network, saliency for the cinguloopercular network, and mentalizing for the DMN. The study by Bellucci, Hahn, et al. (2019) provides evidence that the DMN was the only brain network able to predict individual decisions to trust an anonymous person. Given the need to build mental models of the other person during trust decisions (especially in anonymous settings that abound in occasions for betrayal) (Aimone & Houser, 2013; Van Overwalle & Baetens, 2009) and the role of the DMN in simulating an alternative perspective (Buckner et al., 2008), these results suggest that mentalizing brain regions are pivotal to an individual's propensity to trust, likely because they support simulations of the other person's mind for estimations of her likely future behavior (Fletcher et al., 1995; Van Overwalle, 2009).

In conclusion, these studies indicate specific roles for several brain regions (Figure 8.2). In particular, the STR might be responsible for action–outcome associative learning to identify discrepancies in the other person's behavior. Mentalizing brain regions support the decision-making process in social contexts via simulations of thoughts and behaviors of others. The interplay between the TPJ and OFC underlies the formation of beliefs about others from character trait impressions, with the OFC encoding character trait information and the TPJ representing current beliefs about the other person's likely behavior. Finally, brain regions in the parietal (e.g., IPL), posterior cingulate, and prefrontal cortices (e.g., dlPFC) integrate current feedback about others' actions with other sources of information, such as previous beliefs and reputational knowledge, to guide decisions and prompt behavior change.

8.5   Conclusions

The results discussed in this chapter provide a first overview of the neurocomputational processes underlying trust learning as a form of social learning. Leveraging mathematical formulations of behavior, the core processes of social learning might be uniquely identified and described. Combining these mathematical parameterizations with neuroimaging techniques allows the investigation of the neural instantiations of those cognitive processes underlying social learning. These attempts not only contribute to a better understanding of social cognition in the healthy population but also help tackle the dysfunctioning processes in clinical disorders (Gromann et al., 2013, 2014; King-Casas et al., 2008; Lis et al., 2016; Maurer et al., 2018; Sripada et al., 2009; Xiang et al., 2012) (see also Chapters 16 and 17).

Despite the important advances achieved until now, a unifying neuro-computational theory of social learning is still lacking. To date, many studies investigating social learning have borrowed reinforcement learning and Bayesian models developed in other fields to study other forms of learning (e.g., associative learning). This concerns not only trust learning but also, for example, social dominance learning (Ligneul et al., 2016). Despite their ability to capture some cognitive processes in play in social interactions, their suitability to satisfactorily describe the complexities of social dynamics is yet to be proven. Processes such as strategic thinking, planning, and social comparisons are not formally captured by reinforcement learning and Bayesian models. On the contrary, other models like the Fehr–Schmidt model provide a neat formulation of social comparison computations but lack a framework for belief updating about the interacting agent in repeated interactions that could account for strategy change and behavior revision. A solution might be to use a Bayesian framework based on partially observable Markov decision processes, as recently attempted (Hula et al., 2018; Khalvati et al., 2019; Park et al., 2019). In conclusion, while much progress has been achieved in the last few years, a lot of interesting and fascinating work still awaits future, investigative efforts in the field of computational social neuroscience.

References

Adelstein, J. S., Shehzad, Z., Mennes, M., et al. (2011). Personality is reflected in the brain's intrinsic functional architecture. *PLoS ONE*, 6(11), Article e27633. http://dx.doi.org/10.1371/journal.pone.0027633

Aharon, I., Etcoff, N., Ariely, D., Chabris, C. F., O'Connor, E., & Breiter, H. C. (2001). Beautiful faces have variable reward value: fMRI and behavioral evidence. *Neuron*, 32(3), 537–551. http://dx.doi.org/10.1016/S0896–6273(01)00491-3

Aimone, J. A., & Houser, D. (2013). Harnessing the benefits of betrayal aversion. *Journal of Economic Behavior & Organization*, 89, 1–8. http://dx.doi.org/10.1016/j.jebo.2013.02.001

Alves, P. N., Foulon, C., Karolis, V., et al. (2019). An improved neuroanatomical model of the default-mode network reconciles previous neuroimaging and neuropathological findings. *Communication Biology*, 2, Article 370. http://dx.doi.org/10.1038/s42003–019-0611-3

Ashraf, N., Bohnet, I., & Piankov, N. (2006). Decomposing trust and trustworthiness. *Experimental Economics*, 9(3), 193–208. http://dx.doi.org/10.1007/s10683-006-9122-4

Ashton, M. C., & Lee, K. (2007). Empirical, theoretical, and practical advantages of the HEXACO model of personality structure. *Personality and Social Psychology Review*, 11(2), 150–166. http://dx.doi.org/10.1177/1088868306294907

Ashton, M. C., Lee, K., & de Vries, R. E. (2014). The HEXACO honesty-humility, agreeableness, and emotionality factors: A review of research and theory. *Personality and Social Psychology Review*, 18(2), 139–152. http://dx.doi.org/10.1177/1088868314523838

Ashton, M. C., Lee, K., Perugini, M., et al. (2004). A six-factor structure of personality-descriptive adjectives: Solutions from psycholexical studies in seven languages. *Journal of Personality and Social Psychology*, 86(2), 356–366. http://dx.doi.org/10.1037/0022-3514.86.2.356

Becker, J., Brackbill, D., & Centola, D. (2017). Network dynamics of social influence in the wisdom of crowds. *Proceedings of the National Academy of Sciences of the United States of America*, 114(26), E5070–E5076. http://dx.doi.org/10.1073/pnas.1615978114

Behrens, T. E., Hunt, L. T., Woolrich, M. W., & Rushworth, M. F. (2008). Associative learning of social value. *Nature*, 456(7219), 245–249. http://dx.doi.org/10.1038/nature07538

Bellucci, G., Chernyak, S. V., Goodyear, K., Eickhoff, S. B., & Krueger, F. (2017). Neural signatures of trust in reciprocity: A coordinate-based meta-analysis. *Human Brain Mapping*, 38(3), 1233–1248. http://dx.doi.org/10.1002/hbm.23451

Bellucci, G., Hahn, T., Deshpande, G., & Krueger, F. (2019). Functional connectivity of specific resting-state networks predicts trust and reciprocity in the trust game. *Cognitive, Affective & Behavioral Neuroscience*, 19(1), 165–176. http://dx.doi.org/10.3758/s13415-018-00654-3

Bellucci, G., Molter, F., & Park, S. Q. (2019). Neural representations of honesty predict future trust behavior. *Nature Communications*, 10(1), Article 5184. http://dx.doi.org/10.1038/s41467-019-13261-8

Bellucci, G., Münte, T. F., & Park, S. Q. (2020). Effects of a dopamine agonist on trusting behaviors in females. *Psychopharmacology (Berl)*, 237(6), 1671–1680. http://dx.doi.org/10.1007/s00213-020-05488-x

(in press). Value computations under social uncertainty and serotonin.

Bellucci, G., & Park, S. Q. (2020). Honesty biases trustworthiness impressions. *Journal of Experimental Psychology: General*, 149(8), 1567–1586. http://dx.doi.org/10.1037/xge0000730

(in press). Neurocomputational mechanisms of cognitive biases in impression formation.

Berg, J., Dickhaut, J., & McCabe, K. (1995). Trust, reciprocity, and social history. *Games and Economic Behavior*, 10(1), 122–142. http://dx.doi.org/10.1006/game.1995.1027

Biele, G., Rieskamp, J., & Gonzalez, R. (2009). Computational models for the combination of advice and individual learning. *Cognitive Science*, 33(2), 206–242. http://dx.doi.org/10.1111/j.1551-6709.2009.01010.x

Biele, G., Rieskamp, J., Krugel, L. K., & Heekeren, H. R. (2011). The neural basis of following advice. *PLoS Biology*, 9(6), Article e1001089. http://dx.doi.org/10.1371/journal.pbio.1001089

Bohnet, I., & Zeckhauser, R. (2004). Trust, risk and betrayal. *Journal of Economic Behavior & Organization*, 55(4), 467–484. http://dx.doi.org/10.1016/j.jebo.2003.11.004

Buckner, R. L., Andrews-Hanna, J. R., & Schacter, D. L. (2008). The brain's default network: Anatomy, function, and relevance to disease. *Annals of the New York Academy of Sciences*, 1124, 1–38. http://dx.doi.org/10.1196/annals.1440.011

Burnham, T., McCabe, K., & Smith, V. L. (2000). Friend-or-foe intentionality priming in an extensive form trust game. *Journal of Economic Behavior & Organization*, 43(1), 57–73. http://dx.doi.org/10.1016/s0167-2681(00)00108-6

Burt, R. S., & Knez, M. (1995). Kinds of third-party effects on trust. *Rationality and Society*, 7(3), 255–292.

Camerer, C. F. (2003). Behavioural studies of strategic thinking in games. *Trends in Cognitive Sciences*, 7(5), 225–231. http://dx.doi.org/10.1016/S1364-6613(03)00094-9

Chang, L. J., Doll, B. B., Van't Wout, M., Frank, M. J., & Sanfey, A. G. (2010). Seeing is believing: Trustworthiness as a dynamic belief. *Cognitive Psychology,* 61(2), 87–105. http://dx.doi.org/10.1016/j.cogpsych.2010.03.001

Chaudhuri, A., & Gangadharan, L. (2007). An experimental analysis of trust and trustworthiness. *Southern Economic Journal,* 73(4), 959–985. https://doi.org/10.2307/20111937

Chaudhuri, A., Sopher, B., & Strand, P. (2002). Cooperation in social dilemmas, trust and reciprocity. *Journal of Economic Psychology,* 23(2), 231–249. http://dx.doi.org/10.1016/s0167-4870(02)00065-x

Cheong, J. H., Jolly, E., Sul, S., & Chang, L. J. (2017). Computational models in social neuroscience. In A. A. Moustafa (Ed.), *Computational models of brain and behavior* (1st ed., pp. 229–244). John Wiley & Sons, Ltd.

Coleman, J. (1990). *Foundations of social theory.* The Belknap Press of Harvard University.

Csukás, C., Fracalanza, P., Kovács, T., & Willinger, M. (2008). The determinants of trusting and reciprocal behaviour: Evidence from an intercultural experiment. *Journal of Economic Development,* 33(1), 71–95. http://dx.doi.org/10.35866/caujed.2008.33.1.004

Das, T. K., & Teng, B.-S. (1998). Between trust and control: Developing confidence in partner cooperation in alliances. *Academy of Management Review,* 23(3), 491–512. http://dx.doi.org/10.5465/amr.1998.926623

(2001). Trust, control, and risk in strategic alliances: An integrated framework. *Organization Studies,* 22(2), 251–283. http://dx.doi.org/10.1177/0170840601222004

Delgado, M. R., Frank, R. H., & Phelps, E. A. (2005). Perceptions of moral character modulate the neural systems of reward during the trust game. *Nature Neuroscience,* 8(11), 1611–1618. http://dx.doi.org/10.1038/nn1575

Deutsch, M. (1958). Trust and suspicion. *Journal of Conflict Resolution,* 2(4), 265–279.

Diaconescu, A. O., Mathys, C., Weber, L. A. E., Kasper, L., Mauer, J., & Stephan, K. E. (2017). Hierarchical prediction errors in midbrain and septum during social learning. *Social Cognitive and Affective Neuroscience,* 12(4), 618–634. http://dx.doi.org/10.1093/scan/nsw171

Dosenbach, N. U., Fair, D. A., Miezin, F. M., et al. (2007). Distinct brain networks for adaptive and stable task control in humans. *Proceedings of the National Academy of Sciences of the United States of America,* 104(26), 11073–11078. http://dx.doi.org/10.1073/pnas.0704320104

Dosenbach, N. U., Nardos, B., Cohen, A. L., et al. (2010). Prediction of individual brain maturity using fMRI. *Science,* 329(5997), 1358–1361. http://dx.doi.org/10.1126/science.1194144

Dreher, J. C., Kohn, P., & Berman, K. F. (2006). Neural coding of distinct statistical properties of reward information in humans. *Cerebral Cortex,* 16(4), 561–573. http://dx.doi.org/10.1093/cercor/bhj004

Dunning, D., Anderson, J. E., Schlosser, T., Ehlebracht, D., & Fetchenhauer, D. (2014). Trust at zero acquaintance: More a matter of respect than expectation of reward. *Journal of Personality and Social Psychology*, 107(1), 122–141. http://dx.doi.org/10.1037/a0036673

Dunning, D., Fetchenhauer, D., & Schlösser, T. (2019). Why people trust: Solved puzzles and open mysteries. *Current Directions in Psychological Science*, 28(4), 366–371. http://dx.doi.org/10.1177/0963721419838255

Ekerdt, C. E. M., Kuhn, C., Anwander, A., Brauer, J., & Friederici, A. D. (2020). Word learning reveals white matter plasticity in preschool children. *Brain Structure and Function*, 225(2), 607–619. http://dx.doi.org/10.1007/s00429-020-02024-7

Everett, J. A., Pizarro, D. A., & Crockett, M. J. (2016). Inference of trustworthiness from intuitive moral judgments. *Journal of Experimental Psychology: General*, 145(6), 772–787. http://dx.doi.org/10.1037/xge0000165

Fairley, K., Sanfey, A. G., Vyrastekova, J., & Weitzel, U. (2016). Trust and risk revisited. *Journal of Economic Psychology*, 57, 74–85. http://dx.doi.org/10.1016/j.joep.2016.10.001

Fareri, D. S., Chang, L. J., & Delgado, M. R. (2012). Effects of direct social experience on trust decisions and neural reward circuitry. *Frontiers in Neuroscience*, 6, Article 148. http://dx.doi.org/10.3389/fnins.2012.00148

Fehr, E., & Fischbacher, U. (2003). The nature of human altruism. *Nature*, 425 (6960), 785–791. http://dx.doi.org/10.1038/nature02043

(2004). Social norms and human cooperation. *Trends in Cognitive Sciences*, 8 (4), 185–190. http://dx.doi.org/10.1016/j.tics.2004.02.007

Fehr, E., & Schmidt, K. M. (1999). A theory of fairness, competition, and cooperation. *Quarterly Journal of Economics*, 114(3), 817–868. http://dx.doi.org/10.1162/003355399556151

Fetchenhauer, D., & Dunning, D. (2009). Do people trust too much or too little? *Journal of Economic Psychology*, 30(3), 263–276. http://dx.doi.org/10.1016/j.joep.2008.04.006

Finkl, T., Hahne, A., Friederici, A. D., Gerber, J., Murbe, D., & Anwander, A. (2020). Language without speech: Segregating distinct circuits in the human brain. *Cerebral Cortex*, 30(2), 812–823. http://dx.doi.org/10.1093/cercor/bhz128

Fletcher, P. C., Happe, F., Frith, U., et al. (1995). Other minds in the brain: A functional imaging study of "theory of mind" in story comprehension. *Cognition*, 57(2), 109–128. https://doi.org/10.1016/0010-0277(95)00692-R

Fouragnan, E., Chierchia, G., Greiner, S., Neveu, R., Avesani, P., & Coricelli, G. (2013). Reputational priors magnify striatal responses to violations of trust. *Journal of Neuroscience*, 33(8), 3602–3611. http://dx.doi.org/10.1523/Jneurosci.3086-12.2013

Frost, T., Stimpson, D. V., & Maughan, M. R. (1978). Some correlates of trust. *Journal of Psychology*, 99(1st Half), 103–108. http://dx.doi.org/10.1080/00223980.1978.9921447

Galton, F. (1907). Vox populi. *Nature*, 75(1949), 450–451. http://dx.doi.org/10.1038/075450a0

Gershman, S. J., & Daw, N. D. (2017). Reinforcement learning and episodic memory in humans and animals: An integrative framework. *Annual Review of Psychology*, 68, 101–128. http://dx.doi.org/10.1146/annurev-psych-122414-033625

Gordon, R., & Spears, K. (2012). You don't act like you trust me: Dissociations between behavioural and explicit measures of source credibility judgement. *Quarterly Journal of Experimental Psychology*, 65(1), 121–134. http://dx.doi.org/10.1080/17470218.2011.591534

Gottfried, J. A., & Dolan, R. J. (2004). Human orbitofrontal cortex mediates extinction learning while accessing conditioned representations of value. *Nature Neuroscience*, 7(10), 1144–1152. http://dx.doi.org/10.1038/nn1314

Grèzes, J., Fonlupt, P., Bertenthal, B., Delon-Martin, C., Segebarth, C., & Decety, J. (2001). Does perception of biological motion rely on specific brain regions? *NeuroImage*, 13(5), 775–785. http://dx.doi.org/10.1006/nimg.2000.0740

Gromann, P. M., Heslenfeld, D. J., Fett, A. K., Joyce, D. W., Shergill, S. S., & Krabbendam, L. (2013). Trust versus paranoia: Abnormal response to social reward in psychotic illness. *Brain*, 136(Pt 6), 1968–1975. http://dx.doi.org/10.1093/brain/awt076

Gromann, P. M., Shergill, S. S., de Haan, L., et al. (2014). Reduced brain reward response during cooperation in first-degree relatives of patients with psychosis: An fMRI study. *Psychological Medicine*, 44(16), 3445–3454. http://dx.doi.org/10.1017/S0033291714000737

Hahn, T., Notebaert, K., Anderl, C., Reicherts, P., et al. (2015). Reliance on functional resting-state network for stable task control predicts behavioral tendency for cooperation. *NeuroImage*, 118, 231–236. http://dx.doi.org/10.1016/j.neuroimage.2015.05.093

Hahn, T., Notebaert, K., Anderl, C., Teckentrup, V., Kassecker, A., & Windmann, S. (2015). How to trust a perfect stranger: Predicting initial trust behavior from resting-state brain-electrical connectivity. *Social Cognitive and Affective Neuroscience*, 10(6), 809–813. http://dx.doi.org/10.1093/scan/nsu122

Hampton, A. N., Bossaerts, P., & O'Doherty, J. P. (2008). Neural correlates of mentalizing-related computations during strategic interactions in humans. *Proceedings of the National Academy of Sciences of the United States of America*, 105(18), 6741–6746. http://dx.doi.org/10.1073/pnas.0711099105

Hertz, U., Palminteri, S., Brunetti, S., Olesen, C., Frith, C. D., & Bahrami, B. (2017). Neural computations underpinning the strategic management of influence in advice giving. *Nature Communications*, 8(1), Article 2191. http://dx.doi.org/10.1038/s41467-017-02314-5

Hillebrandt, H., Sebastian, C., & Blakemore, S. J. (2011). Experimentally induced social inclusion influences behavior on trust games. *Cognitive Neuroscience*, 2(1), 27–33. http://dx.doi.org/10.1080/17588928.2010.515020

Ho, T. H., & Weigelt, K. (2005). Trust building among strangers. *Management Science*, 51(4), 519–530. http://dx.doi.org/10.1287/mnsc.1040.0350

Hollerman, J. R., & Schultz, W. (1998). Dopamine neurons report an error in the temporal prediction of reward during learning. *Nature Neuroscience*, 1(4), 304–309. http://dx.doi.org/10.1038/1124

Howard, J. D., & Kahnt, T. (2018). Identity prediction errors in the human midbrain update reward-identity expectations in the orbitofrontal cortex. *Nature Communications*, 9(1), Article 1611. http://dx.doi.org/10.1038/s41467-018-04055-5

Hula, A., Montague, P. R., & Dayan, P. (2015). Monte Carlo planning method estimates planning horizons during interactive social exchange. *PLoS Computational Biology*, 11(6), Article e1004254. http://dx.doi.org/10.1371/journal.pcbi.1004254

Hula, A., Vilares, I., Lohrenz, T., Dayan, P., & Montague, P. R. (2018). A model of risk and mental state shifts during social interaction. *PLoS Computational Biology*, 14(2), Article e1005935. http://dx.doi.org/10.1371/journal.pcbi.1005935

Ingvar, D. H. (1974). *Patterns of brain activity revealed by measurements of regional cerebral blood flow*. Paper presented at the Alfred Benzon Symposium VIII, Copenhagen.

Joiner, J., Piva, M., Turrin, C., & Chang, S. W. C. (2017). Social learning through prediction error in the brain. *NPJ Science of Learning*, 2, Article 8. http://dx.doi.org/10.1038/s41539-017-0009-2

Kahneman, D., & Tversky, A. (1979). Prospect theory: An analysis of decision under risk. *Econometrica*, 47(2), 263–291.

Khalvati, K., Park, S. A., Mirbagheri, S., et al. (2019). Modeling other minds: Bayesian inference explains human choices in group decision making. *Science Advances*, 5(11), Article eaax8783. http://dx.doi.org/10.1126/sciadv.aax8783

King-Casas, B., Sharp, C., Lomax-Bream, L., Lohrenz, T., Fonagy, P., & Montague, P. R. (2008). The rupture and repair of cooperation in borderline personality disorder. *Science*, 321(5890), 806–810. http://dx.doi.org/10.1126/science.1156902

King-Casas, B., Tomlin, D., Anen, C., Camerer, C. F., Quartz, S. R., & Montague, P. R. (2005). Getting to know you: Reputation and trust in a two-person economic exchange. *Science*, 308(5718), 78–83. http://dx.doi.org/10.1126/science.1108062

Koster-Hale, J., Richardson, H., Velez, N., Asaba, M., Young, L., & Saxe, R. (2017). Mentalizing regions represent distributed, continuous, and abstract dimensions of others' beliefs. *NeuroImage*, 161, 9–18. http://dx.doi.org/10.1016/j.neuroimage.2017.08.026

Krueger, F., Grafman, J., & McCabe, K. (2008). Neural correlates of economic game playing. *Philosophical Transactions of the Royal Society B: Biological Sciences*, 363(1511), 3859–3874. http://dx.doi.org/10.1098/rstb.2008.0165

Krueger, F., McCabe, K., Moll, J., et al. (2007). Neural correlates of trust. *Proceedings of the National Academy of Sciences of the United States of*

America, 104(50), 20084–20089. http://dx.doi.org/10.1073/pnas
.0710103104

Kunisato, Y., Okamoto, Y., Okada, G., et al. (2011). Personality traits and the
amplitude of spontaneous low-frequency oscillations during resting state.
Neuroscience Letters, 492(2), 109–113. http://dx.doi.org/10.1016/j.neulet
.2011.01.067

Lamba, A., Frank, M. J., & FeldmanHall, O. (2020). Anxiety impedes adaptive
social learning under uncertainty. *Psychological Science*, 31(5), 592–603.
http://dx.doi.org/10.1177/0956797620910993

Lee, K., & Ashton, M. C. (2004). Psychometric properties of the HEXACO
personality inventory. *Multivariate Behavioral Research*, 39(2), 329–358.
http://dx.doi.org/10.1207/s15327906mbr3902_8

Lewis, J. D., & Weigert, A. (1985). Trust as a social reality. *Social Forces*, 63(4),
967–985. http://dx.doi.org/10.2307/2578601

Li, Y., Vanni-Mercier, G., Isnard, J., Mauguiere, F., & Dreher, J. C. (2016). The
neural dynamics of reward value and risk coding in the human orbitofrontal
cortex. *Brain*, 139(Pt 4), 1295–1309. http://dx.doi.org/10.1093/brain/
awv409

Ligneul, R., Obeso, I., Ruff, C. C., & Dreher, J. C. (2016). Dynamical representation of dominance relationships in the human rostromedial prefrontal
cortex. *Current Biology*, 26(23), 3107–3115. http://dx.doi.org/10.1016/j.cub
.2016.09.015

Lis, S., Baer, N., Franzen, N., et al. (2016). Social interaction behavior in ADHD
in adults in a virtual trust game. *Journal of Attention Disorders*, 20(4),
335–345. http://dx.doi.org/10.1177/1087054713482581

Lockwood, P. L., Apps, M. A., Valton, V., Viding, E., & Roiser, J. P. (2016).
Neurocomputational mechanisms of prosocial learning and links to empa-
thy. *Proceedings of the National Academy of Sciences of the United States of
America*, 113(35), 9763–9768. http://dx.doi.org/10.1073/pnas.1603198113

Lu, X., Li, T., Xia, Z., et al. (2019). Connectome-based model predicts individual
differences in propensity to trust. *Human Brain Mapping*, 40(6),
1942–1954. http://dx.doi.org/10.1002/hbm.24503

Luhmann, N. (1979). Trust: A mechanism for the reduction of social complexity.
In N. Luhmann (Ed.), *Trust and power* (pp. 4–103). Wiley.

Ma, I., Sanfey, A. G., & Ma, W. J. (2020). The social cost of gathering
information for trust decisions. *Scientific Reports*, 10(1), Article 14073.
http://dx.doi.org/10.1038/s41598-020-69766-6

Mahmoodi, A., Bahrami, B., & Mehring, C. (2018). Reciprocity of social
influence. *Nature Communications*, 9(1), Article 2474. http://dx.doi.org/10
.1038/s41467-018-04925-y

Malhotra, D. (2004). Trust and reciprocity decisions: The differing perspectives
of trustors and trusted parties. *Organizational Behavior and Human Decision
Processes*, 94(2), 61–73. http://dx.doi.org/10.1016/j.obhdp.2004.03.001

Malhotra, D., & Murnighan, J. K. (2002). The effects of contracts on interpersonal trust. *Administrative Science Quarterly*, 47(3), 534–559. http://dx.doi.org/10.2307/3094850

Maurer, C., Chambon, V., Bourgeois-Gironde, S., Leboyer, M., & Zalla, T. (2018). The influence of prior reputation and reciprocity on dynamic trust-building in adults with and without autism spectrum disorder. *Cognition*, 172, 1–10. http://dx.doi.org/10.1016/j.cognition.2017.11.007

Mayer, R. C., Davis, J. H., & Schoorman, F. D. (1995). An integrative model of organizational trust. *The Academy of Management Review*, 20(3), 709–734.

McCabe, K. A., Rigdon, M. L., & Smith, V. L. (2003). Positive reciprocity and intentions in trust games. *Journal of Economic Behavior & Organization*, 52 (2), 267–275. http://dx.doi.org/10.1016/s0167-2681(03)00003-9

McGinnies, E., & Ward, C. D. (1980). Better liked than right: Trustworthiness and expertise as factors in credibility. *Personality and Social Psychology Bulletin*, 6(3), 467–472. http://dx.doi.org/10.1177/014616728063023

Mellers, B., Ungar, L., Baron, J., et al. (2014). Psychological strategies for winning a geopolitical forecasting tournament. *Psychological Science*, 25(5), 1106–1115. http://dx.doi.org/10.1177/0956797614524255

Meshi, D., Biele, G., Korn, C. W., & Heekeren, H. R. (2012). How expert advice influences decision making. *PLoS ONE*, 7(11), Article e49748. http://dx.doi.org/10.1371/journal.pone.0049748

Metereau, E., & Dreher, J. C. (2015). The medial orbitofrontal cortex encodes a general unsigned value signal during anticipation of both appetitive and aversive events. *Cortex*, 63, 42–54. http://dx.doi.org/10.1016/j.cortex.2014.08.012

Montague, P. R., Dayan, P., & Sejnowski, T. J. (1996). A framework for mesencephalic dopamine systems based on predictive Hebbian learning. *The Journal of Neuroscience*, 16(5), 1936–1947. http://dx.doi.org/10.1523/jneurosci.16-05-01936.1996

Na, S., Chung, D., Hula, A., et al. (2019). Humans use forward thinking to exert social control. *bioRxiv*. http://dx.doi.org/10.1101/737353

O'Doherty, J., Dayan, P., Schultz, J., Deichmann, R., Friston, K., & Dolan, R. J. (2004). Dissociable roles of ventral and dorsal striatum in instrumental conditioning. *Science*, 304(5669), 452–454. http://dx.doi.org/10.1126/science.1094285

O'Doherty, J., Winston, J., Critchley, H., Perrett, D., Burt, D. M., & Dolan, R. J. (2003). Beauty in a smile: The role of medial orbitofrontal cortex in facial attractiveness. *Neuropsychologia*, 41(2), 147–155. https://doi.org/10.1016/S0028-3932(02)00145-8

Park, S. A., Sestito, M., Boorman, E. D., & Dreher, J. C. (2019). Neural computations underlying strategic social decision making in groups. *Nature Communications*, 10(1), Article 5287. http://dx.doi.org/10.1038/s41467-019-12937-5

Pegors, T. K., Kable, J. W., Chatterjee, A., & Epstein, R. A. (2015). Common and unique representations in pFC for face and place attractiveness. *Journal of Cognitive Neuroscience*, 27(5), 959–973. http://dx.doi.org/10.1162/jocn_a_00777

Phan, K. L., Sripada, C. S., Angstadt, M., & McCabe, K. (2010). Reputation for reciprocity engages the brain reward center. *Proceedings of the National Academy of Sciences of the United States of America*, 107(29), 13099–13104. http://dx.doi.org/10.1073/pnas.1008137107

Pillutla, M. M., Malhotra, D., & Keith Murnighan, J. (2003). Attributions of trust and the calculus of reciprocity. *Journal of Experimental Social Psychology*, 39(5), 448–455. http://dx.doi.org/10.1016/s0022-1031(03)00015-5

Platt, M. L., & Huettel, S. A. (2008). Risky business: The neuroeconomics of decision making under uncertainty. *Nature Neuroscience*, 11(4), 398–403. http://dx.doi.org/10.1038/nn2062

Preuschoff, K., Bossaerts, P., & Quartz, S. R. (2006). Neural differentiation of expected reward and risk in human subcortical structures. *Neuron*, 51(3), 381–390. http://dx.doi.org/10.1016/j.neuron.2006.06.024

Price, C. J. (2012). A review and synthesis of the first 20 years of PET and fMRI studies of heard speech, spoken language and reading. *NeuroImage*, 62(2), 816–847. http://dx.doi.org/10.1016/j.neuroimage.2012.04.062

Raichle, M. E., MacLeod, A. M., Snyder, A. Z., Powers, W. J., Gusnard, D. A., & Shulman, G. L. (2001). A default mode of brain function. *Proceedings of the National Academy of Sciences of the United States of America*, 98(2), 676–682. http://dx.doi.org/10.1073/pnas.98.2.676

Reichelt, J., Sievert, J., & Jacob, F. (2013). How credibility affects eWOM reading: The influences of expertise, trustworthiness, and similarity on utilitarian and social functions. *Journal of Marketing Communications*, 20 (1–2), 65–81. http://dx.doi.org/10.1080/13527266.2013.797758

Rescorla, R. A., & Wagner, A. R. (1972). A theory of Pavlovian conditioning: Variations in the effectiveness of reinforcement and nonreinforcement. *Current Research and Theory*, 64–99, Appleton-Century-Crofts.

Rosenberg, M. D., Finn, E. S., Scheinost, D., et al. (2016). A neuromarker of sustained attention from whole-brain functional connectivity. *Nature Neuroscience*, 19(1), 165–171. http://dx.doi.org/10.1038/nn.4179

Rothbart, M., & Park, B. (1986). On the confirmability and disconfirmability of trait concepts. *Journal of Personality and Social Psychology*, 50(1), 131–142. http://dx.doi.org/10.1037/0022-3514.50.1.131

Rousseau, D. M., Sitkin, S. B., Burt, R. S., & Camerer, C. (1998). Not so different after all: A cross-discipline view of trust. *Academy of Management Review*, 23(3), 393–404. http://dx.doi.org/10.5465/amr.1998.926617

Rudebeck, P. H., & Murray, E. A. (2014). The orbitofrontal oracle: Cortical mechanisms for the prediction and evaluation of specific behavioral outcomes. *Neuron*, 84(6), 1143–1156. http://dx.doi.org/10.1016/j.neuron.2014.10.049

Rudebeck, P. H., Saunders, R. C., Prescott, A. T., Chau, L. S., & Murray, E. A. (2013). Prefrontal mechanisms of behavioral flexibility, emotion regulation and value updating. *Nature Neuroscience*, 16(8), 1140–1145. http://dx.doi .org/10.1038/nn.3440

Sánchez-Pagés, S., & Vorsatz, M. (2007). An experimental study of truth-telling in a sender–receiver game. *Games and Economic Behavior*, 61(1), 86–112. http://dx.doi.org/10.1016/j.geb.2006.10.014

Saxe, R., & Kanwisher, N. (2003). People thinking about thinking people: The role of the temporo-parietal junction in "theory of mind." *NeuroImage*, 19 (4), 1835–1842. http://dx.doi.org/10.1016/s1053-8119(03)00230-1

Schultz, W. (2000). Multiple reward signals in the brain. *Nature Reviews Neuroscience*, 1(3), 199–207. http://dx.doi.org/10.1038/35044563

Schultz, W., Dayan, P., & Montague, P. R. (1997). A neural substrate of prediction and reward. *Science*, 275(5306), 1593–1599. http://dx.doi.org/ 10.1126/science.275.5306.1593

Siegel, J. Z., Estrada, S., Crockett, M. J., & Baskin-Sommers, A. (2019). Exposure to violence affects the development of moral impressions and trust behavior in incarcerated males. *Nature Communications*, 10(1), Article 1942. http://dx.doi.org/10.1038/s41467-019-09962-9

Siegel, J. Z., Mathys, C., Rutledge, R. B., & Crockett, M. J. (2018). Beliefs about bad people are volatile. *Nature Human Behaviour*, 2(10), 750–756. http://dx .doi.org/10.1038/s41562-018-0425-1

Sjöberg, L. (2009). Are all crowds equally wise? A comparison of political election forecasts by experts and the public. *Journal of Forecasting*, 28(1), 1–18. http://dx.doi.org/10.1002/for.1083

Slovic, P. (1993). Perceived risk, trust, and democracy. *Risk Analysis*, 13(6), 675–682. http://dx.doi.org/10.1111/j.1539-6924.1993.tb01329.x

Snijders, C., & Keren, G. (2001). Do you trust? Whom do you trust? When do you trust? *Advances in Group Processes*, 18, 129–160. http://dx.doi.org/10 .1016/S0882-6145(01)18006-9

Sperber, D. A. N., Clément, F., Heintz, C., et al. (2010). Epistemic vigilance. *Mind & Language*, 25(4), 359–393. http://dx.doi.org/10.1111/j.1468-0017 .2010.01394.x

Sripada, C. S., Angstadt, M., Banks, S., Nathan, P. J., Liberzon, I., & Phan, K. L. (2009). Functional neuroimaging of mentalizing during the trust game in social anxiety disorder. *Neuroreport*, 20(11), 984–989. http://dx.doi.org/10 .1097/WNR.0b013e32832d0a67

Stirrat, M., & Perrett, D. I. (2010). Valid facial cues to cooperation and trust: Male facial width and trustworthiness. *Psychological Science*, 21(3), 349–354. http://dx.doi.org/10.1177/0956797610362647

Strickland, L. H. (1958). Surveillance and trust. *Journal of Personality*, 26(2), 200–215. http://dx.doi.org/10.1111/j.1467-6494.1958.tb01580.x

Thielmann, I., & Hilbig, B. E. (2015). The traits one can trust: Dissecting reciprocity and kindness as determinants of trustworthy behavior. *Personality and Social Psychology Bulletin*, 41(11), 1523–1536. http://dx.doi .org/10.1177/0146167215600530

Todorov, A., Pakrashi, M., & Oosterhof, N. N. (2009). Evaluating faces on trustworthiness after minimal time exposure. *Social Cognition*, 27(6), 813–833. http://dx.doi.org/10.1521/soco.2009.27.6.813

Toelch, U., Bach, D. R., & Dolan, R. J. (2014). The neural underpinnings of an optimal exploitation of social information under uncertainty. *Social Cognitive and Affective Neuroscience*, 9(11), 1746–1753. http://dx.doi.org/10.1093/scan/nst173

Tsuchida, A., Doll, B. B., & Fellows, L. K. (2010). Beyond reversal: A critical role for human orbitofrontal cortex in flexible learning from probabilistic feedback. *Journal of Neuroscience*, 30(50), 16868–16875. http://dx.doi.org/10.1523/JNEUROSCI.1958-10.2010

Tversky, A., & Kahneman, D. (1992). Advances in prospect theory: Cumulative representation of uncertainty. *Journal of Risk and Uncertainty*, 5(4), 297–323. http://dx.doi.org/10.1007/Bf00122574

Van Overwalle, F. (2009). Social cognition and the brain: A meta-analysis. *Human Brain Mapping*, 30(3), 829–858. http://dx.doi.org/10.1002/hbm.20547

Van Overwalle, F., & Baetens, K. (2009). Understanding others' actions and goals by mirror and mentalizing systems: A meta-analysis. *NeuroImage*, 48(3), 564–584. http://dx.doi.org/10.1016/j.neuroimage.2009.06.009

Vanni-Mercier, G., Mauguiere, F., Isnard, J., & Dreher, J. C. (2009). The hippocampus codes the uncertainty of cue-outcome associations: An intracranial electrophysiological study in humans. *Journal of Neuroscience*, 29(16), 5287–5294. http://dx.doi.org/10.1523/JNEUROSCI.5298-08.2009

Wardle, M. C., Fitzgerald, D. A., Angstadt, M., Sripada, C. S., McCabe, K., & Phan, K. L. (2013). The caudate signals bad reputation during trust decisions. *PLoS ONE*, 8(6), Article e68884. http://dx.doi.org/10.1371/journal.pone.0068884

Weiner, J. L., & Mowen, J. C. (1986). Source credibility: On the independent effects of trust and expertise. *Advances in Consumer Research*, 13, 306–310.

Wilson, R. K., & Eckel, C. C. (2006). Judging a book by its cover: Beauty and expectations in the trust game. *Political Research Quarterly*, 59(2), 189–202. http://dx.doi.org/10.1177/106591290605900202

Winston, J. S., O'Doherty, J., Kilner, J. M., Perrett, D. I., & Dolan, R. J. (2007). Brain systems for assessing facial attractiveness. *Neuropsychologia*, 45(1), 195–206. http://dx.doi.org/10.1016/j.neuropsychologia.2006.05.009

Wu, H., Liu, X., Hagan, C. C., & Mobbs, D. (2020). Mentalizing during social interaction: A four component model. *Cortex*, 126, 242–252. http://dx.doi.org/10.1016/j.cortex.2019.12.031

Xiang, T., Ray, D., Lohrenz, T., Dayan, P., & Montague, P. R. (2012). Computational phenotyping of two-person interactions reveals differential neural response to depth-of-thought. *PLoS Computational Biology*, 8(12), Article e1002841. http://dx.doi.org/10.1371/journal.pcbi.1002841

Yaniv, I. (2006). The benefit of additional opinions. *Current Directions in Psychological Science*, 13(2), 75–78. http://dx.doi.org/10.1111/j.0963-7214.2004.00278.x

Yaniv, I., & Kleinberger, E. (2000). Advice taking in decision making: Egocentric discounting and reputation formation. *Organizational Behavior and Human Decision Processes*, 83(2), 260–281. http://dx.doi.org/10.1006/obhd.2000.2909

Zatorre, R. J. (2013). Predispositions and plasticity in music and speech learning: Neural correlates and implications. *Science*, 342(6158), 585–589. http://dx.doi.org/10.1126/science.1238414

PART III

Neurocharacteristic Level of Trust

CHAPTER 9

Trust and Distrust
Key Similarities and Differences
Brian W. Haas

9.1 Introduction

How do people form concepts about trust and distrust in their minds? What are the characteristics of trust that are the same or different from the characteristics of distrust? These questions are central to many basic issues within the social sciences, that include economics, marketing, psychology, and neurobiology. Elucidating the way trust works is also highly relevant to better understand the etiology of various forms of psychopathology, such as with borderline personality disorder (Unoka et al., 2009). Across a wide range of different disciplines there exists some agreement as to how trust and distrust are similar to one another and how they are different. Ultimately, working toward a commonly accepted understanding of the workings of trusting each other versus distrusting each other holds the important potential of improving the way people communicate with one another and are able to work effectively within groups. The goal of this chapter is to review scientific literature on what constitutes trust and distrust. Furthermore, this chapter seeks to develop a cohesive model of the neurobiological basis for trust versus distrust. Finally, this chapter will explore several open questions and directions for future research will be discussed.

9.2 Defining Trust and Distrust

It is important to develop a working set of definitions of trust-related concepts. In trust research, several terms have been used. These include trust, untrust, distrust, and mistrust (Marsh & Dibben, 2005). In this chapter, we will focus on the concepts of trust and distrust (Table 9.1). Across a wide range of disciplines trust tends to be conceptualized as

Corresponding author: Brian W. Haas (bhaas@uga.edu).

Table 9.1. *Dissociating trust and distrust as psychological constructs*

Bases for Differentiation	Trust (T)	Distrust (D)	Studies
T and D occur on a single continuum	Willing to be vulnerable	Low trust	Bigley & Pearce, (1998); Mayer et al., (1995)
T and D involve some dissociable attributes	Absence of positive expectations	Presence of negative expectations	Lewicki et al., (1998); Saunders et al., (2014)
T and D involve cognitive calculations	Low probability of risk	High probability of risk	Hill & O'Hara, (2006); Poste et al., (2014)
T and D involve emotional attributes	Compassion	Anger and fear	Beigi et al., (2016)

occurring under conditions of risk or uncertainty that requires one (i.e., trustor) to develop a favorable expectation of the intentions and behaviors of another person or group (i.e., trustee). In turn, this should be sufficient to prompt a willingness to become vulnerable to the trustee's future behaviors (Rousseau et al., 1998; Saunders et al., 2014). This definition accounts for a wide range of different types of scenarios, contexts, and behaviors. For example, within an economic context, a trusting relationship can be conceptualized as involving a person (trustor) being aware of uncertainty in the rate of returns for a retirement investment account. Given the context of risk and uncertainty, the trustor may trust another person (trustee) (e.g., financial advisor) to manage these funds. Another example of a trusting relationship is in a close interpersonal relationship. Good, high quality, interpersonal relationships (romantic or close friends) tend to be characterized by the feeling of comfort while sharing emotions with one another (Johnson-George & Swap, 1982). By trusting one's partner, trustors are within a context of risk and uncertainty, and are willing to be emotionally vulnerable. They anticipate and expect their partners to be responsible and well intentioned throughout the emotional exchange. Ultimately, typical definitions of trust involve a context including risk and an event when the trustor decides how vulnerable they are willing to be and how much responsibility they are willing to allocate to the trustee.

Heterogeneity exists in the way distrust is defined (McKnight & Chervany, 2001). Under some conceptualizations, distrust is directly compared to trust (Saunders et al., 2014). Accordingly, definitions of distrust often simply entail an absence of trust. Under this definition, trust and distrust are thought of as occurring on a single continuum with two poles and rest on the assumption that trust and distrust cannot co-occur (i.e., are mutually exclusive). Several scholarly works support this definition and basically construe distrust as the opposite of trust (Bigley & Pearce, 1998; Mayer et al., 1995). For example, Schoorman et al. (2007), stated: "We can find no credible evidence that a concept of distrust that is conceptually different from trust is theoretically or empirically viable." However, there are exceptions to this definition. Some findings suggest that within a single organization, some people may think about trust and distrust as existing on a continuum, while others do not (Saunders & Thornhill, 2004). Combined, these findings open the door to other ways of conceptualizing distrust. Perhaps trust and distrust are linked but also possess unique components.

Distrust is not always defined as being the exact opposite of trust. For example, Lewicki et al. (1998) described trust and distrust as being linked with one another but also that they are different from one another in some ways. Under this definition, trust and distrust can coexist. People can be characterized as being concurrently high on trust and high on distrust. If trust and distrust are indeed direct opposites, then being low on trust is the same as being high on distrust. However, Lewicki et al. (1998) differentiate low trust from high distrust in the following way. Low trust is characterized by passivity (no hope, faith, or confidence), while high distrust is characterized by fear (skepticism and cynicism). Low trust involves an absence of positive expectations, while high distrust involves the presence of negative exceptions. This theoretical account of the way trust and distrust are differentiated has led to some empirical research on how they tend to be conceptualized.

Saunders et al. (2014) carried out an empirical study on how people think about trust and distrust. In this study, employees in a large organization carried out a card-sorting task. Each card represented a concept or emotion (such as *trusting*, *distrusting*, *confidence*, and *vigilant*). Participants were tasked to organize the cards into piles representing "what they did feel" versus "what they did not feel." Each participant was subsequently interviewed about how they organized their concepts and emotions. The results indicated that within organizational relationships, trust and distrust judgments rarely occur simultaneously. However, the authors also found several incidences where low trust judgments were not necessarily paired with high distrust judgments. Combined, these findings support the idea that trust and distrust are intimately linked but that they also do possess some dissociable attributes (Lewicki et al., 1998; Mal et al., 2018).

Another way that trust and distrust tend to be thought of is with either a focus on cognitive or affective components (Lee, Lee, & Tan, 2010; Morrow Jr. et al., 2004). Several models of trust and distrust exist that are specifically designed to predict how people make economic decisions (Bigley & Pearce, 1998; Kramer, 1999). Often these models focus on the way a person calculates probability and their awareness of level of risk (Posten et al., 2014). In general, these models of trust and distrust tend to focus on the cognitive components underlying the way people make decisions (Hill & O'Hara, 2006). In addition, consistent evidence also exists that trust and distrust judgments are formed, in part, based on how people feel, and/or their emotions. For example, feelings of compassion tend to influence trust-based decisions, and feelings of anger tend to influence distrust-based decisions (Beigi et al., 2016). Taken together, it is important to incorporate both cognitive and affective components, as well as issues related to social and cultural context when describing, measuring, and defining trust and distrust.

9.3   Measuring Trust and Distrust

A wide range of methods tends to be used to measure trust and distrust (Evans & Krueger, 2009; Glaeser et al., 2000; McEvily & Tortoriello, 2011; Sanders et al., 2006). These approaches range from experimental tasks to self-report questionnaires to functional brain-imaging.

Some experimental tasks used to measure trust include the investment (trust) game (TG), the dictator game (DG), the prisoner's dilemma game (PDG), and the public goods game (PGG) (see also Chapter 2). The TG includes two participants, the "sender" and the "returner" (McCabe & Smith, 2000). The sender receives an amount of money and has an opportunity to invest by giving it to the returner. When the returner has tripled the investment, they have a choice as to either be self-interested, and keep the entire sum, or to act in a reciprocal way by sending back most of the earnings. Ultimately, the sender has a choice as to either send money (trust) or hold onto it (distrust). The DG is similar to the TG except that the returner has no opportunity to send back the money to the sender, and it is often played in a single round (Kahneman et al., 1986). The DG game, however, may not involve trust since the receiver has no opportunity to return the money. The PDG involves two players and they are forced to either cooperate or defect (Van Lange & Visser, 1999). If they both opt to cooperate, they will earn a mediocre reward. However, if one defects, and the other does not, then the defector will earn a far greater reward and the other participant will be relatively punished. Navigating through this task effectively requires that the two participants trust each other (Yamagishi et al., 2005). The PGG involves decision making within a group of other participants (Fehr & Gachter, 2000; Ledyard et al., 1995). Each participant decides to invest a portion of money into a fund that will benefit the whole group or keep the money for themselves. The amount of return of the group fund is contingent upon how many group members decide to contribute money. Therefore, one needs to trust that the other group members will also contribute to the fund (Kocher et al., 2015; Parks, 1994). Combined, many different ways exist to measure trust and distrust within experimental laboratory contexts. The majority of these tasks rely on the assessment of how much a person is willing to allocate responsibility to another person to return an expected amount of resources.

Self-report methods are also used to measure trust and distrust. Some of the self-report measures are designed to gauge a person's general and consistent tendency to trust other people. This approach conceptualizes trust as a trait: a stable and enduring characteristic or pattern of behavior. The Big 5 model of personality traits (Neuroticism, Extraversion, Openness to Experience, Agreeableness, and Conscientiousness) can be measured and conceptualized using underlying facet scores (McCrae & Costa Jr., 1992). Agreeableness is a personality trait that consists of several underlying facets, one of which is "trust." The items used to measure the trait of "trust" are designed to characterize the tendency to attribute benevolent intent to others and the disposition to believe that others are honest and well intentioned (Costa Jr. et al., 1991). An example of an item from the trust facet is, "My first reaction is to trust people." Some research demonstrates that greater trust facet self-report scores are associated with an increased tendency to evaluate people's photographs as trustworthy (Haas et al., 2015). In addition, other self-report questionnaires exist that are used to measure trust in others, such as the Trust Inventory (Couch & Jones, 1997) or the Brand Trust Scale to measure trust in brands (Delgado-Ballester, 2004). Combined, there are several ways that self-report techniques can be used to measure the way people think about trust. There are drawbacks to using self-reports, as these measures may be affected by social desirability bias. In addition, the majority of these scales characterize distrust as simply the opposite of trust. Future research is required to develop self-report measures of distrust that conceptualize distrust, in part, as consisting of unique characteristics as compared to trust (Lewicki et al., 1998).

9.4   Neurobiological Basis for Trust versus Distrust

Progress within the social and cognitive neurosciences has yielded a rich understanding of which parts of the brain are involved when people make social cognitive decisions (Bellucci et al., 2017; Krueger & Meyer-Lindenberg, 2019). Functional magnetic resonance imaging (fMRI) is a particularly effective method of characterizing brain activity during psychological processing and provides an excellent opportunity to measure changes in blood oxygenation levels in response to completing psychological tasks.

One way that fMRI has been used to investigate the brain basis for trust is to measure fMRI signal while people make judgments about the trustworthiness of other people as seen in photographs (Rule et al., 2013; Todorov, 2008; Todorov et al., 2009). It should be noted that determining trustworthiness may be only one component of the trust process. Consistent evidence exists that brain regions involved in emotion, attention, and vigilance, such as the amygdala, are engaged when people are making trustworthiness judgments of other people (Engell et al., 2007; Rule et al., 2013; Said et al., 2009; Winston et al., 2002). Bzdok et al., (2011) carried out an activation likelihood estimation meta-analysis on 16 fMRI studies pertaining to facial judgments of trustworthiness and found consistent evidence that the amygdala was engaged during the evaluation of trustworthiness of faces. Some studies have also demonstrated a nonlinear relationship between amygdala activation and trustworthy evaluations of faces. Specifically, fMRI research shows that the amygdala is most engaged when determining faces to be the most trustworthy and untrustworthy (i.e., distrust) (Rule et al., 2013; Said et al., 2009). Furthermore, anatomical MRI research demonstrates that greater right amygdala volume is associated with the tendency to rate faces as more trustworthy and distrustworthy (U-shaped function) (Haas et al., 2015). Interestingly, other research has shown that patients with amygdala damage show a preserved ability to develop and express interpersonal trust (Koscik & Tranel, 2011) (see also Chapter 18). Thought of together, the way the amygdala is often involved in forming trust and distrust judgments tends to support models of trust and distrust as being opposite one another and existing on a continuum (Bigley & Pearce, 1998; Mayer et al., 1995; Schoorman et al., 2007).

Another brain region often found to be activated during trust-based tasks is the ventromedial prefrontal cortex (vmPFC) (Van den Bos & Güroğlu, 2009). Broadly defined, the vmPFC is involved in emotion regulation, social evaluation, and assessing risk (Krawczyk, 2002). Both trust and distrust involve the assessment of risk and, in most cases, also involve some type of social evaluation. Accordingly, fMRI research shows that when participants are playing a modified version of the TG, vmPFC activation is associated with relatively less reciprocation (Li et al., 2009). Other research shows that individual differences in gray matter volume of the vmPFC are associated with the tendency to evaluate faces as more trustworthy and the tendency to trust others in general (i.e., trust facet of Agreeableness) (Haas et al., 2015). Neuropsychological research shows that patients with vmPFC damage tend to be less trusting during the TG (Krawczyk, 2002). Other trust-based tasks such as the PDG (Rilling et al., 2004) and the PGG (Cooper et al., 2010) indicate a link between vmPFC activity and trust-based decision making. These studies support the role of the vmPFC in forming trust- and distrust-based decisions, often during trust-based games that involve the evaluation of economic risk.

The social-cognitive network encompasses several cortical regions involved in integrating and orchestrating social and cognitive information. Within the social-cognitive network, the temporoparietal junction (TPJ) sub-serves an important component of trusting and distrusting others (Krall et al., 2015). The TPJ is involved in theory of mind (Brüne & Brüne-Cohrs, 2006; Carrington & Bailey, 2009; Siegal & Varley, 2002). Theory of mind is the process of understanding that the way another person processes the world is inherently different than the way of oneself (Symons, 2004). This can be within a cognitive context, such as perception. Using theory of mind, one would understand that the way another person perceives the world is different according to who they are, and where they are standing. Theory of mind is also important in terms of understanding the emotions of other people. Using theory of mind, one would understand the way another person feels is different according to who they are. In order to trust another person, one must assess their intentions. Without the ability to understand the perspectives and emotions of other people, one would be severely limited in one's ability to determine if another person is to be trusted or distrusted.

Several empirical studies support the role of the TPJ in trust- and distrust-based decision making. Fujino et al. (2020) showed that temporary lesions of the right TPJ (via transcranial magnetic stimulation) reduce people's intergroup bias during trust decisions. Brain atrophy, including the TPJ, is associated with abnormality in trust-based decision making (Wong et al., 2017). Engelmann et al. (2019) showed that the TPJ is an important node within the neural circuitry linking aversive affect to trust-based decision making. Another study demonstrated that increased vmPFC and TPJ connectivity during an interaction with an honest advisor predicted subsequent trusting behavior (Bellucci et al., 2019). Together, these studies demonstrate that developing trust or distrust of another person is likely contingent upon the healthy functioning of the TPJ. One needs to read another person's state of mind in order to decide whether to trust or distrust them.

Another important brain region to consider within the trust/distrust neural network is the insula. The insula is located deep within the lateral suclus and is involved in monitoring and regulating somatic representation of emotion (Craig, 2011). The anterior region of the insula has been shown to be important for social cognition and reciprocity (Bellucci et al., 2017, 2018). One of the most reliable means to elicit insula activity is via the presentation of disgusting stimuli (Krolak-Salmon et al., 2003; Wicker et al., 2003). When one feels disgusted, it often comes with somatic representations such as nausea and/or disorientation. The insula is important for coding the experience of emotions to visceral, somatic feeling states.

Within the context of trust and distrust, the insula is important for processing how someone feels "in their gut" when making judgments about other people during social interactions. In general, increased insula activation tends to lead to decisions not to trust (i.e., distrust) others. Insula activation increases in response to unfair treatment by one's partner during the ultimatum game (Sanfey et al., 2003; Tabibnia et al., 2008). A study demonstrated that aversive physical temperate, with a cold pack, is associated with increased insula activity and leads to reduced trust-based interpersonal decision making (Kang et al., 2011). Another study showed that unreciprocated trust (or distrust) is associated with greater insula activity (Rilling et al., 2008). Together, this research reveals that the insula acts to incorporate aversive stimuli and somatic feeling states during interpersonal distrust-based decision making.

Few studies have explicitly compared how the brain functions during conditions involving trust versus distrust. In one study, fMRI data were collected while participants were asked to control their feelings of trust or distrust of other people (i.e., photographs of faces) (Filkowski et al., 2016). A direct comparison of the trust and distrust conditions revealed that trust was associated with greater medial PFC activation than during the distrust condition. When compared to the baseline condition (age evaluation), the distrust condition was associated with greater insula activation. Both the trust and distrust conditions (combined) were associated with greater TPJ activation. These results indicate that trust and distrust are constructs possessing shared and unique attributes.

A holistic perspective on the brain mechanisms underlying trust and distrust shows that both constructs tend to be associated with activation within brain regions often termed the social-cognitive network (Lieberman, 2007), which includes the amygdala, the vmPFC, the TPJ, and the insula. These brain regions sub-serve one's ability to process emotions (amygdala), evaluate risk (vmPFC), read other people's mind states (TPJ), and listen to your gut (insula). A limited amount of research indicates that trust and distrust correspond to a U-shaped pattern of amygdala response when making trust- or distrust-based decisions, and that the insula plays a particularly important role during distrust.

9.5 Future Research Questions

There are currently several open research questions on the topic of trust versus distrust. First, more research is required to better understand how many factors contribute to a trust- or distrust-based decision. Currently, it is clear that emotions, risk assessment, and motivation each influence trust-based decision making. However, the way each of these factors influence decision outcomes, under a variety of different contexts, remains poorly understood. Second, the majority of trust- and distrust-based research is based on scenarios that involve an evaluation of trust of another person, and/or risk assessment during an economic-type paradigm. Other forms of trust and distrust clearly also exist, such as trusting oneself, trusting humanity in general, and trusting the natural world. These types of trust and distrust have yet to receive sufficient attention within the research community. One way to explore these topics would be to use psychometric approaches to develop scales to measure the extent to which people trust oneself, humanity in general, or the natural world. Finally, it will be important to develop more ecologically valid methods to investigate the neural underpinnings of trust and distrust. The majority of what we have come to understand about the workings of the social-cognitive brain are derived from fMRI research where participants are not socially engaged with other people. Some novel approaches to improve the ecological validity of trust research would be to include the use of simultaneous, multisubject fMRI data collection and videos as opposed to static images. In order to better understand the workings of the social brain, we must work together to create more valid empirical techniques.

References

Beigi, G., Tang, J., Wang, S., & Liu, H. (2016). *Exploiting emotional information for trust/distrust prediction.* Paper presented at the Proceedings of the 2016 SIAM international conference on data mining. https://doi.org/10 .1137/1.9781611974348.10

Bellucci, G., Chernyak, S. V., Goodyear, K., Eickhoff, S. B., & Krueger, F. (2017). Neural signatures of trust in reciprocity: A coordinate-based meta-analysis. *Human Brain Mapping*, 38(3), 1233–1248. https://doi.org/10 .1002/hbm.23451

Bellucci, G., Feng, C., Camilleri, J., Eickhoff, S. B., & Krueger, F. (2018). The role of the anterior insula in social norm compliance and enforcement: Evidence from coordinate-based and functional connectivity meta-analyses. *Neuroscience & Biobehavioral Reviews*, 92, 378–389. https://doi.org/10 .1016/j.neubiorev.2018.06.024

Bellucci, G., Molter, F., & Park, S. Q. (2019). Neural representations of honesty predict future trust behavior. *Nature Communications*, 10(1), 1–12. https:// doi.org/10.1038/s41467–019-13261-8

Bigley, G. A., & Pearce, J. L. (1998). Straining for shared meaning in organization science: Problems of trust and distrust. *Academy of Management Review*, 23 (3), 405–421. https://doi.org/10.2307/259286

Brüne, M., & Brüne-Cohrs, U. (2006). Theory of mind: Evolution, ontogeny, brain mechanisms and psychopathology. *Neuroscience & Biobehavioral Reviews*, 30(4), 437–455. https://doi.org/10.2307/25928610.1016/j .neubiorev.2005.08.001

Bzdok, D., Langner, R., Caspers, S., et al. (2011). ALE meta-analysis on facial judgments of trustworthiness and attractiveness. *Brain Structure and Function*, 215(3–4), 209–223. https://doi.org/10.1007/s00429–010-0287-4

Carrington, S. J., & Bailey, A. J. (2009). Are there theory of mind regions in the brain? A review of the neuroimaging literature. *Human Brain Mapping*, 30 (8), 2313–2335. https://doi.org/10.1002/hbm.20671

Cooper, J. C., Kreps, T. A., Wiebe, T., Pirkl, T., & Knutson, B. (2010). When giving is good: Ventromedial prefrontal cortex activation for others' intentions. *Neuron*, 67(3), 511–521. https://doi.org/10.1016/j.neuron.2010.06 .030

Costa Jr., P. T., McCrae, R. R., & Dye, D. A. (1991). Facet scales for agreeableness and conscientiousness: A revision of the NEO Personality Inventory. *Personality and Individual Differences*, 12(9), 887–898. https://doi.org/10 .1016/j.neuron.2010.06.030

Couch, L. L., & Jones, W. H. (1997). Measuring levels of trust. *Journal of Research in Personality*, 31(3), 319–336. https://doi.org/10.1006/jrpe.1997 .2186

Craig, A. (2011). Significance of the insula for the evolution of human awareness of feelings from the body. *Annals of the New York Academy of Sciences*, 1225 (1), 72–82. https://doi.org/10.1111/j.1749-6632.2011.05990

Delgado-Ballester, E. (2004). Applicability of a brand trust scale across product categories. *European Journal of Marketing*, 38(5–6), 573–592. https://doi.org/10.1108/03090560410529222

Engell, A. D., Haxby, J. V., & Todorov, A. (2007). Implicit trustworthiness decisions: Automatic coding of face properties in the human amygdala. *Journal of Cognitive Neuroscience*, 19(9), 1508–1519. https://doi.org/10.1162/jocn.2007.19.9.1508

Engelmann, J. B., Meyer, F., Ruff, C. C., & Fehr, E. (2019). The neural circuitry of affect-induced distortions of trust. *Science Advances*, 5(3), Article eaau3413. https://doi.org/10.1126/sciadv.aau3413

Evans, A. M., & Krueger, J. I. (2009). The psychology (and economics) of trust. *Social and Personality Psychology Compass*, 3(6), 1003–1017. https://doi.org/10.1111/j.1751-9004.2009.00232.x

Fehr, E., & Gachter, S. (2000). Cooperation and punishment in public goods experiments. *American Economic Review*, 90(4), 980–994. https://doi.org/10.1257/aer.90.4.980

Filkowski, M. M., Anderson, I. W., & Haas, B. W. (2016). Trying to trust: Brain activity during interpersonal social attitude change. *Cognitive, Affective, & Behavioral Neuroscience*, 16(2), 325–338. https://doi.org/10.3758/s13415-015-0393-0

Fujino, J., Tei, S., Itahashi, T., et al. (2020). Role of the right temporoparietal junction in intergroup bias in trust decisions. *Human Brain Mapping*, 41(6), 1677–1688. https://doi.org/10.1002/hbm.24903

Glaeser, E. L., Laibson, D. I., Scheinkman, J. A., & Soutter, C. L. (2000). Measuring trust. *The Quarterly Journal of Economics*, 115(3), 811–846. https://doi.org/10.1162/003355300554926

Haas, B. W., Ishak, A., Anderson, I. W., & Filkowski, M. M. (2015). The tendency to trust is reflected in human brain structure. *NeuroImage*, 107, 175–181. https://doi.org/10.1016/j.neuroimage.2014.11.060

Hill, C. A., & O'Hara, E. A. (2006). A cognitive theory of trust. *Washington University Law Review*, 84(7), 1717–1796. https://doi.org/10.2139/ssrn.869423

Johnson-George, C., & Swap, W. C. (1982). Measurement of specific interpersonal trust: Construction and validation of a scale to assess trust in a specific other. *Journal of Personality and Social Psychology*, 43(6), 1306–1317. https://doi.org/10.1037/0022-3514.43.6.1306

Kahneman, D., Knetsch, J. L., & Thaler, R. H. (1986). Fairness and the assumptions of economics. *Journal of Business*, 59(4), S285–S300. https://doi.org/10.1086/296367

Kang, Y., Williams, L. E., Clark, M. S., Gray, J. R., & Bargh, J. A. (2011). Physical temperature effects on trust behavior: The role of insula. *Social Cognitive and Affective Neuroscience*, 6(4), 507–515. https://doi.org/10.1093/scan/nsq077

Kocher, M. G., Martinsson, P., Matzat, D., & Wollbrant, C. (2015). The role of beliefs, trust, and risk in contributions to a public good. *Journal of Economic Psychology*, 51, 236–244. https://doi.org//10.1016/j.joep.2015.10.001

Koscik, T. R., & Tranel, D. (2011). The human amygdala is necessary for developing and expressing normal interpersonal trust. *Neuropsychologia*, 49 (4), 602–611. https://doi.org/10.1016/j.neuropsychologia.2010.09.023

Krall, S. C., Rottschy, C., Oberwelland, E., et al. (2015). The role of the right temporoparietal junction in attention and social interaction as revealed by ALE meta-analysis. *Brain Structure and Function*, 220(2), 587–604. https://doi.org/10.1007/s00429–014-0803-z

Kramer, R. M. (1999). Trust and distrust in organizations: Emerging perspectives, enduring questions. *Annual Review of Psychology*, 50(1), 569–598. https://doi.org/10.1146/annurev.psych.50.1.569

Krawczyk, D. C. (2002). Contributions of the prefrontal cortex to the neural basis of human decision making. *Neuroscience & Biobehavioral Reviews*, 26(6), 631–664. https://doi.org/10.1016/S0149–7634(02)00021-0

Krolak-Salmon, P., Hénaff, M. A., Isnard, J., et al. (2003). An attention modulated response to disgust in human ventral anterior insula. *Annals of Neurology: Official Journal of the American Neurological Association and the Child Neurology Society*, 53(4), 446–453. https://doi.org/10.1002/ana.10502

Krueger, F., & Meyer-Lindenberg, A. (2019). Toward a model of interpersonal trust drawn from neuroscience, psychology, and economics. *Trends in Neurosciences*, 42(2), 92–101. https://doi.org/10.1016/j.tins.2018.10.004

Ledyard, J. O., Kagel, J. H., & Roth, A. E. (1995). Public goods: A survey of experimental research. In J. H. Kagel & A. E. Roth (Eds.), *The handbook of experimental economics* (pp. 111–194). Princeton University Press. https://doi.org/RePEc:wpa:wuwppe:9405003

Lee, J., Lee, J.-N., & Tan, B. C. (2010). *Emotional trust and cognitive distrust: From a cognitive-affective personality system theory perspective.* Paper presented at the PACIS. https://doi.org/aisel.aisnet.org/pacis2010/114

Lewicki, R. J., McAllister, D. J., & Bies, R. J. (1998). Trust and distrust: New relationships and realities. *Academy of Management Review*, 23(3), 438–458. https://doi.org/10.2307/259288

Li, J., Xiao, E., Houser, D., & Montague, P. R. (2009). Neural responses to sanction threats in two-party economic exchange. *Proceedings of the National Academy of Sciences*, 106(39), 16835–16840. https://doi.org/10.1073/pnas.0908855106

Lieberman, M. D. (2007). Social cognitive neuroscience: A review of core processes. *Annual Review of Psychology*, 58, 259–289. https://doi.org/10.1146/annurev.psych.58.110405.085654

Mal, C. I., Davies, G., & Diers-Lawson, A. (2018). Through the looking glass: The factors that influence consumer trust and distrust in brands. *Psychology & Marketing*, 35(12), 936–947. https://doi.org/10.1002/mar.21146

Marsh, S., & Dibben, M. R. (2005, May). Trust, untrust, distrust and mistrust: An exploration of the dark(er) side. In P. Herrmann, V. Issarny, & S. Shiu (Eds.), *International conference on trust management* (pp. 17–33). Springer. https://doi.org/10.1007/11429760_2

Mayer, R. C., Davis, J. H., & Schoorman, F. D. (1995). An integrative model of organizational trust. *Academy of Management Review*, 20(3), 709–734. https://doi.org/10.2307/258792

McCabe, K. A., & Smith, V. L. (2000). A comparison of naive and sophisticated subject behavior with game theoretic predictions. *Proceedings of the National Academy of Sciences*, 97(7), 3777–3781. https://doi.org/10.1073/pnas.040577397

McCrae, R. R., & Costa Jr., P. T. (1992). Discriminant validity of NEO-PIR facet scales. *Educational and Psychological Measurement*, 52(1), 229–237. https://doi.org/10.1177/001316449205200128

McEvily, B., & Tortoriello, M. (2011). Measuring trust in organisational research: Review and recommendations. *Journal of Trust Research*, 1(1), 23–63. https://doi.org/10.1080/21515581.2011.552424

McKnight, D. H., & Chervany, N. L. (2001). Trust and distrust definitions: One bite at a time. In R. Falcone, M. Singh, & Y.-H. Tan (Eds.), *Trust in cyber-societies* (pp. 27–54). Springer. https://doi.org/10.1007/3-540-45547-7_3

Morrow Jr., J., Hansen, M. H., & Pearson, A. W. (2004). The cognitive and affective antecedents of general trust within cooperative organizations. *Journal of Managerial Issues*, 16, 48–64. https://doi.org/1G1-115036683

Parks, C. D. (1994). The predictive ability of social values in resource dilemmas and public goods games. *Personality and Social Psychology Bulletin*, 20(4), 431–438. https://doi.org/10.1177/0146167294204010

Posten, A.-C., Ockenfels, A., & Mussweiler, T. (2014). How activating cognitive content shapes trust: A subliminal priming study. *Journal of Economic Psychology*, 41, 12–19. https://doi.org/10.1016/j.joep.2013.04.002

Rilling, J. K., Goldsmith, D. R., Glenn, A. L., et al. (2008). The neural correlates of the affective response to unreciprocated cooperation. *Neuropsychologia*, 46(5), 1256–1266. https://doi.org/10.1016/j.neuropsychologia.2007.11.033

Rilling, J. K., Sanfey, A. G., Aronson, J. A., Nystrom, L. E., & Cohen, J. D. (2004). Opposing BOLD responses to reciprocated and unreciprocated altruism in putative reward pathways. *Neuroreport*, 15(16), 2539–2243. https://doi.org/10.1097/00001756-200411150-00022

Rousseau, D. M., Sitkin, S. B., Burt, R. S., & Camerer, C. (1998). Not so different after all: A cross-discipline view of trust. *Academy of Management Review*, 23(3), 393–404. https://doi.org/10.5465/amr.1998.926617

Rule, N. O., Krendl, A. C., Ivcevic, Z., & Ambady, N. (2013). Accuracy and consensus in judgments of trustworthiness from faces: Behavioral and neural correlates. *Journal of Personality and Social Psychology*, 104(3), 409–426. https://doi.org/10.1037/a0031050

Said, C. P., Baron, S. G., & Todorov, A. (2009). Nonlinear amygdala response to face trustworthiness: Contributions of high and low spatial frequency information. *Journal of Cognitive Neuroscience*, 21(3), 519–528. https://doi.org/10.1162/jocn.2009.21041

Sanders, K., Schyns, B., Dietz, G., & Den Hartog, D. N. (2006). Measuring trust inside organisations. *Personnel Review*, 35(5), 557–588. https://DOI.org/10.1108/00483480610682299

Sanfey, A. G., Rilling, J. K., Aronson, J. A., Nystrom, L. E., & Cohen, J. D. (2003). The neural basis of economic decision making in the ultimatum game. *Science*, 300(5626), 1755–1758. https://doi.org/10.1126/science.1082976

Saunders, M., Dietz, G., & Thornhill, A. (2014). Trust and distrust: Polar opposites, or independent but co-existing? *Human Relations*, 67(6), 639–665. https://doi.org/10.1177/0018726713500831

Saunders, M., & Thornhill, A. (2004). Trust and mistrust in organizations: An exploration using an organizational justice framework. *European Journal of Work and Organizational Psychology*, 13(4), 493–515. https://doi.org/10.1080/13594320444000182

Schoorman, F. D., Mayer, R. C., & Davis, J. H. (2007). An integrative model of organizational trust: Past, present, and future. *Academy of Management Review*, 32(2), 344–354. https://doi.org/10.5465/amr.2007.24348410

Siegal, M., & Varley, R. (2002). Neural systems involved in "theory of mind." *Nature Reviews Neuroscience*, 3(6), 463–471. https://doi.org/10.5465/amr.2007.24348410

Symons, D. K. (2004). Mental state discourse, theory of mind, and the internalization of self–other understanding. *Developmental Review*, 24(2), 159–188. https://doi.org/10.1016/j.dr.2004.03.001

Tabibnia, G., Satpute, A. B., & Lieberman, M. D. (2008). The sunny side of fairness: Preference for fairness activates reward circuitry (and disregarding unfairness activates self-control circuitry). *Psychological Science*, 19(4), 339–347. https://doi.org/10.1111/j.1467-9280.2008.02091.x

Todorov, A. (2008). Evaluating faces on trustworthiness: An extension of systems for recognition of emotions signaling approach/avoidance behaviors. *Annals of the New York Academy of Sciences*, 1124(1), 208–224. https://doi.org/10.1196/annals.1440.012

Todorov, A., Pakrashi, M., & Oosterhof, N. N. (2009). Evaluating faces on trustworthiness after minimal time exposure. *Social Cognition*, 27(6), 813–833. https://doi.org/10.1521/soco.2009.27.6.813

Unoka, Z., Seres, I., Áspán, N., Bódi, N., & Kéri, S. (2009). Trust game reveals restricted interpersonal transactions in patients with borderline personality disorder. *Journal of Personality Disorders*, 23(4), 399–409. https://doi.org/10.1521/pedi.2009.23.4.399

Van den Bos, W., & Güroğlu, B. (2009). The role of the ventral medial prefrontal cortex in social decision making. *Journal of Neuroscience*, 29(24), 7631–7632. https://doi.org/10.1523/JNEUROSCI.1821-09.2009

Van Lange, P. A., & Visser, K. (1999). Locomotion in social dilemmas: How people adapt to cooperative, tit-for-tat, and noncooperative partners. *Journal of Personality and Social Psychology*, 77(4), 762–773. https://doi.org/10.1037/0022-3514.77.4.762

Wicker, B., Keysers, C., Plailly, J., Royet, J.-P., Gallese, V., & Rizzolatti, G. (2003). Both of us disgusted in my insula: The common neural basis of seeing and feeling disgust. *Neuron*, 40(3), 655–664. https://doi.org/10.1016/s0896-6273(03)00679-2

Winston, J. S., Strange, B. A., O'Doherty, J., & Dolan, R. J. (2002). Automatic and intentional brain responses during evaluation of trustworthiness of faces. *Nature Neuroscience*, 5(3), 277–283. https://doi.org/10.1038/nn816

Wong, S., Irish, M., O'Callaghan, C., et al. (2017). Should I trust you? Learning and memory of social interactions in dementia. *Neuropsychologia*, 104, 157–167. https://doi.org/10.1016/j.neuropsychologia.2017.08.016

Yamagishi, T., Kanazawa, S., Mashima, R., & Terai, S. (2005). Separating trust from cooperation in a dynamic relationship: Prisoner's dilemma with variable dependence. *Rationality and Society*, 17(3), 275–308. https://doi.org/10.1177/1043463105055463

Trust and Reciprocity
The Role of Outcome-Based and Belief-Based Motivations

Flora Li, Pearl H. Chiu, and Brooks King-Casas

10.1 Introduction

The sense of trust is an essential part of human development and forms during infancy (Erikson, 1963). Based on a cross-discipline view of trust, Rousseau et al. (1998) define trust as "a psychological state comprising the intention to accept vulnerability based upon positive expectations of the intentions or behavior of another" (p. 395). Like trust, reciprocity is an intrinsic part of cooperative social interactions that is similarly observed within parent–infant interactions (Brazelton et al., 1974). Reciprocity describes humans' propensity to reward generosity (positive reciprocity) and to punish opportunism (negative reciprocity) during social exchanges. Similar to trust, assessing whether to reward or to punish similarly requires decision-makers to interpret others' initial intentions.

As both trust and reciprocity are associated with prosocial behavior, positive reciprocity sometimes displays very similar behavioral and neural signatures as trust, making it particularly challenging to separate the two concepts. Early work in sociology, economics, and neuroscience often discusses trust and reciprocity together as if they are the same (Buchan et al., 2002; Cox, 2004; McCabe et al., 2001). Further, findings in social neuroscience sometimes report similar neural patterns for both trust and reciprocity (Bellucci et al., 2017; Bereczkei et al., 2013), making the two concepts even more difficult to distinguish. However, two features may distinguish trust and reciprocity: (i) vulnerability or risk is associated with trust but not reciprocity, and (ii) punishment is involved in negative reciprocity but not trust.

This work was supported in part by the Department of Veterans Affairs, Office of Research and Development, Rehabilitation Research and Development Grant Nos. D2354R and D7030R (to BK-C), and National Institutes of Health Grant Nos. DA036017, MH115221, and MH122948 (to BK-C), and DA042274 and MH106756 (to PHC). Corresponding authors: Flora Li (florali@nau.edu.cn), Pearl H. Chiu (chiup@vt.edu), and Brooks King-Casas (bkcasas@vt.edu).

In the following sections, we borrow insights from economics and psychology to present various trust- and reciprocity-relevant economic theories and their neural predictions. Subsequently, we review neuroscience studies utilizing the trust game (TG) to draw a neural distinction between trust and reciprocity. Finally, we discuss future directions related to this topic and neuropathologic differences in trust and reciprocity.

10.2 The Trust Game

Both trust and reciprocity are defined differently and examined with diverse methods across disciplines. In this chapter, we constrain our discussion of trust and reciprocity to findings within the TG, a laboratory-controlled two-person monetary exchange developed by Berg et al. (1995) to investigate the concept of trust in their seminal work (see also Chapter 2). Since then, the TG has been used as a standard behavioral economic tool to examine trust and reciprocity experimentally (Bellucci et al., 2019; McCabe et al., 2003; Unoka et al., 2009), and various neuroscience studies have fruitfully exploited variants of the basic TG to explore neural mechanisms underlying cooperative exchange (Robson et al., 2020; Tzieropoulos, 2013).

In the basic TG, two players, an investor and a trustee, make monetary exchanges sequentially (Figure 10.1). With some initial endowment, the game starts with the investor first proposing to invest a portion of her endowment, or not. Any portion invested is multiplied (typically doubled or tripled) before being received by the trustee. The trustee then decides how much of her current holding (the doubled or tripled investment plus any initial endowment) to return. Both players are familiar with the rules of the game, and this setting provides the two players the opportunity for mutual gain, in which the investor invests a positive amount, and the trustee returns a positive amount. Within this exchange, the amount sent by the investor reflects trust, and the amount returned by the trustee reflects positive reciprocity. Although classical economic theory suggests that a rational investor should anticipate a zero return and therefore make zero investment in the first stage, a large economic literature reports mutual cooperation (trust and reciprocity) within TGs, both in the lab and in the field (Cardenas & Carpenter, 2008; Johnson & Mislin, 2011). Typical variations of TGs include varying initial endowments, manipulating the investment return rate, and changing the action space from continuous to discrete or even binary choices.

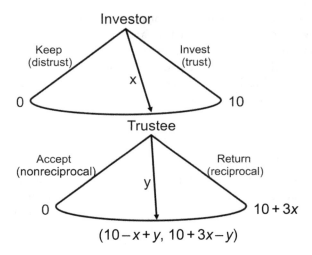

Figure 10.1   Illustration of a trust game.
Both players are endowed with 10 units to start. Investor chooses to share $x \in [0, 10]$. If $x = 0$, the game ends and both players end up with initial endowment. If $x > 0$, then Trustee chooses to return $y \in [0, 10 + 3x]$, and Investor and Trustee's final payoff is $10 - x + y$ and $10 + 3x - y$, respectively. Often the trust game is adjusted with discrete or even binary action spaces to accommodate particular research questions or neuroimaging methods.

The two-step structure of a single-shot TG has a distinctive temporal advantage in both behavioral and neural analyses to separate trust and reciprocity events. Throughout this chapter, trust is defined as the amount invested by the investors or the investors' choice to invest in the TG, and reciprocity is defined as the amount returned by the trustees or the trustees' decision to reciprocate in the TG.

10.3   Economic Theories and Predictions

Various economic theories regarding social preferences have attempted to capture the behavioral motivations behind the TG for each of the players, including both distributional preferences (e.g., inequity aversion [Bolton & Ockenfels, 2000; Fehr & Schmidt, 1999]), and belief-dependent motivations (e.g., guilt aversion [Charness & Dufwenberg, 2006]). However, a fundamental feature that separates the motivations to trust and reciprocate in the TG is the risk inherent in investors' choices embedded naturally in this unique social context (Fehr & Fischbacher,

2003). This risk has been modeled both as a general risk aversion (Lauharatanahirun et al., 2012), as well as betrayal aversion assuming belief-dependent motivations (Aimone et al., 2014; Bohnet & Zeckhauser, 2004) (see also Chapter 5).

10.3.1 Outcome-Based versus Belief-Based Motivations

Both outcome-based and belief-based theories have been used to investigate behavior of investors (trust) and trustees (reciprocity). Distributional preference models or outcome-based models assume individuals care not only about themselves but also about others and describe individuals' preferences over monetary outcome divisions. Examples of distributional preference models include inequality aversion (Bolton & Ockenfels, 2000; Fehr & Schmidt, 1999) and preference for group efficiency (Charness & Rabin, 2002). In contrast to outcome-based models, belief-dependent or belief-based models assume individuals make decisions based on expectations of themselves and others. Economists often model emotions with belief-dependent motivations, such as anger (Battigalli et al., 2019) and guilt (Battigalli & Dufwenberg, 2007). Within these theories, beliefs and expectations about or of others generate emotions, and such emotions influence human actions (Elster, 1998). In this section, we introduce outcome- and belief-based approaches through two classic models: inequality aversion representing distributional preferences and guilt aversion representing belief-dependent motivations.

10.3.2 Outcome-Based Inequality Aversion

Inequity aversion (Fehr & Schmidt, 1999) is a signature model among all distributional preference models, where individuals are assumed to have preferences over equal monetary distributions. In this model, player i receives utility from her own monetary payoff x_i, but receives disutility from unequal monetary payoff compared with player j. Player i dislikes getting not only less (disadvantageous inequality or envy; α) but also more (advantageous inequality or compassion; β) than player j. The model also assumes that $\alpha > \beta$; therefore, player i's disutility from disadvantageous inequality is greater than her disutility from advantageous inequality.

$$U_i(x) = x_i - \alpha[x_j - x_i]^+ - \beta[x_i - x_j]^+, i \neq j$$

Many studies have shown that individuals exhibit distributional preferences when making decisions for themselves and others. Individuals are often willing to sacrifice their own earning to punish opportunists who offer unequal payoffs in ultimatum games (UGs) (Tisserand, 2014). In a UG, a proposer first proposes how to divide a sum of money with a responder. The responder then decides either to accept the division or to reject so that both players receive 0. Fehr and Gächter (2002) report a similar egalitarian preference in a public goods game with punishment, where participants altruistically punish free riders. In this game, a group of players decides how much each player contributes to a public good with a return. Players keep the remaining endowment, and they split the public good return equally. However, players in the group can punish free riders who contributed less with a cost. In an income alteration experiment, where participants have the opportunity to either help or harm any of the group members with their own earnings when playing a public goods game, participants present strong egalitarian preferences to reduce income inequality among group members (Dawes et al., 2007).

Distributional preferences, especially inequality aversion, have been correlated with neural responses in the reward-sensitive neural structures, such that the ventromedial prefrontal cortex (vmPFC) and ventral striatum (vSTR) exhibit stronger activation when disadvantageous and advantageous inequality are diminished (Tricomi et al., 2010). Similarly, in a TG, where participants play as trustees, brain activities in the vSTR and amygdala correlate with decisions that are consistent with distributional preferences quantified within an inequality aversion model (Nihonsugi et al., 2015). In addition, activity in the temporoparietal junction (TPJ), a region implicated in mentalizing or theory of mind (Schurz et al., 2014), has been associated with distributional considerations within social decision making (Hutcherson et al., 2015; Mitchell, 2007). Specifically, Morishima et al. (2012) found that gray matter volume in the right TPJ correlates with individuals' altruistic propensity and predicts the advantageous inequality parameter (β) but not the disadvantageous inequality parameter (α) within a dictator game (DG), where one party (the dictator) determines payoff for both parties. Taking the above studies together, these data suggest that activations within the vmPFC, vSTR, and TPJ reflect the use of outcome-based, distributional preferences when evaluating options during social decision making (Figure 10.2).

10.3.3   Belief-Based Guilt Aversion

Battigalli and Dufwenberg (2007) developed a guilt aversion model based on a straightforward psychological assumption that decision-makers dislike

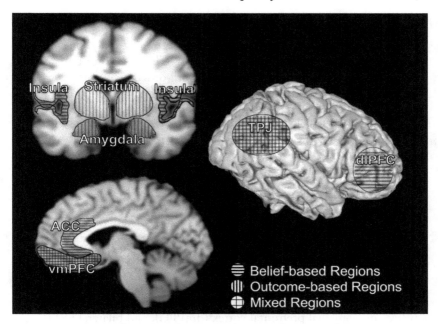

Figure 10.2   Illustration of economic theory-predicted neural outcomes.
Areas labeled with horizontal lines represent brain regions activated during belief-motivated choices. Areas labeled with vertical lines represent brain regions activated during outcome-motivated behavior. Areas labeled with crossed lines indicate brain regions activated during both belief-based and outcome-based decision making.

the negative emotion of guilt. In a TG, both the investor and the trustee might experience guilt, and here we use a trustee's guilt aversion as an illustration. Suppose investor i chooses to invest and expects trustee j to return E'_i (first-order belief), and trustee j believes that investor i expects to receive E''_j (second-order belief). Trustee j does not know the exact value of E'_i, but she uses E''_j instead as a close proxy of investor i's expectation. Guilt is assessed as the positive difference between the amount that trustee j believes investor i expects and the actual amount investor i receives ($[E''_j - x_i]^+$), which corresponds to how much trustee j believes she has hurt investor i. While a guilt-averse trustee j values her own monetary payoff x_j, she also incurs a cost from feeling guilty if she has let investor i down. Parameter γ_j measures how sensitive j is to guilt, and determines trustee j's return amount.

$$U_j(x, E'') = x_j - \gamma_j [E_j'' - x_i]^+, j \neq i$$

Guerra and Zizzo (2004) demonstrated experimentally that trustees exhibit a belief-dependent nature in TGs. Charness and Dufwenberg (2006) further revealed that trustees' second-order beliefs are correlated with their reciprocal decisions in TGs. A survey reports that belief-dependent guilt aversion helps to explain not only reciprocal behavior in TGs but also altruistic behavior in DGs (Cartwright, 2019). In addition to the association between expectations and behavior found in TGs, researchers also observe a correlation between a guilt aversion parameter (γ) evaluated from TGs and guilt sensitivity measured through a self-report questionnaire (Bellemare et al., 2019).

Chang et al. (2011) investigated neural correlates of guilt aversion as participants played as trustees in a TG. Increased neural activity in the mentalizing network, including the insula, anterior cingulate cortex (ACC), TPJ, and right dorsolateral prefrontal cortex (dlPFC), was observed when trustees' repayment matched perceived expectations, reflecting guilt aversion-consistent reciprocal behavior. In contrast, when trustees returned less than expected, increasing neural activations in the vmPFC, dorsomedial prefrontal cortex (dmPFC), and bilateral vSTR were detected. Similar results were shown in another study where authors examined the neural correlates of belief-dependent decision making in UGs (Chang & Sanfey, 2011). This study found that a belief-dependent model outperformed an inequality aversion (outcome-dependent) model in predicting responders' choices to reject or accept offers. That is, when offers increasingly violated responders' expectations, neural responses increased in the left insula and ACC.

Nihonsugi et al. (2015) went a step further to distinguish neural mechanisms for belief-dependent motivations from those reflecting distributional preferences using both neural measurement technique functional magnetic resonance imaging (fMRI) and neural manipulation technique transcranial direct current stimulation (tDCS). This work used both an inequality aversion and a guilt aversion model to capture trustees' behavior in a binary choice TG, where trustees experience disadvantageous inequality when choosing to return more (cooperate), but experience guilt when choosing to return less (defect). Using fMRI, they found that activity in the right dlPFC was associated with the guilt aversion parameter, whereas activity in the vSTR and amygdala was associated with the inequality aversion parameter. Furthermore, a causal relationship was observed, that anodal tDCS over the right dlPFC increases belief-dependent cooperative behavior. Taken together, the work suggests that belief-dependent behavior associated with guilt aversion is supported by activity in a mentalizing network that includes the insula, ACC, TPJ, and dlPFC (Figure 10.2).

10.3.4 Modeling Uncertainty for Investors

While inequality aversion and guilt aversion are commonly used models for examining trust and reciprocity in economics, we also emphasize that an essential feature separating trust from reciprocity is the risk inherent in expressions of trust. Investors face the possibility of nonreciprocation and the associated betrayal, whereas trustees experience no uncertainty over the outcomes of their choice. Decisions to trust or not can be influenced by at least two sources of uncertainty. The first corresponds to a general aversion to risk that is agnostic of the social source of the uncertainty. In addition, a second disutility due to the potential for betrayal can influence an investor's decision to trust.

10.3.4.1 Risk Aversion

Risk aversion describes a phenomenon that individuals often prefer certainty to uncertain outcomes, and sometimes even sacrifice monetary incentives to pick a low value but certain option over a high value but uncertain one. Risk aversion can be modeled as a concavity in the utility function (Bernoulli, 1954). A concave utility function helps to resolve the issue, where traditional expected utility theory assumes that an individual's utility from an increase of earning of \$1,000 is constant regardless of the initial wealth. However, in reality, individuals gain higher utility with lower initial wealth (from \$0 to \$1,000) than with higher initial wealth (from \$999,000 to \$1,000,000). Bernoulli (1954) proposes a power utility function instead of the traditional linear form to capture risk attitude, $U_i(x) = x_i^\theta$. Where risk-averse individuals have parameter $\theta < 1$, risk-neutral individuals have parameter $\theta = 1$, and risk-seeking individuals have parameter $\theta > 1$.

Arrow (1965) and Pratt (1978) propose two measures of risk attitude that are independent of the functional form of the utility function. The first one can be expressed with a constant absolute risk aversion (CARA): $a = -u''(x)/u'(x)$, where $u'(x)$ and $u''(x)$ denote the first and the second derivatives of the utility function $u(x)$. A decision-maker who satisfies CARA is willing to pay the same risk premium to avoid a certain amount of risk regardless of the given wealth. A commonly used CARA utility function is $u(x) = 1 - e^{-ax}$. The second form is constant relative risk aversion (CRRA): $\rho = -(x \cdot u''(x))/u'(x)$, where $\rho \leq 1$ stands for the percentage of wealth that the decision-maker is willing to sacrifice over risk. Bernoulli's power risk aversion function satisfies CRRA. Another commonly used CRRA utility function is $u(x) = \frac{x^{(1-\rho)}}{1-\rho}$.

The majority of the risk aversion literature in economics examines only the individual's decision making (Harrison et al., 2007; Holt & Laury, 2002). Neuroscience literature suggests that risk aversion attitude is associated with activations in the STR and insula (Christopoulos et al., 2009; Preuschoff et al., 2006; Schultz et al., 2008). Extending from risk (known probability) to ambiguity (unknown probability), an fMRI study of risk and ambiguous preferences reported that lateral prefrontal cortex (lPFC) response correlated with ambiguity attitude whereas parietal cortex response correlated with risk attitude (Huettel et al., 2006). Similarly, Schultz et al. (2008) detected a stronger signal in the orbitofrontal cortex (OFC) and amygdala comparing ambiguous to risk gambles. This finding is in line with the results of Hsu et al. (2005), where ambiguous choices were correlated positively with signal in the amygdala and OFC and negatively with the STR. Without cumulative knowledge about partners' preferences, it is unlikely for a player to acquire precise risk probabilities in a TG. Therefore, when decision-makers are influenced by uncertainty to make decisions to trust or not in a TG, we anticipate observing activations in ambiguity-related regions, including the lPFC and amygdala.

Lauharatanahirun et al. (2012) investigated neural mechanisms of processing risk in a nonsocial versus social context using general risk aversion. In a neutral, nonsocial, condition, a participant selected options for herself, and a lottery then determined the payoff; in a social condition, the participant played a TG with real persons who made decisions in previous sessions. The neutral condition was programmed to match the mean, second, and third moments of the social condition. A CRRA utility function $u(x) = \frac{x^{(1-\rho)}}{1-\rho}$ was used to model risky decisions. The authors showed that the amygdala modulated risk-related decisions, such that individuals who were more risk-averse in the social condition displayed a decreased amygdala activity during the neutral condition, but who were more risk-averse in the neutral condition displayed an increased amygdala activity during the social condition. Unfortunately, there exist too few studies utilizing general risk aversion in social contexts to make further predictions about the role of general risk preferences in distinguishing trust from reciprocity.

10.3.4.2   Belief-Dependent Betrayal Aversion

Bohnet and Zeckhauser (2004) proposed the idea of betrayal aversion, in which one's fear of being betrayed by others influences one's willingness to trust. Without a formal model, Bohnet and Zeckhauser (2004) tested the hypothesis that an investor's belief about return security determines her investing decision in a TG, which implies belief-dependent motivations. A stylized belief-dependent betrayal aversion model can be specified as:

$$U_i(x, E) = x_i - \lambda_i [E_i - \min E_i]^+, i \neq j.$$

In a TG (Figure 10.1), investor i's fear of being betrayed can be expressed as a positive discrepancy between the initial expectation of her payoff (E_i) and the potential worst outcome ($\min E_i$). In other words, she fears betrayal when she realizes that it is possible to get less than her initial expectation. Parameter λ_i measures sensitivity to betrayal aversion. Investor i's utility function contains her own payoff x_i and any disutility from the fear of being betrayed. Betrayal aversion is relevant when the decision-maker faces potential risk arising exclusively in a social context, in contrast with general risk aversion that occurs when the outcome is determined by nature, independent from human interactions (Aimone et al., 2015; Cubitt et al., 2017).

Broad behavioral evidence for betrayal aversion can be found across countries among participants with different political, cultural, religious, and historical backgrounds (Bohnet et al., 2008). Aimone and Houser (2012) demonstrate that betrayal aversion alone reduces one-third of the investment in TGs when strategic risk is controlled in the experimental design. Despite the negative impact of betrayal aversion on reducing trust, knowing the presence of betrayal-averse agents increases trustees' reciprocal return (Aimone & Houser, 2013).

There are limited neuroscience studies of betrayal aversion. Aimone et al. (2014) explored the neural correlates of betrayal aversion using a TG setting, in which investors played half of the trials with a human trustee and half with human decisions randomly selected by a computer. Increased neural activity in the right anterior insula, medial frontal cortex, and right dlPFC was reported in human trials contrasted with computer-mediated trials. This work also found that, comparing the choice of trust or not independent of counterparts, participants exhibit increased neural activation in the right anterior insula and ACC. Furthermore, the interaction between the chosen option and the identity of the counterpart revealed enhanced insula activity when participants chose to trust a human partner. It appears that part of the mentalizing network is correlated with betrayal aversion-consistent behavior.

10.4   Neural Distinctions between Trust and Reciprocity

Before discussing neural distinctions between trust and reciprocity, it is worth reiterating that the broad behavioral evidence supports the idea that trust and reciprocity are distinct. The earliest research using the TG found no correlation between decisions to trust and decisions to reciprocate (Berg et al., 1995), and a meta-analysis reviewing 162 TG studies found investors on average sent 50% of their endowment, while trustees reciprocated only 37% of the available amount (Johnson & Mislin, 2011). In addition, data suggest that different factors influence trusting and reciprocal behavior, respectively. Investors' trust decisions are influenced by the randomness of the payment (number of trials paid), whether they are playing against a human, and the geographic or financial regions of the experiment. In comparison, trustees' decisions are affected by the return on investment, whether they played as both roles, and participants' age (Johnson & Mislin, 2011).

While both outcome-dependent motivations and belief-dependent motivations have been hypothesized to contribute to decisions to trust and reciprocate, the neural findings reviewed above suggest a neural distinction between types of motivation, as illustrated in Figure 10.2. The insula, dlPFC, and ACC are consistently associated with concerns about expectations, whereas the STR and amygdala are consistently selected for concerns about distribution. In addition, the TPJ and medial prefrontal cortex seem to play a role in motivating both mentalizing and concern for outcome. In this section, we will focus on the above neural regions as we discuss neural signatures for trust and reciprocity, respectively.

10.4.1   Neural Signatures of Trust

In this section, we discuss several neuroscience articles that focus on neural activity associated with investor decisions within the TG. Delgado et al. (2005) investigated the neural pattern of investors who faced trustees with different moral characters. Participants played a repeated TG with praiseworthy, neutral, and suspect trustees. Not surprisingly, participants trusted "good" partners more and distrusted "bad" partners more. Whole-brain analyses revealed that the vSTR and insula were more active when contrasting trust to distrust decisions. These results are consistent with both the pattern of outcome-dependent and belief-dependent motivations, while insula responses are consistent with the reputation or reciprocal nature of the repeated TG.

Stanley et al. (2012) examined how race influences neural correlates of trust. Participants played a series of one-shot TGs as investors paired with either black, white, or other trustees. A trust-bias score was computed as the normalized difference between mean trust to white and mean trust to black trustees. A positive trust-bias score indicates the investor's mean offer is higher to white trustees than to black trustees, and a negative trust-bias score indicates greater trust of black trustees. The contrast of black relative to white trustees was correlated with trust-bias scores in the STR, meaning that investors show greater responses in the STR to whichever race group they trusted less. In addition, regardless of one's trust bias score, the amygdala was more active when sending money to black versus white trustees. This neural pattern of results is consistent with the idea that trust behavior is driven by concerns for outcome distribution, such as inequality aversion.

Riedl et al. (2014) carried out a TG experiment, in which participants played as investors against human and avatar faces for multiple rounds. The human and avatar faces were rated to be equivalent in trustworthiness. Investors exhibited the same level of trust toward either trustworthy or untrustworthy avatars but displayed a higher level of trust toward trustworthy humans compared to untrustworthy humans. In the decision phase, activity of the vmPFC, dmPFC, and ACC correlated with the contrast of human to avatar. As reviewed above, ACC activity relates to belief-dependent motivations in the TG, and vmPFC and dmPFC activity relates to distributional preferences; therefore, results from Riedl et al. (2014) promote outcome- and belief-dependent motivations in trust.

In an article evaluating developmental differences in the TG, adolescents and young adults (aged 16–27) played repeated TGs as investors with fixed reciprocal and nonreciprocal trustees (Lemmers-Jansen et al., 2017). Behaviorally, males exhibited higher initial trust in their first interaction with a stranger. In the cooperative condition (reciprocal trustee), both males and females increased trust with age. However, when faced with nonreciprocal trustees, older males decreased trust most, while females' trust was independent of age. Activation of the right TPJ and right dlPFC was associated with increasing age during the investment phase while activation of the right caudate was found increasing with age during the repayment phase. As the authors mentioned, since the TG is played repeatedly, investors' decisions in later rounds involve concerns for reputation and reciprocity. As the TPJ has been linked with mentalizing, and inequality aversion, these results suggest trust is motivated by both intention and outcome in developing adolescents and young adults.

Engelmann et al. (2019) conducted an experiment to test how induced aversive affect influences behavioral and neural patterns in the TG. Participants faced prolonged periods of the threat of electric shock (induced aversive affect), while making investment decisions either as investors in a TG or to a TG-equivalent lottery. Negative affect reduced trust and suppressed trust-specific activity in the left TPJ. In addition, aversive affect reduced trust-specific functional connectivity (FC) between the TPJ and the amygdala. Engelmann et al. (2019) further identified a network, including the TPJ, dmPFC, ventrolateral prefrontal cortex, and posterior superior temporal sulcus, that predicted trust behavior. Functional connectivity among the trust network diminished with aversive affect. Based on the dmPFC and TPJ's role in inequality aversion and the amygdala's role in processing risk, Engelmann et al. (2019) provide evidence for outcome-based trust.

In a review of neuroscience studies of TGs, Tzieropoulos (2013) examined factors contributing to trust and reciprocity. She concluded that different cues of trustees, hormones like oxytocin, socioeconomic status, psychiatric disorders, and variations in experimental setups are all factors influencing trusting behaviors. In addition, variations in experimental settings, including whether interactions are one-shot or repeated, can engender learning and reputation. The literature investigating the neural signature of trust demonstrates that behavioral trust is commonly associated with neural responses in brain regions guiding distributional preferences, including the vSTR and amygdala. When TGs are played repeatedly, we also observe trusting behavior in conjunction with activations of belief-based brain regions such as the insula, dlPFC, and ACC. Given current evidence, we cannot rule out the possibility that reciprocal or reputational concerns induced by repeated interaction cause such belief-dependent neural responses.

10.4.2   Neural Signatures of Reciprocity

Compared with research on investors' choices, less research has focused on trustees' behavior. King-Casas et al. (2005) explore the neural dynamics of investors and trustees' repeated interactions. Forty-eight pairs of participants played 10 rounds of a repeated TG during a fMRI scan. Caudate activity among trustees scaled with change in tit-for-tat reciprocity between investors and trustees, with positive deviations in reciprocity eliciting greater enhanced caudate responses relative to negative deviations in reciprocity. Further, caudate activity in trustees predicted increases and decreases in reciprocation. This signal appeared after the revelation of investor's choice in early rounds, but shifted across the repeated exchange, anticipating the revelation of investor's choice in late rounds. While these data suggest reciprocal behavior is, in part, driven by beliefs about expected investor actions, the pattern of neural activity is consistent with outcome-dependent motivations.

In a modified repeated TG, where investors made a back-transfer request and chose whether or not to impose sanctions, Li et al. (2009) investigated trustees' neural responses to potential sanctions during decisions to reciprocate. The sanction was in the form of a fixed fine for not returning the requested amount. Investors imposed sanctions 46% of the time. On average, investors requested two-thirds of the tripled amount, which did not differ from the equal earning split point and did not differ between sanction and no sanction conditions. Interestingly, trustees returned significantly less in the sanction condition than in the no sanction condition. Trustees' neural activity in the right dlPFC during the decision phase negatively correlated with trustees' reciprocation amount, while trustees' neural signal in the vmPFC during investors' choice to sanction positively predicted trustees' reciprocity. These data indicate that sensitivity to sanctions, reflected in the vmPFC response, predicts reciprocal decisions, and the dlPFC response, linked with processing others' intentions, reflects real-time reciprocal behavior.

Van den Bos et al. (2009) explored determinants of reciprocation within the TG. The authors hypothesized that trustee reciprocation is triggered by the amount of risk assumed by investors. The result showed that while trustees reciprocated half of the time, they reciprocated more often when investors took greater risks to trust and as well as when there is a higher potential benefit to trustees for trusting. Trustee decisions to defect over reciprocate resulted in greater activation in the vmPFC and positive activation in the bilateral insula, right TPJ, and ACC. Then together, these results support an intention-based (i.e., belief-based) theory of motivated reciprocity.

The same group of researchers subsequently investigated developmental changes in reciprocity (Van den Bos et al., 2011) (see also Chapter 11). Adolescents and young adults (aged 12–22) played TGs as trustees. As age increased, individuals became more reciprocal, though overall reciprocity was similar to adult behavior in the previous study (Van den Bos et al., 2009). Trustees' decisions to defect over reciprocate was associated with signals in the vmPFC and left insula. In addition, reciprocal behavior was also associated with increased activity in the right dlPFC, bilateral anterior insula, and ACC. The above pattern of activity is consistent with the results of Aimone et al. (2014), suggesting reciprocal behavior to be belief-dependent.

Yet, another study examined how neural correlates of reciprocity are affected by previous experience of reciprocity (Cáceda et al., 2017). Participants played TGs as trustees in a baseline condition and played TGs first as investors and then as trustees in an emotionally challenging condition, where a previous reciprocal experience was evaluated. Behavioral results show that participants reciprocate more often when they are previously reciprocated. Neural results revealed reciprocal behavior in the baseline and the emotional challenge condition to be positively associated with responses of the insula and ACC, again consistent with the theory that reciprocal behavior is motivated by concern for others' intentions.

Though less research has focused on reciprocity than trust, overwhelming evidence suggests that reciprocal behavior is associated with neural responses in belief-dependent brain regions, including the insula, dlPFC, and ACC. That is, of the six articles discussed above, five implicated regions associated with concern for others' intentions.

10.4.3   Comparisons of Trust and Reciprocity

Few neuroscience studies have examined the decisions of both investors and trustees. To directly evaluate distinctions in neural correlates of trust and reciprocity, below we review studies that examine both investors' and trustees' decisions within the same study. In an fMRI experiment where participants play repeated TGs as either investors or trustees, Krueger et al. (2008) identified anterior insula and vmPFC activity to be common to both trust and reciprocity, while stronger right TPJ and lateral frontopolar cortex signal was found for trust when compared to reciprocation. However, during repeated TGs, investors face potential reciprocal concerns or reputation concerns that trustees do not repay well in future interactions, and this concern may manifest in similar neural patterns to those of trustees. Activation in the anterior insula for investors might be driven by this reputation or reciprocal concern, which would be consistent with belief-dependent motivations. Enhanced TPJ activity in the trust condition relative to the reciprocity condition is consistent with distributional motivations.

Bereczkei et al. (2013) conducted a TG experiment to explore the neural correlates of Machiavellian individuals' decision-making process. Machiavellian individuals typically display deception and manipulation for self-interest during social interactions. Based on Machiavellian individuals' ability to exploit others, the authors hypothesized that high Machiavellian (HM) individuals would display elevated activity in brain areas involved in reward-seeking, the anticipation of risky situations, and inference-making compared to low Machiavellian (LM) individuals. Participants played TGs as both investors and trustees during fMRI scanning. HM investors sent less money, HM trustees returned less money, and HM participants accrued greater earnings in the experiment. Increased signal in the thalamus and ACC for investors and the anterior insula and inferior frontal gyrus for trustees was observed among HM relative to LM players. The authors interpreted thalamic responses of investors to be related to processing reward and anticipating risk, while the ACC was related to mentalizing, consistent with trust being driven by both distributional preference and belief-dependent motivations. Insula responses for trustees were associated with mentalizing and making inferences, which suggests reciprocity is driven by concern for others' intentions (belief-based motivation).

A coordinate-based meta-analysis investigating neural correlates of trust and reciprocity in TGs was carried out by Bellucci et al. (2017). Using activation likelihood estimation (ALE), the convergence of foci reported from different neuroimaging studies was determined, and the authors tested whether resulting clusters were above chance. The coordinate-based meta-analysis revealed consistent anterior insula responses during unconditional trust (one-shot TG) and reciprocity, and vSTR during conditional trust (repeated TG). In addition, the fusiform gyrus, intraparietal sulcus, and inferior occipital gyrus were engaged during reciprocal behavior. As discussed earlier, vSTR activity implies concern for inequality in distribution, whereas anterior insula response is consistent with concern for others' intentions. This meta-analysis provides additional support for intention-motivated reciprocity and outcome-motivated trust. However, the strength of evidence should be considered provisional. While 23 studies were included for investor-related results, only 2 of these studies contributed to the unconditional trust result (Aimone et al., 2014; Stanley et al., 2012). Therefore, the unconditional trust result is very likely to be influenced by some unique results from these two articles.

In addition to fMRI studies, differences between trust and reciprocity have been investigated through lesion studies (see also Chapter 18). Krajbich et al. (2009) tested the decision-making performance of vmPFC-damaged patients in a series of economic games, including the TG. Participants included 6 patients with focal damage to the vmPFC, 20 brain-damaged comparisons (BDC, with damage in diverse cortical regions but excluding the vmPFC), and 16 healthy comparisons. Behavioral results showed no difference in trusting behavior across the three groups, but vmPFC-damaged patients returned significantly less compared to healthy comparisons. The authors used an inequality aversion model (Fehr & Schmidt, 1999), where a disadvantageous inequality parameter α and advantageous inequality parameter β were estimated. The computational result demonstrated that vmPFC-damaged patients have significantly lower β compared to both comparison groups, suggesting that vmPFC damage causes patients to become more selfish, caring more about their own payoff. However, no difference in α was found across groups. This result implicates the vmPFC in distributional preferences within the TG.

With minimal research examining neural distinctions between trust and reciprocity, it is extremely challenging to draw definitive conclusions. Current research indicates that reciprocity is belief-dependent as the anterior insula is consistently implicated in reciprocal behavior. In contrast, neural correlates of trust results are mixed in their support of belief-based and outcome-based motivations, with no consistent neural pattern for trust across studies. Clearly, further research examining the behavior of both investors and trustees is required to expand our understanding of motivations of different types of social interactions.

10.4.4   Resting-State Functional Connectivity Differences

In Sections 10.4.1, 10.4.2, and 10.4.3, we discussed brain regions activated during trust and reciprocation within TGs. In addition, FC among these regions can provide additional understanding of potential neural mechanisms separating trust with reciprocity. Task-free resting-state FC (RSFC) has often been used to relate individual-level differences in neural connectivity with personality traits, cognitive capacities, and social preferences (Gordon et al., 2017; Hahn et al., 2015). Here, we discuss two studies that attempt to predict trusting and reciprocal behavior via RSFC (see also Chapter 12).

Cáceda et al. (2015) conducted a TG experiment to predict trustees' reciprocal behavior using RSFC. Participants underwent a 5-minute resting-state functional scan, before playing as trustees in multiple TGs with different opponents. Neural networks were defined with group-level independent component analysis (ICA) during resting state. Ten ICA components were then grouped into six functional networks. This approach found that FC between the salience network (including the ACC, insula, and middle temporal gyrus) and right central-executive network (including the dlPFC, precuneus, superior temporal gyrus, cerebellum, frontal pole, and inferior parietal lobule) was most predictive of trustees' reciprocation decisions (~20%), again consistent with suggestions that reciprocal behavior is motivated by belief-dependent models, possibly guilt aversion.

Another TG experiment using RSFC examines both investors and trustees' behavior (Bellucci et al., 2019). Participants underwent an 11-minute resting-state functional scan, followed by a one-shot TG as either investor or trustee. The authors computed region of interest (ROI) to ROI connectivity and divided all ROIs into five functional neural networks. Investors and trustees were comparable with respect to their social abilities and preferences, and these variables did not predict trust or reciprocity. Level of trust and reciprocation were comparable such that both investors and trustees gave about half of the available share to their opponents. RSFC of different edges within the default-mode network (DMN) predicted trust and reciprocity, respectively. The vmPFC, precuneus, and TPJ predicted trust, whereas the superior frontal gyrus, inferior temporal gyrus, and posterior cingulate cortex (PCC) predicted reciprocity. Besides the DMN, FC of the dlPFC and parietal cortex within the frontoparietal network (FPN) and FC of the insula and ACC within the cingulo-opercular network (CON) also predicted reciprocity.

Though the two studies defined neural networks differently, we see a clear overlap between the FC of the brain regions predicting reciprocity. Again, this result supports the hypothesis that reciprocity is motivated by belief-based theory. However, the distinction of FC within the DMN in predicting trust and reciprocity supports the idea that trust is driven by distributional preferences, such as inequality aversion (Nihonsugi et al., 2015; Tricomi et al., 2010). In addition, the neural evidence disagrees with natural risk aversion (Huettel et al., 2006; Schultz et al., 2008).

10.4.5 Hormone-Level Distinctions

As summarized in the previous subsections, different brain regions react distinctly to trust and reciprocity, and different neural networks predict trust and reciprocity, respectively. At the neuromolecular level, we also find evidence that different neuropeptides and hormones have a distinct effect on trusting and reciprocal behavior (see also Chapter 13).

The neuropeptide oxytocin is known for its unique function in maternal behavior, sexual reproduction, and social bonding (Argiolas & Gessa, 1991; Carter, 1992; Donaldson & Young, 2008; Ross & Young, 2009). Kosfeld et al. (2005) evaluated the effect of intranasal oxytocin on playing the TG. Male participants were randomly assigned to oxytocin or placebo treatments to play as either investors or trustees. Results showed that a single intranasal dose of oxytocin increased investment by 17% compared to the placebo group. Trustees, on average, returned more than invested in both treatments, but the returned amount did not differ between the oxytocin and placebo groups. Therefore, intranasal oxytocin promotes trust but not reciprocity. To control the potential social risk naturally embedded in investors' decisions, the authors ran a TG comparable risk experiment, where investors played against a risk mechanism that replicated trustees' behavior. There was no difference in the investment amount in the risk experiment between the oxytocin and placebo groups. This result further supports oxytocin's effect on social trust.

The steroid hormone testosterone has been linked to gaining or maintaining social status, aggression, antisocial behavior, and peer and family relationships (Booth et al., 2006). Testosterone has been shown to play a role in social competition (Edwards et al., 2006). Because of testosterone's role in aggression and social status, it is natural to hypothesize that investors are more aggressive with testosterone, but trustees in such socially nonchallenging situations obtain a higher social status through prosocial behavior with testosterone. Boksem et al. (2013) conducted a TG experiment with either self-administrated single-dose testosterone or placebo. Female participants played a one-shot TG with anonymous partners, once as investors and once as trustees. The results are consistent with the prior testosterone hypothesis. With testosterone administration, investors decreased investment by 38%, and trustees increased reciprocity by 10%, compared to the placebo group. The authors also showed that testosterone has no impact on risk and ambiguity aversion. This finding supports the idea that testosterone facilitates obtaining high social status in a context-dependent fashion.

Even though the above studies clearly implicate hormones in trust and reciprocal behavior, research on their influence on decision making is mixed. In a randomized controlled trial, researchers observed no difference at all among DG, UG, TG, and risk aversion comparing testosterone and placebo groups (Zethraeus et al., 2009). Whereas in a study using facial trustworthiness evaluations, female participants, especially those who are socially naive, exhibited a decreased trust with testosterone administration relative to placebo (Bos et al., 2010). Like testosterone studies, the effect of oxytocin on trust is similarly not consistent. Some studies find similar results as in Kosfeld et al. (2005) (Heinrichs et al., 2009), but the precise effect of intranasal oxytocin remains debatable (Leng & Ludwig, 2016). Bartz et al. (2011) report that the effect of oxytocin is context-dependent and has great individual differences. A survey on oxytocin affecting trust finds that outcomes of oxytocin studies are highly unstable due to variability in oxytocin administration methods and oxytocin concentration measurement (Nave et al., 2015).

10.5   Discussion and Future Directions

In Section 10.4, we reviewed 18 articles examining the neural behavior of either investors or trustees or both. The overall evidence suggests that reciprocity (trustees' behavior) is more inclined with belief-dependent motivation (Bellucci et al., 2019; Cáceda et al., 2017; Li et al., 2009; Van den Bos et al., 2011). Since trustees face the decision of whether or not to repay investors' good intentions, it is natural to take investors' intentions into consideration when making such decisions; whereas trust (investors' behavior) is more consistent with outcome-based motivation (Bereczkei et al., 2013; Engelmann et al., 2019; Stanley et al., 2012). Because investors in the TG face the decision to divide and invest money, it is natural for them to think about the potential final distribution when making the decision rather than trustees' intention in the future.

Some exceptions indicate that trust and reciprocity are inspired by both outcome and expectations, especially for trust (Bellucci et al., 2017; King-Casas et al., 2005; Krueger et al., 2008; Lemmers-Jansen et al., 2017; Riedl et al., 2014). If we examine the details of those studies with equivocal conclusions, we see that many of those employ the repeated form of TGs, which induce reciprocal concern naturally, when evaluating investors' behavior (Delgado et al., 2005; Krueger et al., 2008; Lemmers-Jansen et al., 2017; Riedl et al., 2014). It is especially important to pay extra attention to the details of the experimental design when we try to distinguish trust and reciprocity (Table 10.1).

Table 10.1. *Outcome-based trust and belief-based reciprocity, evidence from neuroscience literature*

	Trust		
Paper	Repeated Game	Activated Regions	Motivation
Delgado et al. (2005)	yes	insula and ventral striatum	mixed
Stanley et al. (2012)	no	striatum and amygdala	outcome-based
Riedl et al. (2014)	yes	vmPFC, dmPFC, and ACC	mixed
Lemmers-Jansen et al. (2017)	yes	right TPJ, right dlPFC, and right caudate	mixed
Engelmann et al. (2019)	no	left TPJ, dmPFC, and amygdala	outcome-based
Krueger et al. (2008)	yes	anterior insula, right TPJ, and vmPFC	mixed
Bereczkei et al. (2013)	yes	ACC and thalamus	mixed
Bellucci et al. (2017)	both	anterior insula and ventral striatum	mixed
Bellucci et al. (2019)	no	TPJ, vmPFC, and precuneus	outcome-based

	Reciprocity		
Paper	Repeated Game	Activated Regions	Motivation
King-Casas et al. (2005)	yes	ACC and caudate	mixed
Li et al. (2009)	yes	vmPFC and right dlPFC	belief-based
Van den Bos et al. (2009)	no	insula, right TPJ, vmPFC, and ACC	belief-based
Van den Bos et al. (2011)	no	insula, vmPFC, right dlPFC, and ACC	belief-based
Cáceda et al. (2017)	no	insula and ACC	belief-based
Krueger et al. (2008)	yes	anterior insula and vmPFC	belief-based
Bereczkei et al. (2013)	yes	insula	belief-based
Bellucci et al. (2017)	both	anterior insula	belief-based
Cáceda et al. (2015)	no	insula, ACC, and dlPFC	belief-based
Bellucci et al. (2019)	no	insula, ACC, and dlPFC	belief-based

Note: Papers listed under Trust examine investors' neural response, papers listed under Reciprocity examine trustees' neural response, and papers listed under both Trust and Reciprocity examine both players' neural response. Bellucci et al. (2017) is a meta-analysis work. Under Repeated Game, yes if the trust game is played repeatedly, no if the trust game is played as one-shot game, and both if the paper includes multiple experiments and the trust game is played as both formats. Activated Regions lists main regions of interests that identify behavioral motivations, and note that some of the studies listed above also identify activations in other brain regions. Under Motivation, mixed if activation regions include both belief-based regions and outcome-based regions.

10.5.1   Experimental Methodology

In game theory, the same game played repeatedly often derives to divergent outcomes as a one-shot game. Therefore, different neural results are expected regarding how the game is implemented. Repeated TGs create an environment for both investors and trustees to care about social image, reputation, and reciprocity. In addition, repeated TGs also present both players the opportunity to learn their opponents' strategies and the best responses to their opponents' decisions. Therefore, it is reasonable to detect similar neural response for investors and trustees in repeated TGs, such as insula activation in Delgado et al. (2005), dlPFC activity in Lemmers-Jansen et al. (2017), and ACC activity in Riedl et al. (2014), which are regions commonly associated with reciprocal behavior.

Not only is the implementation of the game relevant in distinguishing trust and reciprocity, but whether participants are playing with real humans or computer algorithms matters as well. When participants complete both human and nonhuman opponent treatments, the different treatments prime participants to treat human opponents differently from computer avatars. Therefore, it is natural for participants to consider more about the opponent's intention in the human condition, but consider more about monetary distribution in nonhuman condition. For example, Aimone et al. (2014) observe investors' neural activations in the insula, dlPFC, and ACC when comparing a human to nonhuman condition. Riedl et al. (2014) also find activations in the ACC with a human to avatar contrast in investors' brains. In comparison, in articles without such treatments, investors' decisions are associated with increased activity in the vSTR (Delgado et al., 2005; Lemmers-Jansen et al., 2017; Stanley et al., 2012). The above observation indicates a testable hypothesis that outcome-based or intention-based (i.e., belief-based) social behavior is context-dependent, rather than a stable personality trait.

10.5.2   Future Research Directions

While we conclude that in the TG, reciprocity is more belief-dependent and trust is more outcome-dependent, there are still many unknown features about the two concepts. If social behavior motivation (belief-based, outcome-based, or mixed) is context-dependent, then it is critical to determine the types of context that influence such behavior. It could be the case that the artificial economic game environment enlarges incentives specific to one motivation. Alternatively, it is possible that some experimental designs prime participants to behave in line with a particular motivation. In addition, some neural signatures may be induced by the structure of the TG, and the corresponding behavior or neural signatures may disappear with different strategic games. To elucidate these issues, more research covering different experimental settings and various games in this area is necessary.

One limitation of studying reciprocity with the TG is the lack of negative or loss domain, where trustees can only reward generous investors but are not allowed to punish selfish investors. Therefore, the TG is more suitable for investigating positive but not negative reciprocity. One way to relax the restriction is to play TGs repeatedly, where previous trial choice can be used as a reference point to inform both positive and negative intentions, and tit-for-tat strategies are permitted (King-Casas et al., 2005). However, repeated TGs also bring in reputation and reciprocal concern for investors, making it harder to distinguish trust from reciprocity. The UG, on the other hand, allows punishing malevolent behavior but forbids rewarding benevolent behavior. Also, UGs are less common in exploring negative reciprocity but are often used to explore bargaining and cooperation.

Investigations of both positive and negative reciprocity link our understanding of prosocial and antisocial behavior. Understanding the similarities and differences in domain-specific reciprocities would further enhance our knowledge of human social interaction altogether. Considering the natural propensity of loss aversion (Tversky & Kahneman, 1979), we anticipate that negative and positive reciprocity trigger different sets of brain regions with different intensity (Canessa et al., 2013). To test this hypothesis, researchers should compare the neural differences in trust and UGs to establish benchmarks for understanding positive and negative reciprocity differences, and further develop a new economic game that incorporates both positive and negative reciprocity in the TG to allow direct comparison.

As we reviewed in Section 10.4, there is minimal examination of trust and reciprocity on the network and neuromolecular levels. The literature on the network level often defines its own broad functional networks, which create complications for different articles to compare results. Besides, some of the predefined functional networks might not be ideal frameworks to examine trust and reciprocity. Universal neural networks that reflect both previous findings on trust and reciprocity and anatomical and functional divisions are required to understand the fundamental FC of trust and reciprocity. As we mentioned in Section 10.4.5, on the neuromolecular level, there is not enough investigation to draw useful conclusions, but the existing literature also provides contradicting results. Most of the controversy focuses on the administration method of the hormones, particularly that the same dose of nasal sprays does not translate to consistent neural reactions. In addition, on the hormone level, literature concentrates on the study of oxytocin on trust but neglects the potential effect of many other hormones on trust and reciprocity. There is still much room for future studies on trust and reciprocity utilizing neural network or hormone level methods.

10.5.3   Applications to Psychiatric Disorders

Another future research direction investigating trusting and reciprocal behaviors involves the potential to capture mechanisms of social impairment in psychiatric illnesses (see also Chapters 16 and 17). As we and others have previously reviewed (e.g., King-Casas & Chiu, 2012; Robson et al., 2020), psychiatric illnesses including depression, anxiety, autism, post-traumatic stress disorder (PTSD), and the personality disorders confer substantial interpersonal difficulties. The structure of economic games, including the TG as described here, combined with modern neuroimaging, allows analyses of social behaviors against economic theory and model-derived parameters to clarify mechanistic processes that may be aberrant in individuals with mental illness. To inspire future investigations, we briefly review studies involving TGs in participants with psychopathology and discuss how trusting and reciprocal behavior can be affected by psychiatric disorders.

As just one example, King-Casas et al. (2008) examines individuals with borderline personality disorder (BPD; a personality disorder characterized by unstable social relationships) playing the trustee role in an iterated TG. The authors reported that BPD participants exhibit impaired responses in the insular cortex to trust behaviors such that their neural responses did not vary by magnitude of offers received from the investor. In stark contrast, these participants with BPD showed robust neural responses during reciprocity, wherein a robust signal in the anterior insula was related to the magnitude of repayment to the investors. The specific disruption of neural responses to receiving trust behaviors (and not during reciprocity) facilitates explanatory insights into the unstable relationships and associated neuroscience of BPD. That is, these data suggest aberrant perceptions of social signals from others in BPD rather than an impaired understanding of reciprocity.

Other studies have shown that participants with BPD invest less than healthy controls (HCs) and individuals with major depression in TGs with human opponents, but the difference disappears in a comparable risk game without the social component (Unoka et al., 2009). Also using an iterated TG, Cisler et al. (2015) find that women with assault-related PTSD begin with trust behavior that is comparable to controls, but when this trust is breached with nonreciprocal behavior, they do not return to the initial level of trust. In that work, PTSD was also associated with greater encoding of negative expected social outcomes in the anterior cingulate cortex and medial frontal gyrus, and greater encoding of social prediction errors in the TPJ. In studies of early and chronic psychosis, participants with psychosis and their first-degree relatives demonstrate lower initial trust than controls (Fett et al., 2012, 2016; Gromann et al., 2013). Individuals with psychosis eventually arrive at the same level of trust as controls in the repeated TG when facing reciprocal trustees (Lemmers-Jansen et al., 2019). Still, their trust does not decline as much as HCs when facing nonreciprocal trustees (Fett et al., 2016). In addition, participants with psychosis playing in the investor role display a smaller blood oxygen level-dependent signal in TPJ during trustees' decision and a smaller signal in the caudate facing reciprocal trustees (Gromann et al., 2013). As we discussed earlier, the TPJ and caudate play essential roles in guiding trusting behavior.

In a study where high-functioning males with autism spectrum disorder (ASD) play TGs as trustees, even though participants with ASD demonstrate a similar level of behavioral reciprocity as controls, a weaker signal in the middle cingulate cortex is detected in ASD participants when making decisions to reciprocate (Chiu et al., 2008). Neural responses were intact when ASD participants were viewing investors' trust amounts. The specificity of disruptions in ASD to neural responses during reciprocity and the discrepancy between behavioral and neural reciprocity indicate intact perceptions of trust signals from others and behavioral implementation of reciprocity, but diminished neural processing of this reciprocity. Patients with mild depression symptoms exhibit a similar level of trust as controls (Clark et al., 2013) while both individuals with major depressive disorder and those with bipolar disorder display a higher level of reciprocity than nonpsychiatric controls (Ong, Zaki, & Gruber, 2017). Cáceda et al. (2014) demonstrate that males with depression are more reciprocal than HCs, but females with depression are equal to controls in reciprocity. Investors with high social anxiety and investors with generalized social phobia behave similarly as HCs (Anderl et al., 2018; Sripada et al., 2009;

Sripada et al., 2013). But trustees with high social anxiety present reduced reciprocal behavior compared with controls (Anderl et al., 2018). The medial prefrontal cortex is engaged in the social condition for HCs but not for generalized social phobia investors (Sripada et al., 2009). In addition, activation in the vSTR appears with HCs but not with patients (Sripada et al., 2013).

While studies assessing trust and reciprocity in psychopathology have only begun to scratch the surface, we believe that sufficient evidence exists for the continued use of the TG and other behavioral economic paradigms to parse potential sources of social dysfunction in mental illness.

References

Aimone, J., Ball, S., & King-Casas, B. (2015). The betrayal aversion elicitation task: An individual level betrayal aversion measure. *PLoS ONE*, 10(9), 1–12. https://doi.org/10.1371/journal.pone.0137491

Aimone, J. A., & Houser, D. (2012). What you don't know won't hurt you: A laboratory analysis of betrayal aversion. *Experimental Economics*, 15(4), 571–588. https://doi.org/10.1007/s10683-012-9314-z

(2013). Harnessing the benefits of betrayal aversion. *Journal of Economic Behavior & Organization*, 89, 1–8. https://doi.org/10.1016/j.jebo.2013.02.001

Aimone, J. A., Houser, D., & Weber, B. (2014). Neural signatures of betrayal aversion: An fMRI study of trust. *Proceedings of the Royal Society B: Biological Sciences*, 281(1782), Article 20132127. https://doi.org/10.1098/rspb.2013.2127

Anderl, C., Steil, R., Hahn, T., Hitzeroth, P., Reif, A., & Windmann, S. (2018). Reduced reciprocal giving in social anxiety: Evidence from the trust game. *Journal of Behavior Therapy and Experimental Psychiatry*, 59, 12–18. https://doi.org/10.1016/j.jbtep.2017.10.005

Argiolas, A., & Gessa, G. L. (1991). Central functions of oxytocin. *Neuroscience & Biobehavioral Reviews*, 15(2), 217–231. https://doi.org/10.1016/S0149-7634(05)80002-8

Arrow, K. J. (1965). *Aspects of the theory of risk-bearing*: Yrjö Jahnsson Saatio.

Bartz, J. A., Zaki, J., Bolger, N., & Ochsner, K. N. (2011). Social effects of oxytocin in humans: Context and person matter. *Trends in Cognitive Sciences*, 15(7), 301–309. https://doi.org/10.1016/j.tics.2011.05.002

Battigalli, P., & Dufwenberg, M. (2007). Guilt in games. *American Economic Review*, 97(2), 170–176. https://doi.org/10.1257/aer.97.2.170

Battigalli, P., Dufwenberg, M., & Smith, A. (2019). Frustration, aggression, and anger in leader-follower games. *Games and Economic Behavior*, 117, 15–39. https://doi.org/10.1016/j.geb.2019.06.001

Bellemare, C., Sebald, A., & Suetens, S. (2019). Guilt aversion in economics and psychology. *Journal of Economic Psychology*, 73, 52–59. https://doi.org/10.1016/j.joep.2019.05.002

Bellucci, G., Chernyak, S. V., Goodyear, K., Eickhoff, S. B., & Krueger, F. (2017). Neural signatures of trust in reciprocity: A coordinate-based meta-analysis. *Human Brain Mapping*, 38(3), 1233–1248. https://doi.org/10.1002/hbm.23451

Bellucci, G., Hahn, T., Deshpande, G., & Krueger, F. (2019). Functional connectivity of specific resting-state networks predicts trust and reciprocity in the trust game. *Cognitive, Affective, & Behavioral Neuroscience*, 19(1), 165–176. https://doi.org/10.3758/s13415-018-00654-3

Bereczkei, T., Deak, A., Papp, P., Perlaki, G., & Orsi, G. (2013). Neural correlates of Machiavellian strategies in a social dilemma task. *Brain and Cognition*, 82(1), 108–116. https://doi.org/10.1016/j.bandc.2013.02.012

Berg, J., Dickhaut, J., & McCabe, K. (1995). Trust, reciprocity, and social history. *Games and Economic Behavior*, 10(1), 122–142. https://doi.org/10.1006/game.1995.1027

Bernoulli, D. (1954). Exposition of a new theory on the measurement of risk. *Econometrica*, 22(1), 22–36. https://doi.org/10.2307/1909829

Bohnet, I., Greig, F., Herrmann, B., & Zeckhauser, R. (2008). Betrayal aversion: Evidence from Brazil, China, Oman, Switzerland, Turkey, and the United States. *American Economic Review*, 98(1), 294–310. https://doi.org/10.1257/aer.98.1.294

Bohnet, I., & Zeckhauser, R. (2004). Trust, risk and betrayal. *Journal of Economic Behavior & Organization*, 55(4), 467–484. https://doi.org/10.1016/j.jebo.2003.11.004

Boksem, M. A., Mehta, P. H., Van den Bergh, B., et al. (2013). Testosterone inhibits trust but promotes reciprocity. *Psychological Science*, 24(11), 2306–2314. https://doi.org/10.1177/0956797613495063

Bolton, G. E., & Ockenfels, A. (2000). ERC: A theory of equity, reciprocity, and competition. *American Economic Review*, 90(1), 166–193. https://doi.org/10.1257/aer.90.1.166

Booth, A., Granger, D. A., Mazur, A., & Kivlighan, K. T. (2006). Testosterone and social behavior. *Social Forces*, 85(1), 167–191. https://doi.org/10.1353/sof.2006.0116

Bos, P. A., Terburg, D., & Van Honk, J. (2010). Testosterone decreases trust in socially naive humans. *Proceedings of the National Academy of Sciences*, 107(22), 9991–9995. https://doi.org/10.1073/pnas.0911700107

Brazelton, T. B., Koslowski, B., & Main, M. (1974). The origins of reciprocity: The early mother-infant interaction. In M. Lewis & L. A. Rosenblum (Eds.), *The effect of the infant on its caregiver* (pp. 49–76). Wiley-Interscience.

Buchan, N. R., Croson, R. T., & Dawes, R. M. (2002). Swift neighbors and persistent strangers: A cross-cultural investigation of trust and reciprocity in social exchange. *American Journal of Sociology*, 108(1), 168–206. https://doi.org/10.1086/344546

Cáceda, R., James, G. A., Gutman, D. A., & Kilts, C. D. (2015). Organization of intrinsic functional brain connectivity predicts decisions to reciprocate social behavior. *Behavioural Brain Research*, 292, 478–483. https://doi.org/10.1016/j.bbr.2015.07.008

Cáceda, R., Moskovciak, T., Prendes-Alvarez, S., et al. (2014). Gender-specific effects of depression and suicidal ideation in prosocial behaviors. *PLoS ONE*, 9(9), Article e108733. https://doi.org/10.1371/journal.pone.0108733

Cáceda, R., Prendes-Alvarez, S., Hsu, J.-J., Tripathi, S. P., Kilts, C. D., & James, G. A. (2017). The neural correlates of reciprocity are sensitive to prior experience of reciprocity. *Behavioural Brain Research*, 332, 136–144. https://doi.org/10.1016/j.bbr.2017.05.030

Canessa, N., Crespi, C., Motterlini, M., et al. (2013). The functional and structural neural basis of individual differences in loss aversion. *Journal of Neuroscience*, 33(36), 14307–14317. https://doi.org/10.1523/JNEUROSCI.0497-13.2013

Cardenas, J. C., & Carpenter, J. (2008). Behavioural development economics: Lessons from field labs in the developing world. *The Journal of Development Studies*, 44(3), 311–338. https://doi.org/10.1080/00220380701848327

Carter, C. S. (1992). Oxytocin and sexual behavior. *Neuroscience & Biobehavioral Reviews*, 16(2), 131–144. https://doi.org/10.1016/S0149-7634(05)80176-9

Cartwright, E. (2019). A survey of belief-based guilt aversion in trust and dictator games. *Journal of Economic Behavior & Organization*, 167, 430–444. https://doi.org/10.1016/j.jebo.2018.04.019

Chang, L. J., & Sanfey, A. G. (2011). Great expectations: Neural computations underlying the use of social norms in decision making. *Social Cognitive & Affective Neuroscience*, 8(3), 277–284. https://doi.org/10.1093/scan/nsr094

Chang, L. J., Smith, A., Dufwenberg, M., & Sanfey, A. G. (2011). Triangulating the neural, psychological, and economic bases of guilt aversion. *Neuron*, 70(3), 560–572. https://doi.org/10.1016/j.neuron.2011.02.056

Charness, G., & Dufwenberg, M. (2006). Promises and partnership. *Econometrica*, 74(6), 1579–1601. https://doi.org/10.1111/j.1468-0262.2006.00719.x

Charness, G., & Rabin, M. (2002). Understanding social preferences with simple tests. *The Quarterly Journal of Economics*, 117(3), 817–869. https://doi.org/10.1162/003355302760193904

Chiu, P. H., Kayali, M. A., Kishida, K. T., et al. (2008). Self responses along cingulate cortex reveal quantitative neural phenotype for high-functioning autism. *Neuron*, 57(3), 463–473. https://doi.org/10.1016/j.neuron.2007.12.020

Christopoulos, G. I., Tobler, P. N., Bossaerts, P., Dolan, R. J., & Schultz, W. (2009). Neural correlates of value, risk, and risk aversion contributing to decision making under risk. *Journal of Neuroscience*, 29(40), 12574–12583. https://doi.org/10.1523/JNEUROSCI.2614-09.2009

Cisler, J. M., Bush, K., Steele, J. S., Lenow, J. K., Smitherman, S., & Kilts, C. D. (2015). Brain and behavioral evidence for altered social learning mechanisms among women with assault-related posttraumatic stress disorder. *Journal of Psychiatric Research*, 63, 75–83. https://doi.org/10.1016/j.jpsychires.2015.02.014

Clark, C. B., Thorne, C. B., Hardy, S., & Cropsey, K. L. (2013). Cooperation and depressive symptoms. *Journal of Affective Disorders*, 150(3), 1184–1187. https://doi.org/10.1016/j.jad.2013.05.011

Cox, J. C. (2004). How to identify trust and reciprocity. *Games and Economic Behavior*, 46(2), 260–281. https://doi.org/10.1016/S0899-8256(03)00119-2

Cubitt, R., Gächter, S., & Quercia, S. (2017). Conditional cooperation and betrayal aversion. *Journal of Economic Behavior & Organization*, 141, 110–121. https://doi.org/10.1016/j.jebo.2017.06.013

Dawes, C. T., Fowler, J. H., Johnson, T., McElreath, R., & Smirnov, O. (2007). Egalitarian motives in humans. *Nature*, 446(7137), 794–796. https://doi.org/10.1038/nature05651

Delgado, M. R., Frank, R. H., & Phelps, E. A. (2005). Perceptions of moral character modulate the neural systems of reward during the trust game. *Nature Neuroscience*, 8(11), 1611–1618. https://doi.org/10.1038/nn1575

Donaldson, Z. R., & Young, L. J. (2008). Oxytocin, vasopressin, and the neurogenetics of sociality. *Science*, 322(5903), 900–904. https://doi.org/10.1126/science.1158668

Edwards, D. A., Wetzel, K., & Wyner, D. R. (2006). Intercollegiate soccer: Saliva cortisol and testosterone are elevated during competition, and testosterone is related to status and social connectedness with teammates. *Physiology & Behavior*, 87(1), 135–143. https://doi.org/10.1016/j.physbeh.2005.09.007

Elster, J. (1998). Emotions and economic theory. *Journal of Economic Literature*, 36(1), 47–74. www.jstor.org/stable/2564951

Engelmann, J. B., Meyer, F., Ruff, C. C., & Fehr, E. (2019). The neural circuitry of affect-induced distortions of trust. *Science Advances*, 5(3), Article eaau3413. https://doi.org/10.1126/sciadv.aau3413

Erikson, E. H. (1963). *Childhood and society*. W. W. Norton & Company.

Fehr, E., & Fischbacher, U. (2003). The nature of human altruism. *Nature*, 425 (6960), 785–791. https://doi.org/10.1038/nature02043

Fehr, E., & Gächter, S. (2002). Altruistic punishment in humans. *Nature*, 415 (6868), 137–140. https://doi.org/10.1038/415137a

Fehr, E., & Schmidt, K. M. (1999). A theory of fairness, competition, and cooperation. *The Quarterly Journal of Economics*, 114(3), 817–868. https://doi.org/10.1162/003355399556151

Fett, A.-K. J., Shergill, S. S., Joyce, D. W., et al. (2012). To trust or not to trust: The dynamics of social interaction in psychosis. *Brain*, 135(3), 976–984. https://doi.org/10.1093/brain/awr359

Fett, A.-K., Shergill, S., Korver-Nieberg, N., Yakub, F., Gromann, P., & Krabbendam, L. (2016). Learning to trust: Trust and attachment in early psychosis. *Psychological Medicine*, 46(7), 1437–1447. https://doi.org/10.1017/S0033291716000015

Gordon, E. M., Laumann, T. O., Gilmore, A. W., et al. (2017). Precision functional mapping of individual human brains. *Neuron*, 95(4), 791–807, e797. https://doi.org/10.1016/j.neuron.2017.07.011

Gromann, P. M., Heslenfeld, D. J., Fett, A.-K., Joyce, D. W., Shergill, S. S., & Krabbendam, L. (2013). Trust versus paranoia: Abnormal response to social reward in psychotic illness. *Brain*, 136(6), 1968–1975. https://doi.org/10.1093/brain/awt076

Guerra, G., & Zizzo, D. J. (2004). Trust responsiveness and beliefs. *Journal of Economic Behavior & Organization*, 55(1), 25–30. https://doi.org/10.1016/j.jebo.2003.03.003

Hahn, T., Notebaert, K., Anderl, C., et al. (2015). Reliance on functional resting-state network for stable task control predicts behavioral tendency for cooperation. *NeuroImage*, 118, 231–236. https://doi.org/10.1016/j.neuroimage.2015.05.093

Harrison, G. W., List, J. A., & Towe, C. (2007). Naturally occurring preferences and exogenous laboratory experiments: A case study of risk aversion. *Econometrica*, 75(2), 433–458. https://doi.org/10.1111/j.1468-0262.2006.00753.x

Heinrichs, M., von Dawans, B., & Domes, G. (2009). Oxytocin, vasopressin, and human social behavior. *Frontiers in Neuroendocrinology*, 30(4), 548–557. https://doi.org/10.1016/j.yfrne.2009.05.005

Holt, C. A., & Laury, S. K. (2002). Risk aversion and incentive effects. *American Economic Review*, 92(5), 1644–1655. https://doi.org/10.1257/000282802762024700

Hsu, M., Bhatt, M., Adolphs, R., Tranel, D., & Camerer, C. F. (2005). Neural systems responding to degrees of uncertainty in human decision making. *Science*, 310(5754), 1680–1683. https://doi.org/10.1126/science.1115327

Huettel, S. A., Stowe, C. J., Gordon, E. M., Warner, B. T., & Platt, M. L. (2006). Neural signatures of economic preferences for risk and ambiguity. *Neuron*, 49(5), 765–775. https://doi.org/10.1016/j.neuron.2006.01.024

Hutcherson, C. A., Bushong, B., & Rangel, A. (2015). A neurocomputational model of altruistic choice and its implications. *Neuron*, 87(2), 451–462. https://doi.org/10.1016/j.neuron.2015.06.031

Johnson, N. D., & Mislin, A. A. (2011). Trust games: A meta-analysis. *Journal of Economic Psychology*, 32(5), 865–889. https://doi.org/10.1016/j.joep.2011.05.007

King-Casas, B., & Chiu, P. H. (2012). Understanding interpersonal function in psychiatric illness through multiplayer economic games. *Biological Psychiatry*, 72(2), 119–125. https://doi.org/10.1016/j.biopsych.2012.03.033

King-Casas, B., Sharp, C., Lomax-Bream, L., Lohrenz, T., Fonagy, P., & Montague, P. R. (2008). The rupture and repair of cooperation in borderline personality disorder. *Science*, 321(5890), 806–810. https://doi.org/10.1126/science.1156902

King-Casas, B., Tomlin, D., Anen, C., Camerer, C. F., Quartz, S. R., & Montague, P. R. (2005). Getting to know you: Reputation and trust in a two-person economic exchange. *Science*, 308(5718), 78–83. https://doi.org/10.1126/science.1108062

Kosfeld, M., Heinrichs, M., Zak, P. J., Fischbacher, U., & Fehr, E. (2005). Oxytocin increases trust in humans. *Nature*, 435(7042), 673–676. https://doi.org/10.1038/nature03701

Krajbich, I., Adolphs, R., Tranel, D., Denburg, N. L., & Camerer, C. F. (2009). Economic games quantify diminished sense of guilt in patients with damage to the prefrontal cortex. *Journal of Neuroscience*, 29(7), 2188–2192. https://doi.org/10.1523/JNEUROSCI.5086-08.2009

Krueger, F., Grafman, J., & McCabe, K. (2008). Neural correlates of economic game playing. *Philosophical Transactions of the Royal Society B: Biological Sciences*, 363(1511), 3859–3874. https://doi.org/10.1098/rstb.2008.0165

Lauharatanahirun, N., Christopoulos, G. I., & King-Casas, B. (2012). Neural computations underlying social risk sensitivity. *Frontiers in Human Neuroscience*, 6, Article 213. https://doi.org/10.3389/fnhum.2012.00213

Lemmers-Jansen, I. L., Fett, A.-K. J., Hanssen, E., Veltman, D. J., & Krabbendam, L. (2019). Learning to trust: Social feedback normalizes trust behavior in first-episode psychosis and clinical high risk. *Psychological Medicine*, 49(5), 780–790. https://doi.org/10.1017/S003329171800140X

Lemmers-Jansen, I. L., Krabbendam, L., Veltman, D. J., & Fett, A.-K. J. (2017). Boys vs. girls: Gender differences in the neural development of trust and reciprocity depend on social context. *Developmental Cognitive Neuroscience*, 25, 235–245. https://doi.org/10.1016/j.dcn.2017.02.001

Leng, G., & Ludwig, M. (2016). Intranasal oxytocin: Myths and delusions. *Biological Psychiatry*, 79(3), 243–250. https://doi.org/10.1016/j.biopsych.2015.05.003

Li, J., Xiao, E., Houser, D., & Montague, P. R. (2009). Neural responses to sanction threats in two-party economic exchange. *Proceedings of the National Academy of Sciences*, 106(39), 16835–16840. https://doi.org/10.1073/pnas.0908855106

McCabe, K., Houser, D., Ryan, L., Smith, V., & Trouard, T. (2001). A functional imaging study of cooperation in two-person reciprocal exchange. *Proceedings of the National Academy of Sciences*, 98(20), 11832–11835. https://doi.org/10.1073/pnas.211415698

McCabe, K. A., Rigdon, M. L., & Smith, V. L. (2003). Positive reciprocity and intentions in trust games. *Journal of Economic Behavior & Organization*, 52(2), 267–275. https://doi.org/10.1016/S0167-2681(03)00003-9

Mitchell, J. P. (2007). Activity in right temporo-parietal junction is not selective for theory-of-mind. *Cerebral Cortex*, 18(2), 262–271. https://doi.org/10.1093/cercor/bhm051

Morishima, Y., Schunk, D., Bruhin, A., Ruff, C. C., & Fehr, E. (2012). Linking brain structure and activation in temporoparietal junction to explain the neurobiology of human altruism. *Neuron*, 75(1), 73–79. https://doi.org/10.1016/j.neuron.2012.05.021

Nave, G., Camerer, C., & McCullough, M. (2015). Does oxytocin increase trust in humans? A critical review of research. *Perspectives on Psychological Science*, 10(6), 772–789. https://doi.org/10.1177/1745691615600138

Nihonsugi, T., Ihara, A., & Haruno, M. (2015). Selective increase of intention-based economic decisions by noninvasive brain stimulation to the dorsolateral prefrontal cortex. *Journal of Neuroscience*, 35(8), 3412–3419. https://doi.org/10.1523/JNEUROSCI.3885-14.2015

Ong, D. C., Zaki, J., & Gruber, J. (2017). Increased cooperative behavior across remitted bipolar I disorder and major depression: Insights utilizing a behavioral economic trust game. *Journal of Abnormal Psychology*, 126(1), 1–7. https://doi.org/10.1037/abn0000239

Pratt, J. W. (1978). Risk aversion in the small and in the large. In P. Diamond & M. Rothschild (Eds.), *Uncertainty in economics* (pp. 59–79). Elsevier.

Preuschoff, K., Bossaerts, P., & Quartz, S. R. (2006). Neural differentiation of expected reward and risk in human subcortical structures. *Neuron*, 51(3), 381–390. https://doi.org/10.1016/j.neuron.2006.06.024

Riedl, R., Mohr, P. N., Kenning, P. H., Davis, F. D., & Heekeren, H. R. (2014). Trusting humans and avatars: A brain imaging study based on evolution theory. *Journal of Management Information Systems*, 30(4), 83–114. https://doi.org/10.2753/MIS0742-1222300404

Robson, S. E., Repetto, L., Gountouna, V.-E., & Nicodemus, K. K. (2020). A review of neuroeconomic gameplay in psychiatric disorders. *Molecular Psychiatry*, 25(1), 67–81. https://doi.org/10.1038/s41380-019-0405-5

Ross, H. E., & Young, L. J. (2009). Oxytocin and the neural mechanisms regulating social cognition and affiliative behavior. *Frontiers in Neuroendocrinology*, 30(4), 534–547. https://doi.org/10.1016/j.yfrne.2009.05.004

Rousseau, D. M., Sitkin, S. B., Burt, R. S., & Camerer, C. (1998). Not so different after all: A cross-discipline view of trust. *Academy of Management Review*, 23(3), 393–404. https://doi.org/10.5465/amr.1998.926617

Schultz, W., Preuschoff, K., Camerer, C., et al. (2008). Explicit neural signals reflecting reward uncertainty. *Philosophical Transactions of the Royal Society B: Biological Sciences*, 363(1511), 3801–3811. https://doi.org/10.1098/rstb.2008.0152

Schurz, M., Radua, J., Aichhorn, M., Richlan, F., & Perner, J. (2014). Fractionating theory of mind: A meta-analysis of functional brain imaging studies. *Neuroscience & Biobehavioral Reviews*, 42, 9–34. https://doi.org/10.1016/j.neubiorev.2014.01.009

Sripada, C. S., Angstadt, M., Banks, S., Nathan, P. J., Liberzon, I., & Phan, K. L. (2009). Functional neuroimaging of mentalizing during the trust game in social anxiety disorder. *Neuroreport*, 20(11), 984–989. https://doi.org/10.1097/WNR.0b013e32832d0a67

Sripada, C., Angstadt, M., Liberzon, I., McCabe, K., & Phan, K. L. (2013). Aberrant reward center response to partner reputation during a social exchange game in generalized social phobia. *Depression and Anxiety*, 30(4), 353–361. https://doi.org/10.1002/da.22091

Stanley, D. A., Sokol-Hessner, P., Fareri, D. S., et al. (2012). Race and reputation: Perceived racial group trustworthiness influences the neural correlates of trust decisions. *Philosophical Transactions of the Royal Society B: Biological Sciences*, 367(1589), 744–753. https://doi.org/10.1098/rstb.2011.0300

Tisserand, J.-C. (2014). Ultimatum game: A meta-analysis of the past three decades of experimental research. *Proceedings of the International Academic Conferences, Antibes, France*, 13, 609–609.

Tricomi, E., Rangel, A., Camerer, C. F., & O'Doherty, J. P. (2010). Neural evidence for inequality-averse social preferences. *Nature*, 463(7284), 1089–1091. https://doi.org/10.1038/nature08785

Tversky, A., & Kahneman, D. (1979). Prospect theory: An analysis of decision under risk. *Econometrica*, 47(2), 263–291. https://doi.org/10.2307/1914185

Tzieropoulos, H. (2013). The trust game in neuroscience: A short review. *Social Neuroscience*, 8(5), 407–416. https://doi.org/10.1080/17470919.2013.832375

Unoka, Z., Seres, I., Aspan, N., Bódi, N., & Kéri, S. (2009). Trust game reveals restricted interpersonal transactions in patients with borderline personality disorder. *Journal of Personality Disorders*, 23(4), 399–409. https://doi.org/10.1521/pedi.2009.23.4.399

Van den Bos, W., Van Dijk, E., Westenberg, M., Rombouts, S. A., & Crone, E. A. (2009). What motivates repayment? Neural correlates of reciprocity in the trust game. *Social Cognitive and Affective Neuroscience*, 4(3), 294–304. https://doi.org/10.1093/scan/nsp009

(2011). Changing brains, changing perspectives: The neurocognitive development of reciprocity. *Psychological Science*, 22(1), 60–70. https://doi.org/10.1177/0956797610391102

Zethraeus, N., Kocoska-Maras, L., Ellingsen, T., Von Schoultz, B., Hirschberg, A. L., & Johannesson, M. (2009). A randomized trial of the effect of estrogen and testosterone on economic behavior. *Proceedings of the National Academy of Sciences*, 106(16), 6535–6538. https://doi.org/10.1073/pnas.0812757106

CHAPTER 11

Trust and Demographics
Age and Gender Differences in Trust and Reciprocity Behavior

Hester Sijtsma and Lydia Krabbendam

11.1 Introduction

Trusting others, assessing the reciprocity behavior of others, and adapting trust behavior accordingly are essential components of successful social interactions. It is therefore important to understand the developmental trajectories of trust and reciprocity behavior, as well as the influence of individual characteristics on these developmental patterns. Studies comparing diverse age groups have begun to delineate how trust and reciprocity behavior, and the underlying neural correlates, develop over the life span. Some studies also highlighted differential trajectories for males and females. This chapter gives an overview of the development of trust and reciprocity behavior and the gender differences in trust and reciprocity behavior. Section 11.2 covers a short explanation on what trust entails and a description on suitable methods to examine trust behavior (e.g. the trust game [TG] by Berg et al., 1995). Section 11.3 is about the development of trust and reciprocity behavior and accompanying neural activity. In this section we start by discussing the crucial role that trust plays in early development and how trust is related to adaptive psychosocial functioning and peer relations. Then, studies examining the effect of age on trust and reciprocity behavior using the well-known TG paradigm will be discussed. We then cover a few studies that have used functional neuroimaging to study the development of the neural mechanisms of trust and reciprocity behavior. Section 11.4 covers gender differences in trust and reciprocity behavior and in neural mechanisms of trust and reciprocity behavior. The first part is focused on behavioral studies that have used the TG. The second part discusses the few neuroimaging studies that have examined differences between males and females in brain activity while playing the

Corresponding author: Hester Sijtsma (h.sijtsma@vu.nl).

TG, of which some suggested different strategies between males and females in social interactions where trust plays a role.

11.2   Trust and Measurement of Trust

Trust is evoked in different situations and can have different definitions and, therefore, trust can be measured in several ways. Trust may be present at a micro level (between individuals) and at a macro level (in society) (Kocher, 2017). Two components important for trust are vulnerability and expectation (Evans & Krueger, 2009). Trusting someone else may make you vulnerable because of the risk of a negative outcome (Evans & Krueger, 2009). Trust also signals an expectancy of reciprocity (Evans & Krueger, 2009). Murtin et al. (2018) describe three determinants of trust behavior, namely individual determinants (e.g. a person's social preference to cooperate, demographic characteristics), institutional determinants (e.g. the extent that a government values integrity in society and in its own actions), and societal determinants (e.g. the extent of social connectedness within a society). Lewis and Weigert (1985) argue that trust involves a cognitive, an emotional, and a behavioral dimension. The cognitive aspect is that people decide whether to trust a person based on their knowledge and expectations about the other's trustworthiness (Hill & O'Hara, 2006; Lewis & Weigert, 1985). The emotional component of trust is how people feel about choices and their emotional response to betrayal of trust (Lewis & Weigert, 1985). Trust can also be seen as a social action that involves taking the risk to trust others while not knowing whether this will be reciprocated, which is the behavioral component.

Trust can be measured by questionnaires resulting in self-reported trust behavior or by behavioral games that provide experimental data. Some of the games that are used to examine trust behavior are the public goods game (Ledyard, 1995), the prisoner's dilemma game (Poundstone, 1992), and the TG (Berg et al., 1995) (see also Chapter 2). In this chapter, we focus primarily on studies that used the TG, which is an established experimental paradigm to investigate trust. In the TG, one player (the trustor) shares an amount of money with a second player (the trustee or the partner). The amount shared is multiplied by a predefined factor (often three) and indicates as a measure of trust behavior. After receiving the money from the trustor, the partner decides what part of this amount to return to the trustor. The partner's return is a measure of reciprocity behavior. Showing vulnerability by trusting the partner can be risky for the trustor as there is a chance of receiving a negative return (Evans & Krueger, 2009; Saunders et al., 2014). The TG is focused on trust at the micro level as the interaction is between two individuals (often unknown to one another). Furthermore, it addresses individual determinants of trust such as a person's social preference to cooperate and it allows for the examination of the effect of demographic factors on trust. The cognitive, emotional, and behavioral component of trust as described by Lewis and Weigert (1985) are all addressed during the game. For example, much more than in a self-report questionnaire, the TG assesses the behavioral component of trust as the back-and-forth flow of a social interaction is simulated. In this social interaction, predictions of the trustworthiness of the other person are made (cognitive component of trust) and feelings of reward when trust is reciprocated or feelings of betrayal when trust is not reciprocated are evoked (emotional component of trust). Neuroimaging research can reveal important insights in these cognitive, emotional, and behavioral components of trust and in the effect of demographic factors such as age and gender on the underlying neural mechanisms of trust behavior.

Multiple variations on the TG can be used. For example, studies vary in whether a one-round TG versus a multiple round TG is used. In the one-round game, the investment can be seen as a measure of baseline trust, which is less influenced by the desire to build a social reputation since the interaction is restricted to a single occurrence. In a repeated one-round TG, each round is played with a different partner and thus the investment can be seen as repeated measures of baseline trust. Processes of risk-taking can play a role in one-round TGs particularly, as trusting the unknown partner can be fairly risky (Van den Akker et al., 2018) (see also Chapter 5). In contrast, in a multiple round TG with the same partner, players likely take social reputation into account because trust decisions may influence the next investment or return. This way, the pattern of interactions in a multiple round game may also shed light on the ability to build a mental model of the other player (see also Chapter 8). Studies further vary in whether they use real interactions or interactions with hypothetical partners whose behavior is preprogrammed by computer algorithms. While the first approach provides insight into the naturalistic pattern of evolving trust and reciprocity behavior, using preprogrammed algorithms has the advantage that the response of one player can be standardized and manipulated as being trustworthy or untrustworthy. In addition, using preprogrammed algorithms, it is also possible to investigate how a priori information on reputation and actual responses together influence decisions in the TG. Examples of such a priori information are to provide a cover story about the moral character of the hypothetical other player or to reveal the facial appearance of the partner (which can be trustworthy or untrustworthy) (see also Chapter 7).

As mentioned, trust is a multifaceted concept tapping into cognitive, emotional, and behavioral components (Lewis & Weigert, 1985). Neuroimaging research has suggested that key cognitive and affective processes involved in the multiple round TG are processes of mentalizing, social reward learning, cognitive control, and conflict monitoring (Alós-Ferrer & Farolfi, 2019; Bellucci et al., 2017; Krueger & Meyer-Lindenberg, 2019; Tzieropoulos, 2013). Mentalizing processes are recruited as one assesses the mental states of the partner and attempts to understand their intentions. This way, partners develop a mental model of each other and are increasingly able to predict the response in the next round (King-Casas et al., 2005). Processing the feedback of the interaction partner additionally involves (social) reward learning, especially when this feedback is better (or worse) than expected and subsequent behavior has to be adapted accordingly. Conflict monitoring processes may come into play when one has to override one's own response tendency based on the behavior of the partner. Specifically, untrustworthy returns may conflict with a default tendency to trust, making interactions with untrustworthy partners more cognitively demanding than interactions with trustworthy partners (Bailey & Leon, 2019). These reward and conflict monitoring processes also help to predict the trustworthiness and behavior of the partner. Neuroimaging studies have shown that areas that are part of the so-called social brain, such as the temporoparietal junction (TPJ) and medial prefrontal cortex (Blakemore, 2008, 2012), and areas previously related to reward and cognitive control processes, such as the caudate and the anterior cingulate cortex (ACC) (Bellucci et al., 2017; Fett, Gromann, et al., 2014), play a role during the TG. We will cover these studies in Section 11.3.2 and Section 11.4.

11.3   Age Differences in Trust and Reciprocity Behavior

In this section we first discuss the development of initial, baseline trust in a one-round TG and in the first round in a multiple round TG. This will be followed by studies outlining the effect of context on single investments during development and studies examining the progression of the ability to adapt trust in interactions with trustworthy and untrustworthy partners. Finally, we discuss the age-related change of reciprocity behavior.

11.3.1 Behavioral Studies

Learning whom to trust is important from an early age. In Erikson's model of the different stages of psychosocial functioning, the first stage ("trust versus mistrust") delineates that early trust development is crucial for adaptive psychosocial functioning (Erikson, 1963). In their first stage of life (0–12 months), infants are fully dependent on adults for their basic needs and, therefore, infants must learn to trust adults (Erikson, 1963). Later in development, children are guided by adults to learn about the world and, in this process, the child needs to find out whether the person who provides the information is trustworthy or not (Corriveau et al., 2009). For example, in a study with children of 4 and 5 years old, it was shown that children at this age distinguished between information provided by their mother and information provided by a stranger in different ways, depending on their attachment style (Corriveau et al., 2009). In another study, it was found that children who receive secure support from their mother have more state trust in their mother compared to children whose mother is absent (Vandevivere et al., 2018). These studies point toward the idea that the trust relationship between children and parents is related to the attachment between the child and the parent (Rotenberg et al., 2013; Thompson, 2008). The attachment theory posits that a child's cognitive representation, called the internal working model, describes their expectations regarding the accessibility and responsiveness of the caregiver (Thompson, 2008). These trust expectations and beliefs in parents affect the child's trust beliefs and behavior toward peers (Rotenberg et al., 2013). Studies show that trust is a critical component of peer relationships (Betts & Rotenberg, 2008; Betts et al., 2014) and that childhood trust behavior is related to the development of prosocial behavior (Malti et al., 2016), social competence (Chin, 2014), and being liked by peers more often (Chin, 2014).

Examining trust using the TG is mostly done in children from 8 years and older. In the early stages of development, studies have reported an increase in baseline trust from childhood to young adulthood (Derks et al., 2014 [ages 14–17]; Fett, Gromann, et al., 2014 [ages 13–49]; Van den Bos et al., 2012 [ages 11–23]). It is thought that this increase in baseline trust during development is related to an increase in risk-taking (Steinberg, 2008) and ongoing maturation of mentalizing skills during adolescence (Bosco et al., 2014; Dumontheil et al., 2010), in conjunction with an increase in the breadth and complexity of social interactions

(Erdley & Day, 2017). However, more research is needed, as several studies investigating children, adolescents, and young adults could not replicate the increase in baseline trust (Fett, Shergill, et al., 2014 [ages 13–18]; Güroğlu et al., 2014 [ages 9–18]; Lemmers-Jansen et al., 2019 [ages 13–19]; Lemmers-Jansen et al., 2017 [ages 16–27]; Van de Groep et al., 2018 [ages 12–18]). In sum, baseline trust is present in young children, some (but not all) studies report an increase from childhood to young adulthood, after which baseline trust remains relatively stable.

Not all trust is the same. Manipulations of the TG can elucidate the extent to which individuals take risks and benefits for both players into account. This was done in a repeated one-round TG study by Van den Bos et al. (2010) in four age groups (children: mean age 9; young adolescents: mean age 12; mid-adolescents: mean age 16; and late adolescents: mean age 22). In high risk rounds the trustor could potentially lose many coins when trusting the partner whereas in low risk rounds the loss was small relative to not trusting the partner. In high benefit rounds, the partner received more coins when being trusted in comparison to not being trusted whereas the gain was small in low benefit rounds. No age differences were found for the risk manipulation as all age groups showed less trust behavior during high risk rounds compared to low risk rounds (see Van de Groep et al., 2018 for similar findings in adolescents aged 12–18). In contrast, age differences were found for the benefit manipulation (Van den Bos et al., 2010). Children, young adolescents, and mid-adolescents did not differentiate between the high and low benefit rounds, but the late adolescents trusted more often in high compared to low benefit rounds. This may indicate that the late adolescents' trust decisions were based on both their own outcome and the partner's outcome, which can potentially be explained by their better developed perspective-taking abilities (Van den Bos et al., 2010).

Multiple round TGs may highlight the ability to fine-tune and adapt trust behavior toward the partner's behavior, indexed by the change in investments over the course of the game. The ability to fine-tune trust behavior toward the trustworthiness of the partner is related to perspective-taking skills (Fett, Shergill, et al., 2014). Adolescents that have a higher score on perspective-taking skills showed more trust behavior toward a trustworthy partner and less benevolent behavior and more malevolent behavior toward an untrustworthy partner compared to adolescents with a lower score on perspective-taking skills (Fett, Shergill, et al., 2014). Concerning the effect of age on the fine-tuning of trust behavior, another study showed that older participants adapted investments over the course of trustworthy versus untrustworthy interactions more so than younger participants did (Fett, Gromann, et al., 2014 [ages 13–49]). Relatedly, in another study, mid-adolescents (ages 15–17) and late adolescents (ages 19–23) showed an increase of trust behavior during trustworthy interactions and a decrease of trust during untrustworthy interactions while young adolescents (ages 11–12) did not show a change of trust behavior during the course of the games (Van den Bos et al., 2012). Two other studies in adolescence and young adulthood, however, did not report better adaptation to the interaction partner with age (Fett, Shergill, et al., 2014 [ages 13–18]; Lemmers-Jansen et al., 2017 [ages 16–27]). In another study, the design of the TG was adapted in such a way that a priori trust-related information about the partner was provided to investigate how this influences trust behavior (Lee et al., 2016). Adolescents received a priori information that was inconsistent with the actual behavior of the partner during the game. When the partner was less trustworthy or more trustworthy than a priori information suggested, mid-adolescents (ages 14–15) and late adolescents (ages 16–18) were more flexible in changing their trust behavior accordingly compared to young adolescents (ages 12–13) (Lee et al., 2016). In sum, the skills to fine-tune one's own behavior toward the partner seem to develop from adolescence into (young) adulthood, which may be related to more advanced mentalizing skills.

Only a few studies using the TG have included older adults when examining trust behavior and reciprocity behavior. A one-round TG was used to study baseline trust which appeared to increase linearly from age 8 to age 22 after which it stayed more or less stable to age 68 (Sutter & Kocher, 2007). In another study in which a one-round mail-based design TG was used, 20-year-old and 70-year-old participants did not show different baseline trust behavior, although both groups did show a preference to interact with a person of similar age (Holm & Nystedt, 2005). A meta-analysis showed age differences in the way people responded to information about the partner's trustworthiness that was provided prior to the game (Bailey & Leon, 2019). It was shown that older adults (>60 years) were more trusting toward a partner who, according to a priori information, was untrustworthy, compared to younger adults (>30 years) (Bailey & Leon, 2019). In contrast, no effect of age on trust behavior was found in interactions with partners for whom neutral or trustworthy a priori information was provided (Bailey & Leon, 2019). Furthermore, one study shows that the ability to adapt to partner feedback during the TG may deteriorate in old age (Rasmussen & Gutchess, 2019). Furthermore, a study examining reciprocity behavior showed an increase in reciprocity behavior from ages 8 to 68 (Sutter & Kocher, 2007). Other studies have used questionnaire data to examine age differences in how much trust is placed in people in general and in specific groups like family and friends. For example, Li and Fung (2013) found that age was positively associated with generalized trust and with trust that is placed in family, friends, neighbors, and strangers (ages 15–98). The effect of age on trust placed in neighbors and strangers was bigger than the age effects on trust placed in friends and family. One of the explanations that Li and Fung (2013) give is that older people have a limited time perspective and, therefore, connectedness with others becomes more important for them, which enhances placing trust in others. A cross-sectional and longitudinal study by Poulin and Haase (2015) replicated these findings and showed that trust and well-being were positively associated, especially for older adults. In the same line, generalized trust was found to be positively associated with health, happiness, and life satisfaction and negatively associated with the likelihood of illnesses in a sample of older adults (Chan et al., 2017 [mean age: 63.5]). So, trust is essential for an adaptive psychosocial development in the early days of life (Erikson, 1963), but also later in life, trust seems to be associated with better psychosocial functioning and health.

The development of reciprocity behavior during a TG has also been examined. Findings from studies in adolescent samples showed an increase in reciprocity behavior. In the cross-sectional study by Van den Bos et al. (2010), described above, a linear increase in reciprocity behavior from childhood up to mid-adolescence (ages 9–16) was found and this stabilized during late adolescence (mean age 22). Furthermore, late adolescents were better able to differentiate between different types and perspectives of trustors. For example, in the study by Van den Bos et al. (2010) described before, mid-adolescents (mean age 16) and late adolescents (mean age 22) who played the role of the partner showed more reciprocity behavior in the rounds in which the trustor took a high risk by trusting. Children (mean age 9) and young adolescents (mean age 12) did not show this differentiation. Also, young adolescents, mid-adolescents, and late adolescents who played the role of the partner showed more reciprocity behavior when their benefit to be trusted by the trustor was high compared to low. Again, children playing the role of the partner did not show this difference in reciprocity behavior. The age-related increase in understanding the risk that the trustor took by trusting the partner was also observed in another study (Van den Bos et al., 2011) and may be explained by increased mentalizing skills or increased sensitivity to social reward during adolescence. In another study, older adolescents (ages 15–18) showed less reciprocity behavior toward anonymous and disliked partners compared to neutral partners while younger adolescents (ages 9–12) did not differentiate between partners, supporting the notion that differentiation between trustors increases with age (Güroğlu et al., 2014).

To summarize, trust behavior is essential and present at a young age. Already at 8 years of age, children show baseline trust behavior in the TG and there is evidence that baseline trust behavior increases up till young adulthood, although this latter finding is not very robust. In addition, adaptation toward both trustworthy and untrustworthy partners continues to mature throughout adolescence and adulthood. This age-related increase in adaptation behavior can be explained by development of mentalizing (Fett, Shergill, et al., 2014; Tzieropoulos, 2013) and an increased sensitivity to social reward, which occur in parallel with the increasing complexity of the social environment during adolescence. In line with this, the ability to adapt trust behavior when expectations about a partner's reciprocity behavior appear to be incorrect develops further from childhood to young adulthood. Furthermore, reciprocity behavior seems to increase throughout adolescence, as well as understanding the situation of the trustor when social risk was involved.

There are only a few TG studies on the elderly. A meta-analysis showed that the ability to adapt trust behavior may change again later in life, as older adults (>60 years) were more trusting than younger adults (>30 years) when according to a priori information the partner is untrustworthy (Bailey & Leon, 2019). A possible explanation for this finding may be that untrustworthy interactions are more cognitively demanding compared to trustworthy ones. Alternatively, older adults may be more inclined to restore trust. Some studies that used questionnaire data to examine trust have also found more trust with increasing age, possibly because social connectedness with others becomes increasingly important when people get older; however, trust behavior in the elderly requires further studies.

11.3.2 *Neuroimaging Studies*

Section 11.3.1 suggests that adolescence is an important maturational phase for the development of trust. During adolescence, the social context becomes more complex and peers become increasingly important. This aligns with the current conceptualization of adolescence as a window of opportunity for social and cultural learning (Van Hoorn et al., 2019). The development of social decision making is accompanied by changes in the developing brain. Overall, converging evidence points to the notion of an anterior-to-posterior developmental shift of activity in brain regions associated with social cognition. That is, adolescents have more anterior activity such as in the dorsomedial prefrontal cortex (dmPFC), while in adults activity increases in posterior areas such as the posterior superior temporal sulcus (Pfeifer & Blakemore, 2012). However, up till now, only a few studies have specifically investigated the development of the neural mechanisms of trust and reciprocity behavior. We will first discuss the development of brain activation associated with interactions with a trustworthy partner, followed by interactions with an untrustworthy partner. Finally, the development of the neural mechanisms of reciprocity behavior will be discussed.

For trustworthy interactions, age has been associated with increased activity in the TPJ, the posterior cingulate cortex, the precuneus, the precentral gyri, and the middle frontal gyri when making investment decisions (Fett, Gromann, et al., 2014 [ages 13–49]). The TPJ, posterior cingulate cortex, and the precuneus have previously been associated with mentalizing processes and the age-related changes in activity may be associated with an increased understanding of social signals of interactions partners, although it is important to note that these brain areas are involved in multiple functions, and this interpretation relies on reverse inference. During the period of making investment decisions, age-related increases in the right TPJ activity and in the right dorsolateral prefrontal cortex (dlPFC) activity, related to cognitive control, were also found in another study (Lemmers-Jansen et al., 2017 [ages 16–27]). Together with other areas, the TPJ is part of the so-called social brain and, in concurrence to a development in social behavior, these areas show great functional and structural changes throughout adolescence (Blakemore, 2008, 2012).

Besides mentalizing processes, the TG has been linked to processes of reward. The study by Fett, Gromann, et al. (2014) showed that age was found to be negatively associated with activity in reward-related areas such as the orbitofrontal cortex, the bilateral caudate, and the bilateral dmPFC during investment decisions with a trustworthy partner (ages 13–49). Earlier studies showed that activity in these areas is important for learning and that activity is reduced when outcomes and expectations match (Delgado et al., 2005; Schiffer & Schubotz, 2011), as might be the case for trustworthy behavior. This may speculatively imply that learning may have become less important with age, as the older participants had a higher baseline trust that may indicate they expected a trustworthy interaction partner (Fett, Gromann, et al., 2014). In contrast, in a study with a smaller age range, right caudate activity increased with age during the processing of the partner's response, suggesting that further studies are needed to investigate the development of caudate activity during trustworthy interactions (Lemmers-Jansen et al., 2017 [ages 16–27]). Finally, in another study in adolescents, no main effect of age on the neural correlates of trust when playing with a trustworthy partner was found, even though at the level of the behavior, there was a positive association between age and overall trust (Lemmers-Jansen et al., 2019 [ages 13–19]). In sum, there is some evidence that during adolescence and up to adulthood activity in areas related to mentalizing increase and activity in areas related to reward and learning processes decrease when engaging in trustworthy interactions; however, there is a paucity of research and these findings await replication.

During investment decisions in TGs with an untrustworthy partner, age was associated with a stronger decline of trust throughout the game and with increased activity in the left TPJ and the ACC (Fett, Gromann, et al., 2014 [ages 13–49]). The TPJ may be involved in mentalizing processes needed to adjust to the behavior of the partner, and the increase in activity may underlie the better adaptation with increasing age, although this interpretation relies on reverse inference and should be treated with caution. The ACC is involved in conflict monitoring processes, and the involvement of the ACC may tentatively reflect the expectation of a trustworthy partner while the actual partner's behavior was untrustworthy (Fett, Gromann, et al., 2014). This may be stronger in older individuals, as the increase in baseline trust with age may reflect stronger expectations of trustworthy returns (Fett, Gromann, et al., 2014). A similar (trend-level) result was seen in an adolescent sample in which, compared to younger adolescents, older adolescents showed more ACC and dlPFC activity, related to cognitive control, during investment decisions in a game with an untrustworthy partner (Lemmers-Jansen et al., 2019 [ages 13–19]). No effect of age on neural activity during investments was found in a slightly older adolescent sample (Lemmers-Jansen et al., 2017 [ages 16–27]). When receiving the partner's response, right caudate activity increased with age in older adolescents (Lemmers-Jansen et al., 2017 [ages 16–27]) while no main effect of age was found in the younger adolescent sample (Lemmers-Jansen et al., 2019 [ages 13–19]). In sum, similar to the findings for trustworthy interactions, during untrustworthy interactions activity in areas associated with mentalizing increase with age from adolescence to adulthood. In addition, age-related increases in activity in areas associated with cognitive control and conflict monitoring have been reported (see Table 11.1 for an overview of studies that examined the effect of age on the neural mechanisms of trust).

Table 11.1. *Overview of studies that examined the effect of age on the neural mechanisms of trust*

Partner	Relation between Process and Age*	Phase of Game	Brain Areas	Ages	Study
Trustworthy	Mentalizing +	Investment	TPJ, posterior cingulate cortex, precuneus	13–49	Fett, Gromann, et al., (2014)
Trustworthy	Mentalizing +	Investment	TPJ	16–27	Lemmers-Jansen et al., (2017)
Trustworthy	Cognitive control +	Investment	dlPFC	16–27	Lemmers-Jansen et al., (2017)
Trustworthy	Reward –	Investment	Orbitofrontal cortex, caudate, dmPFC	13–49	Fett, Gromann, et al., (2014)
Trustworthy	Reward +	Feedback	Caudate	16–27	Lemmers-Jansen et al., (2017)
Trustworthy		Investment, feedback	No relation activity and age	13–19	Lemmers-Jansen et al., (2019)
Untrustworthy	Mentalizing +	Investment	TPJ	13–49	Fett, Gromann, et al., (2014)
Untrustworthy	Conflict monitoring +	Investment	ACC	13–49	Fett, Gromann, et al., (2014)
Untrustworthy	Conflict monitoring, cognitive control +	Investment	ACC, dlPFC	13–19	Lemmers-Jansen et al., (2019)
Untrustworthy	Reward +	Feedback	Caudate	16–27	Lemmers-Jansen et al., (2017)
Untrustworthy		Investment	No relation activity and age	16–27	Lemmers-Jansen et al., (2017)
Untrustworthy		Feedback	No relation activity and age	13–19	Lemmers-Jansen et al., (2019)

Note: A plus sign (+) indicates a positive relationship with age, a minus sign (−) a negative relationship with age.

When playing the role of the partner, young adults (ages 18–22) and mid-adolescents (ages 15–17) showed increased activity in the left TPJ and increased activity in the right dlPFC compared to younger adolescents (ages 12–14) during the phase in which the trustor investment is shown (Van den Bos et al., 2011). For the young adults and mid-adolescents, it was shown that this increased activity was accompanied by a greater understanding of the risk that the trustor took by trusting the partner. The behavioral and neural results may indicate a shift of attention from the self to the other, perhaps driven by better mentalizing abilities of the older adolescents compared to the younger ones. The increased dlPFC activity with age may signal increased cognitive control processes during the task. Furthermore, when reciprocating trust decisions, younger adolescents (ages 12–14) showed more activity in the anterior medial prefrontal cortex (amPFC) compared to mid-adolescents (ages 15–17) and young adults (ages 18–22) (Van den Bos et al., 2011). As the amPFC plays a role in self-referential processing and in mentalizing processes, it is suggested that self-referential thoughts play a bigger role during young adolescence when reciprocating trust toward others compared to late adolescence. These findings are consistent with the anterior-to-posterior developmental shift of activity in areas associated with mentalizing (Pfeifer & Blakemore, 2012).

11.3.3 Summary

Baseline trust behavior is present in young children, although not all studies show an increase of baseline trust throughout adolescence. The adaptation of trust behavior and fine-tuning skills seem to develop throughout adolescence and adulthood and this might be explained by better mentalizing skills across age. Furthermore, the patterns of activity in areas associated with mentalizing and self-other processing change from adolescence to adulthood, which can be related to the behavioral pattern of age-related increases in overall trust behavior and age-related fine-tuning of trust behavior. Activity in reward-related areas decreases from adolescence to adulthood when interacting with trustworthy partners, which may possibly indicate that trustworthy interactions match with expectations to a greater degree in adults compared to adolescence. During interactions with untrustworthy partners, activity in areas related to conflict monitoring increases from adolescence to adulthood, possibly suggesting that with age untrustworthy returns elicit greater conflict. When reciprocating trust, activity in areas associated with mentalizing increases during adolescence, in conjunction with trust behavior that increasingly takes the perspective of the trustor into account. It is important to note the challenges inherent to studies in developmental cognitive neuroscience. One challenge is that neurodevelopmental processes should always be seen in light of structural brain developments in white matter and grey matter (Crone et al., 2010). To examine how functional brain processes relate to developments in brain structure such as synaptic changes is a complicated field of study with continuous ongoing research (Crone et al., 2010). Also, several issues related to the technique of functional imaging have been the subject of debate. Examples of such issues are selecting an appropriate task that is related to both behavioral and brain processes and selecting a suitable control task to which the cognitive processes of interests can be compared to. Another challenge is to choose age groups that are meaningful for the cognitive processes being studied while developmental trajectories in brain and behavior are different for cognitive processes and across individuals (Crone et al., 2010; Luna et al., 2010). In addition, there is still limited research investigating age differences in the neural correlates of trust and reciprocity behavior. There is increasing attention on this topic from researchers in adolescence and young adults, which could be complemented by research in old age to obtain a comprehensive understanding of changes in trust and reciprocity behavior over the life span.

11.4   Gender Differences in Trust and Reciprocity Behavior

In this section, we review the evidence for gender differences in trust and reciprocity behavior as well as differential developmental trajectories for males and females. First, we discuss gender differences in baseline trust behavior, followed by the influence of gender on trust behavior when interacting with a trustworthy or an untrustworthy partner. Next, gender differences in reciprocity behavior will be discussed. Finally, we will outline the few studies on the effect of gender on the underlying neural mechanisms of trust and reciprocity behavior.

11.4.1   Behavioral Studies

A meta-analysis consisting of 94 TG studies that examined trust behavior in adults showed that males are more trusting at baseline compared to females, although the effect size of this gender difference was small (Van den Akker et al., 2018). The authors examined several moderators related to the experimental setup of the TG but none were significant, although this could be related to lack of statistical power. These moderators included the factor that was used to multiply the investment before sending it to the partner, whether a monetary compensation was given for participation, whether the participants played both the role of the trustor and the partner, whether the partner revealed its returned amount on the first trial, whether the strategy method was used in which conditional decisions were made, and the number of times the TG was administered. Studies that examined adolescent samples generally confirmed that males show more baseline trust compared to females (Derks et al., 2014 [ages 14–17]; Lemmers-Jansen et al., 2017 [ages 16–27]; Van de Groep et al., 2018 [ages 12–18]), although one study did not report higher baseline trust in male adolescents compared to female ones (Lemmers-Jansen et al., 2019 [ages 13–19]). A recent study in students showed that gender differences in baseline trust may perhaps be subtler such as that males and females tend to take and avoid risks in different situations (Takahashi et al., 2020). In sum, most studies report that males show more baseline trust compared to females, but the difference is small and may be dependent on context.

The meta-analysis of Van den Akker et al. (2018) showed that the number of rounds did not moderate the finding that student and adult males show more trust behavior compared to student and adult females, indicating that males show more trust behavior during both one-round TGs and during multiple round TGs than females (Van den Akker et al., 2018). However, two studies investigating this in adolescent samples did not report gender differences in trust during multiple round TGs with a trustworthy partner, suggesting that this difference is either less robust or emerges later in development (Lemmers-Jansen et al., 2019 [ages 13–19]; Lemmers-Jansen et al., 2017 [ages 16–27]).

Few studies investigated gender differences during TGs with an untrustworthy partner, and these studies suggest that there may be developmental differences for males and females. During untrustworthy interactions, males decreased their trust behavior throughout the game and this decline became stronger with age (Lemmers-Jansen et al., 2017 [ages 16–27]). However, in a slightly younger sample, contradictory results were found as younger males showed a stronger decline in trust behavior compared to older males (Lemmers-Jansen et al., 2019 [ages 13–19]). In the older adolescent sample, females showed a decrease of trust during untrustworthy interactions but there was no age effect found on this decrease of trust behavior (Lemmers-Jansen et al., 2017 [ages 16–27]). In the other study, younger females did not show adaption of trust behavior (Lemmers-Jansen et al., 2019 [ages 13–19]). Results of a different study indicated that female students showed more trust behavior compared to male students in response to trust violations by the partner (Haselhuhn et al., 2015). Also, when the partner tries to rebuild trust after untrustworthy behavior, females showed a greater tendency to restore trust than males (Haselhuhn et al., 2015). This was mediated by a greater motivation of females to have and preserve social relationships (Haselhuhn et al., 2015).

On balance, studies investigating reciprocity behavior indicate small or no differences between males and females. No differences were observed in the meta-analysis of Van den Akker et al. (2018) in which 80 studies were included. This was confirmed in adolescent samples in repeated one-round TGs (Derks et al., 2014 [ages 14–17]; Van de Groep et al., 2018 [ages 12–18]) and in the study by Van den Bos et al. (2010) (ages 9–22) described above. Some other studies found gender differences but only in specific situations or in a certain age group. For example, in the study by Sutter and Kocher (2007) in which people in different age groups participated (ages 8–68), only in the youngest group it was shown that girls showed more reciprocity behavior compared to boys (mean age 8). Two other studies found that female students showed more reciprocity behavior during the first round of a TG compared to male students but this gender difference disappeared throughout the course of the game (Chaudhuri et al., 2013; Chaudhuri & Sbai, 2011). Furthermore, Garbarino and Slonim (2009) found in their study that in the youngest age group (age <25), females showed more reciprocity behavior when the returned amount from the trustor was high, while males showed more reciprocity behavior when the trustor's returned amount was low. This effect was not present in older age groups (ages 25–49 and age >50).

11.4.2 Neuroimaging Studies

Only a few studies examined gender differences in the underlying neural mechanisms of trust and reciprocity behavior. During the phase in which the response of a trustworthy partner was shown to the trustor, males had more TPJ activity compared to females while females showed more caudate activity (Lemmers-Jansen et al., 2017 [ages 16–27]). There were no gender differences in neural activity when making investment decisions (Lemmers-Jansen et al., 2017 [ages 16–27]). This study reported no gender differences in average trust behavior across the game, which makes it difficult to interpret the observed neural differences. Lemmers-Jansen et al. (2017) speculate that the increased caudate activity of females may signal greater social learning by females compared to males, especially since females in this study showed a lower baseline trust at the beginning of the interaction. In a younger sample (Lemmers-Jansen et al., 2019 [ages 13–19]), males showed more left TPJ activity compared to females while females showed more left caudate activity compared to males during the period that the participants received the trustworthy partner's response; however, both results were at trend level. Also, when female participants made trust decisions, activity in the left TPJ and the right caudate were negatively associated with age while this relationship was opposite for male participants (Lemmers-Jansen et al., 2019 [ages 13–19]). No behavioral gender differences in trust behavior were found in this study. Lemmers-Jansen et al. (2019) suggest that the gender differences in neural activity in the absence of behavioral differences may suggest males and females use different cognitive strategies in these social interactions.

When interacting with an untrustworthy partner, no gender differences were found in neural activity during investment decisions and when receiving the partner's response in an older adolescent sample (Lemmers-Jansen et al., 2017 [ages 16–27]). In a younger sample, no gender differences in neural activity were found when making investments while a slight age-related increase of left TPJ activity when receiving the untrustworthy partner's response was found for females and an age-related decrease in left TPJ activity was found for males (Lemmers-Jansen et al., 2019 [ages 13–19]). No gender differences in trust behavior were found. Overall, the limited number of studies indicate some gender differences in patterns of brain activity during the TG; however, the absence of associations with behavioral differences hinders the interpretation of the findings.

In a different study, an interactive TG was used in which two adults played multiple TG rounds that involved varying levels of social risk (Wu et al., 2020). Gender differences were found as males showed more activity in the ventrolateral prefrontal cortex and in the precuneus than females. These results were interpreted to mean that males used increased cognitive control processes to inhibit social risk information and made more use of strategic choices by using self-referencing to maximize their profit (Wu et al., 2020). Furthermore, females showed increased subgenual ACC activity when social risk in the TG round increased, while males did not show differing activity for different levels of social risk. This was interpreted as increased sensitivity by females for the social risk of getting betrayed, and consequently, females deciding to have less concern for the interaction partner (Wu et al., 2020). In contrast, in their strategic choices, males seem to be less sensitive to the social risk attached to these choices compared to females (Wu et al., 2020).

11.4.3   *Summary*

The most robust behavioral gender difference seems to be in baseline trust, with males investing more than females, a difference which is already apparent in adolescence. It is possible that the difference in baseline trust is associated with gender differences in risk-taking behavior. Van den Akker et al. (2018) suggest that, based on the evolutionary theory, males may be more risk-taking compared to females and this may result in acquiring goods and achieving a higher social status, which suggest one to be a good partner for offspring. The second, more tentative, observation that emerges from this review is that when interacting with an untrustworthy partner, males decrease their trust more than females. This gender difference may indicate that females prioritize maintaining a social relationship with the interaction partner (Lemmers-Jansen et al., 2017). In contrast, reciprocity behavior seems to be largely similar for males and females. The few studies that have examined gender differences in the neural mechanisms of trust show increased activity in the TPJ, for males compared to females, while females show more activity in the caudate. Also, males and females seem to handle social risks differently when trusting others and when receiving reciprocity behavior of others. This may tentatively point to different strategies that males and females employ during the TG; however, much more research is needed before conclusions can be drawn.

11.5   Conclusion and Future Directions

This chapter gave an overview of the research on the development of trust and reciprocity behavior and on the gender differences in trust and reciprocity behavior. Developmental studies show that baseline trust is present at a young age and increases until young adulthood, although this increase is not found consistently. Studies further show an increase in fine-tuning and in the ability to adapt trust behavior in response to the reciprocity behavior of the interaction partner throughout adolescence. Furthermore, an increase in reciprocity behavior throughout adolescence is found. This conclusion fits the general idea that adolescence is an important phase for the development of social behavior, characterized by an increased sensitivity to others' perspectives and an increased ability to adapt their own behavior accordingly (Eisenberg et al., 2005; Van den Bos et al., 2011). In conjunction with this conclusion, some studies show an increase of activity in mentalizing-related areas during adolescence and young adulthood. In addition, activity in reward-related areas and areas related to conflict monitoring decrease during adolescence and young adulthood. However, the (developmental) neuroimaging literature is scarce and future, preferably longitudinal, research is needed to replicate and expand these findings. Trust in the elderly has not been investigated extensively but some studies, including studies using questionnaire data, suggest trust increases across the life span. As trust behavior is an essential component within social relationships, these studies could usefully take into account the dynamics of the social environment later in life.

Concerning gender differences in baseline trust, males seem to show more baseline trust toward others compared to females, more trust toward a trustworthy partner in a multiple round TG, and to decrease their trust more so when interacting with an untrustworthy partner, but overall the differences are small. Furthermore, a meta-analysis did not report gender differences in reciprocity behavior. Few studies examined gender differences in the neural mechanisms of trust and suggested that males have more activity in areas that have been associated with mentalizing while females show more activity in areas that have been associated with reward and learning processes. Furthermore, when choices imply social risks, neuroimaging results suggested males are more strategic and less sensitive to these risks compared to females. These studies highlight how functional neuroimaging can potentially elucidate differences in the strategies that males and females employ during the TG, and provide testable hypotheses for future studies.

A suggestion for future research is to examine the effect of culture or geographical location on trust behavior and reciprocity behavior. So far, only a few behavioral studies have suggested that there may be some meaningful differences in TG behavior associated with cultural factors. A robust finding of a meta-analysis by Johnson and Mislin (2011) is that less trust is shown by people in studies conducted in Africa compared to studies conducted in North America (Johnson & Mislin, 2011). In the future, the emerging field of cultural neuroscience could build on this database as a starting point for investigating the neural correlates associated with these differences.

References

Alós-Ferrer, C., & Farolfi, F. (2019). Trust games and beyond. *Frontiers in Neuroscience*, 13, 887. DOI: https://doi.org/10.3389/fnins.2019.00887

Bailey, P. E., & Leon, T. (2019). A systematic review and meta-analysis of age-related differences in trust. *Psychology and Aging*, 34(5), 674–685. https://doi.org/10.1037/pag0000368

Bellucci, G., Chernyak, S. V., Goodyear, K., Eickhoff, S. B., & Krueger, F. (2017). Neural signatures of trust in reciprocity: A coordinate-based meta-analysis. *Human Brain Mapping*, 38(3), 1233–1248. https://doi.org/10.1002/hbm.23451

Berg, J., Dickhaut, J., & McCabe, K. (1995). Trust, reciprocity, and social history. *Games and Economic Behavior*, 10(1), 122–142. https://doi.org/10.1006/game.1995.1027

Betts, L. R., & Rotenberg, K. J. (2008). A social relations analysis of children's trust in their peers across the early years of school. *Social Development*, 17(4), 1039–1055. https://doi.org/10.1111/j.1467-9507.2008.00479.x

Betts, L. R., Rotenberg, K. J., Petrocchi, S., et al. (2014). An investigation of children's peer trust across culture: Is the composition of peer trust universal? *International Journal of Behavioral Development*, 38(1), 33–41. https://doi.org/10.1177/0165025413505248

Blakemore, S.-J. (2008). The social brain in adolescence. *Nature Reviews Neuroscience*, 9(4), 267–277. https://doi.org/10.1038/nrn2353

   (2012). Development of the social brain in adolescence. *Journal of the Royal Society of Medicine*, 105(3), 111–116. https://doi.org/10.1258/jrsm.2011.110221

Bosco, F. M., Gabbatore, I., & Tirassa, M. (2014). A broad assessment of theory of mind in adolescence: The complexity of mindreading. *Consciousness and Cognition*, 24, 84–97. https://doi.org/10.1016/j.concog.2014.01.003

Chan, D., Hamamura, T., Li, L. M. W., & Zhang, X. (2017). Is trusting others related to better health? An investigation of older adults across six non-western countries. *Journal of Cross-Cultural Psychology*, 48(8), 1288–1301. https://doi.org/10.1177/0022022117722632

Chaudhuri, A., Paichayontvijit, T., & Shen, L. (2013). Gender differences in trust and trustworthiness: Individuals, single sex and mixed sex groups. *Journal of Economic Psychology*, 34, 181–194. https://doi.org/10.1016/j.joep.2012.09.013

Chaudhuri, A., & Sbai, E. (2011). Gender differences in trust and reciprocity in repeated gift exchange games. *New Zealand Economic Papers*, 45(1–2), 81–95. https://doi.org/10.1080/00779954.2011.556072

Chin, J.-C. (2014). Young children's trust beliefs in peers: Relations to social competence and interactive behaviors in a peer group. *Early Education and Development*, 25(5), 601–618. https://doi.org/10.1080/10409289.2013.836698

Corriveau, K. H., Harris, P. L., Meins, E., et al. (2009). Young children's trust in their mother's claims: Longitudinal links with attachment security in infancy. *Child Development*, 80(3), 750–761. https://doi.org/10.1111/j.1467-8624.2009.01295.x

Crone, E. A., Poldrack, R. A., & Durston, S. (2010). Challenges and methods in developmental neuroimaging. *Human Brain Mapping*, 31(6), 835–837. https://doi.org/10.1002/hbm.21053

Delgado, M. R., Frank, R. H., & Phelps, E. A. (2005). Perceptions of moral character modulate the neural systems of reward during the trust game. *Nature Neuroscience*, 8(11), 1611–1618. https://doi.org/10.1038/nn1575

Derks, J., Lee, N. C., & Krabbendam, L. (2014). Adolescent trust and trustworthiness: Role of gender and social value orientation. *Journal of Adolescence*, 37 (8), 1379–1386. https://doi.org/10.1016/j.adolescence.2014.09.014

Dumontheil, I., Apperly, I. A., & Blakemore, S. J. (2010). Online usage of theory of mind continues to develop in late adolescence. *Developmental Science*, 13 (2), 331–338. https://doi.org/10.1111/j.1467-7687.2009.00888.x

Eisenberg, N., Cumberland, A., Guthrie, I. K., Murphy, B. C., & Shepard, S. A. (2005). Age changes in prosocial responding and moral reasoning in adolescence and early adulthood. *Journal of Research on Adolescence*, 15(3), 235–260. https://doi.org/10.1111/j.1532-7795.2005.00095.x

Erdley, C. A., & Day, H. J. (2017). Friendship in childhood and adolescence. In M. Hojjat & A. Moyer (Eds.), *The psychology of friendship* (pp. 3–19). Oxford University Press. https://doi.org/10.1093/acprof:oso/9780190222024.001.0001

Erikson, E. H. (1963). *Childhood and society*. W. W. Norton & Company. https://doi.org/10.30965/9783657768387_048

Evans, A. M., & Krueger, J. I. (2009). The psychology (and economics) of trust. *Social and Personality Psychology Compass*, 3(6), 1003–1017. https://doi.org/10.1111/j.1751-9004.2009.00232.x

Fett, A.-K. J., Gromann, P. M., Giampietro, V., Shergill, S. S., & Krabbendam, L. (2014). Default distrust? An fMRI investigation of the neural development of trust and cooperation. *Social Cognitive and Affective Neuroscience*, 9 (4), 395–402. https://doi.org/10.1093/scan/nss144

Fett, A.-K. J., Shergill, S. S., Gromann, P. M., et al. (2014). Trust and social reciprocity in adolescence: A matter of perspective-taking. *Journal of Adolescence*, 37(2), 175–184. https://doi.org/10.1016/j.adolescence.2013.11.011

Garbarino, E., & Slonim, R. (2009). The robustness of trust and reciprocity across a heterogeneous U.S. population. *Journal of Economic Behavior & Organization*, 69(3), 226–240. https://doi.org/10.1016/j.jebo.2007.06.010

Güroğlu, B., Van den Bos, W., & Crone, E. A. (2014). Sharing and giving across adolescence: An experimental study examining the development of prosocial behavior. *Frontiers in Psychology*, 5, 1–13. https://doi.org/10.3389/fpsyg.2014.00291

Haselhuhn, M. P., Kennedy, J. A., Kray, L. J., Van Zant, A. B., & Schweitzer, M. E. (2015). Gender differences in trust dynamics: Women trust more than men following a trust violation. *Journal of Experimental Social Psychology*, 56, 104–109. https://doi.org/10.1016/j.jesp.2014.09.007

Hill, C. A., & O'Hara, E. A. (2006). A cognitive theory of trust. *Washington University Law Review*, 84, 1717–1796. https://doi.org/10.2139/ssrn.869423

Holm, H., & Nystedt, P. (2005). Intra-generational trust: A semi-experimental study of trust among different generations. *Journal of Economic Behavior & Organization*, 58(3), 403–419. https://doi.org/10.1016/j.jebo.2003.10.013

Johnson, N. D., & Mislin, A. A. (2011). Trust games: A meta-analysis. *Journal of Economic Psychology*, 32(5), 865–889. https://doi.org/10.1016/j.joep.2011.05.007

King-Casas, B., Tomlin, D., Anen, C., Camerer, C. F., Quartz, S. R., & Montague, P. R. (2005). Getting to know you: Reputation and trust in a two-person economic exchange. *Science*, 308(5718), 78–83. https://doi.org/10.1126/science.1108062

Kocher, M. G. (2017). How trust in social dilemmas evolves with age. In P. A. M. Van Lange, B. Rockenbach, & T. Yamagishi (Eds.), *Trust in social dilemmas* (pp. 101–118). Oxford University Press. https://doi.org/10.1093/oso/9780190630782.003.0006

Krueger, F., & Meyer-Lindenberg, A. (2019). Toward a model of interpersonal trust drawn from neuroscience, psychology, and economics. *Trends in neurosciences*, 42(2), 92–101. DOI: https://doi.org/10.1016/j.tins.2018.10.004

Ledyard, J. O. (1995). Public goods: A survey of experimental research. In J. Kagel & A. Roth (Eds.), *Handbook of experimental economics* (pp. 111–194). Princeton University Press. https://doi.org/10.2307/j.ctvzsmff5

Lee, N. C., Jolles, J., & Krabbendam, L. (2016). Social information influences trust behaviour in adolescents. *Journal of Adolescence*, 46, 66–75. https://doi.org/10.1016/j.adolescence.2015.10.021

Lemmers-Jansen, I. L., Fett, A.-K. J., Shergill, S. S., Van Kesteren, M. T., & Krabbendam, L. (2019). Girls-boys: An investigation of gender differences in the behavioral and neural mechanisms of trust and reciprocity in adolescence. *Frontiers in Human Neuroscience*, 13, 1–12. https://doi.org/10.3389/fnhum.2019.00257

Lemmers-Jansen, I. L., Krabbendam, L., Veltman, D. J., & Fett, A.-K. J. (2017). Boys vs. girls: Gender differences in the neural development of trust and reciprocity depend on social context. *Developmental Cognitive Neuroscience*, 25, 235–245. https://doi.org/10.1016/j.dcn.2017.02.001

Lewis, J. D., & Weigert, A. (1985). Trust as a social reality. *Social Forces*, 63(4), 967–985. https://doi.org/10.1093/sf/63.4.967

Li, T., & Fung, H. H. (2013). Age differences in trust: An investigation across 38 countries. *Journals of Gerontology Series B: Psychological Sciences and Social Sciences*, 68(3), 347–355. https://doi.org/10.1093/geronb/gbs072

Luna, B., Velanova, K., & Geier, C. F. (2010). Methodological approaches in developmental neuroimaging studies. *Human Brain Mapping*, 31(6), 863–871. https://doi.org/10.1002/hbm.21073

Malti, T., Averdijk, M., Zuffianò, A., et al. (2016). Children's trust and the development of prosocial behavior. *International Journal of Behavioral Development*, 40(3), 262–270. https://doi.org/10.1177/0165025415584628

Murtin, F., Fleischer, L., Siegerink, V., et al. (2018). *Trust and its determinants: Evidence from the Trustlab experiment*. OECD Statistics Working Papers, 2018/02. https://doi.org/10.1787/869ef2ec-en

Pfeifer, J. H., & Blakemore, S.-J. (2012). Adolescent social cognitive and affective neuroscience: Past, present, and future. *Social Cognitive and Affective Neuroscience*, 7(1), 1–10. https://doi.org/10.1093/scan/nsr099

Poulin, M. J., & Haase, C. M. (2015). Growing to trust: Evidence that trust increases and sustains well-being across the life span. *Social Psychological and Personality Science*, 6(6), 614–621. https://doi.org/10.1177/1948550615574301

Poundstone, W. (1992). *Prisoner's dilemma.* Doubleday.

Rasmussen, E. C., & Gutchess, A. (2019). Can't read my broker face: Learning about trustworthiness with age. *The Journals of Gerontology: Series B*, 74(1), 82–86. https://doi.org/10.1093/geronb/gby012

Rotenberg, K. J., Petrocchi, S., Lecciso, F., & Marchetti, A. (2013). Children's trust beliefs in others and trusting behavior in peer interaction. *Child Development Research*, 2013, 1–8. https://doi.org/10.1155/2013/806597

Saunders, M. N., Dietz, G., & Thornhill, A. (2014). Trust and distrust: Polar opposites, or independent but co-existing? *Human Relations*, 67(6), 639–665. https://doi.org/10.1177/0018726713500831

Schiffer, A.-M., & Schubotz, R. I. (2011). Caudate nucleus signals for breaches of expectation in a movement observation paradigm. *Frontiers in Human Neuroscience*, 5, 1–12. https://doi.org/10.3389/fnhum.2011.00038

Steinberg, L. (2008). A social neuroscience perspective on adolescent risk-taking. *Developmental Review*, 28(1), 78–106. https://doi.org/10.1016/j.dr.2007.08 .002

Sutter, M., & Kocher, M. G. (2007). Trust and trustworthiness across different age groups. *Games and Economic Behavior*, 59(2), 364–382. https://doi.org/ 10.1016/j.geb.2006.07.006

Takahashi, H., Shen, J., & Ogawa, K. (2020). Gender-specific reference-dependent preferences in the experimental trust game. *Evolutionary and Institutional Economics Review*, 17, 25–38. https://doi.org/10.1007/ s40844–019-00155-z

Thompson, R. A. (2008). Early attachment and later development: Familiar questions, new answers. In J. Cassidy & P. R. Shaver (Eds.), *Handbook of attachment: Theory, research, and clinical applications* (pp. 348–365). The Guilford Press. https://doi.org/10.1002/imhj.21730

Tzieropoulos, H. (2013). The trust game in neuroscience: A short review. *Social Neuroscience*, 8(5), 407–416. https://doi.org/10.1080/17470919.2013 .832375

Van de Groep, S., Meuwese, R., Zanolie, K., Güroğlu, B., & Crone, E. A. (2018). Developmental changes and individual differences in trust and reciprocity in adolescence. *Journal of Research on Adolescence*, 30, 192–208. https://doi.org/ 10.1111/jora.12459

Van den Akker, O., Van Vugt, M., Van Assen, M. A., & Wicherts, J. M. (2018). Sex differences in trust and trustworthiness: A meta-analysis of the trust game and the gift-exchange game. *Pre-print on PsyArXiv.*

Van den Bos, W., Van Dijk, E., & Crone, E. A. (2012). Learning whom to trust in repeated social interactions: A developmental perspective. *Group Processes*

& *Intergroup Relations*, 15(2), 243–256. https://doi.org/10.1177/ 1368430211418698

Van den Bos, W., Van Dijk, E., Westenberg, M., Rombouts, S. A., & Crone, E. A. (2011). Changing brains, changing perspectives: The neurocognitive development of reciprocity. *Psychological Science*, 22(1), 60–70. https://doi .org/10.1177/0956797610391102

Van den Bos, W., Westenberg, M., Van Dijk, E., & Crone, E. A. (2010). Development of trust and reciprocity in adolescence. *Cognitive Development*, 25(1), 90–102. https://doi.org/10.1016/j.cogdev.2009.07.004

Van Hoorn, J., Shablack, H., Lindquist, K. A., & Telzer, E. H. (2019). Incorporating the social context into neurocognitive models of adolescent decision making: A neuroimaging meta-analysis. *Neuroscience & Biobehavioral Reviews*, 101, 129–145. https://doi.org/10.1016/j.neubiorev .2018.12.024

Vandevivere, E., Bosmans, G., Roels, S., Dujardin, A., & Braet, C. (2018). State trust in middle childhood: An experimental manipulation of maternal support. *Journal of Child and Family Studies*, 27(4), 1252–1263. https://doi.org/ 10.1007/s10826-017-0954-7

Wu, Y., Hall, A. S., Siehl, S., Grafman, J., & Krueger, F. (2020). Neural signatures of gender differences in interpersonal trust. *Frontiers in Human Neuroscience*, 14, 1–11. https://doi.org/10.3389/fnhum.2020.00225

CHAPTER 12

Trust and Brain Dynamics
Insights from Task-Based and Task-Free Neuroimaging Investigations

Yan Wu and Frank Krueger

12.1 Introduction

Interpersonal trust – a willingness to tolerate disadvantage or insecurity based on assumptions about the actions of another person (Seppänen et al., 2007) – plays a fundamental role in our diverse social life and relationships. Its widespread need in human relations has led to comprehensive studies in neuroscience, psychology, and economics (Krueger & Meyer-Lindenberg, 2019).

One of the most common research approaches to measure interpersonal trust is through the use of variants of the two-person sequential trust game (TG) (Berg et al., 1995; Camerer & Weigelt, 1988). In the TG, one player is the trustor and the other one the trustee. Both players are endowed with monetary units that they can exchange for real money at an established exchange rate following the completion of the game. The trustor decides whether or not to pass some of her/his endowment to the trustee (*trust stage*). If the trustor chooses to send money to the trustee, the transferred amount is then multiplied by the experimenter (usually doubled or tripled) and sent to the trustee. The trustee decides then either to reciprocate (or to betray) by returning some money back to the trustor (*trustworthiness stage*). The trustor is notified at the end of the game about the decision of the trustee and the total gains (*feedback stage*). In general, the sum of money sent by the trustor usually measures trust, while trustworthiness represents the amount returned by the trustee.

Variations of the TG exist. In the binary TG, for example, the trustor (or trustee) makes a binary choice, reflecting a "yes" or "no" decision to trust (or reciprocate) as in most situations in real life – instead of sending a variable amount as in the standard TG (Bohnet & Zeckhauser, 2004; Eckel & Wilson, 2004). Further, a risk game – involving a computer

Corresponding author: Frank Krueger (fkrueger@gmu.edu).

counterpart instead of a human partner returning a random amount to the trustor – is used as a control condition that taps into whether the trustor's performance in the TG is truly a reflection of trust rather than just a reflection of risk-taking behavior (Bohnet & Zeckhauser, 2004; Eckel & Wilson, 2004; Kosfeld et al., 2005). The TG can be played out over single or multiple iterations (Johnson & Mislin, 2011): The trustor plays either with a different trustee (one-shot) or with the same trustee (multi-shot) each time. In the one-shot game version, the observed trust behavior can be seen as a *propensity* or *preference* to trust strangers. In contrast, in the multi-shot game version, trust is modulated either based on prior information on the reputation (i.e., prior-based trust) (Fouragnan et al., 2013) (see also Chapter 7) or the actual behavior (i.e., interaction-based trust) of the counterpart (King-Casas et al., 2005; Krueger et al., 2007) (see also Chapter 8) –reflecting processes of *trust dynamics.*

Several neuroscience methodologies have helped to identify brain regions involved in trust. Such approaches include the use of brain lesions patient studies (Belfi et al., 2015; Koscik & Tranel, 2011; Moretto et al., 2013), exogenous oxytocin (Baumgartner et al., 2008; Kosfeld et al., 2005; Nave et al., 2015) or testosterone studies (Boksem et al., 2013; Bos et al., 2010) (see Chapter 13), and neuroimaging studies such as electroencephalography (EEG) (Fu et al., 2019; Hahn, Notebaert, Anderl, Teckentrup, et al., 2015; Sun et al., 2019) and functional magnetic resonance imaging (fMRI) (Bellucci et al., 2018; Fehr, 2009; Riedl & Javor, 2012; Tzieropoulos, 2013).

Although a plethora of fMRI studies have been conducted that explore the brain's functional activities in interpersonal trust (Krueger & Meyer-Lindenberg, 2019); little effort has been made to elucidate the commonalities and differences on varying fMRI approaches – that is, task-based fMRI (tb-fMRI) versus task-free fMRI (tf-fMRI). During tb-fMRI, participants complete the TG inside the MRI scanner to locate brain regions associated with interpersonal trust (Friston et al., 1995), whereas during tf-fMRI they undergo a resting-state fMRI scan (also called rs-fMRI scan) to link spontaneous brain fluctuations of rs networks with trust behavior that is measured outside of the scanner (Biswal et al., 1995).

Although tb- and tf-fMRI studies have provided valuable information on the neural mechanisms related to trust, it remains unknown whether both fMRI techniques provide consistent brain activities and how these techniques reveal unique aspects of neuropsychological processes underlying interpersonal trust. The goal of this chapter is to compare the commonalities and differences between tb- and tf-fMRI studies on interpersonal trust and discuss how these two techniques can make unique contributions to our understanding of the psychoneurobiological underpinnings of trust.

12.2 Task-Based Neural Signatures of Trust

Tb-fMRI detects relative changes in the blood oxygen level-dependent (BOLD) hemodynamic response to neural activity of certain presented stimuli (Ogawa et al., 1992) – a valid but indirect measure of neural activity (Logothetis, 2008). BOLD imaging is based on neural activity-dependent changes in local magnetic fields. A stable infusion of oxygenated hemoglobin is accompanied by neural activity, which shifts the ratio of de-/oxygenated hemoglobin molecules in the local blood supply to activated brain regions. The BOLD contrast is based on this local change in the magnetic field – allowing the detection of differences in signals between two psychological states (e.g., trust vs. distrust) or two groups (e.g., patients vs. healthy controls) (Bush & Cisler, 2013).

Tb-fMRI studies, usually testing about 18–30 participants, employ different types of designs to enhance the order and timing of the stimuli to find an optimization among estimation efficiency, detection power, and predictability (Durnez et al., 2017): event-related designs (i.e., separable trials of varying task-types), block designs (i.e., equivalent trial types to build a task-specific block), or mixed block with event-related designs (i.e., a combination of event-related and block designs) (Petersen & Dubis, 2011). A typical trust tb-fMRI study employs visual stimuli to cue participants to play TGs (or risk games as control games) – as one-shot TGs evaluating trust propensity or multi-shot TG evaluating trust dynamics – while acquiring BOLD contrast images for the duration of about two to three runs (with each run about 10–15 minutes). To analyze interbrain activity between two players, hyperscanning can be employed (Montague, 2002) in which trustor and trustee interact with each other in a different MRI scanner as their brains are simultaneously scanned (e.g., King-Casas et al., 2005; Krueger et al., 2007; Tomlin, 2006).

Tb-fMRI often employs univariate methods such as general linear model analysis (Worsley & Friston, 1995) to examine brain activations related to trust by estimating the temporal synchrony between experimental observations and the predicted brain responses during the different TG stages: the trust stage (e.g., contrast: trust vs. distrust), trustworthiness stage (e.g., contrast: reciprocity vs. betrayal), and feedback stage (e.g., contrast: trust [reciprocate] vs. trust [betrayal]). Moreover, a multivariate pattern analysis approach can be applied (Haxby, 2012), that is, a pattern classification approach that seeks to characterize the combination of activities among multiple voxels (regions) in a TG fMRI experiment to differentiate between experimental conditions (e.g., contrast: trust vs. distrust) (Bellucci, Molter, & Park, 2019). To evaluate functional connectivity (FC) among brain regions engaged in interpersonal trust, a psychophysiological interaction (PPI) analysis approach can also be employed to identify voxels in which activity is more correlated with activity from a seed region of interest (ROI) in a given psychological context (O'Reilly et al., 2012). Since PPI analyses cannot determine directionality (i.e., causality) between functionally connected regions, approaches measuring effective connectivity such as dynamic causal modeling (DCM) (Friston et al., 2011) or Granger causality mapping (GCM) (Roebroeck et al., 2005) can be employed. Whereas DCM is based upon a deterministic model that produces predicted crossed spectra from the biophysically feasible model of coupled neural fluctuations in a distributed neuronal network (Friston et al., 2011), GCM does not depend on a priori specification of a network model comprising preselected regions and connections between them (Roebroeck et al., 2005).

The fMRI literature on human trust behavior has identified several essential subcortical and cortical brain regions (for reviews see Fehr, 2009; Riedl & Javor, 2012; Rilling & Sanfey, 2011; Tzieropoulos, 2013). A recent coordinate-based meta-analysis of fMRI studies employing the TG identified consistent activation patterns across fMRI studies (Bellucci et al., 2017). On the one hand, one- versus multi-shot TGs for the trust phase consistently activate the right anterior insula (AI) – a brain region probably encoding aversive feelings such as betrayal aversion (Aimone et al., 2014; Bohnet et al., 2008) (see also Chapter 5). In contrast, multi-shot versus one-shot TGs consistently engage the ventral striatum (vSTR, nucleus accumbens) – a brain region possibly involved in reward prediction such as in learning a partner's reputation (Delgado et al., 2005; Fareri et al., 2012; King-Casas et al., 2005).

On the other hand, contrasting multi-shot TGs for the decision versus feedback phase constantly activate the vSTR (nucleus accumbens), while the dorsal striatum (dSTR, caudate nucleus) is coherently engaged for the reverse contrast. According to actor–critic models of reinforcement learning, two distinct components are involved (Joel et al., 2002): a "critic" likely represented by the vSTR that learns to predict future reward by updating the temporal difference error between the predicted and the actual rewards (O'Doherty et al., 2004), and an "actor" possibly encoded by the dSTR that maintains knowledge on rewarding consequences of acts to optimize potential future rewards (Baumgartner et al., 2008; King-Casas et al., 2005).

The activation pattern between one- and multi-shot games during the trust phase indicates a transition from uncertainty about betrayal aversion (i.e., AI) in one-shot TGs to reward expectation (i.e., vSTR) in multi-shot TGs mediated by optimizing action–outcome association (i.e., dSTR) during the feedback phase. Through repeated interactions, trustors may form clear opinions about the trustees and base their decisions on the credibility that the partner has gained from previous experiences. In this sense, the initial uncertainty about the outcomes of a decision to trust is minimized as the behavior of the partner is no longer unpredictable and the betrayal aversion is diminished.

A plethora of evidence exists that other key regions belonging to domain-general large-scale networks are also involved in trust decisions. Besides the striatum (dSTR, vSTR), the ventral tegmental area (VTA) is another region of the *reward network* (RWN) that mediates trust decisions (Krueger et al., 2007) – a region associated with the evaluation of expected and realized reward (Hollerman & Schultz, 1998). Besides the AI, the amygdala and dorsal anterior cingulate cortex (dACC) – regions associated with the salience network (SAN) – are associated with interpersonal trust. For example, amygdala damage contributes to increased trust (Koscik & Tranel, 2011; Van Honk et al., 2013) – supporting this brain region's role in the processing of emotional consequences following trust decisions (see also Chapter 18). Activity in the dACC parametrically tracks increases in outgroup (but not ingroup) trust (Hughes et al., 2017) and enhances when trustors interact iteratively with an untrustworthy partner (Fett et al., 2014) – supporting the role of this brain region in monitoring the social dilemma of the trustor.

Brain regions belonging to other networks such as the central-executive network (CEN, e.g., lateral prefrontal cortex, lPFC) also play a crucial role in trust decisions. For example, activity in the right ventrolateral prefrontal cortex (vlPFC) is positively associated with general trust (Yanagisawa et al., 2011). Further, the dorsolateral PFC (dlPFC) responds differently to cooperative versus noncooperative counterparts when prior reputation information about counterparts are available – suggesting that this brain region monitors contextually modulated decision values over trials, thereby enhancing participants' performance (Fouragnan et al., 2013).

Moreover, decisions to trust are based on inferences of others' trustworthiness, engaging the default-mode network (DMN), including the dorsomedial prefrontal cortex (dmPFC) and temporoparietal junction

(TPJ) – generally implicated in mentalizing and theory of mind (Gallagher & Frith, 2003; Spreng et al., 2009). Whereas activity in the dmPFC is high during the initial trust-building stage, it declines once trust has been established (Krueger et al., 2007), suggesting that this region may be involved in encoding whether someone is trustworthy. TPJ activity increases during trust decisions (Fett et al., 2014) but reduces through aversive affect due to threat of shock (Engelmann et al., 2019), suggesting that this area may reflect a participant's capacity to mentalize the intention and choice of the partner and ultimately adopt the participants' trust behavior toward their partner (Engelmann et al., 2019; Van Overwalle, 2009).

Taken together, activation patterns during task-based fMRI studies have been recently summarized in a neuropsychoeconomic model of trust (Krueger & Meyer-Lindenberg, 2019). In this model, trust emerges from the interactions of motivation, affect, and cognition systems that engage key regions rooted in domain-general large-scale brain networks: RWN (e.g., vSTR, dSTR), SAN (e.g., AI, amygdala, dACC), CEN (e.g., dlPFC, vlPFC), and DMN (e.g., dmPFC, TPJ). The motivation system involves the RWN to signal the expected reward for trusting another person, while the affective system engages the SAN to integrate the aversion of the risk of betrayal by another person. The cognitive system includes the CEN to implement context-based decision strategies and the DMN to determine relationship-based trustworthiness for trusting a partner (Krueger & Meyer-Lindenberg, 2019).

Tb-fMRI findings suggest that through repeated interactions, interpersonal trust may develop from calculus-based trust (i.e., conducting rational costs and benefits calculations of trust decisions driven primarily by the SAN), through knowledge-based trust (i.e., using contextual information and feedback to learn trustees' behavior and promote their trust relationships, driven primarily by the CEN to implement a strategy or the DMN to assess the trustworthiness of the partner), to identification-based trust (i.e., establishing a rewarding identification with trustees, driven primarily by the RWN) (Krueger & Meyer-Lindenberg, 2019).

12.3   Task-Free Neural Signatures of Trust

Tf-fMRI is based on spontaneous low-frequency (<0.1 Hz) BOLD signal fluctuations at rest (Biswal et al., 1995), where some regions are more highly correlated with one another than with others (Raichle & Snyder, 2007). Tf-fMRI can be acquired with an independent rs-fMRI scan lasting between 5 and 20 minutes: individuals are advised to relax (with eyes open or closed), remain still and awake, and not to think systematically about anything (Biswal et al., 1995; Lee et al., 2013; Rosazza & Minati, 2011). Individuals complete the TG after rs acquisition to guarantee the independence of tf-fMRI from trust behavior measures. The anatomically separated but functionally related regions exhibit patterns of intrinsic connectivity termed as rs networks (Fox & Raichle, 2007; Power et al., 2011; Van den Heuvel & Pol, 2010) – for example, the SAN, DMN, and CEN – that are stable over time and surprisingly close to the networks activated by a wide variety of tb-fMRI studies (Bressler & Menon, 2010; Damoiseaux et al., 2006; Smitha et al., 2017). Concerns about the impact of individuals' current state, mood, instruction (i.e., maintain eyes open or closed), preprocessing approaches, scanning length, and other factors (e.g., substance withdrawal, drowsiness, and sleep) on the intrinsic activity and resting-state functional connectivity (RSFC) of those networks have been addressed by moderate-to-high test-retest reliability (Andellini et al., 2015; D. M. Cole et al., 2010; Heine et al., 2012; Patanaik et al., 2018; Patriat et al., 2013; Wong et al., 2012; Zuo et al., 2010).

Multiple approaches have been proposed to analyze tf-fMRI data. For assessing RSFC, commonly used methods include seed-based analysis, functional connectivity density mapping (FCDM), independent component analysis (ICA), and graph analysis (Smitha et al., 2017). Seed-based analysis is the simplest analysis technique for identifying FC networks for which the BOLD time course from voxels in an ROI (i.e., seed region) is extracted and its temporal correlation with the time course of all other brain voxels is determined (Azeez & Biswal, 2017). ICA is a data-driven analysis that separates a series of signals into independent components and extracts statistically independent spatial maps and their associated time courses (Fox & Raichle, 2007). FCDM enables the measurement of individual FC maps with a higher spatial resolution (≥ 3 mm isotropic) to take maximum advantage of fMRI datasets' native resolution (Tomasi & Volkow, 2010). Graph analysis shows a highly effective organization of the brain network optimized toward a high degree of local and global efficiency, also called small-world topology (Sporns et al., 2007).

RSFC analysis can be conducted alone or in combination with a prediction-analytics framework – shifting the focus from correlational to predictive brain-behavior relationships. In a prediction-analytics framework, relating whole-brain RSFC patterns to phenotypic variables such as trust behavior via multivariate prediction analyses (e.g., multivariate classification and regression methods through machine learning) is crucial in turning FC into biomarkers that predict individual variability in phenotypes of interest and generalize those results to novel samples (Dosenbach et al., 2010; Orrù et al., 2012; Yarkoni & Westfall, 2017). RSFC activity acts as a neural "fingerprint" – accounting for variability in tb-fMRI activity (Tavor et al., 2016; Tobyne et al., 2018) as well as behavioral and psychological dispositions (Dubois & Adolphs, 2016). For example, RSFC of large-scale brain networks predicts personality traits (Dubois et al., 2018; Hsu et al., 2018; Nostro et al., 2018), creativity (Beaty et al., 2018), impulsivity (Li et al., 2013), social value orientation (Hahn, Notebaert, Anderl, Reicherts, et al., 2015), costly punishment (Feng et al., 2018), deception (Tang et al., 2018), brain maturity (Dosenbach et al., 2010), and brain disorders including autism (Plitt et al., 2015), schizophrenia (Mwansisya et al., 2017), and obsessive-compulsive disorder (Reggente et al., 2018).

RSFC fMRI in combination with a prediction-analytics framework has been increasingly utilized to predict trust propensity over the past five years. Bellucci et al. (2019) investigated whether specific RSFC networks predict individual differences in trust tendency utilizing a one-shot TG. RSFC within the DMN predicted individual differences in initial trust behavior (i.e., trust propensity) supporting previous evidence from an EEG-based RSFC study. Hahn, Notebaert, Anderl, Teckentrup, et al. (2015) showed that the trustor's initial trust can only be predicted from RSFC (connections of electrodes located over the right frontal cortex and the parietal cortex) in the first round but not from later rounds of the TG that represents a measure of trust dynamics established through social learning.

Lu et al. (2019) demonstrated that interindividual variations in trust propensity are predicted by RSFC of the distributed key nodes within and between domain-general large-scale networks: the SAN (amygdala), CEN (lateral PFC, lPFC), DMN (TPJ, temporal pole), and RWN (caudate). These findings indicate that the affective system of trust (i.e., the SAN) possibly comprises aversive feelings associated with the risk of betrayal by the partner; the motivational system of trust (i.e., the RWN) probably determines the predicted reward for trusting another person; and the cognitive systems such as the CEN conceivably adopt context-based strategies and the DMN plausibly evaluates a partner's trustworthiness to transform the risk of betrayal into a positive expectation of reciprocity.

Feng et al. (2020) showed that individual variations in trust propensity can be predicted by node strength (based on tf-fMRI) and gray matter volume (based on structural MRI) across parts of three identified modules within large-scale brain networks: the DMN (e.g., dmPFC, superior temporal gyrus) probably helping to simulate the trustworthiness of an anonymous partner based on implementing a calculus-based trust strategy; the CEN (e.g., vlPFC, dlPFC) likely providing the cognitive capacity to overcome the conflict of uncertainty and to inhibit knowledge on the risk of treachery; and the action-perception network (APN, e.g., supramarginal gyrus, superior parietal lobule, precuneus) possibly conducting a cost-benefit analysis when determining the amount of money to be sent and the amount to be received back from the partner.

To summarize, tf-fMRI studies can examine the prediction of individual variations in trust propensity based on rs brain measures. Multivariate prediction analyses have shown that individual variations in trust propensity can be predicted by intrinsic functional features across multiple regions that have been previously implicated as modules of domain-general large-scale brain networks (i.e., SAN, CEN, DMN, RWN) – supporting psychological mechanisms that partially determine the trust propensity of an individual. Importantly, intrinsic FC patterns only predict an individual's trust behavior measured at the first round (i.e., trust propensity perceived as a personality trait expressed in the underlying RSFC) but not at later rounds (i.e., experience-based trust due to social learning based on the feedback input per round not reflected in RSFC).

12.4 Summary and Conclusion

In this chapter, we compared the commonalities and differences between tb- and tf-fMRI approaches for studying trust and explored how these two approaches can make unique contributions in our understanding of the psychoneurobiological underpinnings of this phenomenon (Table 12.1). Overall, tb-fMRI trust studies typically involve the completion of the TG inside the scanner to capture online the neural correlates of distinct psychological processes related to the different stages of the TG (i.e., trust, trustworthiness, feedback) in localized brain regions engaged in trust propensity (i.e., one-shot TG) and trust dynamics (i.e., multi-shot TG) behavior at the group level. In contrast, tf-fMRI trust studies involve scanning at rest with the completion of the TG afterward outside of the scanner to capture the FC organized among brain regions to predict trust propensity at the individual level.

Importantly, tb-fMRI (Bellucci et al., 2017; Krueger & Meyer-Lindenberg, 2019) and tf-fMRI (Bellucci, Hahn, Deshpande, & Krueger,

Table 12.1. *Comparison between task-based and task-free neuroimaging approaches*

	Task-Based	Task-Free
BOLD signal	task evoked signal changes	intrinsic spontaneous low-frequency signal oscillations (<0.1 Hz)
Trust measures	trust propensity & dynamics at the group level	trust propensity at the individual level
TG paradigm	one- or multi-shot TG inside MRI scanner(s) (hyperscanning)	rest (eyes open or closed) inside and one-shot TG outside MRI scanner
Control condition	lottery game	no control game
Data acquisition	30–60 minutes	5–20 minutes
Subject recruitment	~20-40	>50
Analysis techniques	univariate: GLM, PPI; multivariate: MVPA	univariate: RSFC, graph-based network analysis; multivariate: CPM

Notes: TG, trust game; GLM, general linear model; PPI, psychophysiological interaction; MVPA, multi-voxel pattern analysis; RSFC, resting-state functional connectivity, CPM, connectome-based predictive modeling.

2019; Feng et al., 2020; Lu et al., 2019) studies revealed converging evidence for the underlying neural signatures of trust. While tb-fMRI studies have indicated activity of single crucial brain regions – engaging both subcortical (e.g., AI, amygdala, STR) and cortical (e.g., TPJ, vmPFC, lPFC, and vlPFC) regions – related to the psychological components of trust at the group level, tf-fMRI studies highlight the role of RSFC of those brain regions belonging to domain-general large-scale brain networks – SAN, CEN, DMN, and RWN – accounting for the individual differences in trust propensity (Krueger & Meyer-Lindenberg, 2019).

However, more work remains to be done to prove a direct link between these two approaches to further uncover the neuropsychological mechanisms of trust. On the one hand, a combination of tb- and tf-fMRI approaches within the same study session can offer a new kind of solution by unveiling the predictive power of both task-free and task-based FC to individual variations in trust behavior (M. W. Cole et al., 2016; Tavor et al., 2016). There has been no published combined research using both approaches for the exploration of interpersonal trust behavior. To date, connectome-based analyses usually focus on tf-fMRI; however, rest is an unrestricted condition that does not capture the full spectrum of individual differences in RSFC (Finn et al., 2017). For example, predictive models constructed from tb-fMRI data outperform models constructed from tf-fMRI data for predicting fluid intelligence (Greene et al., 2018), encouraging a paradigm switch from tf- to tb-fMRI FC (e.g., PPI) and effective connectivity (e.g., DCM, GCM) analyses for trust research. Although tb-fMRI studies provide a medium for the practical and objective modulation of brain states – allowing to explore their impact on FC patterns and individual differences in these patterns – the majority of tb-fMRI studies use correlation analysis (i.e., relying on in-sample population inferences) to establish individual differences of trust (Lo et al., 2015; Whelan & Garavan, 2014). It will be appropriate to switch to a predictive machine-learning framework to improve generalizability and to understand fMRI-derived statistics at the individual subject level (Gabrieli et al., 2015; Linden, 2012).

On the other hand, independently of both approaches, we should strive for normative fMRI research (Dubois & Adolphs, 2016). The reliability for both fMRI approaches should be improved for studying the neural correlates of trust, in which a relationship between the statistical and neuropsychological trust measure derived from fMRI should be acquired consistently at various locations for different people over multiple sessions, likely using slightly distinct trust paradigms (e.g., developing additional tasks to measure trust behavior to provide convergent validity to ensure a more accurate estimate of human trust) and control games (e.g., including the lottery game to control for general risk-taking behavior and the dictator game to decompose trust from altruism). Further, larger sample sizes (N>100) would be beneficial to increase statistical power and to ensure out-of-sample reliability in a predictive framework (Button et al., 2013; Yarkoni & Braver, 2010). Finally, heterogeneous samples would be helpful to classify between control and clinical samples (Fett et al., 2012; King-Casas et al., 2008) (see also Chapters 16 and 17). For example, it could be beneficial to include participants with a greater range of trust propensity – even including those with problems in social functioning (Lemmers-Jansen et al., 2019). These functional pathological changes could be considered as potential reliable biomarkers for a more biologically orientated science of human neuropsychiatric disease (Crawford & Garthwaite, 2008; Cuthbert & Insel, 2013).

Not far from now, it may be possible to interpret the tb/rf-fMRI-derived statistics of an individual in terms of their distribution in a normative sample, leading to a more neurobiology-based science of interpersonal trust; therefore contributing to the understanding of the central question of systems social neuroscience: How the brain gives rise to the mind that determines social behaviors such as interpersonal trust.

References

Aimone, J. A., Houser, D., & Weber, B. (2014). Neural signatures of betrayal aversion: An fMRI study of trust. *Proceedings. Biological Sciences*, 281(1782), 1–6. https://doi.org/10.1098/rspb.2013.2127

Andellini, M., Cannatà, V., Gazzellini, S., Bernardi, B., & Napolitano, A. (2015). Test-retest reliability of graph metrics of resting state MRI functional brain networks: A review. *Journal of Neuroscience Methods*, 253, 183–192. https://doi.org/10.1016/j.jneumeth.2015.05.020

Azeez, A. K., & Biswal, B. B. (2017). A review of resting-state analysis methods. *Neuroimaging Clinics of North America*, 27(4), 581–592. https://doi.org/10.1016/j.nic.2017.06.001

Baumgartner, T., Heinrichs, M., Vonlanthen, A., Fischbacher, U., & Fehr, E. (2008). Oxytocin shapes the neural circuitry of trust and trust adaptation in humans. *Neuron*, 58(4), 639–650. https://doi.org/10.1016/j.neuron.2008.04.009

Beaty, R. E., Kenett, Y. N., Christensen, A. P., et al. (2018). Robust prediction of individual creative ability from brain functional connectivity. *Proceedings of the National Academy of Sciences*, 115(5), 1087–1092. https://doi.org/10.1073/pnas.1713532115

Belfi, A. M., Koscik, T. R., & Tranel, D. (2015). Damage to the insula is associated with abnormal interpersonal trust. *Neuropsychologia*, 71, 165–172. https://doi.org/10.1016/j.neuropsychologia.2015.04.003

Bellucci, G., Chernyak, S. V., Goodyear, K., Eickhoff, S. B., & Krueger, F. (2017). Neural signatures of trust in reciprocity: A coordinate-based meta-analysis. *Human Brain Mapping*, 38(3), 1233–1248. https://doi.org/10.1002/hbm.23451

Bellucci, G., Feng, C., Camilleri, J., Eickhoff, S. B., & Krueger, F. (2018). The role of the anterior insula in social norm compliance and enforcement: Evidence from coordinate-based and functional connectivity meta-analyses. *Neuroscience & Biobehavioral Reviews*, 92, 378–389. https://doi.org/10.1016/j.neubiorev.2018.06.024

Bellucci, G., Hahn, T., Deshpande, G., & Krueger, F. (2019). Functional connectivity of specific resting-state networks predicts trust and reciprocity in the trust game. *Cognitive, Affective & Behavioral Neuroscience*, 19(1), 165–176. https://doi.org/10.3758/s13415-018-00654-3

Bellucci, G., Molter, F., & Park, S. Q. (2019). Neural representations of honesty predict future trust behavior. *Nature Communications*, 10(1), Article 5184. https://doi.org/10.1038/s41467-019-13261-8

Berg, J., Dickhaut, J., & McCabe, K. (1995). Trust, reciprocity, and social history. *Games and Economic Behavior*, 10(1), 122–142. https://doi.org/10.1006/game.1995.1027

Biswal, B., Zerrin Yetkin, F., Haughton, V. M., & Hyde, J. S. (1995). Functional connectivity in the motor cortex of resting human brain using echo-planar MRI. *Magnetic Resonance in Medicine*, 34(4), 537–541. https://doi.org/10.1002/mrm.1910340409

Bohnet, I., Greig, F., Herrmann, B., & Zeckhauser, R. (2008). Betrayal aversion: Evidence from Brazil, China, Oman, Switzerland, Turkey, and the United States. *American Economic Review*, 98(1), 294–310. https://doi.org/10.1257/aer.98.1.294

Bohnet, I., & Zeckhauser, R. (2004). Trust, risk and betrayal. *Journal of Economic Behavior & Organization*, 55(4), 467–484. https://doi.org/10.1016/j.jebo.2003.11.004

Boksem, M. A. S., Mehta, P. H., Van den Bergh, B., et al. (2013). Testosterone inhibits trust but promotes reciprocity. *Psychological Science*, 24(11), 2306–2314. https://doi.org/10.1177/0956797613495063

Bos, P. A., Terburg, D., & Van Honk, J. (2010). Testosterone decreases trust in socially naive humans. *Proceedings of the National Academy of Sciences*, 107(22), 9991–9995. https://doi.org/10.1073/pnas.0911700107

Bressler, S. L., & Menon, V. (2010). Large-scale brain networks in cognition: Emerging methods and principles. *Trends in Cognitive Sciences*, 14(6), 277–290. https://doi.org/10.1016/j.tics.2010.04.004

Bush, K., & Cisler, J. (2013). Decoding neural events from fMRI BOLD signal: A comparison of existing approaches and development of a new algorithm. *Magnetic Resonance Imaging*, 31(6), 976–989. https://doi.org/10.1016/j.mri.2013.03.015

Button, K. S., Ioannidis, J. P. A., Mokrysz, C., et al. (2013). Power failure: Why small sample size undermines the reliability of neuroscience. *Nature Reviews Neuroscience*, 14(5), 365–376. https://doi.org/10.1038/nrn3475

Camerer, C., & Weigelt, K. (1988). Experimental tests of a sequential equilibrium reputation model. *Econometrica*, 56(1), 1–36. https://doi.org/10.2307/1911840

Cole, D. M., Smith, S. M., & Beckmann, C. F. (2010). Advances and pitfalls in the analysis and interpretation of resting-state fMRI data. *Frontiers in Systems Neuroscience*, 4(8), 1–8. https://doi.org/10.3389/fnsys.2010.00008

Cole, M. W., Ito, T., Bassett, D. S., & Schultz, D. H. (2016). Activity flow over resting-state networks shapes cognitive task activations. *Nature Neuroscience*, 19(12), 1718–1726. https://doi.org/10.1038/nn.4406

Crawford, J. R., & Garthwaite, P. H. (2008). On the "optimal" size for normative samples in neuropsychology: Capturing the uncertainty when normative data are used to quantify the standing of a neuropsychological test score.

Child Neuropsychology, 14(2), 99–117. https://doi.org/10.1080/09297040801894709

Cuthbert, B. N., & Insel, T. R. (2013). Toward the future of psychiatric diagnosis: The seven pillars of RDoC. *BMC Medicine*, 11(1), Article 126. https://doi.org/10.1186/1741-7015-11-126

Damoiseaux, J. S., Rombouts, S. A. R. B., Barkhof, F., et al. (2006). Consistent resting-state networks across healthy subjects. *Proceedings of the National Academy of Sciences*, 103(37), 13848–13853. https://doi.org/10.1073/pnas.0601417103

Delgado, M. R., Frank, R. H., & Phelps, E. A. (2005). Perceptions of moral character modulate the neural systems of reward during the trust game. *Nature Neuroscience*, 8(11), 1611–1618. https://doi.org/10.1038/nn1575

Dosenbach, N. U. F., Nardos, B., Cohen, A. L., et al. (2010). Prediction of individual brain maturity using fMRI. *Science*, 329(5997), 1358–1361. https://doi.org/10.1126/science.1194144

Dubois, J., & Adolphs, R. (2016). Building a science of individual differences from fMRI. *Trends in Cognitive Sciences*, 20(6), 425–443. https://doi.org/10.1016/j.tics.2016.03.014

Dubois, J., Galdi, P., Han, Y., Paul, L. K., & Adolphs, R. (2018). Resting-state functional brain connectivity best predicts the personality dimension of openness to experience. *Personality Neuroscience*, 1, Article e6. https://doi.org/10.1017/pen.2018.8

Durnez, J., Blair, R., & Poldrack, R. A. (2017). Neurodesign: Optimal experimental designs for task fMRI [Preprint]. *Neuroscience*. https://doi.org/10.1101/119594

Eckel, C. C., & Wilson, R. K. (2004). Is trust a risky decision? *Journal of Economic Behavior & Organization*, 55(4), 447–465. https://doi.org/10.1016/j.jebo.2003.11.003

Engelmann, J. B., Meyer, F., Ruff, C. C., & Fehr, E. (2019). The neural circuitry of affect-induced distortions of trust. *Science Advances*, 5(3), Article eaau3413. https://doi.org/10.1126/sciadv.aau3413

Fareri, D. S., Chang, L. J., & Delgado, M. R. (2012). Effects of direct social experience on trust decisions and neural reward circuitry. *Frontiers in Neuroscience*, 6, Article 148. https://doi.org/10.3389/fnins.2012.00148

Fehr, E. (2009). On the economics and biology of trust. *Journal of the European Economic Association*, 7(2–3), 235–266. https://doi.org/10.1162/JEEA.2009.7.2-3.235

Feng, C., Zhu, Z., Cui, Z., et al. (2020). Prediction of trust propensity from intrinsic brain morphology and functional connectome. *Human Brain Mapping*, Article hbm.25215. https://doi.org/10.1002/hbm.25215

Feng, C., Zhu, Z., Gu, R., Wu, X., Luo, Y.-J., & Krueger, F. (2018). Resting-state functional connectivity underlying costly punishment: A machine-learning approach. *Neuroscience*, 385, 25–37. https://doi.org/10.1016/j.neuroscience.2018.05.052

Fett, A.-K. J., Shergill, S. S., Gromann, P. M., et al. (2014). Trust and social reciprocity in adolescence: A matter of perspective-taking. *Journal of Adolescence*, 37(2), 175–184. https://doi.org/10.1016/j.adolescence.2013.11.011

Fett, A.-K. J., Shergill, S. S., Joyce, D. W., et al. (2012). To trust or not to trust: The dynamics of social interaction in psychosis. *Brain*, 135(3), 976–984. https://doi.org/10.1093/brain/awr359

Finn, E. S., Scheinost, D., Finn, D. M., Shen, X., Papademetris, X., & Constable, R. T. (2017). Can brain state be manipulated to emphasize individual differences in functional connectivity? *NeuroImage*, 160, 140–151. https://doi.org/10.1016/j.neuroimage.2017.03.064

Fouragnan, E., Chierchia, G., Greiner, S., Neveu, R., Avesani, P., & Coricelli, G. (2013). Reputational priors magnify striatal responses to violations of trust. *The Journal of Neuroscience*, 33(8), Article 3602. https://doi.org/10.1523/JNEUROSCI.3086-12.2013

Fox, M. D., & Raichle, M. E. (2007). Spontaneous fluctuations in brain activity observed with functional magnetic resonance imaging. *Nature Reviews Neuroscience*, 8(9), 700–711. https://doi.org/10.1038/nrn2201

Friston, K. J., Frith, C. D., Turner, R., & Frackowiak, R. S. J. (1995). Characterizing evoked hemodynamics with fMRI. *NeuroImage*, 2(2), 157–165. https://doi.org/10.1006/nimg.1995.1018

Friston, K. J., Li, B., Daunizeau, J., & Stephan, K. E. (2011). Network discovery with DCM. *NeuroImage*, 56(3), 1202–1221. https://doi.org/10.1016/j.neuroimage.2010.12.039

Fu, C., Yao, X., Yang, X., Zheng, L., Li, J., & Wang, Y. (2019). Trust game database: Behavioral and EEG data from two trust games. *Frontiers in Psychology*, 10, Article 2656. https://doi.org/10.3389/fpsyg.2019.02656

Gabrieli, J. D. E., Ghosh, S. S., & Whitfield-Gabrieli, S. (2015). Prediction as a humanitarian and pragmatic contribution from human cognitive neuroscience. *Neuron*, 85(1), 11–26. https://doi.org/10.1016/j.neuron.2014.10.047

Gallagher, H. L., & Frith, C. D. (2003). Functional imaging of "theory of mind." *Trends in Cognitive Sciences*, 7(2), 77–83. https://doi.org/10.1016/S1364-6613(02)00025-6

Greene, A. S., Gao, S., Scheinost, D., & Constable, R. T. (2018). Task-induced brain state manipulation improves prediction of individual traits. *Nature Communications*, 9(1), Article 2807. https://doi.org/10.1038/s41467-018-04920-3

Hahn, T., Notebaert, K., Anderl, C., Reicherts, P., et al. (2015). Reliance on functional resting-state network for stable task control predicts behavioral tendency for cooperation. *NeuroImage*, 118, 231–236. https://doi.org/10.1016/j.neuroimage.2015.05.093

Hahn, T., Notebaert, K., Anderl, C., Teckentrup, V., Kaßecker, A., & Windmann, S. (2015). How to trust a perfect stranger: Predicting initial trust behavior from resting-state brain-electrical connectivity. *Social*

Cognitive and Affective Neuroscience, 10(6), 809–813. https://doi.org/10.1093/scan/nsu122

Haxby, J. V. (2012). Multivariate pattern analysis of fMRI: The early beginnings. *NeuroImage*, 62(2), 852–855. https://doi.org/10.1016/j.neuroimage.2012.03.016

Heine, L., Soddu, A., Gómez, F., et al. (2012). Resting state networks and consciousness. *Frontiers in Psychology*, 3, Article 295. https://doi.org/10.3389/fpsyg.2012.00295

Hollerman, J. R., & Schultz, W. (1998). Dopamine neurons report an error in the temporal prediction of reward during learning. *Nature Neuroscience*, 1(4), 304–309. https://doi.org/10.1038/1124

Hsu, W.-T., Rosenberg, M. D., Scheinost, D., Constable, R. T., & Chun, M. M. (2018). Resting-state functional connectivity predicts neuroticism and extraversion in novel individuals. *Social Cognitive and Affective Neuroscience*, 13(2), 224–232. https://doi.org/10.1093/scan/nsy002

Hughes, B. L., Ambady, N., & Zaki, J. (2017). Trusting outgroup, but not ingroup members, requires control: Neural and behavioral evidence. *Social Cognitive and Affective Neuroscience*, 12(3), 372–381. https://doi.org/10.1093/scan/nsw139

Joel, D., Niv, Y., & Ruppin, E. (2002). Actor–critic models of the basal ganglia: New anatomical and computational perspectives. *Neural Networks*, 15(4–6), 535–547. https://doi.org/10.1016/S0893-6080(02)00047-3

Johnson, N. D., & Mislin, A. A. (2011). Trust games: A meta-analysis. *Journal of Economic Psychology*, 32(5), 865–889. https://doi.org/10.1016/j.joep.2011.05.007

King-Casas, B., Sharp, C., Lomax-Bream, L., Lohrenz, T., Fonagy, P., & Montague, P. R. (2008). The rupture and repair of cooperation in borderline personality disorder. *Science*, 321(5890), 806–810. https://doi.org/10.1126/science.1156902

King-Casas, B., Tomlin, D., Anen, C., Camerer, C. F., Quartz, S. R., & Read Montague, P. (2005). Getting to know you: Reputation and trust in a two-person economic exchange. *Science*, 308(5718), 78–83. https://doi.org/10.1126/science.1108062

Koscik, T. R., & Tranel, D. (2011). The human amygdala is necessary for developing and expressing normal interpersonal trust. *Neuropsychologia*, 49(4), 602–611. https://doi.org/10.1016/j.neuropsychologia.2010.09.023

Kosfeld, M., Heinrichs, M., Zak, P. J., Fischbacher, U., & Fehr, E. (2005). Oxytocin increases trust in humans. *Nature*, 435(7042), 673–676. https://doi.org/10.1038/nature03701

Krueger, F., McCabe, K., Moll, J., et al. (2007). Neural correlates of trust. *Proceedings of the National Academy of Sciences*, 104(50), 20084–20089. https://doi.org/10.1073/pnas.0710103104

Krueger, F., & Meyer-Lindenberg, A. (2019). Toward a model of interpersonal trust drawn from neuroscience, psychology, and economics. *Trends in Neurosciences*, 42(2), 92–101. https://doi.org/10.1016/j.tins.2018.10.004

Lee, M. H., Smyser, C. D., & Shimony, J. S. (2013). Resting-state fMRI: A review of methods and clinical applications. *American Journal of Neuroradiology*, 34(10), 1866–1872. https://doi.org/10.3174/ajnr.A3263

Lemmers-Jansen, I. L. J., Fett, A.-K. J., Hanssen, E., Veltman, D. J., & Krabbendam, L. (2019). Learning to trust: Social feedback normalizes trust behavior in first-episode psychosis and clinical high risk. *Psychological Medicine*, 49(5), 780–790. https://doi.org/10.1017/S003329171800140X

Li, N., Ma, N., Liu, Y., et al. (2013). Resting-state functional connectivity predicts impulsivity in economic decision-making. *Journal of Neuroscience*, 33(11), 4886–4895. https://doi.org/10.1523/JNEUROSCI.1342-12.2013

Linden, D. E. J. (2012). The challenges and promise of neuroimaging in psychiatry. *Neuron*, 73(1), 8–22. https://doi.org/10.1016/j.neuron.2011.12.014

Lo, A., Chernoff, H., Zheng, T., & Lo, S.-H. (2015). Why significant variables aren't automatically good predictors. *Proceedings of the National Academy of Sciences*, 112(45), 13892–13897. https://doi.org/10.1073/pnas.1518285112

Logothetis, N. K. (2008). What we can do and what we cannot do with fMRI. *Nature*, 453(7197), 869–878. https://doi.org/10.1038/nature06976

Lu, X., Li, T., Xia, Z., et al. (2019). Connectome-based model predicts individual differences in propensity to trust. *Human Brain Mapping*, 40(6), 1942–1954. https://doi.org/10.1002/hbm.24503

Montague, P. (2002). Hyperscanning: Simultaneous fMRI during linked social interactions. *NeuroImage*, 16(4), 1159–1164. https://doi.org/10.1006/nimg.2002.1150

Moretto, G., Sellitto, M., & di Pellegrino, G. (2013). Investment and repayment in a trust game after ventromedial prefrontal damage. *Frontiers in Human Neuroscience*, 7, Article 593. https://doi.org/10.3389/fnhum.2013.00593

Mwansisya, T. E., Hu, A., Li, Y., et al. (2017). Task and resting-state fMRI studies in first-episode schizophrenia: A systematic review. *Schizophrenia Research*, 189, 9–18. https://doi.org/10.1016/j.schres.2017.02.026

Nave, G., Camerer, C., & McCullough, M. (2015). Does oxytocin increase trust in humans? A critical review of research. *Perspectives on Psychological Science*, 10(6), 772–789. https://doi.org/10.1177/1745691615600138

Nostro, A. D., Müller, V. I., Varikuti, D. P., et al. (2018). Predicting personality from network-based resting-state functional connectivity. *Brain Structure and Function*, 223(6), 2699–2719. https://doi.org/10.1007/s00429-018-1651-z

O'Doherty, J., Dayan, P., Schultz, J., Deichmann, R., Friston, K., & Dolan, R. J. (2004). Dissociable roles of ventral and dorsal striatum in instrumental conditioning. *Science*, 304(5669), 452–454. https://doi.org/10.1126/science.1094285

Ogawa, S., Tank, D. W., Menon, R., et al. (1992). Intrinsic signal changes accompanying sensory stimulation: Functional brain mapping with magnetic resonance imaging. *Proceedings of the National Academy of Sciences*, 89(13), 5951–5955. https://doi.org/10.1073/pnas.89.13.5951

O'Reilly, J. X., Woolrich, M. W., Behrens, T. E. J., Smith, S. M., & Johansen-Berg, H. (2012). Tools of the trade: Psychophysiological interactions and functional connectivity. *Social Cognitive and Affective Neuroscience*, 7(5), 604–609. https://doi.org/10.1093/scan/nss055

Orrù, G., Pettersson-Yeo, W., Marquand, A. F., Sartori, G., & Mechelli, A. (2012). Using Support Vector Machine to identify imaging biomarkers of neurological and psychiatric disease: A critical review. *Neuroscience & Biobehavioral Reviews*, 36(4), 1140–1152. https://doi.org/10.1016/j.neubiorev.2012.01.004

Patanaik, A., Tandi, J., Ong, J. L., Wang, C., Zhou, J., & Chee, M. W. L. (2018). Dynamic functional connectivity and its behavioral correlates beyond vigilance. *NeuroImage*, 177, 1–10. https://doi.org/10.1016/j.neuroimage.2018.04.049

Patriat, R., Molloy, E. K., Meier, T. B., et al. (2013). The effect of resting condition on resting-state fMRI reliability and consistency: A comparison between resting with eyes open, closed, and fixated. *NeuroImage*, 78, 463–473. https://doi.org/10.1016/j.neuroimage.2013.04.013

Petersen, S. E., & Dubis, J. W. (2011). The mixed block/event design. *NeuroImage*, 62(2), 1177–1184. https://doi.org/10.1016/j.neuroimage.2011.09.084

Plitt, M., Barnes, K. A., Wallace, G. L., Kenworthy, L., & Martin, A. (2015). Resting-state functional connectivity predicts longitudinal change in autistic traits and adaptive functioning in autism. *Proceedings of the National Academy of Sciences*, 112(48), E6699–E6706. https://doi.org/10.1073/pnas.1510098112

Power, J. D., Cohen, A. L., Nelson, S. M., et al. (2011). Functional network organization of the human brain. *Neuron*, 72(4), 665–678. https://doi.org/10.1016/j.neuron.2011.09.006

Raichle, M. E., & Snyder, A. Z. (2007). A default mode of brain function: A brief history of an evolving idea. *NeuroImage*, 37(4), 1083–1090. https://doi.org/10.1016/j.neuroimage.2007.02.041

Reggente, N., Moody, T. D., Morfini, F., et al. (2018). Multivariate resting-state functional connectivity predicts response to cognitive behavioral therapy in obsessive–compulsive disorder. *Proceedings of the National Academy of Sciences*, 115(9), 2222–2227. https://doi.org/10.1073/pnas.1716686115

Riedl, R., & Javor, A. (2012). The biology of trust: Integrating evidence from genetics, endocrinology, and functional brain imaging. *Journal of Neuroscience, Psychology, and Economics*, 5(2), 63–91. https://doi.org/10.1037/a0026318

Rilling, J. K., & Sanfey, A. G. (2011). The neuroscience of social decision making. *Annual Review of Psychology*, 62(1), 23–48. https://doi.org/10.1146/annurev.psych.121208.131647

Roebroeck, A., Formisano, E., & Goebel, R. (2005). Mapping directed influence over the brain using Granger causality and fMRI. *NeuroImage*, 25(1), 230–242. https://doi.org/10.1016/j.neuroimage.2004.11.017

Rosazza, C., & Minati, L. (2011). Resting-state brain networks: Literature review and clinical applications. *Neurological Sciences*, 32(5), 773–785. https://doi.org/10.1007/s10072-011-0636-y

Seppänen, R., Blomqvist, K., & Sundqvist, S. (2007). Measuring interorganizational trust: A critical review of the empirical research in 1990–2003. *Industrial Marketing Management*, 36(2), 249–265. https://doi.org/10.1016/j.indmarman.2005.09.003

Smitha, K., Akhil Raja, K., Arun, K., et al. (2017). Resting state fMRI: A review on methods in resting state connectivity analysis and resting state networks. *The Neuroradiology Journal*, 30(4), 305–317. https://doi.org/10.1177/1971400917697342

Sporns, O., Honey, C. J., & Kötter, R. (2007). Identification and classification of hubs in brain networks. *PLoS ONE*, 2(10), Article e1049. https://doi.org/10.1371/journal.pone.0001049

Spreng, R. N., Mar, R. A., & Kim, A. S. N. (2009). The common neural basis of autobiographical memory, prospection, navigation, theory of mind, and the default mode: A quantitative meta-analysis. *Journal of Cognitive Neuroscience*, 21(3), 489–510. https://doi.org/10.1162/jocn.2008.21029

Sun, H., Verbeke, W. J. M. I., Pozharliev, R., Bagozzi, R. P., Babiloni, F., & Wang, L. (2019). Framing a trust game as a power game greatly affects interbrain synchronicity between trustor and trustee. *Social Neuroscience*, 14(6), 635–648. https://doi.org/10.1080/17470919.2019.1566171

Tang, H., Lu, X., Cui, Z., et al. (2018). Resting-state functional connectivity and deception: Exploring individualized deceptive propensity by machine learning. *Neuroscience*, 395, 101–112. https://doi.org/10.1016/j.neuroscience.2018.10.036

Tavor, I., Jones, O. P., Mars, R. B., Smith, S. M., Behrens, T. E., & Jbabdi, S. (2016). Task-free MRI predicts individual differences in brain activity during task performance. *Science*, 352(6282), 216–220. https://doi.org/10.1126/science.aad8127

Tobyne, S. M., Somers, D. C., Brissenden, J. A., Michalka, S. W., Noyce, A. L., & Osher, D. E. (2018). Prediction of individualized task activation in sensory modality-selective frontal cortex with "connectome fingerprinting." *NeuroImage*, 183, 173–185. https://doi.org/10.1016/j.neuroimage.2018.08.007

Tomasi, D., & Volkow, N. D. (2010). Functional connectivity density mapping. *Proceedings of the National Academy of Sciences*, 107(21), 9885–9890. https://doi.org/10.1073/pnas.1001414107

Tomlin, D. (2006). Agent-specific responses in the cingulate cortex during economic exchanges. *Science*, 312(5776), 1047–1050. https://doi.org/10.1126/science.1125596

Tzieropoulos, H. (2013). The trust game in neuroscience: A short review. *Social Neuroscience*, 8(5), 407–416. https://doi.org/10.1080/17470919.2013.832375

Van den Heuvel, M. P., & Hulshoff Pol, H. E. (2010). Exploring the brain network: A review on resting-state fMRI functional connectivity. *European*

Neuropsychopharmacology, 20(8), 519–534. https://doi.org/10.1016/j
.euroneuro.2010.03.008

Van Honk, J., Eisenegger, C., Terburg, D., Stein, D. J., & Morgan, B. (2013).
Generous economic investments after basolateral amygdala damage.
Proceedings of the National Academy of Sciences, 110(7), 2506–2510.
https://doi.org/10.1073/pnas.1217316110

Van Overwalle, F. (2009). Social cognition and the brain: A meta-analysis.
Human Brain Mapping, 30(3), 829–858. https://doi.org/10.1002/hbm
.20547

Whelan, R., & Garavan, H. (2014). When optimism hurts: Inflated predictions
in psychiatric neuroimaging. *Biological Psychiatry,* 75(9), 746–748. https://
doi.org/10.1016/j.biopsych.2013.05.014

Wong, C. W., Olafsson, V., Tal, O., & Liu, T. T. (2012). Anti-correlated
networks, global signal regression, and the effects of caffeine in resting-
state functional MRI. *NeuroImage,* 63(1), 356–364. https://doi.org/10
.1016/j.neuroimage.2012.06.035

Worsley, K. J., & Friston, K. J. (1995). Analysis of fMRI time-series revisited –
again. *NeuroImage,* 2(3), 173–181. https://doi.org/10.1006/nimg.1995
.1023

Yanagisawa, K., Masui, K., Furutani, K., Nomura, M., Ura, M., & Yoshida, H.
(2011). Does higher general trust serve as a psychosocial buffer against social
pain? An NIRS study of social exclusion. *Social Neuroscience,* 6(2), 190–197.
https://doi.org/10.1080/17470919.2010.506139

Yarkoni, T., & Braver, T. S. (2010). Cognitive neuroscience approaches to
individual differences in working memory and executive control:
Conceptual and methodological issues. In A. Gruszka, G. Matthews, & B.
Szymura (Eds.), *Handbook of individual differences in cognition* (pp. 87–107).
Springer. https://doi.org/10.1007/978-1-4419-1210-7_6

Yarkoni, T., & Westfall, J. (2017). Choosing prediction over explanation in
psychology: Lessons from machine learning. *Perspectives on Psychological
Science,* 12(6), 1100–1122. https://doi.org/10.1177/1745691617693393

Zuo, X.-N., Kelly, C., Adelstein, J. S., Klein, D. F., Castellanos, F. X., &
Milham, M. P. (2010). Reliable intrinsic connectivity networks: Test–retest
evaluation using ICA and dual regression approach. *NeuroImage,* 49(3),
2163–2177. https://doi.org/10.1016/j.neuroimage.2009.10.080

PART IV

Neuromolecular Level of Trust

CHAPTER 13

Trust and Oxytocin
Context-Dependent Exogenous and Endogenous Modulation of Trust

Zhimin Yan and Peter Kirsch

13.1 Introduction

Oxytocin (OXT) is a rather ancient peptide hormone and neuropeptide, which has been found in many kinds of species ranging from invertebrates to mammals (Donaldson & Young, 2008). It has been traditionally associated with parturition and lactation (Dale, 1906; Ott & Scott, 1910). However, in the late twentieth century, increasing number of studies discovered the link between oxytocin and maternal behavior (Pedersen & Prange, 1979), as well as social bonds (see review [Kovács, 1986]). A seminal study by Kosfeld and colleagues in 2005 revealed exogenous OXT administration increases interpersonal trust between humans (Kosfeld et al., 2005), which initiated overwhelming interest and led to further studies investigating the administered OXT effects on social behaviors, especially trust. However, recent findings failed to disclose such a straightforward "trust-promoting" OXT effect (Declerck et al., 2020; Nave et al., 2015), challenging the role of OXT in trusting behavior.

This chapter provides a comprehensive review of studies on the connections between OXT and trust. We start with a short introduction of OXT and its exogenous administration and endogenous assessments. Then we review studies investigating the effects of both exogenous and endogenous OXT on trust, and also shed light on the emerging assumption of context-dependent social effects of OXT in the context of OXT – trust connection. Further, we discuss the OXT treatments that are implemented to alleviate deficits in interpersonal trust in mental disorders and the OXT effect on the neural correlates of trust. Finally, we discuss major limitations and confusions in studies exploring the OXT effects on trust.

Corresponding author: Peter Kirsch (peter.kirsch@zi-mannheim.de).

13.2   Oxytocin

OXT is a peptide hormone consisting of nine amino acids (Gimpl & Fahrenholz, 2001). It is synthesized along with its sister neuropeptide arginine vasopressin in the magnocellular and parvocellular neurons of the supraoptic, paraventricular, and accessory nuclei of the hypothalamus (Grinevich et al., 2016). OXT acts in both the peripheral and central nervous systems. In the peripheral nervous system, OXT is released by the posterior pituitary into blood circulation. It plays a crucial role as a hormone, facilitating uterine contractions during parturition and milk ejection during lactation (Keverne & Kendrick, 1992). In the central nervous system, OXT can act as a neurotransmitter as it is released from axon terminals of oxytocinergic neurons that project from the hypothalamus to the mesocorticolimbic system that is composed of a group of brain regions associated with social and emotional processing (Donaldson & Young, 2008; Knobloch et al., 2012). Accordingly, numerous mechanistic studies using optogenetics, viral vectors, etc. have demonstrated the effects of endogenous and exogenous OXT on the salience network (including the insula and amygdala), reward system (including nucleus accumbens [NAcc], ventral tegmental area [VTA], and orbitofrontal cortex [OFC]), and default mode network (such as medial prefrontal cortex; for details read Kendrick et al., 2017; Quintana et al., 2019).

In general, two approaches are widely used to evaluate OXT's effects on social cognition: exogenous OXT administration and the endogenous OXT system. Exogenous OXT through intranasal delivery is the most commonly used approach to directly manipulate the OXT level in the central nervous system with randomized double-blind placebo-controlled experimental designs (MacDonald et al., 2011), where causal effects of OXT on social behaviors can be examined (Campbell, 2010). Most of these studies were conducted with male participants only given the confound of the interaction between OXT and menstrual cycle stage on social behaviors (Salonia et al., 2005) as well as the risk of exogenous OXT causing uterine contractions in women.

The endogenous OXT system can be probed through measuring OXT peripherally (plasma, urine, saliva) or centrally (cerebrospinal fluid or postmortem brain samples). OXT concentrations then can be correlated with behavioral and imaging measures (McCullough et al., 2013), but this fails to establish causality (Nave et al., 2015). Further, given that social behaviors are centrally mediated, peripheral measurement of OXT is of questionable value as a marker of central OXT signaling, as it is still unclear how these two domains of OXT coordinate or interact with each other (Valstad et al., 2017).

Additionally, genetic approaches have also been leveraged to probe the function of the endogenous OXT system. For example, models of OXT or OXT receptor gene knockout have been used to investigate the OXT effect on social behaviors (DeVries et al, 1997) (see also Chapter 15). In human research, mainly single-nucleotide polymorphisms (SNPs) in the gene coding for the oxytocin receptors (OXTR) and other genes related to the OXT system have been employed to test the correlations of the genetic variability with differences in social behaviors (Nave et al., 2015; Quintana et al., 2019). The merit of a genetic approach is that it can directly detect the relations between OXT and behaviors from the perspective of genetics (Kumsta & Heinrichs, 2013). However, resembling the approach assessing the peripheral OXT, the genetic approach applied to human research enables merely associations of OXTR and social processes to be revealed (Kumsta & Heinrichs, 2013; Nave et al., 2015).

13.3   Oxytocin and Trust

Research on trust has attracted many scholars working in different academic fields. In the current chapter, we define trust as an internal mental state in which one appraises another as "trustworthy," such that one will make oneself vulnerable to the uncertainty of another's response (Nave et al., 2015; Watson, 2005). This indicates that trust involves two domains: intention to trust others and trusting behavior. The intention to trust is the result of a series of implicit cognitive processes including the individual's trust trait / propensity to trust and trustworthiness perception, whereas the trusting behavior is presented in an explicit manner that is observable and measurable. Accordingly, the connection between OXT and trust will be elaborated from the trusting intention and trusting behavior respectively in Section 13.3.1.

13.3.1   Oxytocin and Trusting Behavior

Previous studies conducted a series of well-designed experimental paradigms to measure trusting behavior (Watson, 2005). The trust game (TG) is the most common one, which was developed by Camerer and Weigelt (1988) and simplified by Berg and colleagues (1995) (see Chapter 2 for details). The game can be played with the subject assuming one or both roles: investor and trustee. The amount of investment from the investor is a measure of trusting behavior, and the amount of money returned to the investor from the trustee is an indicator of trustworthiness. It can be played as series of single moves with different partners on each trial or with same partners throughout the game where the reputation of partners' trustworthiness could be considered as an additional variable influencing trusting behavior.

13.3.1.1   Exogenous OXT Administration and Trusting Behavior

The TG was applied in the seminal study of Kosfeld and colleagues (Kosfeld et al., 2005) using a double-blind, between-subjects, placebo-controlled design. Intranasal OXT compared to placebo administered before playing the TG increased the amount of money transferred from the investor to the trustee. The control task in this study was a risk game where the subjects invested into a project instead of a trustee compared to the TG and OXT did not affect investors' transfer levels compared to placebo. Since the TG used in this study was the single mover version, one potential conclusion from this study was that OXT could promote "blind trust." However, this assumption was not completely supported by the subsequent studies using intranasal OXT administration with the trust task (Barraza et al., 2011; Baumgartner et al., 2008; Klackl et al., 2013).

Baumgartner and colleagues (Baumgartner et al., 2008) further examined if the OXT administration could diminish mistrust under the context of others' betrayal. They inserted a feedback screen into the middle of the TG informing the subjects that only 50% of their investment would yield a return from the trustees. Although they failed to contribute to replicate the general "trust-promoting" effect of OXT during the prefeedback session, their results showed the OXT group maintaining their trusting behavior in comparison to the placebo group in the postfeedback session. These findings suggest an OXT effect on trust adaptation, which reinforced the idea that OXT might counteract the trust-inhibiting force of betrayal aversion (Bohnet & Zeckhauser, 2004), but the finding could not be replicated by a subsequent study using the same experimental design (Klackl et al., 2013). Further, a critical review of six studies using the TG with intranasal OXT delivery concluded that no significant "trust-promoting" effect of OXT was found (Nave et al., 2015).

Very recently, a research group led by Ernst Fehr, the senior author of the Kosfeld et al. study, reported results of a registered replication study (Declerck et al., 2020) that used the same task as their previous study (Kosfeld et al., 2005). In this follow-up study, no significant effect of OXT on trusting behavior was found for the entire sample of 677 participants with more than 95% statistical power. However, in an exploratory post-hoc analysis, splitting the sample into participants with high versus low trait trust, the OXT effect to augment trust behavior was statistically significant for the group with a low disposition to trust other people. Therefore, these results further support the assumption that OXT cannot promote "blind trust" but may work on trusting behavior modulated by individual factors, such as personalality traits.

In addition to the TG, Mikolajczak and colleagues established a so-called envelope task to examine if OXT promotes one's trust concerning personal confidential information (Mikolajczak, Pinon, et al., 2010). Subjects in this task were required to complete a survey concerning questions about their sexual practices and fantasies. Before the survey, they were informed that all their data will be coded pseudonymously and read via a recognition device rather than by the experimenters. After completing the survey, participants were asked to place the form into an envelope and then decide whether they wanted to seal it or even use sticky tape to cover their answers before they were read by a device. Compared to the participants in the placebo group, those in the OXT group sealed the envelope significantly less frequently, supporting the "trust-promoting" effect of OXT (Mikolajczak, Pinon, et al., 2010). This study, however, did not use a double-blind approach to manipulate intranasal OXT administration. In their later replication study using a randomized double-blind placebo-controlled approach, the "trust-promoting" effect of OXT was not reproduced (Lane et al., 2015).

13.3.1.2 Endogenous OXT System and Trusting Behavior

Studies correlating peripheral OXT levels with trusting behavior also revealed inconsistent results. A study by Zak and colleagues was the first to report the associations of peripheral OXT and trusting behavior (Zak et al., 2005). They applied the TG to a small-scale sample and found a significant positive correlation between the peripheral OXT level and the trusting behavior. However, these findings could not be replicated by Zhong and colleagues with a rather larger sample size (Zhong et al., 2012). Instead, Zhong and colleagues revealed a U-shaped relation between the peripheral OXT concentration and trusting behavior where individuals with higher or lower levels of OXT performed more trusting behaviors in comparison to those with intermediate OXT levels. Another study used a prisoners' dilemma game and was not able to find any significant associations between peripheral OXT level and trusting behavior (Christensen et al., 2014).

Genetic association studies (see also Chapter 15) that correlated the OXTR SNPs with trusting behavior were also subject to inconsistent conclusions. Krueger and colleagues (Krueger et al., 2012) used a candidate gene approach to investigate the effect of OXT on trust task behavior in healthy male Caucasian participants. They discovered a positive association of a common variation (OXTR rs53576) with trusting behavior. This finding was reproduced by a study by Nishina and colleagues in a Japanese male sample, but not in Japanese female participants (Nishina et al., 2015). This might be one reason for other studies failing to replicate the associations between OXRT SNPs and trusting behavior combining both sexes for their analyses (Apicella et al., 2010; Bakermans-Kranenburg & Van IJzendoorn, 2014; Tabak et al., 2014). Unfortunately, the validity of these genetic association studies suffers from low statistical power. Benjamin and colleagues found that different genetic variations of the OXTR account for a substantial proportion of the variability in many economic behaviors (including trusting behavior), but they also pointed out that the effect sizes of these findings were dramatically small (Benjamin et al., 2012). Thus, interpretation of the results of studies with a genetic association approach has to be made with caution.

Taken together, these studies on the association between the endogenous OXT system and trusting behavior yield inconsistent results and suffer from lack of replication.

13.3.2 Oxytocin and Intention to Trust

Most studies researching the relationship between OXT and intention to trust conducted the exogenous OXT administration approach. To study the appraisal of trustworthiness, Theodoridou and colleagues (Theodoridou et al., 2009) conducted a double-blind placebo-controlled study and utilized a trustworthiness rating task in which participants were required to rate the trustworthiness of a series of neutral facial expressions. Participants in the OXT group rated neutral expressions as more trustworthy than those in the placebo group. With the same experimental design, another study (Lambert et al., 2014) applied a trustworthiness judgment task with a series of artificially generated neutral faces and failed to replicate the intranasal OXT effect on trustworthiness perception. However, with their second task of this study that required subjects to judge the trustworthiness of artificial faces manipulated by changes in trustworthiness while comparing with natural neutral faces, they found the OXT group performed more accurately at recognizing untrustworthy faces. Although the findings of these two studies indicated that OXT might influence the perception of trustworthiness, some more recent studies using trustworthiness ratings failed to replicate these effects of OXT on the perception of trustworthiness (Grainger et al., 2019; Quintana et al., 2015; Teed et al., 2019; Woolley et al., 2017).

In addition, a few studies also investigated the intranasal OXT effect on responses to self-report questionnaires examining one's propensity to trust. They consistently reported that the administration of OXT increases the perception of one's own propensity to trust (Cardoso et al., 2012, 2013), which may indicate that an increased propensity to trust caused by the OXT administration moderates the OXT effect on trusting behavior.

Regarding the endogenous OXT system, only one study investigated the associations between OXTR SNPs and self-reported trust perception, but it failed to reveal any significant associations of self-reported trust with OXTR rs53576 or with Serravalle OXTR rs2268490 (Fang et al., 2020). Thus, it is still obscure if the endogenous OXT system exerts an influence on trust perception.

In short, previous findings investigating the effect of OXT on the intention to trust as well as on trusting behavior do not support the initial conclusion that OXT could promote "blind trust" (Kosfeld et al., 2005). Increasing evidence has pointed out that the social effects of OXT are not straightforward, but rely more on the social context and the features of social communicators (Bartz, Zaki, et al., 2011). In Section 13.4, we review the possible modulators of the "trust-promoting" OXT effect.

13.4 The Context-Dependent Oxytocin Effects on Trust

13.4.1 *Oxytocin and Trust in the Social Context*

As OXT can foster in-group favoritism leading to in-group altruism (Zhang, Gross, et al., 2019), social affiliation has been considered as one of the most influential factors modulating the OXT effects on trust. Social affiliation refers to a desire to interact and pleasure in being with others (McClelland, 1987), which may result in intergroup conflict by implicitly developing the bias of in-group favoritism and out-group derogation (Balliet et al., 2014). De Dreu and colleagues (De Dreu et al., 2010) applied an intergroup prisoners' dilemma game to male participants who were assigned to two three-person groups using a double-blind, between-subjects, placebo-controlled design. In comparison to the placebo group, more money was transferred to the in-group account than the out-group account in the OXT group. This finding was supported by a subsequent meta-analysis that evidenced that intranasal OXT administration can augment in-group trusting behavior (Van IJzendoorn & Bakermans-Kranenburg, 2012). A more recent study further suggested such in-group trusting behavior caused by OXT administration may be independent of cognitive control, seemingly to be intuitive instead of consciously deliberated (Ten Velden et al., 2017). Additionally, this OXT-induced in-group trusting behavior was also found under the context of ethnicity-based social affiliation (Kret & De Dreu, 2017).

Besides, prior social experience is another type of context that also modulates the effect of OXT on trusting behavior. Declerck and colleagues (Declerck et al., 2010) employed a coordination game and manipulated the personal contact prior to the task using a double-blind, between-subjects, placebo-controlled design. They found that OXT promoted trust-based cooperative behavior only in the personal contact group. In the absence of prior personal contact, OXT enhanced risk aversion and caution behavior by reducing trust-based cooperation. Moreover, prior social experience also affects the OXT effects on self-reported trust perception. In a double-blind placebo-controlled design, subjects were randomly assigned to either the OXT or placebo group, then were subject to a live social rejection paradigm followed by assessments of mood and self-reported trust (Cardoso et al., 2013). The results illustrated an interaction between mood and drug (oxytocin/placebo) on trust perception where OXT (compared to placebo) significantly increased self-reported trust perception only in the participants who suffered more negative moods after social rejection.

13.4.2   *Personal Features Modulating the Oxytocin–Trust Relation*

The effects of OXT administration on trust may be modulated by one's baseline trust level. Merolla and colleagues randomly assigned their subjects to receive intranasal OXT or placebo administration to explore the OXT effects on trustworthiness in the context of political systems (Merolla et al., 2013). They applied a series of questionnaires in terms of interpersonal trust and political figures and actions before and after drug treatments. They disclosed an obvious OXT effect on improving political trustworthiness perception in participants with lower-level initial interpersonal trust. This is consistent with the recent exploratory finding of Declerk and colleagues that the trust-enhancing effect of OXT can only be observed in participants with lower trait trust (Declerck et al., 2020).

Exogenous OXT may also have different effects on trusting behavior varying between males and females. In a double-blind, between-subjects, placebo-controlled design study, Yao and colleagues investigated the OXT administration effect on modulating trust restoration in a TG where all participants suffered unfair treatments by the other four virtual players during the first-round game and underwent four types of repair strategies (financial compensation, apologies, fair, and nothing) sent by virtual players before the second-round game (Yao et al., 2014). The results displayed that only female participants performed less trusting behavior in the second-round game under OXT compared to placebo administration, especially in the context of attempted trust repair using financial compensation. This modulatory effect of gender on the trust-promoting OXT effect was also reported in a study assessing the endogenous OXT system. Nishina and colleagues investigated the associations among OXTR rs53576, attitudinal trust, and trusting behavior and revealed GG carriers of rs53576 performing more trusting behavior and reporting higher attitudinal scores than AA carriers only in men, but not in women (Nishina et al., 2015). They further revealed that the OXTR genotype affects trusting behavior in men through the general attitudinal trust.

13.4.3 Features of the Trustees Modulating the Oxytocin–Trust Relation

Previous studies suggested the features of the trustee also modulate the OXT administration effect on trusting behavior. First, Mikolajczak and colleagues (Mikolajczak, Gross, et al., 2010) administered either intranasal OXT or a placebo to their participants and conducted a modified TG in which they manipulated the trustees' trustworthiness/reliability. Their results showed that subjects in the OXT group tended to transfer more money to the reliable trustees, emphasizing that the trustees' features matter while discussing the trust-promoting effects of OXT. This conclusion has been supported and extended by a subsequent study of de Visser and colleagues (de Visser et al., 2017). In this randomized double-blind placebo-controlled study, de Visser and colleagues found the reliability of trustees modulates the effects of OXT on trusting behavior regardless of the trustee being human or nonhuman. Moreover, the trustees' gender may influence the OXT effects on trusting behavior as well. Luo and colleagues (Luo et al., 2017) manipulated the trustees' trustworthiness and gender in a decision-making task in which intranasal OXT and placebo were administered randomly. Their findings demonstrated that people in the OXT group preferred to accept social advice given by trusted female but not male advisors, indicating an interaction between the individual trustworthiness and gender of the trustee modulates the promoting OXT effect on trusting behavior.

Taken together, the considerable findings of previous studies have demonstrated that the effect of OXT administration on trust is not straightforward, but context-dependent. Specifically, it may be modulated by social context and the features of participants (including investors and trustees). These findings refine our understanding of in whom and when OXT affects trusting behavior, which further underlines OXT as a putative treatment for neuropsychiatric disorders, including mood disorders, substance use disorders, and psychotic disorders.

13.5   Oxytocin and Trust in the Context of Mental Disorders

The most-investigated disorder in the context of the effect of OXT treatment on social cognitive function is autism spectrum disorder (ASD), which is marked by deficits in social interaction and communication, aberrant social function, and repetitive behaviors (Lord, Cook, Leventhal, & Amaral, 2000). Since previous evidence suggested negative associations of ASD with plasma OXT (Green et al., 2001; Modahl et al., 1998), as well as with OXTR SNPs (e.g., rs7632287, rs237887, rs2268491, and rs2254298 (LoParo & Waldman, 2015), the OXT administration effects on social cognition have been widely investigated in ASD (Ooi et al., 2017). Only one of these studies tested the effects of OXT on trusting behavior in patients with ASD. Andari and colleagues administrated intranasal OXT or placebo to highly functioning participants with ASD in a crossover within-subject design (Andari et al., 2010). In this design, they used a modified Cyberball game that manipulated the trustworthiness level of the simulated co-players by defining different probabilities of reciprocation. They found that patients with ASD showed more trusting behavior (ball tosses) to the most trustworthy player compared to the untrustworthy player under OXT administration. These findings highlighted a therapeutic potential of oxytocin on social-cognitive training for patients with ASD. However, a recent meta-analysis included seven studies that tested the effects of OXT on different domains of social cognition in ASD, which reported no significant effects of OXT on social cognition (Ooi et al., 2017). As limited studies were included in this meta-analysis, more OXT treatment studies in ASD are still needed.

Apart from ASD, other studies have examined the effect of OXT on trust in patients with borderline personality disorder (BPD). Interpersonal difficulties and impairments in evaluating others' trustworthiness are well documented for BPD patients (see for review Lazarus et al., 2014). Bartz and colleagues applied a social dilemma game to patients with BPD and healthy participants who received intranasal OXT or placebo treatments (Bartz, Simeon, et al., 2011). Under OXT, patients with BPD demonstrated less trusting behavior and a reduced likelihood of cooperative responses compared to healthy participants, which was modulated by the highly anxiously attached and rejection-sensitive participants. A subsequent study used a classic TG and replicated the trust-decreasing effects of OXT in patients with BPD and added the history of childhood trauma of the patients to be one of the possible modulators of such OXT effects in BPD (Ebert et al., 2013). These consistent findings in patients with BPD might suggest that OXT treatment probably is not a promising treatment to improve interpersonal trust in patients with BPD due to the features of disorganized attachment in BPD (Bartz, Simeon, et al., 2011).

Moreover, as OXT may allay positive symptoms and even alleviate the negative symptoms and the deficits in social cognition in schizophrenia (see for review Feifel, Shilling, & MacDonald, 2016), there is an increasing interest in administrating exogenous OXT for patients with schizophrenia to improve their social cognition level regardless of the state of the endogenous OXT system. However, no significant "trust-promoting" OXT effects were found in patients with schizophrenia. In a study by Wooley and colleagues, OXT did not promote trust in patients with schizophrenia who were required to complete a facial trustworthiness rating task after intranasal OXT administration (Woolley et al., 2017). Studies with long-term OXT administration did not demonstrate increased trusting behavior in individuals with schizophrenia either. In a double-blind crossover design, Pedersen and colleagues (Pedersen et al., 2011) manipulated the OXT and placebo administration twice per day for 14 days to test the long-term OXT administration effects on ratings of trustworthiness. As a result, they did not reveal any significant OXT effects on trust perception. Lee and colleagues implemented a three-week trial with OXT treatments and measured four domains of social cognition and social functioning and reported nonsignificant OXT effects on social cognition (Lee et al., 2019). These studies mentioned above examined the domain of trust perception in patients with schizophrenia; future studies would test the OXT effects on the trusting behavior by carrying out the various trust-related tasks and further discuss the possible modulators that might affect the OXT effects on trust in schizophrenia.

Finally, one study (Tauber et al., 2011) examined the "trust-promoting" OXT effects in patients with Prader-Willi syndrome, a genetic neurodevelopmental disorder affecting hypothalamic functioning including OXT-producing neurons of the paraventricular nucleus. Under OXT, the authors found increased self-reported trust scores in patients with Prader-Willi syndrome. Another study was conducted to explore the OXT effects on trust in patients with pain following OXT and placebo administration (Long & Freeman, 2019). Their findings suggested that OXT can not only reduce pain sensitivity in patients with pain but also can improve the trust ratings.

13.6   Oxytocin and the Neural Correlates of Trust

Considerable imaging studies have revealed a large-scale brain network associated with trust involving the reward system, the salience network, the default mode network as well as the central executive network (for more details see Krueger & Meyer-Lindenberg, 2019). These brain regions associated with trust highly overlap with the oxytocin pathway in the human brain, such as the subcortical and temporal brain structures, along with the olfactory region (Quintana et al., 2019), indicating possible effects of OXT on the neural correlates of trust.

As mentioned before, Baumgartner and colleagues (Baumgartner et al., 2008) used the TG with a response of the trustee reflecting a betrayal of trust in half of the trials and reported a lack of trust adaptation after the betrayal of trust under OXT but not under placebo. Using functional magnetic resonance imaging (fMRI), they found the absence of trust adaptation under OXT is associated with reduced activation of the amygdala, the midbrain regions, as well as the dorsal striatum (dSTR). The decreased activation in the amygdala and midbrain regions under OXT has been well documented (Kirsch et al., 2005; Sauer et al., 2019 and the dSTR activation is linked to feedback processing and reward learning (O'Doherty et al., 2004). Thus, the OXT effect on trusting behavior is probably interpreted as an interplay of fear processing and behavioral adaptations.

However, a subsequent study challenged the conclusion of Baumgartner et al. (2008). Ide and colleagues (Ide et al., 2018) conducted a TG during fMRI scans after applying intranasal OXT or placebo. They modeled the participants' performance during the task. Their results yielded an effect of OXT in terms of a reduction of feedback learning resulting in "unjustified distrust," which was associated with decreased connectivity of OFC with the amygdala and NAcc. Thus, the authors concluded that the "unjustified distrust" is probably attributed to the neural effects of OXT on attenuating social reward learning. Such a learning-attenuating effect of OXT requires more empirical replications.

In terms of the neural correlates of the intention to trust, a study applied a facial rating task in which participants were required to judge the trustworthiness and the dominance of a series of neutral faces during fMRI scans (Teed et al., 2019). On the behavioral level, they found no effect of OXT on trustworthiness ratings but an increased dominance rating under OXT administration. However, on the neural level, they found a positive association between the trustworthiness rating and the connectivity of the VTA with the fusiform gyrus and hippocampus. This result suggests a potential effect of OXT on the encoding of trustworthy faces facilitating familiarity and making them more memorable (Rimmele et al., 2009).

Also, a genetic imaging study investigated the role of amygdala volume in the association between OXTR rs53576 and attitudinal trust (Nishina et al., 2018). The results showed that the left amygdala volume mediated the association of rs53576 genotypes and attitudinal trust only in males. This extended the assumption to the neural level that there is a gender effect on the association between OXTR and trust (Kendrick et al., 2017).

Although limited studies explored the OXT effect on the neural correlates of trust, there is a consistency that OXT can influence the brain processes related to trust, mainly in regions associated with emotional processing and reward. However, additional research is needed to enlighten the neural basis of the associations between OXT and trust, especially in patients with mental disorders associated with reduced interpersonal trust.

13.7 Limitations and Future Studies

A large body of studies has drawn its attention to discussing the associations of OXT and trust in the past decade, leading to a fruitful achievement. However, there are still some limitations calling for future attention. First, the low reproducibility of certain landmark findings has become the biggest concern. For example, the initiated findings of the OXT effect on trust behavior (Kosfeld et al., 2005) and on rating trustworthiness (Krueger et al., 2012) partly failed to be replicated by subsequent studies. Since the effects of OXT on trust are probably context-dependent, future studies could focus more on exploring the variables mediating or moderating the associations between OXT and trust.

Besides, most of these studies have suffered from methodological weaknesses of assaying OXT, which could also contribute to the interpretation of the low reproducibility. For example, the administration of intranasal OXT is the most frequently implemented approach in investigating the effects of OXT on trust, but its usage in previous studies yields three limitations. First, most studies using intranasal OXT administration only recruited male participants, limiting the generalizability of the findings. Second, although two seminal papers by Lee and colleagues stressed that intranasal OXT administration can reach the cerebrospinal fluid and parts of brain regions in rhesus macaques (Lee et al., 2018, 2020), clear evidence that the OXT delivery actually reaches those brain targets involved in social cognition in humans is missing in previous studies (Nave et al., 2015). Third, a commonly used protocol of administering intranasal OXT is still missing, leading to variability between studies regarding the doses of intranasal OXT applied and the latency between the application and the test of its effect. A few studies endeavored to address this issue, but the results are mixed. Quintana and colleagues (Quintana et al., 2015) stated that a low dose of OXT (8 IU) could be more effective in reducing the perception of anger than a higher dose (24 IU), whereas a more recent study underlined the effectiveness of the administration of a 24 IU dose (Spengler et al., 2017). Thus, a gold standard of administering intranasal OXT is warranted for future studies.

Moreover, there has been an explosion of interest in studying social interaction from the perspective of the interactions of genes with the environment in the past decade (Manuck & McCaffery, 2014). Based on this notion, a recent genetic study reported an effect of the interaction between job stress and OXTR rs53576 or rs2268490 on general trust perception (Fang et al., 2020) where high job stress was related to low general trust in homozygotic carriers (GG/AA) of the OXTR rs53576 polymorphism and heterocygotic (CT) carriers for the OXTR rs2268490 polymorphism. The findings emphasized that the possible effects of the interactions of genes with the environment can also be extended onto trust perception. Future studies could use a gene–environment interaction approach conceiving variant models to gain a deeper understanding of interpersonal trust.

Finally, the neuroendocrine modulation of trust must not be restricted to OXT but other neuropeptides and neurotransmitters as well as the interrelation between different substances may also be relevant. For example, it has been shown that testosterone (TES) also plays an important role in the context of trust, mainly by reducing interpersonal trust (Boksem et al., 2013; Bos et al., 2010). Bos and colleagues (2010) argue that TES plays an antagonistic role to OXT in the neurohumoral modulation of trust that might be particularly relevant in competitive contexts. Carre et al. (2014) found that an increase of endogenous TES release during competition predicts the reduction of interpersonal trust in terms of trust ratings of neutral faces in males but not females. Interestingly, there is some evidence that the trust-reducing effect of TES is related to its impact on the amygdala (Bos et al., 2012) and therefore a neural system that has been related to the trust-increasing effect of OXT. However, the effect of testosterone on trust might also be influenced by neurodevelopmental and environmental effects. Buskens et al., 2016 found that the trust-reducing effect of TES during a multi-round TG was only observable in females with a high prenatal testosterone-to-estradiol ratio as indexed by the second-to-fourth digit (2D–4D) ratio. Therefore, much more research is needed to draw a more complete picture of the neurohumoral and neuro-biological mechanisms underlying trust and trusting behavior taking TES and other potential modulators as well as their interaction with biological and environmental influences into account.

13.8   Final Conclusions

Taking the evidence reported above together, although the association between OXT and trust has been widely investigated during the past decades, a direct trust-promoting effect of OXT as proposed by early studies has not been found. Instead, there is evidence that the relationship between OXT and trust is modulated by manifold factors that are closely interrelated, for example social affiliation, personality traits, gender, mental disorders, and genetic disposition. Although findings of imaging studies support the idea that brain regions are modulated by OXT in the context of tasks probing trust behavior, more empirical evidence is still warranted to extend the knowledge of OXT effects on neural correlates of trust.

Future research should aim to conceive models of the OXT–trust connection considering the interactions between genes, brain functioning, and the environment, advancing the knowledge of understanding inter-personal trust. However, all these arguments are also valid for the more general, prosocial effect of OXT. While there is still a lot of evidence for the role of OXT as a prosocial neuropeptide (Meyer-Lindenberg et al., 2011) it becomes more and more obvious that this effect is modulated by contextual factors like the social environment and the personality traits of the individuals involved in a particular social interaction (Bartz, Zaki, et al., 2011). According to Bartz and colleagues these contextual factors influence basic social mechanisms like anxiety reduction, social salience, and affiliative motivation that themselves contribute to a more general social-cognitive and prosocial effect of OXT. While the factors that have been described to influence the effect of OXT on trust are very similar to those found for other social domains, one could argue that there is no specific trust-promoting effect of OXT but, depending on the social situation and the individual dispositions, the prosocial effect of OXT is also reflected in increased trusting behavior or the intention to trust.

References

Andari, E., Duhamel, J.-R., Zalla, T., Herbrecht, E., Leboyer, M., & Sirigu, A. (2010). Promoting social behavior with oxytocin in high-functioning autism spectrum disorders. *Proceedings of the National Academy of Sciences*, 107(9), 4389–4394. https://doi.org/10.1073/pnas.0910249107

Apicella, C. L., Cesarini, D., Johannesson, M., et al. (2010). No association between oxytocin receptor (OXTR) gene polymorphisms and experimentally elicited social preferences. *PLoS ONE*, 5(6), Article e11153. https://doi.org/10.1371/journal.pone.0011153

Bakermans-Kranenburg, M. J., & Van IJzendoorn, M. H. (2014). A sociability gene? Meta-analysis of oxytocin receptor genotype effects in humans. *Psychiatric Genetics*, 24(2), 45–51. https://doi.org/10.1097/YPG.0b013e3283643684

Balliet, D., Wu, J., & De Dreu, C. K. (2014). Ingroup favoritism in cooperation: A meta-analysis. *Psychological Bulletin*, 140(6), 1556–1581. https://doi.org/10.1037/a0037737

Barraza, J. A., McCullough, M. E., Ahmadi, S., & Zak, P. J. (2011). Oxytocin infusion increases charitable donations regardless of monetary resources. *Hormones and Behavior*, 60(2), 148–151. https://doi.org/10.1016/j.yhbeh.2011.04.008

Bartz, J., Simeon, D., Hamilton, H., et al. (2011). Oxytocin can hinder trust and cooperation in borderline personality disorder. *Social Cognitive and Affective Neuroscience*, 6(5), 556–563. https://doi.org/10.1093/scan/nsq085

Bartz, J., Zaki, J., Bolger, N., & Ochsner, K. (2011). Social effects of oxytocin in humans: Context and person matter. *Trends in Cognitive Sciences*, 15(7), 301–309. https://doi.org/10.1016/j.tics.2011.05.002

Baumgartner, T., Heinrichs, M., Vonlanthen, A., Fischbacher, U., & Fehr, E. (2008). Oxytocin shapes the neural circuitry of trust and trust adaptation in humans. *Neuron*, 58(4), 639–650. https://doi.org/10.1016/j.neuron.2008.04.009

Benjamin, D. J., Cesarini, D., Van Der Loos, M. J., et al. (2012). The genetic architecture of economic and political preferences. *Proceedings of the National*

Academy of Sciences, 109(21), 8026–8031. https://doi.org/10.1073/pnas.1120666109

Berg, J., Dickhaut, J., & McCabe, K. (1995). Trust, reciprocity, and social history. *Games and Economic Behavior*, 10(1), 122–142. https://doi.org/10.1006/game.1995.1027

Bohnet, I., & Zeckhauser, R. (2004). Trust, risk and betrayal. *Journal of Economic Behavior & Organization*, 55(4), 467–484. https://doi.org/10.1016/j.jebo.2003.11.004

Boksem, M. A. S., Mehta, P. H., Van den Bergh, B., et al. (2013). Testosterone inhibits trust but promotes reciprocity. *Psychological Science*, 24(11), 2306–2314. https://doi.org/10.1177/0956797613495063

Bos, P. A., Hermans, E. J., Ramsey, N. F., & Van Honk, J. (2012). The neural mechanisms by which testosterone acts on interpersonal trust. *NeuroImage*, 61(3), 730–737. https://doi.org/10.1016/j.neuroimage.2012.04.002

Bos, P. A., Terburg, D., & Van Honk, J. (2010). Testosterone decreases trust in socially naive humans. *Proceedings of the National Academy of Sciences*, 107(22), 9991–9995. https://doi.org/10.1073/pnas.0911700107

Buskens, V., Raub, W., Van Miltenburg, N., Montoya, E. R., & Van Honk, J. (2016). Testosterone administration moderates effect of social environment on trust in women depending on second-to-fourth digit ratio. *Scientific Reports*, 6(1), Article 27655. https://doi.org/10.1038/srep27655

Camerer, C., & Weigelt, K. (1988). Experimental tests of a sequential equilibrium reputation model. *Econometrica*, 56(1), 1–36. https://doi.org/10.2307/1911840

Campbell, A. (2010). Oxytocin and human social behavior. *Personality and Social Psychology Review: An Official Journal of the Society for Personality and Social Psychology, Inc.*, 14(3), 281–295. https://doi.org/10.1177/1088868310363594

Cardoso, C., Ellenbogen, M. A., & Linnen, A.-M. (2012). Acute intranasal oxytocin improves positive self-perceptions of personality. *Psychopharmacology*, 220(4), 741–749. https://doi.org/10.1007/s00213-011-2527-6

Cardoso, C., Ellenbogen, M. A., Serravalle, L., & Linnen, A. M. (2013). Stress-induced negative mood moderates the relation between oxytocin administration and trust: Evidence for the tend-and-befriend response to stress? *Psychoneuroendocrinology*, 38(11), 2800–2804. https://doi.org/10.1016/j.psyneuen.2013.05.006

Carre, J. M., Baird-Rowe, C. D., & Hariri, A. R. (2014). Testosterone responses to competition predict decreased trust ratings of emotionally neutral faces. *Psychoneuroendocrinology*, 49, 79–83. https://doi.org/10.1016/j.psyneuen.2014.06.011

Christensen, J. C., Shiyanov, P. A., Estepp, J. R., & Schlager, J. J. (2014). Lack of association between human plasma oxytocin and interpersonal trust in a prisoner's dilemma paradigm. *PLoS ONE*, 9(12), Article e116172. https://doi.org/10.1371/journal.pone.0119691

Dale, H. H. (1906). On some physiological actions of ergot. *The Journal of Physiology*, 34(3), 163–206. https://doi.org/10.1113/jphysiol.1906.sp001148

De Dreu, C. K., Greer, L. L., Handgraaf, M. J., et al. (2010). The neuropeptide oxytocin regulates parochial altruism in intergroup conflict among humans. *Science*, 328(5984), 1408–1411. https://doi.org/10.1126/science.1189047

de Visser, E. J., Monfort, S. S., Goodyear, K., et al. (2017). A little anthropomorphism goes a long way: Effects of oxytocin on trust, compliance, and team performance with automated agents. *Human Factors*, 59(1), 116–133. https://doi.org/10.1177/0018720816687205

Declerck, C. H., Boone, C., & Kiyonari, T. (2010). Oxytocin and cooperation under conditions of uncertainty: The modulating role of incentives and social information. *Hormones and Behavior*, 57(3), 368–374. https://doi.org/10.1016/j.yhbeh.2010.01.006

Declerck, C. H., Boone, C., Pauwels, L., Vogt, B., & Fehr, E. (2020). A registered replication study on oxytocin and trust. *Nature Human Behaviour*, 4, 646–655. https://doi.org/10.1038/s41562-020-0878-x

DeVries, A. C., Young III, W. S., & Nelson, R. J. (1997). Reduced aggressive behaviour in mice with targeted disruption of the oxytocin gene. *Journal of Neuroendocrinology*, 9(5), 363–368. https://doi.org/10.1046/j.1365-2826.1997.t01-1-00589.x

Donaldson, Z. R., & Young, L. J. (2008). Oxytocin, vasopressin, and the neurogenetics of sociality. *Science*, 322(5903), 900–904. https://doi.org/10.1126/science.1158668

Ebert, A., Kolb, M., Heller, J., Edel, M.-A., Roser, P., & Brüne, M. (2013). Modulation of interpersonal trust in borderline personality disorder by intranasal oxytocin and childhood trauma. *Social Neuroscience*, 8(4), 305–313. https://doi.org/10.1080/17470919.2013.807301

Fang, Y., Li, Z., Wu, S., Wang, C., Dong, Y., & He, S. (2020). Oxytocin receptor gene polymorphisms moderate the relationship between job stress and general trust in Chinese Han university teachers. *Journal of Affective Disorders*, 260, 18–23. https://doi.org/10.1016/j.jad.2019.08.080

Feifel, D., Shilling, P. D., & MacDonald, K. (2016). A review of oxytocin's effects on the positive, negative, and cognitive domains of schizophrenia. *Biological Psychiatry*, 79(3), 222–233. https://doi.org/10.1016/j.biopsych.2015.07.025

Gimpl, G., & Fahrenholz, F. (2001). The oxytocin receptor system: Structure, function, and regulation. *Physiological Reviews*, 81(2), 629–683. https://doi.org/10.1152/physrev.2001.81.2.629

Grainger, S. A., Henry, J. D., Steinvik, H. R., & Vanman, E. J. (2019). Intranasal oxytocin does not alter initial perceptions of facial trustworthiness in younger or older adults. *Journal of Psychopharmacology*, 33(2), 250–254. https://doi.org/10.1177/0269881118806303

Green, L., Fein, D., Modahl, C., et al. (2001). Oxytocin and autistic disorder: Alterations in peptide forms. *Biological Psychiatry*, 50(8), 609–613. https://doi.org/10.1016/s0006-3223(01)01139-8

Grinevich, V., Knobloch-Bollmann, H. S., Eliava, M., Busnelli, M., & Chini, B. (2016). Assembling the puzzle: Pathways of oxytocin signaling in the brain. *Biological Psychiatry*, 79(3), 155–164. https://doi.org/10.1016/j.biopsych .2015.04.013

Ide, J. S., Nedic, S., Wong, K. F., et al. (2018). Oxytocin attenuates trust as a subset of more general reinforcement learning, with altered reward circuit functional connectivity in males. *NeuroImage*, 174, 35–43. https://doi.org/ 10.1016/j.neuroimage.2018.02.035

Kendrick, K. M., Guastella, A. J., & Becker, B. (2017). Overview of human oxytocin research. In R. Hurlemann & V. Grinevich (Eds.), *Behavioral pharmacology of neuropeptides: Oxytocin* (pp. 321–348). Springer. https:// doi.org/10.1007/7854_2017_19

Keverne, E. B., & Kendrick, K. M. (1992). Oxytocin facilitation of maternal behavior in sheep. *Annals of the New York Academy of Sciences*, 652(1), 83–101. https://doi.org/10.1111/j.1749-6632.1992.tb34348.x

Kirsch, P., Esslinger, C., Chen, Q., et al. (2005). Oxytocin modulates neural circuitry for social cognition and fear in humans. *Journal of Neuroscience*, 25 (49), 11489–11493. https://doi.org/10.1523/JNEUROSCI.3984-05.2005

Klackl, J., Pfundmair, M., Agroskin, D., & Jonas, E. (2013). Who is to blame? Oxytocin promotes nonpersonalistic attributions in response to a trust betrayal. *Biological Psychology*, 92(2), 387–394. https://doi.org/10.1016/j .biopsycho.2012.11.010

Knobloch, H. S., Charlet, A., Hoffmann, L. C., et al. (2012). Evoked axonal oxytocin release in the central amygdala attenuates fear response. *Neuron*, 73 (3), 553–566. https://doi.org/10.1016/j.neuron.2011.11.030

Kosfeld, M., Heinrichs, M., Zak, P. J., Fischbacher, U., & Fehr, E. (2005). Oxytocin increases trust in humans. *Nature*, 435(7042), 673–676. https:// doi.org/10.1038/nature03701

Kovács, G. L. (1986). Oxytocin and behavior. In D. Ganten & D. Pfaff (Eds.), *Neurobiology of oxytocin* (pp. 91–128). Springer. https://doi.org/10.1007/ 978-3-642-70414-7_4

Kret, M. E., & De Dreu, C. K. (2017). Pupil-mimicry conditions trust in partners: Moderation by oxytocin and group membership. *Proceedings of the Royal Society B: Biological Sciences*, 284(1850), Article 20162554. https:// doi.org/10.1098/rspb.2016.2554

Krueger, F., & Meyer-Lindenberg, A. (2019). Toward a model of interpersonal trust drawn from neuroscience, psychology, and economics. *Trends in Neurosciences*, 42(2), 92–101. https://doi.org/10.1016/j.tins.2018.10.004

Krueger, F., Parasuraman, R., Iyengar, V., et al. (2012). Oxytocin receptor genetic variation promotes human trust behavior. *Frontiers in Human Neuroscience*, 6, Article 4. https://doi.org/10.3389/fnhum.2012.00004

Kumsta, R., & Heinrichs, M. (2013). Oxytocin, stress and social behavior: Neurogenetics of the human oxytocin system. *Current Opinion in Neurobiology*, 23(1), 11–16. https://doi.org/10.1016/j.conb.2012.09.004

Lambert, B., Declerck, C. H., & Boone, C. (2014). Oxytocin does not make a face appear more trustworthy but improves the accuracy of trustworthiness judgments. *Psychoneuroendocrinology*, 40, 60–68. https://doi.org/10.1016/j.psyneuen.2013.10.015

Lane, A., Mikolajczak, M., Treinen, E., et al. (2015). Failed replication of oxytocin effects on trust: The envelope task case. *PLoS ONE*, 10(9), Article e0137000. https://doi.org/10.1371/journal.pone.0137000

Lazarus, S. A., Cheavens, J. S., Festa, F., & Rosenthal, M. Z. (2014). Interpersonal functioning in borderline personality disorder: A systematic review of behavioral and laboratory-based assessments. *Clinical Psychology Review*, 34(3), 193–205. https://doi.org/10.1016/j.cpr.2014.01.007

Lee, M. R., Scheidweiler, K. B., Diao, X. X., et al. (2018). Oxytocin by intranasal and intravenous routes reaches the cerebrospinal fluid in rhesus macaques: Determination using a novel oxytocin assay. *Molecular Psychiatry*, 23(1), 115–122. https://doi.org/10.1038/mp.2017.27

Lee, M. R., Shnitko, T. A., Blue, S. W., et al. (2020). Labeled oxytocin administered via the intranasal route reaches the brain in rhesus macaques. *Nature Communications*, 11(1), Article 2783. https://doi.org/10.1038/s41467-020-15942-1

Lee, M. R., Wehring, H. J., McMahon, R. P., et al. (2019). The effect of intranasal oxytocin on measures of social cognition in schizophrenia: A negative report. *Journal of Psychiatry and Brain Science*, 4(1), Article e190001. https://doi.org/10.20900/jpbs.20190001

Long, P. A., & Freeman, H. (2019). Patients in pain: The effects of oxytocin on trust and decision making. *Proceedings of the International Symposium on Human Factors and Ergonomics in Health Care*, 8(1), 164–166. https://doi.org/10.1177/2327857919081040

LoParo, D., & Waldman, I. (2015). The oxytocin receptor gene (OXTR) is associated with autism spectrum disorder: A meta-analysis. *Molecular Psychiatry*, 20(5), 640–646. https://doi.org/10.1038/mp.2014.77

Lord, C., Cook, E. H., Leventhal, B. L., & Amaral, D. G. (2000). Autism spectrum disorders. *Neuron*, 28(2), 355–363. https://doi.org/10.1016/s0896-6273(00)00115-x

Luo, R., Xu, L., Zhao, W., et al. (2017). Oxytocin facilitation of acceptance of social advice is dependent upon the perceived trustworthiness of individual advisors. *Psychoneuroendocrinology*, 83, 1–8. https://doi.org/10.1016/j.psyneuen.2017.05.020

MacDonald, E., Dadds, M. R., Brennan, J. L., Williams, K., Levy, F., & Cauchi, A. J. (2011). A review of safety, side-effects and subjective reactions to intranasal oxytocin in human research. *Psychoneuroendocrinology*, 36(8), 1114–1126. https://doi.org/10.1016/j.psyneuen.2011.02.015

Manuck, S. B., & McCaffery, J. M. (2014). Gene-environment interaction. *Annual Review of Psychology*, 65, 41–70. https://doi.org/10.3389/fpsyg.2018.02036

McClelland, D. C. (1987). *Human motivation*. Cambridge University Press. https://doi.org/10.1017/CBO9781139878289

McCullough, M. E., Churchland, P. S., & Mendez, A. J. (2013). Problems with measuring peripheral oxytocin: Can the data on oxytocin and human behavior be trusted? *Neuroscience & Biobehavioral Reviews*, 37(8), 1485–1492. https://doi.org/10.1016/j.neubiorev.2013.04.018

Merolla, J. L., Burnett, G., Pyle, K. V., Ahmadi, S., & Zak, P. J. (2013). Oxytocin and the biological basis for interpersonal and political trust. *Political Behavior*, 35(4), 753–776. https://doi.org/10.1007/s11109-012-9219-8

Meyer-Lindenberg, A., Domes, G., Kirsch, P., & Heinrichs, M. (2011). Oxytocin and vasopressin in the human brain: Social neuropeptides for translational medicine. *Nature Reviews Neuroscience*, 12(9), 524–538. https://doi.org/10.1038/nrn3044

Mikolajczak, M., Gross, J. J., Lane, A., Corneille, O., de Timary, P., & Luminet, O. (2010). Oxytocin makes people trusting, not gullible. *Psychological Science*, 21(8), 1072–1074. https://doi.org/10.1177/0956797610377343

Mikolajczak, M., Pinon, N., Lane, A., de Timary, P., & Luminet, O. (2010). Oxytocin not only increases trust when money is at stake, but also when confidential information is in the balance. *Biological Psychology*, 85(1), 182–184. https://doi.org/10.1016/j.biopsycho.2010.05.010

Modahl, C., Green, L. A., Fein, D., et al. (1998). Plasma oxytocin levels in autistic children. *Biological Psychiatry*, 43(4), 270–277. https://doi.org/10.1016/s0006-3223(97)00439-3

Nave, G., Camerer, C., & McCullough, M. (2015). Does oxytocin increase trust in humans? A critical review of research. *Perspectives on Psychological Science: A Journal of The Association for Psychological Science*, 10(6), 772–789. https://doi.org/10.1177/1745691615600138

Nishina, K., Takagishi, H., Fermin, A., et al. (2018). Association of the oxytocin receptor gene with attitudinal trust: Role of amygdala volume. *Social Cognitive and Affective Neuroscience*, 13(10), 1091–1097. https://doi.org/10.1093/scan/nsy075

Nishina, K., Takagishi, H., Inoue-Murayama, M., Takahashi, H., & Yamagishi, T. (2015). Polymorphism of the oxytocin receptor gene modulates behavioral and attitudinal trust among men but not women. *PLoS ONE*, 10(10), Article e0137089. https://doi.org/10.1371/journal.pone.0137089

O'Doherty, J., Dayan, P., Schultz, J., Deichmann, R., Friston, K., & Dolan, R. J. (2004). Dissociable roles of ventral and dorsal striatum in instrumental conditioning. *Science*, 304(5669), 452–454. https://doi.org/10.1126/science.1094285

Ooi, Y. P., Weng, S.-J., Kossowsky, J., Gerger, H., & Sung, M. (2017). Oxytocin and autism spectrum disorders: A systematic review and meta-analysis of randomized controlled trials. *Pharmacopsychiatry*, 50(1), 5–13. https://doi.org/10.1055/s-0042-109400

Ott, I., & Scott, J. C. (1910). The action of infundibulin upon the mammary secretion. *Proceedings of the Society for Experimental Biology and Medicine*, 8 (2), 48–49. https://doi.org/10.3181/00379727-8-27

Pedersen, C. A., Gibson, C. M., Rau, S. W., et al. (2011). Intranasal oxytocin reduces psychotic symptoms and improves theory of mind and social perception in schizophrenia. *Schizophrenia Research*, 132(1), 50–53. https://doi .org/10.1016/j.schres.2011.07.027

Pedersen, C. A., & Prange, A. J. (1979). Induction of maternal behavior in virgin rats after intracerebroventricular administration of oxytocin. *Proceedings of the National Academy of Sciences*, 76(12), 6661–6665. https://doi.org/10 .1073/pnas.76.12.6661

Quintana, D. S., Rokicki, J., Van der Meer, D., et al. (2019). Oxytocin pathway gene networks in the human brain. *Nature Communications*, 10(1), 1–12. https://doi.org/10.1038/s41467-019-08503-8

Quintana, D. S., Westlye, L. T., Rustan, Ø. G., et al. (2015). Low-dose oxytocin delivered intranasally with Breath Powered device affects social-cognitive behavior: A randomized four-way crossover trial with nasal cavity dimension assessment. *Translational Psychiatry*, 5(7), Article e602. https://doi.org/10 .1038/tp.2015.93

Rimmele, U., Hediger, K., Heinrichs, M., & Klaver, P. (2009). Oxytocin makes a face in memory familiar. *Journal of Neuroscience*, 29(1), 38–42. https://doi .org/10.1523/JNEUROSCI.4260-08.2009

Salonia, A., Nappi, R. E., Pontillo, M., et al. (2005). Menstrual cycle-related changes in plasma oxytocin are relevant to normal sexual function in healthy women. *Hormones and Behavior*, 47(2), 164–169. https://doi.org/10.1016/j .yhbeh.2004.10.002

Sauer, C., Montag, C., Reuter, M., & Kirsch, P. (2019). Oxytocinergic modulation of brain activation to cues related to reproduction and attachment: Differences and commonalities during the perception of erotic and fearful social scenes. *International Journal of Psychophysiology: Official Journal of the International Organization of Psychophysiology*, 136, 87–96. https://doi.org/ 10.1016/j.ijpsycho.2018.06.005

Spengler, F. B., Schultz, J., Scheele, D., et al. (2017). Kinetics and dose dependency of intranasal oxytocin effects on amygdala reactivity. *Biological Psychiatry*, 82(12), 885–894. https://doi.org/10.1016/j.biopsych.2017.04 .015

Tabak, B. A., McCullough, M. E., Carver, C. S., Pedersen, E. J., & Cuccaro, M. L. (2014). Variation in oxytocin receptor gene (OXTR) polymorphisms is associated with emotional and behavioral reactions to betrayal. *Social Cognitive and Affective Neuroscience*, 9(6), 810–816. https://doi.org/10 .1093/scan/nst042

Tauber, M., Mantoulan, C., Copet, P., et al. (2011). Oxytocin may be useful to increase trust in others and decrease disruptive behaviours in patients with Prader-Willi syndrome: A randomised placebo-controlled trial in 24 patients. *Orphanet Journal of Rare Diseases*, 6(1), Article 47. https://doi.org/10.1186/1750-1172-6-47

Teed, A. R., Han, K., Rakic, J., Mark, D. B., & Krawczyk, D. C. (2019). The influence of oxytocin and vasopressin on men's judgments of social dominance and trustworthiness: An fMRI study of neutral faces. *Psychoneuroendocrinology*, 106, 252–258. https://doi.org/10.1016/j.psyneuen.2019.04.014

Ten Velden, F. S., Daughters, K., & De Dreu, C. K. (2017). Oxytocin promotes intuitive rather than deliberated cooperation with the in-group. *Hormones and Behavior*, 92, 164–171. https://doi.org/10.1016/j.yhbeh.2016.06.005

Theodoridou, A., Rowe, A. C., Penton-Voak, I. S., & Rogers, P. J. (2009). Oxytocin and social perception: Oxytocin increases perceived facial trustworthiness and attractiveness. *Hormones and Behavior*, 56(1), 128–132. https://doi.org/10.1016/j.yhbeh.2009.03.019

Valstad, M., Alvares, G. A., Egknud, M., et al. (2017). The correlation between central and peripheral oxytocin concentrations: A systematic review and meta-analysis. *Neuroscience & Biobehavioral Reviews*, 78, 117–124. https://doi.org/10.1016/j.neubiorev.2017.04.017

Van IJzendoorn, M. H., & Bakermans-Kranenburg, M. J. (2012). A sniff of trust: Meta-analysis of the effects of intranasal oxytocin administration on face recognition, trust to in-group, and trust to out-group. *Psychoneuroendocrinology*, 37(3), 438–443. https://doi.org/10.1016/j.psyneuen.2011.07.008

Watson, M. L. (2005). *Can there be just one trust? A cross-disciplinary identification of trust definitions and measurement.* The Institute for Public Relations, 1–25.

Woolley, J., Chuang, B., Fussell, C., et al. (2017). Intranasal oxytocin increases facial expressivity, but not ratings of trustworthiness, in patients with schizophrenia and healthy controls. *Psychological Medicine*, 47(7), 1311–1322. https://doi.org/10.1017/S0033291716003433

Yao, S., Zhao, W., Cheng, R., Geng, Y., Luo, L., & Kendrick, K. M. (2014). Oxytocin makes females, but not males, less forgiving following betrayal of trust. *The International Journal of Neuropsychopharmacology*, 17(11), 1785–1792. https://doi.org/10.1017/s1461145714000090x

Zak, P. J., Kurzban, R., & Matzner, W. T. (2005). Oxytocin is associated with human trustworthiness. *Hormones and Behavior*, 48(5), 522–527. https://doi.org/10.1016/j.yhbeh.2005.07.009

Zhang, H., Gross, J., De Dreu, C., & Ma, Y. (2019). Oxytocin promotes coordinated out-group attack during intergroup conflict in humans. *eLife*, 8, Article e40698. https://doi.org/10.7554/eLife.40698.001

Zhong, S., Monakhov, M., Mok, H. P., et al. (2012). U-shaped relation between plasma oxytocin levels and behavior in the trust game. *PLoS ONE*, 7(12), Article e51095. https://doi.org/10.1371/journal.pone.0051095

CHAPTER 14

Trust and Psychopharmaca:
Neuromodulation of the Signaling Pathways Underlying Trust Behavior

Mary R. Lee, Apoorva Veerareddy, and Frank Krueger

14.1 Introduction

Trust penetrates relationships in all aspects of human life. As humans trust, communities become more egalitarian, economies grow, and perceived well-being thrives (Rothstein & Uslaner, 2005). Researchers from a large variety of scholarly disciplines, including psychology, economics, and neuroscience, have studied trust in reciprocity. This has allowed for a transdisciplinary integration of knowledge from economic behaviors (i.e., trust game, TG), psychological states (i.e., motivational, affective, and cognitive), and neurobiological systems (i.e., brain networks, hormones/neurotransmitters, and genes). While other chapters in this volume concentrate on linking the behavioral, psychological, neural, and genetic levels of trust, we emphasize here the neurochemical level of trust – that is, the pharmacological manipulation of neurotransmitter systems implicated in the neurocircuitry of trust behavior (note that neuropeptide hormones [e.g., oxytocin] and steroid hormones [e.g., testosterone] are addressed in Chapter 13).

In this chapter, we review research that used pharmacological agents to examine processes of neural signaling systems influencing trust behavior. Identifying the neurochemical level of trust can shed light on trust impairment, which is a crucial feature of several neuropsychiatric disorders (see also Chapters 16 and 17). Our chapter consists of three parts. In Section 14.2, we describe the laboratory measurements, the underlying neural networks, and the related target neurotransmitter systems that probe trust behavior. In Section 14.3, we examine the psychopharmacological studies focusing first on studies that implemented the TG and second on studies that applied trust ratings after completing other cooperative exchange games. In Section 14.4, we draw attention to shortcomings in the present

Corresponding authors: Mary R. Lee (mary.lee3@va.gov) and Frank Krueger (fkrueger@gmu.edu).

psychopharmacological research and provide recommendations that can direct future multidisciplinary studies toward a deeper understanding of trust's neuropsychoeconomic foundations.

14.2 Game Types, Brain Networks, and Neuromodulators of Trust

Pharmacologic manipulation of trust behavior involves three components. First, reliable laboratory measures of trust behavior such as the TG are employed that are standardized and reproducible (Berg et al., 1995; Camerer, 2003). Second, the TG has been widely employed in neuroimaging studies including functional magnetic resonance imaging (fMRI), electroencephalography (EEG), and brain lesions that allow the identification of key regions of the underlying domain-general large-scale brain networks driving trust behavior. Third, pharmacologic agents are administered that selectively target receptors of neurotransmitters that are known to modulate brain regions of those domain-general large-scale networks involved in trust behavior.

14.2.1 Game Types of Trust

A quantitative and accurate laboratory measure of trust behavior is the two-player TG, where one player is the trustor (or investor) and the other one is the trustee (Berg et al., 1995; Camerer, 2003) (see also Chapter 2). In the trust stage, the trustor receives an initial endowment of money from the experimenter and decides whether to share (trust) or not share (nontrust) some of his/her endowment with the trustee. If the trustor decides to share, then the money transferred to the trustee is compounded (usually doubled or tripled) and forwarded to the trustee by the experimenter. In the reciprocity stage, the trustee determines to repay some part of the transferred money to the trustor (i.e., reciprocity) or to keep the received money (i.e., betrayal). In the feedback stage, the trustor is notified about the trustee's transferred amount. The trustor's transferred money measures trust behavior, while the trustee's returned money measures trustworthiness behavior. The trustor must decide between a sure gain of keeping all of the initial endowment (not sharing) or taking a social risk and sharing the money, which then increases in magnitude and promises to reward the trustor with a greater sum of money compared to the initial endowment that the trustor is given. To control whether the amount sent truly reflects trust rather than risk-taking behavior, a lottery game is often implemented as a control condition that applies the same rules as the TG but involves a computer instead of a human counterpart that returns a random amount of money back to the trustor (Johnson & Mislin, 2011).

The TG can be played in single (one-shot) or multiple (multi-shot) interactions with the same partner whose trustworthiness may be unknown or known. The one-shot TG with an anonymous partner measures a person's propensity-based trust, that is, a trait-based characteristic for one to trust others (Mayer et al., 1995). Without details about the partner's trustworthiness, the trust decision presumably relies on the trustor's general inclination to trust that an unknown other will reciprocate (McKnight et al., 1998). A one-shot TG in which the trustor is given some information about the trustee such as physical appearance (e.g., trustee's facial features) (Burnham et al., 2000; Todorov et al., 2009; Van't Wout & Sanfey, 2008; Willis & Todorov, 2006; Winston et al., 2002) and/or prior behavior (e.g., benevolence and integrity) (Delgado et al., 2005; Mayer et al., 1995) measures impression-based trust (Fouragnan et al., 2013) (see also Chapter 7).

In contrast, the multi-round TG with the same anonymous partner measures trust dynamics; the trustor learns by dynamically updating the beliefs about the partner's trustworthiness over successive interactions (i.e., reinforcement learning) based on the round-to-round behavior of the partner (i.e., experience-based trust) (Fett et al., 2012; King-Casas et al., 2005; Krueger et al., 2007) (see also Chapter 8). Individuals integrate these three key components of trust – that is, their propensity to trust, their initial impression of the reliability of others, and their capacity to learn from experiential feedback – to inform their trust decisions (Alarcon et al., 2018; Bonnefon et al., 2013; Chang et al., 2010).

14.2.2   Networks of Trust

The TG has been widely employed in behavioral and neuroimaging studies such as in studies of patients with brain lesions (Belfi et al., 2015; Koscik & Tranel, 2011; Moretto et al., 2013) as well as those employing EEG (Fu et al., 2019; Hahn et al., 2015; Sun et al., 2019) and fMRI (Bellucci et al., 2018; Fehr, 2009; Krueger & Meyer-Lindenberg, 2019; Riedl & Javor, 2012; Tzieropoulos, 2013). The latter have elucidated the fundamental neural networks underlying trust behavior that have been confirmed by coordinate-based meta-analyses (Bellucci et al., 2017; Bellucci et al., 2018). The trust phase for the one-shot TG consistently activates the right dorsal anterior insula (AI) – a brain region that is a crucial brain region of the salience network (SAN) – known to encode aversive feelings (disgust) that may be generated by risking a subsequent breach of trust (Aimone et al., 2014; Bohnet et al., 2008). In contrast, the multi-shot TG reliably activates the ventral striatum (vSTR, nucleus accumbens) – a brain region of the mesolimbic reward network (RWN) that is activated in response to reward prediction. This reward prediction occurs with learning based on one's partner's behavior on successive trials (Delgado et al., 2005; Fareri et al., 2012; King-Casas et al., 2005). Finally, in the multi-shot TG, contrasting the decision versus feedback phase reliably activates the vSTR (nucleus accumbens), while the dorsal STR (dSTR, caudate nucleus) is coherently engaged for the reverse contrast – a key region of the nigrostriatal RWN involved in reinforcement learning to maximize the future rewards (Baumgartner et al., 2008; King-Casas et al., 2005).

Hence, different versions of the TG, as well as the different stages therein, activate distinct brain regions that may represent context-specific psychological (motivational, affective, cognitive) processes. A recent proposed neuropsychoeconomic trust model explains how trust develops – starting from calculus-based, over knowledge-based, ending with identification-based trust (Lewicki & Bunker, 1995) – through repeated social interactions and its associated domain-general large-scale networks (Krueger & Meyer-Lindenberg, 2019). During the calculus-based trust stage, guided mainly by SAN (i.e., risk of betrayal), trustors face ambiguous circumstances with little knowledge about the partner's trustworthiness (i.e., the unknown unknowns) and conduct rational cost-benefit calculations for establishing and retaining a trust relationship. Advancing to the knowledge-based trust stage, driven primarily by the central-executive network (CEN, adoption of strategy) or default-mode network (DMN, evaluation of trustworthiness), trustors encounter uncertain circumstances (i.e., the known unknowns as well as the unknown knowns) and gain information about the situations and the trustees to anticipate their actions reliably to enhance their trust relationships. Finally, proceeding to the identification-based trust phase steered preeminently by the RWN (presumption of reward), trustors confront certain situations (i.e., the known knowns) and establish a rewarding identification with trustees and appreciate their motivations to trust them with confidence.

Overall, a switch in engagement from SAN (AI) to RWN (vSTR) can be identified when transferring from one- to multi-shot TGs exchanges – probably representing a shift from calculus-based (i.e., ambiguity about possible betrayal) to identification-based (i.e., assurance about expected reward) trust (Bellucci et al., 2017). Pharmacologic agents, acting at endogenous receptors, can modulate these networks and alter downstream trust behaviors, as described next.

14.2.3   Neuromodulators of Trust

At the neurochemical level, while traditional neurotransmitters may bind to receptors for only fractions of a millisecond before being inactivated, neuromodulators adjust neuronal activity in a context-sensitive manner and remain active for intervals ranging from seconds to hours (Crockett & Fehr, 2014). These neuromodulators regulate the levels of neurochemicals in the brain in response to events in the environment and subsequently influence information processing in local brain regions of domain-general large-scale brain networks, and are therefore sensitive to psychopharmacological drug manipulation (Robbins & Arnsten, 2009). In particular, pharmacological agents can stimulate or block endogenous receptors directly by targeting a receptor type with varying degrees of specificity. Pharmacologic agents can also intervene in the cellular reuptake or synaptic metabolism of endogenous neuromodulators. For example, the effects of those agents – acting as agonists or antagonists – on neuromodulator function depends on whether they activate pre- or post-synaptic receptors. When binding to post-synaptic receptors, agonists (vs. antagonists) mimic (vs. block) the actions of the endogenous neuromodulator to have a net effect of increasing (vs. decreasing) neuromodulator function. However, agonists have a net effect of decreasing neuromodulator function when binding to autoreceptors located on presynaptic receptors, since autoreceptors inhibit synthesis and release neurotransmitters when activated. By contrast, autoreceptor antagonism can stimulate neurotransmitter synthesis and release by blocking negative feedback caused by endogenous neurotransmitters. Brain regions that lie in the neurocircuitry of trust behavior (reviewed in Crockett & Fehr, 2014) (e.g., insular cortex, STR) express receptors for neuromodulators that modulate trust behavior, including opiates, monoamine neurotransmitters (e.g., serotonin, dopamine, norepinephrine), as well as pharmacologic agents such as 3,4-Methyl-enedioxy-methamphetamine (MDMA) that increases the activity of all three of these monoamine neurotransmitters. In Section 14.3 we will describe psychopharmacological studies that utilized the TG (Berg et al., 1995; Camerer, 2003), followed by studies that employed trust ratings after completing other cooperative exchange games.

14.3 Review of Psychopharmacological Studies

14.3.1 Combining TG with the Administration of Pharmacological Agents

In our review of the literature over the last ten years, five studies combined a version of the TG with the administration of pharmacological agents – including pramipexole (dopaminergic modulation), methylphenidate (dopaminergic modulation), naltrexone (opioidergic modulation), minocycline (microglial modulation), and acetaminophen (analgesic and antipyretic modulation) – to study their impact on trust behavior.

Pramipexole. Bellucci et al. (2020) examined the relationship between the dopaminergic system on the impression-based trust behavior of unknown partners' facial trustworthiness by employing a within-subjects, double-blind, placebo-controlled, crossover design. On two different days, healthy female participants (n = 28) were administered either pramipexole (0.5 mg) (i.e., dopamine D2/D3 receptor agonist) or placebo orally before playing one-shot TGs as trustors with different anonymous partners whose faces varied maximally on trustworthiness with minimal differences in attractiveness. Participants received no feedback about the partner's reciprocity to avoid social learning, and facial trustworthiness and attractiveness ratings were collected after playing the TG with all partners.

As expected, estimations of trustworthiness (based solely on viewing the partner's face) were positively correlated with trust behavior, and this relationship endured even when controlling for the influence of attractiveness. Partners who were judged more trustworthy were entrusted with more money. After administration of pramipexole, participants entrusted less money with their partners overall compared to placebo. Importantly, there was no main effect of pramipexole on judgments of trustworthiness, nor was there a pramipexole by trustworthiness interaction on trusting behavior. Given that trustworthiness is strongly linked to trust behavior, the effect of pramipexole to reduce trust behavior without reducing estimations of trustworthiness (or attractiveness) is puzzling and raises the question of what mechanisms the drug is acting on to impact trust behavior. The results indicate that pramipexole is acting on behavioral constructs distinct from estimations of trustworthiness; for example, it could be acting to increase risk aversion or to reduce impulsivity. Finally, an interaction of pramipexole with hormonal contraception was identified where trust behavior significantly decreased in hormonal contraceptive nonusers only. In addition, participants who used hormonal contraceptives as compared to nonusers perceived partners with higher levels of facial trustworthiness as more attractive.

The mechanism by which pramipexole, a dopamine D2/D3 receptor agonist, modulates impression-based trust behavior probably involves the interplay of different neuromodulator systems and regions, including dopaminergic brain regions in the STR and the medial prefrontal cortex (PFC) (Ishibashi et al., 2011; Riba et al., 2008). A dopamine agonist effect of pramipexole may explain the decrease of impression-based trust due to saturating one's need to belong as well as limiting one's willingness to relate to and associate with others (Baumeister & Leary, 1995). The reduction in impression-based trust may be related to pramipexole's agonist action on presynaptic D3 receptors, resulting in reduced dopaminergic signaling (Gurevich & Joyce, 1999; Hall et al., 1996; Ishibashi et al., 2011; Murray et al., 1994; Riba et al., 2008). Activation of the D3 autoreceptor inhibits the phasic reward-related firing of dopaminergic neurons (Riba et al., 2008; Sokoloff et al., 2006), and this inhibition is present in individuals with disorders of social functioning and avoidance (Caceda et al., 2014; Cacioppo et al., 2009; Fernandez-Theoduloz et al., 2019). Therefore, pramipexole administration might have reduced an individual's willingness to trust, perhaps by reducing meso-dopaminergic pathway signaling during anticipation of reward (Knutson et al., 2005). In the context of reduced reward signaling, the uncertainty or risk may become more prominent, resulting in a reduction of trust.

Of note, the study sample was limited to female participants (due to gender differences in dopaminergic response to reward stimuli) (Munro et al., 2006; Soutschek et al., 2017) and did not control for the menstrual cycle phase, therefore, reducing the generalizability of the reported results. Further, the interpretation of results is limited by the absence of a comparison condition, such as a lottery game that would control for risk-taking behavior. Finally, there was a lack of data on contraceptive type used by the female sample since different types of hormonal contraceptives may interact with pharmacological modulations of brain dynamics in different ways (Petersen et al., 2014).

Methylphenidate. Ratala and colleagues (2019) examined the function of catecholamine (dopamine [DA] and noradrenaline [NA]) transmission on both impression-based trust (i.e., facial features) and experience-based trust (i.e., learning via repeated interaction with the same partner) utilizing a within-subjects, double-blind, placebo-controlled crossover design. Methylphenidate (MPH) is a psychostimulant drug that blocks the dopamine transporter, and to a lesser degree, the noradrenaline transporter, thereby elevating synaptic catecholamine levels (Volkow et al., 2005). After administering MPH (20 mg) and placebo, healthy female (n = 24) and male (n = 11) participants played multi-shot TGs under the following conditions: partners (represented by photos of faces) with high and low trustworthiness and partners with high and low reciprocity. The partner faces were assigned to high and low trustworthiness groups based on results from a previous study with different participants who rated the appearance of faces on trustworthiness. Reciprocity was preprogrammed into partners in the multi-shot TG. A nonsocial control condition (slot machine game) was implemented to control for risk-taking behavior. The TG was played as a multi-shot game with each partner type, so impression-based trust could be determined separately for each partner type from experienced-based trust behavior (during the multiple rounds played with each partner).

As expected, there was a main effect of facial trustworthiness on impression-based trust, where trust behavior was highest with partners who were previously rated high in trustworthiness, followed by partners rated low in trustworthiness. Trust behavior was the lowest with the control (slot machine) game. In contrast, judgments of trustworthiness based on facial appearance did not transfer to predict experience-based trust behavior. For experience-based trust, experienced reciprocity was the salient factor where trustors invested more in partners showing high compared to low reciprocity over repeated trials. Logically, a shift from impression- to experience-based trust emerged, where trust was initially driven by facial cues and with experience was driven by experiences with the partner.

How did MPH affect this pattern of behavior? There was a three-way interaction among MPH (compared to placebo), trustworthiness, and reciprocity on trust behavior. MPH decreased trust behavior specifically for low trustworthy partners who were also low on reciprocity, indicating that MPH may promote learning selectively in the setting of negative consequences (i.e., low trustworthiness and low reciprocity). In addition, the lack of a drug effect in the high reciprocator partner trials may have been due to a ceiling effect as participants trusted high reciprocators (as determined by the experiment) at least 75% of the time.

MPH modulated trust in a context-specific fashion. Learning from rewards and punishments is mediated by catecholamine transmission

(Collins & Frank, 2013). Catecholamines influence the degree to which instructions and experience interact and modulate reinforcement learning as well as biased choice (Bodi et al., 2009; Frank et al., 2004; Pessiglione et al., 2006). MPH may have increased motivation for experience-based trust (Hysek et al., 2014; Maoz et al., 2014; Wardle & de Wit, 2012) by increasing extracellular dopamine levels in the STR (Campbell-Meiklejohn, Simonsen, Jensen, et al., 2012). As an alternative explanation, MPH could also have changed risk perception since it has been linked to riskier decision tendencies in clinical compared with healthy populations (Campbell-Meiklejohn, Simonsen, Scheel-Kruger, et al., 2012; DeVito et al., 2008; Rahman et al., 2006; Shiels et al., 2009).

Naltrexone. Schweiger et al. (2014) examined the opioid system in relation to the "warm liking" (WL) consummatory phase of reward processing (Depue & Morrone-Strupinsky, 2005) and its effect on trust behavior – implementing a between-subjects, double-blind, placebo-controlled design. Female participants (n = 95) were administered either naltrexone (i.e., mu opioid receptor [μ-OR] antagonist; 25 mg) or placebo orally and were assigned to one of two emotion-induction groups: WL or neutral emotion. Before and after the emotion induction (through personal memories and short film clips), they played as trustors in one-shot TGs with different unknown partners (whose photo appeared at the start of each trial) without receiving feedback per trial. Subsequently, participants completed a control game – a real-estate game apportioning money to buildings rather than people – to distinguish interpersonal trust from the mere risk-taking effects. Further, at different times during the session, participants provided ratings of several states of emotion (e.g., WL) and rated the trustworthiness of the various partners encountered in the TG. Frontal asymmetry (an EEG predictor of approach motivation/behavioral activation) was recorded during the initial rest period and emotion induction.

The findings indicated a significantly lower left-frontal asymmetry in WL compared to the neutral condition, supporting the assumption of a decreased approach motivation. Further, μ-OR blockade by naltrexone reduced induction of WL, and levels of self-report of WL decreased accordingly under naltrexone compared to placebo. Trust increased after administering of naltrexone under the neutral emotion-induction condition, but the same effect was observed for the decisions in the control game (i.e., real-estate game), indicating that the drug effect was likely targeting risk-taking rather than social risk (i.e., trust). Naltrexone further reduced trustworthiness because trustworthiness ratings were positively associated with trust decisions.

The impact of changes in opioidergic neurotransmission on the effects of WL – for self-report (i.e., WL rating) and behavioral (i.e., trust) measures – supports an association between opioid receptors activation and perceptions of interpersonal warmth and affection (Depue & Morrone-Strupinsky, 2005). Naltrexone inhibition of μ-ORs minimized the personal perception of WL and trust behavior caused by affiliative stimuli, indicating that μ-OR stimulation has a critical impact on social behaviors in humans besides animals (Depue & Morrone-Strupinsky, 2005; Nelson & Panksepp, 1998; Trezza et al., 2011). Whereas the "seeking-expectancy-wanting" system – mainly based on the mesolimbic dopamine system (Berridge & Robinson, 2003) – enables incentive-motivated actions (accompanied by wanting-expectancy), the "care-liking" system – primarily based on opioidergic rather than dopaminergic neuro-transmission in the vSTR (Berridge & Robinson, 2003) – encourages affiliation and caring to support the goal of attachment (accompanied by WL) (Depue & Morrone-Strupinsky, 2005), facilitated by the neuropeptide oxytocin (Depue & Morrone-Strupinsky, 2005; Nelson & Panksepp, 1998).

Opiates play a role in primate sociality (Depue & Morrone-Strupinsky, 2005; Nelson & Panksepp, 1998), and μ-ORs have been associated with feelings of interpersonal warmth and reduced incentive motivation for interpersonal relations (Depue & Morrone-Strupinsky, 2005). Nucleus accumbens μ-OR blockade prevents play-enhancing effects of opioid agonist morphine implementation, and morphine stimulation is necessary and sufficient to improve social play (Trezza et al., 2011). Finally, naltrex-one adversely affects animal mother–child attachment, implying that opiate activity is essential for social decision making (Panksepp, 2009). Since trust increased under naltrexone in the neutral emotion-induction condition and the same effect was observed for the decisions in the real-estate game (i.e., control game), the observed drug effect was likely target-ing risk-taking rather than trust. Of note, only young female participants in heterosexual relationships using oral contraceptives were tested, limiting the generalizability of these results.

Minocycline. Watabe and colleagues (2012) studied how minocycline works on human social decision making in a double-blind, randomized trial. Male healthy participants (n = 49) with college/university-level education were administered minocycline (100 mg) or placebo orally over four days before playing one-shot versions of the TG and the dictator game (DG, measuring generosity) (Kahneman et al., 1986) with two anonymous male partners. At pre-and post-treatment, participants completed a self-report general trust scale – measuring respondents' estimation of others' human trustworthiness (i.e., benevolence) (Yamagishi & Yamagishi, 1994).

Minocycline did not promote trusting behavior or more altruistic resource allocation. However, the more participants trusted others as measured by the general trust scale, the more trust behavior they displayed (but no more altruistic resource allocation) – depending on whether they received minocycline but not placebo. Minocycline contributed to more rational decision-making strategies, likely by increasing emotion regulation. Participants in the minocycline treatment took a more rational strategy (constructing their decision primarily on how much they generally trusted people), attending to the lack of information about the partner rather than to their fears about that lack of information being potentially exploited in a risky situation by their anonymous partners.

Minocycline has traditionally been used as a tetracycline antibiotic to treat various infectious diseases and has recently found a new use in the treatment of brain diseases (e.g., stroke, multiple sclerosis) and may have therapeutic potential in psychiatric diseases (Levkovitz et al., 2010; Munzar et al., 2002). Minocycline inhibits activation of microglia, that is, a glial cell type with immunological functions. Activated microglia release cytokines, free radicals, and neurotransmitters that contribute to homeostasis and brain pathologies, including neurodegenerative disorders and neuropathic pain (Block et al., 2007; Hanisch & Kettenmann, 2007). Further, microglial activation appears in the brains of patients with acute-phase schizophrenia (Doorduin et al., 2009; Van Berckel et al., 2008), methamphetamine users (Sekine et al., 2008), alcoholics (He & Crews, 2008; Wu et al., 2011), and patients that have completed suicide (Steiner et al., 2006, 2008). Moreover, animal studies demonstrated that stressors (e.g., physical pain, isolation) might induce microglial activation (Frank et al., 2007; Schiavone et al., 2009), leading to anxiety that can be minimized by minocycline (Neigh et al., 2009). Overall, the results may indicate that anxiety resulting from risk-taking in the TG may have been blunted by minocycline via inhibition of microglia.

It remains to be explained, however, whether not only microglial modulation but also other CNS effects – for example, interaction with brain glutamate and dopamine neurotransmission and potentiation of neurite outgrowth in neuronal cells leading to neuronal plasticity

(Hashimoto & Ishima, 2010) – could have been involved in the observed trust-related behavioral effects. In addition, a small sample size, male-specific interactions, and low dose-dependent effects may have affected the obtained results. Finally, although a DG (decomposing trust from altruism behavior) was utilized, the implementation of a lottery game (decomposing social risk [trust behavior] from general risk behavior) was lacking – reducing, therefore, the specificity of the administrated drug and its underlying neural effects.

Acetaminophen. Roberts et al. (2019) explored the impact of an over-the-counter drug acetaminophen (1,000 mg) (i.e., paracetamol [the active ingredient in Tylenol] known to be analgesic and antipyretic) on social and economic trust – utilizing a between-subjects, double-blind, and placebo-controlled design. Besides analyzing data from a national population-based survey, the authors conducted a series of laboratory experiments in which healthy female (n = 118) and male (n = 73) participants played multi-shot TGs as trustors with different anonymous partners without receiving any feedback on their decisions. In the first series of experiments, participants were not informed about their partner's past behavior (i.e., propensity-based trust) and had to say how much they would expect back from their partner (i.e., expected return) after making their trust decisions. In the second series of experiments, participants' expectations were manipulated by informing them about their partner's actual past behavior completing the same task as a trustee (i.e., impression-based trust).

The study found for the national community sample evidence that use of acetaminophen negatively correlated with neighborhood trust and feelings of social integration. Further, for the first series of TG experiments, acetaminophen decreased the influence of self-generated expectations on economic trust (i.e., investments) such that the association between expected return and investment was less on acetaminophen compared to placebo. Finally, a marginal effect of acetaminophen compared to placebo was found for the second series of TG experiments: Economic trust behavior increased when investors were informed regarding the trustee's prior reciprocity behavior with a different partner.

How can a negative association between the use of acetaminophen and neighborhood trust in the survey be explained, whereas in the second set of TG experiments, an immediate dose of acetaminophen improved behavioral trust? Because survey data is correlational, low levels of neighborhood trust could lead to greater illness or pain, which could increase acetaminophen consumption. Further, although the laboratory research used an immediate dosage of acetaminophen, the survey research assessed chronic usage – potentially leading to an adaptation in receptor density and to the decline in neighborhood trust. Finally, acetaminophen acutely administered enhanced trust behavior with partners expressly supposed to abuse that trust. Regular intake of acetaminophen may raise the risk of people misplacing trust in others, and increased experiences of treachery could eventually lead to a more distrustful view of the world.

Although acetaminophen's underlying molecular mechanisms are unknown, it can reduce extremes of emotion (Durso et al., 2015), distress about another person's physical and social misfortunes (Mischkowski et al., 2016), and distress related to social rejection (Dewall et al., 2010) – leading to a reduction of neural activation in regions of the SAN (e.g., AI) previously associated with physical, social pain (Dewall et al., 2010; Fung & Alden, 2017). One psychological mechanism of acetaminophen could be to influence general risk-taking behavior but not social risk (i.e., trust) behavior. The TG measures both general risk-taking behavior (related to a person's propensity to see risks) as well as social risk behavior (related to betrayal aversion toward the other partner) (Bohnet & Zeckhauser, 2004; Kosfeld et al., 2005). For the first series of TG experiments, acetaminophen dampens emotional processing and leads to higher risk but not trust behavior, which results in a mismatch of expected return and trust behavior. However, for the second series of TG experiments, knowing about the trustworthiness of the other partner reduced betrayal aversion plus general risk-taking due to acetaminophen, which leads to greater trust behavior compared to placebo. A diminished betrayal aversion would cause an overall increase in the invested amounts and, therefore, could explain the impact of acetaminophen in the second series of TG experiments. A recent coordinate-based meta-analysis on fMRI TG studies has associated the AI with betrayal aversion (Bellucci et al., 2017), and acetaminophen has been shown to dampen AI responses related to social pain (Dewall et al., 2010). However, since the study did not include a lottery game that controls general risk-taking behavior, the proposed mechanisms for the first and second series of TGs cannot be disentangled.

14.3.2 Combining a Trust Scale with Exchange Games and Administration of Pharmacological Agents

Two studies have examined the effect of MDMA (i.e., ecstasy, a releasing agent of monoamines) and risperidone (an atypical antipsychotic drug: a dopamine D2 and serotonin 5HT2A receptor antagonist with 5HT2 > D2 antagonist activity) versus trifluoperazine (a D1 and D2 antagonist) on trust by combining a trust scale with the performance of other exchange games, which can be completed in one- or multi-shot formats to measure cooperative behavior as a precursor of trust.

MDMA. Gabay et al. (2019) combined a prisoner's dilemma game (PDG) (Flood, 1952) measuring cooperation with fMRI to study the neurobehavioral effects of MDMA (100 g) (often used for neuroenhancement and as a party drug) on cooperation and trust by implementing a double-blind, placebo-controlled, crossover study. While being scanned, healthy male participants (n = 21) played repeated rounds of the PDG game (with real monetary consequences) with the same partners (referred to by the first name but not by the picture) – choosing to compete or cooperate and to rate their trust in each other player on each iteration – under three partner conditions: trustworthy partner (mostly cooperative), untrustworthy partner (mostly uncooperative), and computer partner (control condition).

The results showed MDMA's context-specific modification of cooperative behavior. MDMA improved cooperation with trustworthy but not untrustworthy or nonsocial control opponents – mirrored by evaluated activity in brain regions commonly linked with social interactions after feedback about the trustworthy opponent's decisions. Trust ratings were greater for the trustworthy compared to the untrustworthy partner (or computer control); however, no effect of the drug on trust or drug by partner condition interaction was observed. At the neural level, an interaction between MDMA treatment and opponent type was identified during the trust rating phase: When dealing with trustworthy opponents, the dorsal caudate showed increased activity on MDMA in comparison to placebo. The activity of the dorsal caudate has been interpreted as a reward signal when receiving feedback of reciprocal cooperation (King-Casas et al., 2005; Rilling et al., 2002) and associated with developing a model of partner reputation through signaling an "intention to trust" (King-Casas et al., 2005). When considering trust in trustworthy but not untrustworthy opponents, higher activity of this brain region on MDMA might reflect a greater subjective reward from this evaluation – leading to a stronger building of reputation and greater future cooperation.

MDMA induces a transition in social relations and assessment of others' actions – culminating in greater cooperation with trustworthy partners despite being betrayed. Immediate use of ecstasy is linked with both increased face trustworthiness ratings and cooperative behaviors measured with monetary exchange games gauging cooperation (e.g., DG [as proposer], ultimatum game [as proposer]) (Stewart et al., 2014). Further, MDMA enhances empathy for positively valenced stimuli and reduces accuracy of identifying negative facial emotions as well as produces subjective "empathogenic" effects such as trust, closeness to others, openness, and drug liking as well as increased plasma levels of oxytocin and prolactin (Schmid et al., 2014). Finally, MDMA enhances prosocial feelings such as increased subjective ratings of friendliness, closeness, openness, and understanding toward others (Bedi et al., 2010; Cami et al., 2000; Kolbrich et al., 2008; Liechti et al., 2000; Tancer & Johanson, 2003) – which likely contributes to the high popularity of ecstasy and its use for psychotherapy (Mithoefer et al., 2011; Oehen et al., 2013).

The neuropharmacological mechanisms of MDMA are mixed, including not only an increase of oxytocin levels but also synaptic availability of DA, NA, and serotonin (5-HT stimulation) (de la Torre et al., 2004). Among MDMA's multiple neurotransmitter actions, its serotonergic effects are far larger than those of DA and NA and are thought to produce its major neuropsychological consequences (Carhart-Harris & Nutt, 2017) that are primarily responsible for its social and euphoric effects (Kuypers et al., 2014; Rudnick & Wall, 1992). MDMA acts as a substrate for the serotonin-transporter – causing serotonin to be released by nerve terminals and preventing its reuptake (Schmidt et al., 1986). Overall, increased serotonin function is associated with prosocial and affiliative behaviors and reduced serotonin function with antisocial and aggressive behaviors (Young et al., 2001). Moreover, MDMA elevates levels of oxytocin (Wolff et al., 2006), which is thought to mediate the prosocial effects of MDMA (Thompson et al., 2007). Oxytocin is known to induce the release of serotonin, which consecutively increases the availability of the serotonin 1A receptor in key brain areas (e.g., amygdala, insula) for social behavior (Lefevre et al., 2017). Oxytocin's links to social bonding, attachment, and trust have been observed in humans (Dumont et al., 2009; Heinrichs et al., 2003; Kosfeld et al., 2005) (see also Chapter 13).

However, the specific effects of MDMA across these different mechanisms cannot be disentangled within this study. Without blocking serotonin and other target receptors, the effects of MDMA cannot be causally assigned to particular receptor subtypes. Another drawback of this study is the use of an inactive placebo because participants are conscious of whether they have been administered psychedelic and dissociative drugs. Finally, only male participants were enrolled, but psychopharmacological investigations are especially susceptible to hormonal variations among participants. However, gender variations were found in MDMA's subjective effects (Allott & Redman, 2007), and the reported findings may not be universal between genders, whereas single-sex studies have more power to detect a given effect.

Antipsychotic Drugs. Tse et al. (2016) used an interactive puzzle game without monetary incentives to investigate how social interactions improve social functioning through contrasting schizophrenic patients undergoing atypical (i.e., risperidone) with standard (i.e., trifluoperazine) antipsychotic treatments. Schizophrenic patients (n = 24) first completed measures about positive and negative symptoms as well as executive and social functioning. Then, patients within groups (risperidone-treated, trifluoperazine-treated) were paired up to play the interactive tangrams game, that is, a standardized dyadic puzzle task that required the formation of as many as possible given target shapes within a time limit (Knutson et al., 1998). Finally, participants completed ratings to measure interpersonal trust (Johnson-George & Swap, 1982) and rejection (Coyne, 1976) toward their game partners.

The results revealed that patients receiving risperidone (an atypical antipsychotic treatment) compared to trifluoperazine (a typical antipsychotic treatment) demonstrated significant improvement in overall symptom levels, executive functioning, social support, social engagement, cooperative behavior, and trust toward a stranger game partner – independently of various potential confounding factors (e.g., age, drug dosage differences, years of medication received) and without affecting basic personality dimensions, affiliative index, or social rejection. Lower affiliative behavior was associated with positive symptoms, and interpersonal trust affected social engagement, although executive functioning did not explain lower interpersonal trust or social disengagement.

Enhancing social competence with risperidone may be linked to the improvement of social behaviors, interpersonal trust, and symptoms. Studies of psychopharmacological mechanisms have proposed that antipsychotics can not only treat distressing symptoms but can also improve affiliative behaviors by the enhancement of interpersonal trust via an alternative route. Atypical antipsychotic treatment – blocking the serotonin ($5HT2A$) receptor site, lowering the transmission of $5HT2A$ receptor – increases the gene expression of oxytocin, which has been associated with the enhancement of social cognition and affiliation, including interpersonal trust (Keri et al., 2009). Previous research has shown that the

5HT2A receptor gene is linked to cooperative behaviors (Schroeder et al., 2013). Moreover, the atypical antipsychotic treatment effectively reduces aggressive behavior (Gerretsen et al., 2010), improves social competence in patients with schizophrenia (Harvey et al., 2006), and enhances prosocial behavior in children with disruptive behavior and sub-average IQ (Snyder et al., 2002). However, no randomized placebo-controlled study design was implemented – new patients were likely to receive typical compared to atypical antipsychotic treatments due to an improved side-effect profile – that potentially could result in confounding variables such as a placebo effect.

14.4 Summary and Future Directions

We reviewed a group of methodologically and pharmacologically diverse small studies either employing the TG as an objective measure of trusting behavior or exchange games combined with a trust scale. Overall, some preliminary evidence exists that the modulation of the opiate, serotonergic, and dopaminergic systems impacts trust behavior as measured by paradigms that have face validity as laboratory measures of trust. However, many essential questions on how neuromodulators impact trust remain. First, what is the mechanism by which these pharmacologic agents change trust behavior? What psychological constructs are they acting on as they do change estimations of trustworthiness? Further, what is the interaction between these pharmacologic agents and context? How do these pharmacologic agents modulate trust behavior in the context of, for example, a paradigm that models trust propensity versus trust dynamics?

Beyond external beliefs of whether a partner is trustworthy, internal beliefs about expectation of reciprocity also affect trusting behavior (Fairley et al., 2019). This could also be a nidus for exploration if changing beliefs about one's own trustworthiness can modulate reward processing and prime the system to change trust behavior with or without pharmacologic intervention. Future research is needed to resolve those questions considering the limitations listed for each reviewed study.

An advantage of using pharmacological manipulations to study the neurobiology of trust is that such manipulations can establish causal mechanisms – as long as the experiment is designed properly. In addition to implementing a double-blind, placebo-controlled design, a positive control such as a second pharmacological agent ideally should be added to control for side effects related to the drug of interest. Even if the difference between drug and placebo can be distinguished (potentially due to physical side effects), some degree of blindness can be maintained as long as no distinction between experimental treatment and positive control is possible.

Larger and more heterogeneous samples, including both females and males, need to replicate previous findings. When possible, within-subjects designs should be applied because genetic polymorphisms that influence the signaling properties within neuromodulator systems (e.g., the function of specific types of neuromodulator receptors) could create potentially large variation between individuals in terms of their physiological response to pharmacological treatment. When using a between-subjects design, experimental and placebo groups should be matched not only on characteristics such as sex, age, and education but also on personality traits and genetic polymorphisms relevant to the neuromodulator system under study. Moreover, it may be more fruitful to use patient populations where trust behavior is altered (e.g., posttraumatic stress disorder, borderline personality disorder, autism spectrum disorder). In these populations, the effect of these pharmacologic agents may be more apparent (Robson et al., 2020) (see also Chapters 16 and 17).

A more ecological measure of the drug effect on trust behavior would be repeated dosing (instead of a single dose of the drug) to steady-state followed by administration of the laboratory measures. Collecting blood samples to measure plasma levels of the drug can serve as important covariates in behavioral and neuroimaging analyses. In addition, collecting subjective beliefs at the end of the experiment, such as treatment received, the veracity of the experimental set-up, engagement with the task, and desire to please experimenters, allows controlling for possible neuromodulator effects on these measures. Since pharmacological manipulations can have physical side effects or influence mood, subjective rating scales (e.g., Visual Analogue Scales [Bond & Lader, 1974]; Positive and Negative Affect Scales [Watson et al., 1988]) are useful tools to assess the causal effects of neuromodulators on subjective feelings (e.g., alertness, anxiety, nausea), which can be included as regressors of no interest in statistical models.

Trust behavior is a complex contruct comprised of several basic motivational, affective, and cognitive processes. Each of these may be sensitive to the pharmacologic agent itself. Therefore, it is essential to include experimental conditions to control for these processes. In particular, studies should include the lottery game for controlling general risk-taking behavior. However, evidence has shown that besides measuring aspects of social risk behavior (trust) and general risk behavior, the TG also measures aspects of altruistic behavior. Therefore, a two-player DG (Kahneman et al., 1986) – that is, the first player (i.e., dictator) is given an endowment and can unilaterally decide how much from this money to give to the second player (i.e., receiver) – can be utilized to decompose trust from altruism (Cox, 2004). Another obstacle is taking control of basic motivational processes, which can be impacted by the neuromodulator of investigation. In the TG, monetary reward is confounded with the social factor trust because neuro-modulators (e.g., serotonin and dopamine) impact the encoding of rewards (Jocham et al., 2011; Seymour et al., 2012). Accordingly, a transposition to a nonmonetary TG would be helpful in future research.

Finally, it is simple to investigate how drug therapies modify behavior and brain hemodynamic responses; however, these measures reflect the downstream effects of the changes in neurotransmission at the molecular level. Future studies should combine pharmacological manipulations with positron emission tomography, fMRI, and behavioral measurements to link the drug treatment to changes in endogenous neurotransmitter synthesis and release, to changes in neural activity, and to changes in behavior (Martinez et al., 2003; Selvaraj et al., 2012). The integration of pharmacological manipulations with neuroimaging will ease the identification of the brain networks that are causally involved in producing trust behavior. As systems social neuroscience progresses, it will become imperative to combine those methods that allow inferences about cause and effect not only for cross-sectional but also longitudinal drug studies – potentially leading the current research toward an innovative path of investigations aiming at unrevealing the psychoneurobiological underpinnings of trust.

References

Aimone, J. A., Houser, D., & Weber, B. (2014). Neural signatures of betrayal aversion: An fMRI study of trust. *Proceedings: Biological Sciences*, 281(1782), Article 20132127. https://doi.org/10.1098/rspb.2013.2127

Alarcon, G. M., Lyons, J. B., Christensen, J. C., et al. (2018). The effect of propensity to trust and perceptions of trustworthiness on trust behaviors in dyads. *Behavioral Research Methods*, 50(5), 1906–1920. https://doi.org/10.3758/s13428-017-0959-6

Allott, K., & Redman, J. (2007). Are there sex differences associated with the effects of ecstasy/3,4-methylenedioxymethamphetamine (MDMA)? *Neuroscience & Biobehavioral Reviews*, 31(3), 327–347. https://doi.org/10.1016/j.neubiorev.2006.09.009

Baumeister, R. F., & Leary, M. R. (1995). The need to belong: Desire for interpersonal attachments as a fundamental human motivation.

Psychological Bulletin, 117(3), 497–529. https://doi.org/10.1037/0033-2909.117.3.497

Baumgartner, T., Heinrichs, M., Vonlanthen, A., Fischbacher, U., & Fehr, E. (2008). Oxytocin shapes the neural circuitry of trust and trust adaptation in humans. *Neuron*, 58(4), 639–650. https://doi.org/10.1016/j.neuron.2008.04.009

Bedi, G., Hyman, D., & de Wit, H. (2010). Is ecstasy an "empathogen"? Effects of +/-3,4-methylenedioxymethamphetamine on prosocial feelings and identification of emotional states in others. *Biological Psychiatry*, 68(12), 1134–1140. https://doi.org/10.1016/j.biopsych.2010.08.003

Belfi, A. M., Koscik, T. R., & Tranel, D. (2015). Damage to the insula is associated with abnormal interpersonal trust. *Neuropsychologia*, 71, 165–172. https://doi.org/10.1016/j.neuropsychologia.2015.04.003

Bellucci, G., Chernyak, S. V., Goodyear, K., Eickhoff, S. B., & Krueger, F. (2017). Neural signatures of trust in reciprocity: A coordinate-based meta-analysis. *Human Brain Mapping*, 38(3), 1233–1248. https://doi.org/10.1002/hbm.23451

Bellucci, G., Feng, C., Camilleri, J., Eickhoff, S. B., & Krueger, F. (2018). The role of the anterior insula in social norm compliance and enforcement: Evidence from coordinate-based and functional connectivity meta-analyses. *Neuroscience & Biobehavoral Reviews*, 92, 378–389. https://doi.org/10.1016/j.neubiorev.2018.06.024

Bellucci, G., Munte, T. F., & Park, S. Q. (2020). Effects of a dopamine against on trusting behaviors in females. *Psychopharmacology (Berl)*, 237(6), 1671–1680. https://doi.org/10.1007/s00213-020-05488-x

Berg, J., Dickhaut, J., & McCabe, K. (1995). Trust, reciprocity, and social history. *Games and Economic Behavior*, 10(1), 122–142. https://doi.org/10.1006/game.1995.1027

Berridge, K. C., & Robinson, T. E. (2003). Parsing reward. *Trends in Neuroscience*, 26(9), 507–513. https://doi.org/10.1016/s0166-2236(03)00233-9

Block, M. L., Zecca, L., & Hong, J. S. (2007). Microglia-mediated neurotoxicity: Uncovering the molecular mechanisms. *Nature Reviews Neuroscience*, 8(1), 57–69. https://doi.org/10.1038/nrn2038

Bodi, N., Keri, S., Nagy, H., et al. (2009). Reward-learning and the novelty-seeking personality: A between- and within-subjects study of the effects of dopamine agonists on young Parkinson's patients. *Brain*, 132(Pt 9), 2385–2395. https://doi.org/10.1093/brain/awp094

Bohnet, I., Greig, F., Herrmann, B., & Zeckhauser, R. (2008). Betrayal aversion: Evidence from Brazil, China, Oman, Switzerland, Turkey, and the United States. *American Economic Review*, 98(1), 294–310. https://doi.org/10.1257/aer.98.1.294

Bohnet, I., & Zeckhauser, R. (2004). Trust, risk and betrayal. *Journal of Economic Behavior & Organization*, 55(4), 467–484. https://doi.org/10.1016/j.jebo.2003.11.004

Bond, A., & Lader, M. (1974). The use of analogue scales in rating subjective feelings. *British Journal of Medical Psychology*, 47, 211–218. https://doi.org/10.1111/j.2044-8341.1974.tb02285.x

Bonnefon, J. F., Hopfensitz, A., & De Neys, W. (2013). The modular nature of trustworthiness detection. *Journal of Experimental Psychology: General*, 142(1), 143–150. https://doi.org/10.1037/a0028930

Burnham, T., McCabe, K., & Smith, V. L. (2000). Friend-or-foe intentionality priming in an extensive form trust game. *Journal of Economic Behavior & Organization*, 43(1), 57–73. https://doi.org/10.1016/s0167–2681(00)00108-6

Caceda, R., Moskovciak, T., Prendes-Alvarez, S., et al. (2014). Gender-specific effects of depression and suicidal ideation in prosocial behaviors. *PLoS ONE*, 9(9), Article e108733. https://doi.org/10.1371/journal.pone.0108733

Cacioppo, J. T., Norris, C. J., Decety, J., Monteleone, G., & Nusbaum, H. (2009). In the eye of the beholder: Individual differences in perceived social isolation predict regional brain activation to social stimuli. *Journal of Cognitive Neuroscience*, 21(1), 83–92. https://doi.org/10.1162/jocn.2009.21007

Camerer, C. F. (2003). Behavioural studies of strategic thinking in games. *Trends in Cognitive Sciences*, 7(5), 225–231. https://doi.org/10.1016/S1364–6613(03)00094-9

Cami, J., Farre, M., Mas, M., et al. (2000). Human pharmacology of 3,4-methylenedioxymethamphetamine ("ecstasy"): Psychomotor performance and subjective effects. *Journal of Clinical Psychopharmacology*, 20(4), 455–466. https://doi.org/10.1097/00004714-200008000-00010

Campbell-Meiklejohn, D. K., Simonsen, A., Jensen, M., et al. (2012). Modulation of social influence by methylphenidate. *Neuropsychopharmacology*, 37(6), 1517–1525. https://doi.org/10.1038/npp.2011.337

Campbell-Meiklejohn, D., Simonsen, A., Scheel-Kruger, J., et al. (2012). In for a penny, in for a pound: Methylphenidate reduces the inhibitory effect of high stakes on persistent risky choice. *Journal of Neuroscience*, 32(38), 13032–13038. https://doi.org/10.1523/jneurosci.0151-12.2012

Carhart-Harris, R. L., & Nutt, D. J. (2017). Serotonin and brain function: A tale of two receptors. *Journal of Psychopharmacology*, 31(9), 1091–1120. https://doi.org/10.1177/0269881117725915

Chang, L. J., Doll, B. B., Van 't Wout, M., Frank, M. J., & Sanfey, A. G. (2010). Seeing is believing: Trustworthiness as a dynamic belief. *Cognitive Psychology*, 61(2), 87–105. https://doi.org/10.1016/j.cogpsych.2010.03.001

Collins, A. G., & Frank, M. J. (2013). Cognitive control over learning: Creating, clustering, and generalizing task-set structure. *Psychological Review*, 120(1), 190–229. https://doi.org/10.1037/a0030852

Cox, J. C. (2004). How to identify trust and reciprocity. *Games and Economic Behavior*, 46(2), 260–281. https://doi.org/10.1016/s0899–8256(03)00119-2

Coyne, J. (1976). Depression and the response of others. *Journal of Abnormal Psychology*, 85, 186–193. https://doi.org/10.1037/0021-843x.85.2.186

Crockett, M. J., & Fehr, E. (2014). Pharmacology of economic and social decision making. In P. W. Glimcher & E. Fehr (Eds.), *Neuroeconomics* (2nd ed., pp. 259–279). Academic Press.

de la Torre, R., Farre, M., Roset, P. N., et al. (2004). Human pharmacology of MDMA: Pharmacokinetics, metabolism, and disposition. *Therapeutic Drug Monitoring*, 26(2), 137–144. https://doi.org/10.1097/00007691-200404000-00009

Delgado, M. R., Frank, R. H., & Phelps, E. A. (2005). Perceptions of moral character modulate the neural systems of reward during the trust game. *Nature Neuroscience*, 8(11), 1611–1618. https://doi.org/10.1038/nn1575

Depue, R. A., & Morrone-Strupinsky, J. V. (2005). A neurobehavioral model of affiliative bonding: Implications for conceptualizing a human trait of affiliation. *Behavioral and Brain Sciences*, 28(3), 313–350; discussion 350–395. https://doi.org/10.1017/s0140525x05000063

DeVito, E. E., Blackwell, A. D., Kent, L., et al. (2008). The effects of methylphenidate on decision making in attention-deficit/hyperactivity disorder. *Biological Psychiatry*, 64(7), 636–639. https://doi.org/10.1016/j.biopsych.2008.04.017

Dewall, C. N., Macdonald, G., Webster, G. D., et al. (2010). Acetaminophen reduces social pain: Behavioral and neural evidence. *Psychological Science*, 21(7), 931–937. https://doi.org/10.1177/0956797610374741

Doorduin, J., de Vries, E. F., Willemsen, A. T., de Groot, J. C., Dierckx, R. A., & Klein, H. C. (2009). Neuroinflammation in schizophrenia-related psychosis: A PET study. *Journal of Nuclear Medicine*, 50(11), 1801–1807. https://doi.org/10.2967/jnumed.109.066647

Dumont, G. J., Sweep, F. C., Van der Steen, R., et al. (2009). Increased oxytocin concentrations and prosocial feelings in humans after ecstasy (3,4-methylenedioxymethamphetamine) administration. *Social Neuroscience*, 4(4), 359–366. https://doi.org/10.1080/17470910802649470

Durso, G. R., Luttrell, A., & Way, B. M. (2015). Over-the-counter relief from pains and pleasures alike: Acetaminophen blunts evaluation sensitivity to both negative and positive stimuli. *Psychological Science*, 26(6), 750–758. https://doi.org/10.1177/0956797615570366

Fairley, K., Vyrastekova, J., Weitzel, U., & Sanfey, A. G. (2019). Subjective beliefs about trust and reciprocity activate an expected reward signal in the ventral striatum. *Frontiers in Neuroscience*, 13, Article 660. https://doi.org/10.3389/fnins.2019.00660

Fareri, D. S., Chang, L. J., & Delgado, M. R. (2012). Effects of direct social experience on trust decisions and neural reward circuitry. *Frontiers in Neuroscience*, 6, Article 148. https://doi.org/10.3389/fnins.2012.00148

Fehr, E. (2009). On the economics and biology of trust. *Journal of the European Economic Association*, 7(2–3), 235–266. https://doi.org/10.1162/jeea.2009.7.2-3.235

Fernandez-Theoduloz, G., Paz, V., Nicolaisen-Sobesky, E., et al. (2019). Social avoidance in depression: A study using a social decision making task. *Journal of Abnormal Psychology*, 128(3), 234–244. https://doi.org/10.1037/abn0000415

Fett, A. K., Shergill, S. S., Joyce, D. W., et al. (2012). To trust or not to trust: The dynamics of social interaction in psychosis. *Brain*, 135(Pt 3), 976–984. https://doi.org/10.1093/brain/awr359

Flood, M. M. (1952). *Some experimental games: Research memorandum RM-789*. RAND Corporation.

Fouragnan, E., Chierchia, G., Greiner, S., Neveu, R., Avesani, P., & Coricelli, G. (2013). Reputational priors magnify striatal responses to violations of trust. *Journal of Neuroscience*, 33(8), 3602–3611. https://doi.org/10.1523/jneurosci.3086-12.2013

Frank, M. G., Baratta, M. V., Sprunger, D. B., Watkins, L. R., & Maier, S. F. (2007). Microglia serve as a neuroimmune substrate for stress-induced potentiation of CNS pro-inflammatory cytokine responses. *Brain, Behavior, and Immunity*, 21(1), 47–59. https://doi.org/10.1016/j.bbi.2006.03.005

Frank, M. J., Seeberger, L. C., & O'Reilly R. C. (2004). By carrot or by stick: Cognitive reinforcement learning in parkinsonism. *Science*, 306(5703), 1940–1943. https://doi.org/10.1126/science.1102941

Fu, C., Yao, X., Yang, X., Zheng, L., Li, J., & Wang, Y. (2019). Trust game database: Behavioral and EEG data from two trust games. *Frontiers in Psychology*, 10, Article 2656. https://doi.org/10.3389/fpsyg.2019.02656

Fung, K., & Alden, L. E. (2017). Once hurt, twice shy: Social pain contributes to social anxiety. *Emotion*, 17(2), 231–239. https://doi.org/10.1037/emo0000223

Gabay, A. S., Kempton, M. J., Gilleen, J., & Mehta, M. A. (2019). MDMA increases cooperation and recruitment of social brain areas when playing trustworthy players in an iterated prisoner's dilemma. *Journal of Neuroscience*, 39(2), 307–320. https://doi.org/10.1523/jneurosci.1276-18.2018

Gerretsen, P., Graff-Guerrero, A., Menon, M., et al. (2010). Is desire for social relationships mediated by the serotonergic system in the prefrontal cortex? An [(18)F]setoperone PET study. *Social Neuroscience*, 5(4), 375–383. https://doi.org/10.1080/17470911003589309

Gurevich, E. V., & Joyce, J. N. (1999). Distribution of dopamine D3 receptor expressing neurons in the human forebrain: Comparison with D2 receptor expressing neurons. *Neuropsychopharmacology*, 20(1), 60–80. https://doi.org/10.1016/s0893-133x(98)00066-9

Hahn, T., Notebaert, K., Anderl, C., Teckentrup, V., Kassecker, A., & Windmann, S. (2015). How to trust a perfect stranger: Predicting initial trust behavior from resting-state brain-electrical connectivity. *Social Cognitive and Affective Neuroscience*, 10(6), 809–813. https://doi.org/10.1093/scan/nsu122

Hall, H., Halldin, C., Dijkkstra, D., et al. (1996). Autoradiographic localisation of D 3 - dopamine receptors in the human brain using the selective D 3 -

dopamine receptor agonist (+)-[3] PD 128907. *Psychopharmacology*, 128, 240–247. https://doi.org/10.1007/s002130050131

Hanisch, U. K., & Kettenmann, H. (2007). Microglia: Active sensor and versatile effector cells in the normal and pathologic brain. *Nature Neuroscience*, 10 (11), 1387–1394. https://doi.org/10.1038/nn1997

Harvey, P. D., Patterson, T. L., Potter, L. S., Zhong, K., & Brecher, M. (2006). Improvement in social competence with short-term atypical antipsychotic treatment: A randomized, double-blind comparison of quetiapine versus risperidone for social competence, social cognition, and neuropsychological functioning. *American Journal of Psychiatry*, 163(11), 1918–1925. https://doi .org/10.1176/ajp.2006.163.11.1918

Hashimoto, K., & Ishima, T. (2010). A novel target of action of minocycline in NGF-induced neurite outgrowth in PC12 cells: Translation initiation [corrected] factor eIF4AI. *PLoS ONE*, 5(11), Article e15430. https://doi.org/10 .1371/journal.pone.0015430

He, J., & Crews, F. T. (2008). Increased MCP-1 and microglia in various regions of the human alcoholic brain. *Experimental Neurology*, 210(2), 349–358. https://doi.org/10.1016/j.expneurol.2007.11.017

Heinrichs, M., Baumgartner, T., Kirschbaum, C., & Ehlert, U. (2003). Social support and oxytocin interact to suppress cortisol and subjective responses to psychosocial stress. *Biological Psychiatry*, 54(12), 1389–1398. https://doi.org/ 10.1016/s0006-3223(03)00465-7

Hysek, C. M., Simmler, L. D., Schillinger, N., et al. (2014). Pharmacokinetic and pharmacodynamic effects of methylphenidate and MDMA administered alone or in combination. *International Journal of Neuropsychopharmacology*, 17(3), 371–381. https://doi.org/10.1017/S1461145713001132

Ishibashi, K., Ishii, K., Oda, K., Mizusawa, H., & Ishiwata, K. (2011). Binding of pramipexole to extrastriatal dopamine D2/D3 receptors in the human brain: A positron emission tomography study using 11C-FLB 457. *PLoS ONE*, 6 (3), Article e17723. https://doi.org/10.1371/journal.pone.0017723

Jocham, G., Klein, T. A., & Ullsperger, M. (2011). Dopamine-mediated reinforcement learning signals in the striatum and ventromedial prefrontal cortex underlie value-based choices. *Journal of Neuroscience*, 31(5), 1606–1613. https://doi.org/10.1523/jneurosci.3904-10.2011

Johnson, N. D., & Mislin, A. A. (2011). Trust games: A meta-analysis. *Journal of Economic Psychology*, 32(5), 865–889. https://doi.org/10.1016/j.joep.2011.05.007

Johnson-George, C., & Swap, W. C. (1982). Measurement of specific interpersonal trust: Construction and validation of a scale to assess trust in a specific other. *Journal of Personality and Social Psychology*, 43(6), 1306–1317. https:// doi.org/10.1037/0022-3514.43.6.1306

Kahneman, D., Knetsch, J. L., & Thaler, R. H. (1986). Fairness and the assumptions of economics. *Journal of Business*, 59(4), S285–S300. https:// doi.org/10.2307/2352761

Keri, S., Kiss, I., & Kelemen, O. (2009). Sharing secrets: Oxytocin and trust in schizophrenia. *Social Neuroscience*, 4(4), 287–293. https://doi.org/10.1080/ 17470910802319710

King-Casas, B., Tomlin, D., Anen, C., Camerer, C. F., Quartz, S. R., & Montague, P. R. (2005). Getting to know you: Reputation and trust in a two-person economic exchange. *Science*, 308(5718), 78–83. https://doi.org/10.1126/science.1108062

Knutson, B., Taylor, J., Kaufman, M., Peterson, R., & Glover, G. (2005). Distributed neural representation of expected value. *Journal of Neuroscience*, 25(19), 4806–4812. https://doi.org/10.1523/jneurosci.0642-05.2005

Knutson, B., Wolkowitz, O. M., Cole, S. W., et al. (1998). Selective alteration of personality and social behavior by serotonergic intervention. *American Journal of Psychiatry*, 155(3), 373–379. https://doi.org/10.1176/ajp.155.3.373

Kolbrich, E. A., Goodwin, R. S., Gorelick, D. A., Hayes, R. J., Stein, E. A., & Huestis, M. A. (2008). Plasma pharmacokinetics of 3,4-methylenedioxymethamphetamine after controlled oral administration to young adults. *Therapeutic Drug Monitoring*, 30(3), 320–332. https://doi.org/10.1097/ftd.0b013e3181684fa0

Koscik, T. R., & Tranel, D. (2011). The human amygdala is necessary for developing and expressing normal interpersonal trust. *Neuropsychologia*, 49(4), 602–611. https://doi.org/10.1016/j.neuropsychologia.2010.09.023

Kosfeld, M., Heinrichs, M., Zak, P. J., Fischbacher, U., & Fehr, E. (2005). Oxytocin increases trust in humans. *Nature*, 435(7042), 673–676. https://doi.org/10.1038/nature03701

Krueger, F., McCabe, K., Moll, J., et al. (2007). Neural correlates of trust. *Proceedings of the National Academy of Sciences USA*, 104(50), 20084–20089. https://doi.org/10.1073/pnas.0710103104

Krueger, F., & Meyer-Lindenberg, A. (2019). Toward a model of interpersonal trust drawn from neuroscience, psychology, and economics. *Trends in Neuroscience*, 42(2), 92–101. https://doi.org/10.1016/j.tins.2018.10.004

Kuypers, K. P., de la Torre, R., Farre, M., et al. (2014). No evidence that MDMA-induced enhancement of emotional empathy is related to peripheral oxytocin levels or 5-HT1a receptor activation. *PLoS ONE*, 9(6), Article e100719. https://doi.org/10.1371/journal.pone.0100719

Lefevre, A., Richard, N., Jazayeri, M., et al. (2017). Oxytocin and serotonin brain mechanisms in the nonhuman primate. *Journal of Neuroscience*, 37(28), 6741–6750. https://doi.org/10.1523/jneurosci.0659-17.2017

Levkovitz, Y., Mendlovich, S., Riwkes, S., et al. (2010). A double-blind, randomized study of minocycline for the treatment of negative and cognitive symptoms in early-phase schizophrenia. *Journal of Clinical Psychiatry*, 71(2), 138–149. https://doi.org/10.4088/jcp.08m04666yel

Lewicki, R., & Bunker, B. (1995). Trust in relationships. *Administrative Science Quarterly*, 5(1), 583–601. https://doi.org/10.2307/259288

Liechti, M. E., Baumann, C., Gamma, A., & Vollenweider, F. X. (2000). Acute psychological effects of 3,4-methylenedioxymethamphetamine (MDMA, "ecstasy") are attenuated by the serotonin uptake inhibitor citalopram.

Neuropsychopharmacology, 22(5), 513–521. https://doi.org/10.1016/S0893-133x(99)00148-7

Maoz, H., Tsviban, L., Gvirts, H. Z., et al. (2014). Stimulants improve theory of mind in children with attention deficit/hyperactivity disorder. *Journal of Psychopharmacology*, 28(3), 212–219. https://doi.org/10.1177/0269881113492030

Martinez, D., Slifstein, M., Broft, A., et al. (2003). Imaging human mesolimbic dopamine transmission with positron emission tomography. Part II: amphetamine-induced dopamine release in the functional subdivisions of the striatum. *Journal of Cerebral Blood Flow & Metabolism*, 23(3), 285–300. https://doi.org/10.1097/01.wcb.0000048520.34839.1a

Mayer, R. C., Davis, J. H., & Schoorman, F. D. (1995). An integrative model of organizational trust. *Academy of Management Review*, 20(3), 709–734. https://doi.org/10.2307/258792

McKnight, D., Cummings, L., & Chervany, N. (1998). Initial trust formation in new organizational relationships. *Academy of Management Review*, 23, 473–490. https://doi.org/10.2307/259290

Mischkowski, D., Crocker, J., & Way, B. M. (2016). From painkiller to empathy killer: Acetaminophen (paracetamol) reduces empathy for pain. *Social, Cognitive and Affective Neuroscience*, 11(9), 1345–1353. https://doi.org/10.1093/scan/nsw057

Mithoefer, M. C., Wagner, M. T., Mithoefer, A. T., Jerome, L., & Doblin, R. (2011). The safety and efficacy of {+/-}3,4-methylenedioxymethamphetamine-assisted psychotherapy in subjects with chronic, treatment-resistant posttraumatic stress disorder: The first randomized controlled pilot study. *Journal of Psychopharmacology*, 25(4), 439–452. https://doi.org/10.1177/0269881110378371

Moretto, G., Sellitto, M., & di Pellegrino, G. (2013). Investment and repayment in a trust game after ventromedial prefrontal damage. *Frontiers in Human Neuroscience*, 7, Article 593. https://doi.org/10.3389/fnhum.2013.00593

Munro, C. A., McCaul, M. E., Wong, D. F., et al. (2006). Sex differences in striatal dopamine release in healthy adults. *Biological Psychiatry*, 59(10), 966–974. https://doi.org/10.1016/j.biopsych.2006.01.008

Munzar, P., Li, H., Nicholson, K. L., Wiley, J. L., & Balster, R. L. (2002). Enhancement of the discriminative stimulus effects of phencyclidine by the tetracycline antibiotics doxycycline and minocycline in rats. *Psychopharmacology (Berl)*, 160(3), 331–336. https://doi.org/10.1007/s00213-001-0989-7

Murray, A. M., Ryoo, H. L., Gurevich, E., & Joyce, J. N. (1994). Localization of dopamine D3 receptors to mesolimbic and D2 receptors to mesostriatal regions of human forebrain. *Proceedings of the National Academy of Sciences USA*, 91(23), 11271–11275. https://doi.org/10.1073/pnas.91.23.11271

Neigh, G. N., Karelina, K., Glasper, E. R., et al. (2009). Anxiety after cardiac arrest/cardiopulmonary resuscitation: Exacerbated by stress and prevented by minocycline. *Stroke*, 40(11), 3601–3607. https://doi.org/10.1161/strokeaha.109.564146

Nelson, E. E., & Panksepp, J. (1998). Brain substrates of infant-mother attachment: Contributions of opioids, oxytocin, and norepinephrine. *Neuroscience & Biobehavioral Reviews*, 22(3), 437–452. https://doi.org/10.1016/s0149-7634(97)00052-3

Oehen, P., Traber, R., Widmer, V., & Schnyder, U. (2013). A randomized, controlled pilot study of MDMA (+/- 3,4-Methylenedioxymethamphetamine)-assisted psychotherapy for treatment of resistant, chronic post-traumatic stress disorder (PTSD). *Journal of Psychopharmacology*, 27(1), 40–52. https://doi.org/10.1177/0269881112464827

Panksepp, J. (2009). *Affective neuroscience*. Oxford University Press.

Pessiglione, M., Seymour, B., Flandin, G., Dolan, R. J., & Frith, C. D. (2006). Dopamine-dependent prediction errors underpin reward-seeking behaviour in humans. *Nature*, 442(7106), 1042–1045. https://doi.org/10.1038/nature05051

Petersen, N., Kilpatrick, L. A., Goharzad, A., & Cahill, L. (2014). Oral contraceptive pill use and menstrual cycle phase are associated with altered resting state functional connectivity. *NeuroImage*, 90, 24–32. https://doi.org/10.1016/j.neuroimage.2013.12.016

Rahman, S., Robbins, T. W., Hodges, J. R., et al. (2006). Methylphenidate ("Ritalin") can ameliorate abnormal risk-taking behavior in the frontal variant of frontotemporal dementia. *Neuropsychopharmacology*, 31(3), 651–658. https://doi.org/10.1038/sj.npp.1300886

Ratala, C. E., Fallon, S. J., Van der Schaaf, M. E., Ter Huurne, N., Cools, R., & Sanfey, A. G. (2019). Catecholaminergic modulation of trust decisions. *Psychopharmacology (Berl)*, 236(6), 1807–1816. https://doi.org/10.1007/s00213-019-5165-z

Riba, J., Kramer, U. M., Heldmann, M., Richter, S., & Munte, T. F. (2008). Dopamine agonist increases risk taking but blunts reward-related brain activity. *PLoS ONE*, 3(6), Article e2479. https://doi.org/10.1371/journal.pone.0002479

Riedl, R., & Javor, A. (2012). The biology of trust: Integrating evidence from genetics, endocrinology, and functional brain imaging. *Journal of Neuroscience, Psychology, and Economics*, 5(2), 63–91. https://doi.org/10.1037/a0026318

Rilling, J., Gutman, D., Zeh, T., Pagnoni, G., Berns, G., & Kilts, C. (2002). A neural basis for social cooperation. *Neuron*, 35(2), 395–405. https://doi.org/10.1016/s0896-6273(02)00755-9

Robbins, T. W., & Arnsten, A. F. (2009). The neuropsychopharmacology of fronto-executive function: Monoaminergic modulation. *Annual Review of Neuroscience*, 32, 267–287. https://doi.org/10.1146/annurev.neuro.051508.135535

Roberts, I. D., Krajbich, I., & Way, B. M. (2019). Acetaminophen influences social and economic trust. *Scientific Reports*, 9(1), Article 4060. https://doi.org/10.1038/s41598-019-40093-9

Robson, S. E., Repetto, L., Gountouna, V. E., & Nicodemus, K. K. (2020). A review of neuroeconomic gameplay in psychiatric disorders. *Molecular Psychiatry*, 25(1), 67–81. https://doi.org/10.1038/s41380-019-0405-5

Rothstein, B., & Uslaner, E. M. (2005). All for all: Equality, corruption, and social trust. *World Politics*, 58, 41–72. https://doi.org/10.1353/wp.2006.0022

Rudnick, G., & Wall, S. C. (1992). The molecular mechanism of "ecstasy" [3,4-methylenedioxy-methamphetamine (MDMA)]: Serotonin transporters are targets for MDMA-induced serotonin release. *Proceedings of the National Academy of Sciences USA*, 89(5), 1817–1821. https://doi.org/10.1073/pnas.89.5.1817

Schiavone, S., Sorce, S., Dubois-Dauphin, M., et al. (2009). Involvement of NOX2 in the development of behavioral and pathologic alterations in isolated rats. *Biological Psychiatry*, 66(4), 384–392. https://doi.org/10.1016/j.biopsych.2009.04.033

Schmid, Y., Hysek, C. M., Simmler, L. D., Crockett, M. J., Quednow, B. B., & Liechti, M. E. (2014). Differential effects of MDMA and methylphenidate on social cognition. *Journal of Psychopharmacology*, 28(9), 847–856. https://doi.org/10.1177/0269881114542454

Schmidt, C. J., Wu, L., & Lovenberg, W. (1986). Methylenedioxymethamphetamine: A potentially neurotoxic amphetamine analogue. *European Journal of Pharmacology*, 124(1–2), 175–178. https://doi.org/10.1016/0014-2999(86)90140-8

Schroeder, K. B., McElreath, R., & Nettle, D. (2013). Variants at serotonin transporter and 2A receptor genes predict cooperative behavior differentially according to presence of punishment. *Proceedings of the National Academy of Sciences USA*, 110(10), 3955–3960. https://doi.org/10.1073/pnas.1216841110

Schweiger, D., Stemmler, G., Burgdorf, C., & Wacker, J. (2014). Opioid receptor blockade and warmth-liking: Effects on interpersonal trust and frontal asymmetry. *Social, Cognitive and Affective Neuroscience*, 9(10), 1608–1615. https://doi.org/10.1093/scan/nst152

Sekine, Y., Ouchi, Y., Sugihara, G., et al. (2008). Methamphetamine causes microglial activation in the brains of human abusers. *Journal of Neuroscience*, 28(22), 5756–5761. https://doi.org/10.1523/jneurosci.1179-08.2008

Selvaraj, S., Turkheimer, F., Rosso, L., et al. (2012). Measuring endogenous changes in serotonergic neurotransmission in humans: A [11C]CUMI-101 PET challenge study. *Molecular Psychiatry*, 17(12), 1254–1260. https://doi.org/10.1038/mp.2012.78

Seymour, B., Daw, N. D., Roiser, J. P., Dayan, P., & Dolan, R. (2012). Serotonin selectively modulates reward value in human decision making. *Journal of Neuroscience*, 32(17), 5833–5842. https://doi.org/10.1523/jneurosci.0053-12.2012

Shiels, K., Hawk, L. W., Reynolds, B., et al. (2009). Effects of methylphenidate on discounting of delayed rewards in attention deficit/hyperactivity disorder. *Experimental and Clinical Psychopharmacology*, 17(5), 291–301. https://doi.org/10.1037/a0017259

Snyder, R., Turgay, A., Aman, M., et al. (2002). Effects of risperidone on conduct and disruptive behavior disorders in children with subaverage IQs. *Journal of the American Academy of Child and Adolescent Psychiatry*, 41(9), 1026–1036. https://doi.org/10.1097/00004583-200209000-00002

Sokoloff, P., Diaz, J., Le Foll, B., et al. (2006). The dopamine D3 receptor: A therapeutic target for the treatment of neuropsychiatric disorders. *CNS & Neurological Disorders Drug Targets*, 5(1), 25–43. https://doi.org/10.2174/187152706784111551

Soutschek, A., Burke, C. J., Raja Beharelle, A., et al. (2017). The dopaminergic reward system underpins gender differences in social preferences. *Nature Human Behavior*, 1(11), 819–827. https://doi.org/10.1038/s41562-017-0226-y

Steiner, J., Bielau, H., Brisch, R., et al. (2008). Immunological aspects in the neurobiology of suicide: Elevated microglial density in schizophrenia and depression is associated with suicide. *Journal of Psychiatric Research*, 42(2), 151–157. https://doi.org/10.1016/j.jpsychires.2006.10.013

Steiner, J., Mawrin, C., Ziegeler, A., et al. (2006). Distribution of HLA-DR-positive microglia in schizophrenia reflects impaired cerebral lateralization. *Acta Neuropathologica*, 112(3), 305–316. https://doi.org/10.1007/s00401-006-0090-8

Stewart, L. H., Ferguson, B., Morgan, C. J., et al. (2014). Effects of ecstasy on cooperative behaviour and perception of trustworthiness: A naturalistic study. *Journal of Psychopharmacology*, 28(11), 1001–1008. https://doi.org/10.1177/0269881114544775

Sun, H., Verbeke, W., Pozharliev, R., Bagozzi, R. P., Babiloni, F., & Wang, L. (2019). Framing a trust game as a power game greatly affects interbrain synchronicity between trustor and trustee. *Social Neuroscience*, 14(6), 635–648. https://doi.org/10.1080/17470919.2019.1566171

Tancer, M., & Johanson, C. E. (2003). Reinforcing, subjective, and physiological effects of MDMA in humans: A comparison with d-amphetamine and mCPP. *Drug and Alcohol Dependence*, 72(1), 33–44. https://doi.org/10.1016/s0376-8716(03)00172-8

Thompson, M. R., Callaghan, P. D., Hunt, G. E., Cornish, J. L., & McGregor, I. S. (2007). A role for oxytocin and 5-HT(1A) receptors in the prosocial effects of 3,4 methylenedioxymethamphetamine ("ecstasy"). *Neuroscience*, 146(2), 509–514. https://doi.org/10.1016/j.neuroscience.2007.02.032

Todorov, A., Pakrashi, M., & Oosterhof, N. (2009). Evaluating faces on trustworthiness after minimal time exposure. *Social Cognition*, 27(6), 813–833. https://doi.org/10.1521/soco.2009.27.6.813

Trezza, V., Damsteegt, R., Achterberg, E. J., & Vanderschuren, L. J. (2011). Nucleus accumbens mu-opioid receptors mediate social reward. *Journal of Neuroscience*, 31(17), 6362–6370. https://doi.org/10.1523/jneurosci.5492-10.2011

Tse, W. S., Wong, A. S., Chan, F., Pang, A. H., Bond, A. J., & Chan, C. K. (2016). Different mechanisms of risperidone result in improved interpersonal trust, social engagement and cooperative behavior in patients with schizophrenia compared to trifluoperazine. *Psychiatry and Clinical Neurosciences*, 70(5), 218–226. https://doi.org/10.1111/pcn.12382

Tzieropoulos, H. (2013). The trust game in neuroscience: A short review. *Social Neuroscience*, 8(5), 407–416. https://doi.org/10.1080/17470919.2013.832375

Van't Wout, M., & Sanfey, A. G. (2008). Friend or foe: The effect of implicit trustworthiness judgments in social decision making. *Cognition*, 108(3), 796–803. https://doi.org/10.1016/j.cognition.2008.07.002

Van Berckel, B. N., Bossong, M. G., Boellaard, R., et al. (2008). Microglia activation in recent-onset schizophrenia: A quantitative (R)-[11C]PK11195 positron emission tomography study. *Biological Psychiatry*, 64(9), 820–822. https://doi.org/10.1016/j.biopsych.2008.04.025

Volkow, N. D., Wang, G. J., Fowler, J. S., & Ding, Y. S. (2005). Imaging the effects of methylphenidate on brain dopamine: New model on its therapeutic actions for attention-deficit/hyperactivity disorder. *Biological Psychiatry*, 57(11), 1410–1415. https://doi.org/10.1016/j.biopsych.2004.11.006

Wardle, M. C., & de Wit, H. (2012). Effects of amphetamine on reactivity to emotional stimuli. *Psychopharmacology (Berl)*, 220(1), 143–153. https://doi.org/10.1007/s00213-011-2498-7

Watabe, M., Kato, T. A., Monji, A., Horikawa, H., & Kanba, S. (2012). Does minocycline, an antibiotic with inhibitory effects on microglial activation, sharpen a sense of trust in social interaction? *Psychopharmacology (Berl)*, 220(3), 551–557. https://doi.org/10.1007/s00213-011-2509-8

Watson, D., Clark, L. A., & Tellegen, A. (1988). Development and validation of brief measures of positive and negative affect: The PANAS scales. *Journal of Personality and Social Psychology*, 54(6), 1063–1070. https://doi.org/10.1037//0022-3514.54.6.1063

Willis, J., & Todorov, A. (2006). First impressions: Making up your mind after a 100-ms exposure to a face. *Psychological Science*, 17(7), 592–598. https://doi.org/10.1111/j.1467-9280.2006.01750.x

Winston, J. S., Strange, B. A., O'Doherty, J., & Dolan, R. J. (2002). Automatic and intentional brain responses during evaluation of trustworthiness of faces. *Nature Neuroscience*, 5(3), 277–283. https://doi.org/10.1038/nn816

Wolff, K., Tsapakis, E. M., Winstock, A. R., et al. (2006). Vasopressin and oxytocin secretion in response to the consumption of ecstasy in a clubbing population. *Journal of Psychopharmacology*, 20(3), 400–410. https://doi.org/10.1177/0269881106061514

Wu, Y., Lousberg, E. L., Moldenhauer, L. M., et al. (2011). Attenuation of microglial and IL-1 signaling protects mice from acute alcohol-induced sedation and/or motor impairment. *Brain, Behavior, and Immunity*, 25 (Suppl. 1), S155–164. https://doi.org/10.1016/j.bbi.2011.01.012

Yamagishi, T., & Yamagishi, M. (1994). Trust and commitment in the United States and Japan. *Motivation and Emotion*, 18, 129–166. https://doi.org/10.1007/bf02249397

Young, L. J., Lim, M. M., Gingrich, B., & Insel, T. R. (2001). Cellular mechanisms of social attachment. *Hormones and Behavior*, 40(2), 133–138. https://doi.org/10.1006/hbeh.2001.1691

CHAPTER 15

Trust and Genetics
Genetic Basis of Trust Behavior and Trust Attitude

Qiulu Shou, Kuniyuki Nishina, and Haruto Takagishi

15.1 Introduction

Trust plays a pivotal role in human societies as a lubricant in interpersonal relationships, facilitating economic transactions (Humphrey & Schmitz, 1998; Simpson, 2007). Studies in various fields, such as economics, social psychology, and sociology, have provided evidence that high trust has a positive association with individual, interpersonal, and social factors (for a review, see Yamagishi, 2011). For example, a high level of trust is associated with high social intelligence (Yamagishi et al., 1999), and trust is a predictor of a country's economic level (Zak & Knack, 2001). Moreover, trust is also a form of social capital and an indicator of a society's maturity (Putnam et al., 1994). It has also been clarified that the degree of trust greatly depends on the social environment and is shaped as a result of adaptation to it (Yamagishi & Yamagishi, 1994).

Although research on trust has been conducted mainly in the social sciences, it has been treated as an important issue in the life sciences in recent years. Over the last 15 years, a great deal of research has been accumulated, and the biological basis for trust has become clear. This chapter focuses on the study of the biological basis of trust, especially the genetic basis. Are individual differences in trust subject to genetic influences, and thus possibly heritable, and which specific gene is associated with trust? To answer these questions, this chapter will review previous related studies and introduce the genetic basis of trust, including behavior and attitude level. First, we will introduce methods for measuring trust behavior and attitude. Next, we will describe previous studies that used twin methods to examine whether genetic factors affect trust.

The studies (Nishina et al., 2015, 2018, 2019) mentioned in this chapter were supported by JSPS KAKENHI Grant Numbers JP19H04915, JP15H05730, and JP25118004. We honor the series of trust studies by Dr. Toshio Yamagishi and thank him for supporting the research reported in this chapter. Corresponding author: Haruto Takagishi (haruharry@gmail.com).

Furthermore, we will review various studies that have examined the relationship between trust and polymorphism of some specific genes such as the oxytocin receptor gene (*OXTR*), arginine vasopressin receptor 1A gene (*AVPR1A*), dopamine D4 receptor gene (*DRD4*), and serotonin transporter gene (*SLC6A4*) using molecular biological techniques. Finally, we will discuss the future direction of studies on the genetic basis of trust.

15.2   Measuring Trust

Research on trust has so far been conducted using two distinct methods: (1) the trust game (TG) (also referred to as the investment game; Berg et al., 1995) to measure trust behavior; (2) questionnaires to measure the trust attitudes of others (Yamagishi & Yamagishi, 1994) (see also Chapter 2). The TG is a two-person task of exchanging financial rewards. The first player receives a certain amount of money from the experimenter and decides how much of it to transfer to the other player. The amount transferred is multiplied (e.g., three times) by the experimenter, and the second player receives it. Subsequently, the second player decides how to divide the money between the two players. The game finishes after the second player has decided. The amount transferred from the first player is defined as trust behavior: The amount that the first player transfers to the second player depends on how much the former trusts the latter. The TG has been used as a method of measuring trust behavior in various fields, such as experimental economics (Berg et al., 1995; Camerer, 2011), neuroscience (Delgado et al., 2005; King-Casas et al., 2005; Krueger et al., 2007; McCabe et al., 2001), and social psychology (Kiyonari et al., 2006; Romano et al., 2017; Yamagishi et al., 2017).

Trust attitudes measured by questionnaires reflect the tendency of beliefs toward people's trustworthiness in general (Yamagishi, 2011). Individual differences exist in trust attitudes, which influence trust behaviors (Mifune & Li, 2018; Yamagishi et al., 2015). Many psychological scales have been developed to measure trust attitudes. Rotter's (1967) *Interpersonal Trust Scale* is widely used to measure trust attitudes in the field of social psychology. The *General Trust Scale*, developed by Yamagishi and Yamagishi (1994), is used to measure one's general expectation of the trustworthiness of others. Moreover, the *World Value Survey* (e.g., Inglehart, 1997), a global research project, includes an exploration of people's trust attitudes over time across almost 100 countries. In this chapter, we separately discuss trust behavior measured using the TG and trust attitude measured using questionnaires.

15.3 Twin Studies

One method for investigating the genetic basis of trust is through conducting twin studies (Cesarini et al., 2008; Hiraishi et al., 2008; Oskarsson et al., 2012). Twin studies apply a traditional way of comparing monozygotic and dizygotic twin pairs to investigate the influence of genetic and environmental factors on psychological traits and behaviors. The genetic effect on trust behavior has been shown to be as low as 10%–20% (Cesarini et al., 2008), whereas trust attitude has been reported to have a higher genetic effect. Sturgis et al. (2010) found a 66% genetic effect on trust attitude. Similarly, the genetic effect on trust attitude for men and women is 33% and 39%, respectively, in Oskarsson et al. (2012), and 31% in Hiraishi et al. (2008). Moreover, Reimann et al. (2017) demonstrated that, except for the environment, trust shows significant genetic influences, whereas distrust does not.

15.4 Research on Genetic Polymorphisms

Another method for investigating the genetic basis of trust is through conducting studies on genetic polymorphisms (Apicella et al., 2010; Krueger et al., 2012; Nishina et al., 2015). The human genome has approximately 3.2 billion base pairs, of which approximately 21,000 genes have been identified (e.g., Arney, 2018). Base pairs have many individual differences, and those in one base pair are called single-nucleotide polymorphisms. The majority of studies have focused on genes involved in the synthesis of hormones and neurotransmitters that have been reported to be associated with trust, and examined the association of single-nucleotide polymorphisms within those genes with trust.

15.4.1 Oxytocin and Trust

Oxytocin is one of the candidates for the biological basis of human trust. It is a neuropeptide synthesized in the paraventricular nucleus and supraoptic nucleus of the hypothalamus (Meyer-Lindenberg et al., 2011) (see also Chapter 13). It is secreted into the blood from the posterior lobe of the pituitary gland and acts in various organs in the body. In addition, oxytocin neurons in the paraventricular nucleus project axons to various areas of the brain (e.g., amygdala, hippocampus, and nucleus accumbens) and function as neuromodulators.

Human studies have shown that oxytocin regulates social cognition and social behavior, such as facial recognition (Kirsch et al., 2005), ingroup favoritism (De Dreu et al., 2010), parenting behavior (Feldman, 2015), social bonding (Feldman, 2012), social stress (Heinrichs et al., 2003), and the theory of mind (Domes et al., 2007). In particular, pioneering research examining the effects of intranasally administered oxytocin on trust revealed that oxytocin promotes trust behavior in the TG (Kosfeld et al., 2005). To determine the effect of oxytocin on brain function, Baumgartner et al. (2008) conducted a pharmaco-imaging study and found that intranasal administration of oxytocin attenuates the activity of the amygdala, resulting in increased trust behavior even in situations with a high probability of betrayal by other players.

Recently, some studies have cast doubt on the robustness of intranasal oxytocin administration studies (e.g., Walum et al., 2016). Walum et al. (2016) pointed out that because of the small sample size and low statistical power, it is possible that published intranasal oxytocin findings do not represent true effects. Moreover, there is no eloquent theory explaining how oxytocin affects human sociality (e.g., Bartz et al., 2011). For example, the hypothesis that oxytocin reduces anxiety, especially social anxiety, could explain the promotion effect of oxytocin on trust, as oxytocin increases prosocial behavior by reducing anxiety toward betrayal (Bartz et al., 2011). However, this hypothesis could not explain other effects of oxytocin on sociality (e.g., ingroup bias). Specifically, Nave et al. (2015) reviewed previous studies and pointed out six studies that failed to replicate the findings reported by Kosfeld et al. (2005) and Baumgartner et al. (2008). Moreover, Declerck et al. (2020) conducted a double-blind, placebo-controlled direct replication of Kosfeld et al.'s (2005) study using a large sample size. This study also failed to demonstrate the same promotion effect of oxytocin on trust behavior as Kosfeld et al. (2005), but found that oxytocin is associated with increased trust behavior among people with a low level of trust attitude measured by Yamagishi's General Trust Scale. Based on this finding, it is possible that the trust attitude that researchers always ignore plays an important role in the effect of oxytocin on trust. Or rather, oxytocin is more likely to affect one's attitude as opposed to behavior, which needs to be examined in the future.

15.4.2   Oxytocin Receptor Gene

The oxytocin receptor is encoded by the *OXTR*, which is localized to chromosome 3 in humans. The *OXTR* has approximately 17,000 base

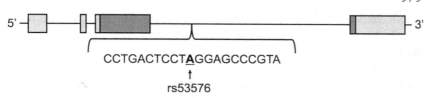

Figure 15.1   Structure of the oxytocin receptor gene.
The *OXTR* rs53576 is a single-nucleotide polymorphism in the third intron of the oxytocin receptor gene. Light gray shows the noncoding region and dark gray shows the coding region (Takagishi, 2020).

pairs and contains three introns and four exons (Inoue et al., 1994). It has multiple single-nucleotide polymorphisms. Remarkably, the *OXTR* variant rs53576, a single-nucleotide polymorphism involving a silent guanine (G) to adenine (A) change in intron 3 of the *OXTR* (Figure 15.1), is associated with trust behavior in young men (Krueger et al., 2012). Using the TG, Krueger et al. (2012) found that men with the GG genotype show higher levels of trust behavior than men with the AG or AA genotype. However, Apicella et al. (2010) did not find any association between the *OXTR* rs53576 genotypes and trust behavior in men nor women. According to Nishina et al. (2015), a possible reason for this difference between the two studies is the variation in participants' demographic attributes. First, the two studies recruited participants from different age groups. Krueger et al. (2012) recruited male college students aged approximately 20 years, whereas Apicella et al. (2010) recruited men and women aged between 20 and 50 years. Second, the two studies differed in the sex ratio of participants: The ratio of men was 100% in Krueger et al. (2012) and about 20% in Apicella et al. (2010). The bias in sex ratio might have reduced the power of detection regarding the relationship between the *OXTR* rs53576 genotypes and trust in men.

Therefore, Nishina et al. (2015) examined the relationship between the *OXTR* rs53576 genotypes and behavioral trust in 427 Japanese adults with a wide range of ages (20s to 50s) and an almost even sex ratio. Their study succeeded in replicating the findings of Krueger et al. (2012): Men with the GG genotype showed higher trust behavior in the TG than men with the AA genotype. Additionally, regarding women, no significant relationship was found between the *OXTR* rs53576 genotypes and trust behavior, as in Apicella et al. (2010). Nishina et al. (2015) also examined the relationship between the *OXTR* rs53576 genotypes and trust attitudes. To measure the participants' level of trust attitude, they used the *World*

Value Survey question: "Generally speaking, would you say that most people can be trusted or that you need to be very careful in dealing with people?" The same results were observed: Men with the GG genotype showed higher levels of trust attitude compared to men with the AA or AG genotype, whereas in women, there was no relation between the *OXTR* rs53576 genotypes and trust attitude. Further, trust attitude mediates the relationship between the *OXTR* rs53576 genotypes and trust behavior. The results imply that the *OXTR* is directly related to trust attitude, not trust behavior, and indirectly related to trust behavior through trust attitude.

Nishina et al. (2015) and Krueger et al. (2012) demonstrated a significant relationship between the *OXTR* rs53576 genotypes and trust only in men. One possible reason may be the higher level of estrogen in women compared to men. Estrogen modulates the secretion of oxytocin (Champagne et al., 2001). Moreover, its secretion changes with the menstrual cycle (Crockford et al., 2014). Therefore, the absence of a relationship between *OXTR* rs53576 and trust in women may result from individual differences in estrogen secretion levels.

In addition, the participants in Nishina et al. (2015) were East Asians. Studies comparing American and East Asian samples have indicated that the frequency of the GG genotype in East Asians is lower than that in Americans, whereas the frequency of the AA genotype in East Asians is higher than that in Americans (Kim et al., 2010, 2011; Sasaki et al., 2011). According to previous studies (Krueger et al., 2012; Nishina et al., 2015), men with the GG genotype have a higher level of trust behavior and trust attitude than men with the AG or AA genotype. This result is consistent with Yamagishi's (2011) emancipation theory of trust, which proposes and explains the phenomenon of Americans having a higher level of trust compared to the Japanese (Yamagishi & Yamagishi, 1994). Yamagishi (2011) discussed that high levels of trust in Americans are formed to adapt to the social environment, with a major advantage of increased interaction with others. Their findings imply that a higher ratio of people with the GG genotype who tend to be more trustful, especially men, are in America, where they need to have higher trust levels. The effects of cultural factors on these relations must also be examined.

Many studies have examined the mechanism between genotypes and phenotypes, with brain function and brain structure as intermediate phenotypes. Such an approach is called imaging genetics. In the human brain, oxytocin receptors are predominantly distributed in the amygdala (Barberis & Tribollet, 1996; Loup et al., 1991; Tribollet et al., 1992).

Moreover, intranasal oxytocin administration attenuates amygdala activity toward untrustworthy opponents in the TG (Baumgartner et al., 2008). Plasma oxytocin and the volume of the right amygdala have an inverse correlation (Andari et al., 2014). As such, some studies on imaging genetics have attempted to examine the association between the *OXTR* rs53576 genotypes and the function and structure of the amygdala (Tost et al., 2010; Wang et al., 2014). Tost et al. (2010) found that men with the GG genotype have a smaller amygdala volume compared to men with the AG or AA genotype, whereas women with the GG genotype have a larger amygdala volume compared to women with the AG or AA genotype. Wang et al. (2014) reported that women with the GG and AG genotypes have larger amygdala volumes than women with the AA genotype. Based on these findings, the *OXTR* rs53576 genotypes may be associated with the amygdala, which affects the level of trust.

Nishina et al. (2018) analyzed the data of the same participants in Nishina et al. (2015), which included magnetic resonance imaging data. Nishina et al. (2018) examined the relationship between trust, the *OXTR* rs53576 genotypes, and amygdala volume. The results showed that the volume of the left amygdala was significantly smaller in men with the GG genotype than in men with the AA or AG genotype, whereas in women, the volume was significantly smaller in those with the AA or AG genotype than in those with the GG genotype. In addition, the volume of the left amygdala was negatively associated with trust attitude in men, whereas no such association was observed in women. Nishina et al. (2018) also found a significant mediation effect of the volume of the left amygdala on the association between the *OXTR* rs53576 genotypes and trust attitude in men. These results indicate that the volume of the left amygdala plays an important role in the association between the *OXTR* rs53576 genotypes and trust attitude in men. Subsequent analysis, not reported in the paper (Nishina et al., 2018), revealed that the volume of the left amygdala was not associated with trust behavior. Given that oxytocin is considered to play an important role in reducing anxiety-like behavior in animals (Blume et al., 2008; Windle et al., 1997), Bartz et al. (2011) proposed the "anxiety-reduction hypothesis" that oxytocin reduces anxiety and fear by reducing amygdala activity. Men with the GG genotype in terms of the *OXTR* rs53576 variants have a large distribution of oxytocin receptors in the amygdala, which suppresses amygdala activity and may have a high anxiety-suppressing effect. Such long-term relations are presumed to influence the volume and level of trust in the amygdala. However, some recent studies (e.g., Marek et al., 2020) criticize the low replicability of brain-behavior research; it is better to conduct a replication study by Nishina et al. (2018) with a larger sample size (e.g., over 2,000 samples) in the future.

In addition, Zheng et al. (2020) recently examined the relationship among trust, *OXTR* rs53576, and the environment. The study found that childhood adversity had a negative association with trust attitude measured by Yamagishi's General Trust Scale, and that *OXTR* rs53576 moderated the impact of childhood adversity on trust attitude. Specifically, the negative association between childhood adversity and general trust is only significant among those with the AA genotype. This implies that *OXTR* rs53576 moderates the relationship between childhood experiences and trust. It is necessary to examine the interaction between the environment and *OXTR* rs53576 on trust in the future.

15.4.3   *Arginine Vasopressin Receptor 1A Gene*

Arginine vasopressin is a hormone similar to oxytocin; it differs from oxytocin in only one of the nine amino acids. Arginine vasopressin is a peptide hormone synthesized in the hypothalamus and acts in the central nervous system (Meyer-Lindenberg et al., 2011), which affects human behaviors, like oxytocin (Heinrichs & Domes, 2008). However, unlike oxytocin, arginine vasopressin is associated with typical male social behaviors, including aggression and pair-bond formation, and mediates anxiety-inducing effects (Heinrichs & Domes, 2008). Indeed, arginine vasopressin promotes anxiety and fearful responses to emotional stimuli (Brunnlieb et al., 2013; Shalev et al., 2011). As previously stated, oxytocin can promote trust by reducing the fear of betrayal. Therefore, arginine vasopressin may be associated with avoidance and distrust behavior rather than with trust behavior (Riedl & Javor, 2012).

Some studies provide evidence that the length of a promoter region in the *AVPR1A* is associated with human sociality (e.g., Hopkins et al., 2012; Walum et al., 2008). *AVPR1A* is located on chromosome 12 in humans; it has approximately 8,400 base pairs with two exons (Thibonnier et al., 1996). Microsatellite polymorphisms in the promoter region are associated with human prosocial behavior. The repeat length in RS3, a complex repeat of (CT)4-TT-(CT)8-(GT)24, is associated with allocation behavior in economic games (Avinun et al., 2012; Knafo et al., 2008; Wang et al., 2016). Considering that trust behavior and trust attitude are associated with human prosocial behaviors (e.g., Mifune & Li, 2018), Riedl and Javor (2012) predicted that the length of a promoter region in *AVPR1A* is

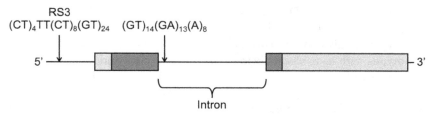

Figure 15.2   Structure of the arginine vasopressin receptor 1A gene.
There are microsatellite polymorphisms in the promoter region and intron. Light gray
shows the noncoding region and dark gray shows the coding region.

associated with trust. However, to date, this hypothesis has not been examined.

Microsatellite polymorphisms are present in the promoter and intron regions of *AVPR1A* (Figure 15.2). Microsatellite polymorphisms in the intron region have also been found in common marmosets (*Callithrix jacchus*) and reported to be associated with sociality and neuroticism (Inoue-Murayama et al., 2018). Nishina et al. (2019) examined whether the repeat lengths of microsatellite polymorphism in the intron of *AVPR1A* are associated with trust, and found that people with a short form of *AVPR1A* show a high level of trust behavior compared to people with a long form. An animal study (Inoue-Murayama et al., 2018) found associations between the short form and high levels of sociality and low levels of neuroticism. The cross-species commonality seems to indicate that arginine vasopressin has an evolutionary old regulatory function with respect to social behavior.

15.4.4   Dopamine D4 Receptor Gene

Dopamine is a neurotransmitter that is mainly associated with reward processes. Animal studies have provided evidence that the release of oxytocin can be induced by a positive social stimulus (Liu & Wang, 2003), subsequently promoting midbrain dopamine release and social interaction behavior (Hung et al., 2017; Shahrokh et al., 2010). As trust is associated with expectation of a reward (reciprocity level of the trustee; King-Casas et al., 2005), the level of trust may be influenced by oxytocin–dopamine interactions, which may be affected by the number of dopamine receptors. The level of trust may also be associated with the dopamine receptor gene.

Dreber et al. (2012) examined the relationship between trust behavior observed in the TG and the *DRD4*, located on chromosome 11. The polymorphism in *DRD4* is a 48 base-pair tandem repeat in exon 3 that consists of 2–11 repeats (Ding et al., 2002). In Dreber et al. (2012), genotypes are divided into two dichotomous classes, 7R— and 7R+, where genotypes with 2–6 repeats belong to the 7R— class and genotypes with 7–11 repeats belong to the 7R+ class. The results revealed that people with 7R— *DRD4* have higher trust behavior compared to people with 7R+ *DRD4* in the TG. It should be noted that the sample size of the 7R+ class is extremely small in this study: N = 17 of 122 belong to the 7R+ class.

15.4.5   *Serotonin Transporter Gene*

Serotonin (5-HT) is a neurotransmitter that affects emotional and cognitive processes (Savitz & Ramesar, 2004). The *SLC6A4* contains a polymorphism in the promoter region (5-HTTLPR), which has short (S) and long (L) genotypes (Lesch et al., 1997). The S-genotype (SS/SL) of the 5-HTTLPR polymorphism has been associated with individuals' attention toward negative stimuli and emotions (Fox et al., 2009). Kong (2015) proposed a gene–environment interaction model of the relationship between trust attitude and 5-HTTLPR polymorphism. He analyzed the data of 58 societies, particularly the average level of trust attitude in each society, the degree of democracy in society, and the prevalence of the 5-HTTLPR S-genotype. The data were collected from various worldwide surveys, such as the *World Value Survey* and other related studies. The results showed that the prevalence of the 5-HTTLPR S-genotype is a critical moderator for the linkage between democracy and trust attitude. Specifically, the positive relationship between democracy and trust attitude exists only in societies with a lower prevalence of the 5-HTTLPR S-genotype and is absent in societies with a higher prevalence level. This model implicated the possibility of an interaction between genetic and societal factors. However, it is a study on the relationship between the 5-HTTLPR and the level of attitudinal trust at the societal level, not at the individual level.

15.5   Future Directions

According to the gene–environment interaction theory proposed by Manuck and McCaffery (2014), both genetics and the environment influence trust behavior and trust attitude. Previous studies using the twin method have demonstrated that some trust is influenced by genes (about 10%–20% in trust behavior and above 30% in trust attitude). Specifically, researchers found that some genes, such as *OXTR*, *AVPR1A*, *DRD4*, and *SLC6A4* (so far), particularly influence the level of trust. However, the interaction effect between genes and the environment has not been studied extensively. In the future, it will be necessary to further examine the interaction effect between genes and the environment on trust. For example, based on Yamagishi's emancipation theory of trust, there is a cultural difference between East Asians and Americans regarding the level of trust; it is therefore valuable to examine the effect of genes on this cultural difference. Moreover, researchers have considered the brain as an intermediate phenotype to explain the association between genes and behavior (Nishina et al., 2018). For example, it is possible that variations in genes, such as *OXTR* rs53576, in encoding their receptors contribute to individual differences in trust by altering brain structure and function. Therefore, Nishina et al. (2018) examined the relationship between trust, genes, and brain structure. However, there are few studies focusing on the relationship between trust, the brain, and genes such as *AVPR1A*, which should be examined in the future.

References

Andari, E., Schneider, F. C., Mottolese, R., Vindras, P., & Sirigu, A. (2014). Oxytocin's fingerprint in personality traits and regional brain volume. *Cerebral Cortex*, 24(2), 479–486. https://doi.org/10.1093/cercor/bhs328

Apicella, C. L., Cesarini, D., Johannesson, M., et al. (2010). No association between oxytocin receptor (OXTR) gene polymorphisms and experimentally elicited social preferences. *PLoS ONE*, 5(6), Article e11153. https://doi.org/10.1371/journal.pone.0011153

Arney, K. (2018). *How to code a human: Exploring the DNA blueprints that make us who we are.* Andre Deutsch.

Avinun, R., Ebstein, R. P., & Knafo, A. (2012). Human maternal behaviour is associated with arginine vasopressin receptor 1A gene. *Biology Letters*, 8(5), 894–896. https://doi.org/10.1098/rsbl.2012.0492

Barberis, C., & Tribollet, E. (1996). Vasopressin and oxytocin receptors in the central nervous system. *Critical Reviews in Neurobiology*, 10(1), 119–154. https://doi.org/10.1615/CritRevNeurobiol.v10.i1.60

Bartz, J. A., Zaki, J., Bolger, N., & Ochsner, K. N. (2011). Social effects of oxytocin in humans: Context and person matter. *Trends in Cognitive Sciences*, 15(7), 301–309. https://doi.org/10.1016/j.tics.2011.05.002

Baumgartner, T., Heinrichs, M., Vonlanthen, A., Fischbacher, U., & Fehr, E. (2008). Oxytocin shapes the neural circuitry of trust and trust adaptation in humans. *Neuron*, 58(4), 639–650. https://doi.org/10.1016/j.neuron.2008.04.009

Berg, J., Dickhaut, J., & McCabe, K. (1995). Trust, reciprocity, and social history. *Games and Economic Behavior*, 10(1), 122–142. https://doi.org/10.1006/game.1995.1027

Blume, A., Bosch, O. J., Miklos, S., et al. (2008). Oxytocin reduces anxiety via ERK1/2 activation: Local effect within the rat hypothalamic paraventricular nucleus. *European Journal of Neuroscience*, 27(8), 1947–1956. https://doi.org/10.1111/j.1460-9568.2008.06184.x

Brunnlieb, C., Münte, T. F., Tempelmann, C., & Heldmann, M. (2013). Vasopressin modulates neural responses related to emotional stimuli in the right amygdala. *Brain Research*, 1499, 29–42. https://doi.org/10.1016/j.brainres.2013.01.009

Camerer, C. F. (2011). *Behavioral game theory: Experiments in strategic interaction*. Princeton University Press.

Cesarini, D., Dawes, C. T., Fowler, J. H., Johannesson, M., Lichtenstein, P., & Wallace, B. (2008). Heritability of cooperative behavior in the trust game. *Proceedings of the National Academy of Sciences*, 105(10), 3721–3726. https://doi.org/10.1073/pnas.0710069105

Champagne, F., Diorio, J., Sharma, S., & Meaney, M. J. (2001). Naturally occurring variations in maternal behavior in the rat are associated with differences in estrogen-inducible central oxytocin receptors. *Proceedings of the National Academy of Sciences*, 98(22), 12736–12741. https://doi.org/10.1073/pnas.221224598

Crockford, C., Deschner, T., Ziegler, T. E., & Wittig, R. M. (2014). Endogenous peripheral oxytocin measures can give insight into the dynamics of social relationships: A review. *Frontiers in Behavioral Neuroscience*, 8, Article 68. https://doi.org/10.3389/fnbeh.2014.00068

De Dreu, C. K., Greer, L. L., Handgraaf, M. J., et al. (2010). The neuropeptide oxytocin regulates parochial altruism in intergroup conflict among humans. *Science*, 328(5984), 1408–1411. https://doi.org/10.1126/science.1189047

Declerck, C. H., Boone, C., Pauwels, L., Vogt, B., & Fehr, E. (2020). A registered replication study on oxytocin and trust. *Nature Human Behaviour*, 4, 646–655. https://doi.org/10.1038/s41562-020-0878-x

Delgado, M. R., Frank, R. H., & Phelps, E. A. (2005). Perceptions of moral character modulate the neural systems of reward during the trust game. *Nature Neuroscience*, 8(11), 1611–1618. https://doi.org/10.1038/nn1575

Ding, Y. C., Chi, H. C., Grady, D. L., et al. (2002). Evidence of positive selection acting at the human dopamine receptor D4 gene locus. *Proceedings of the National Academy of Sciences*, 99(1), 309–314. https://doi.org/10.1073/pnas.012464099

Domes, G., Heinrichs, M., Michel, A., Berger, C., & Herpertz, S. C. (2007). Oxytocin improves "mind-reading" in humans. *Biological Psychiatry*, 61(6), 731–733. https://doi.org/10.1016/j.biopsych.2006.07.015

Dreber, A., Rand, D. G., Wernerfelt, N., Montgomery, C., & Malhotra, D. K. (2012). Genetic correlates of economic and social risk taking. *SSRN*. https://doi.org/10.2139/ssrn.2141601

Feldman, R. (2012). Oxytocin and social affiliation in humans. *Hormones and Behavior*, 61(3), 380–391. https://doi.org/10.1016/j.yhbeh.2012.01.008

——— (2015). Sensitive periods in human social development: New insights from research on oxytocin, synchrony, and high-risk parenting. *Development and Psychopathology*, 27(2), 369–395. https://doi.org/10.1017/S0954579415000048

Fox, E., Ridgewell, A., & Ashwin, C. (2009). Looking on the bright side: Biased attention and the human serotonin transporter gene. *Proceedings of the Royal Society B: Biological Sciences*, 276(1663), 1747–1751. https://doi.org/10.1098/rspb.2008.1788

Heinrichs, M., Baumgartner, T., Kirschbaum, C., & Ehlert, U. (2003). Social support and oxytocin interact to suppress cortisol and subjective responses to psychosocial stress. *Biological Psychiatry*, 54(12), 1389–1398. https://doi.org/10.1016/S0006-3223(03)00465-7

Heinrichs, M., & Domes, G. (2008). Neuropeptides and social behaviour: Effects of oxytocin and vasopressin in humans. *Progress in Brain Research*, 170, 337–350. https://doi.org/10.1016/S0079-6123(08)00428-7

Hiraishi, K., Yamagata, S., Shikishima, C., & Ando, J. (2008). Maintenance of genetic variation in personality through control of mental mechanisms: A test of trust, extraversion, and agreeableness. *Evolution and Human Behavior*, 29(2), 79–85. https://doi.org/10.1016/j.evolhumbehav.2007.07.004

Hopkins, W. D., Donaldson, Z. R., & Young, L. J. (2012). A polymorphic indel containing the RS3 microsatellite in the 5′ flanking region of the vasopressin V1a receptor gene is associated with chimpanzee (*Pan troglodytes*) personality. *Genes, Brain and Behavior*, 11(5), 552–558. https://doi.org/10.1111/j.1601-183X.2012.00799.x

Humphrey, J., & Schmitz, H. (1998). Trust and inter-firm relations in developing and transition economies. *The Journal of Development Studies*, 34(4), 32–61. https://doi.org/10.1080/00220389808422528

Hung, L. W., Neuner, S., Polepalli, J. S., et al. (2017). Gating of social reward by oxytocin in the ventral tegmental area. *Science*, 357(6358), 1406–1411. https://doi.org/10.1126/science.aan4994

Inglehart, R. (1997). *Modernization and postmodernization: Cultural, economic, and political change in 43 societies*. Princeton University Press. https://doi.org/10.2307/j.ctv10vm2ns

Inoue, T., Kimura, T., Azuma, C., et al. (1994). Structural organization of the human oxytocin receptor gene. *The Journal of Biological Chemistry*, 269(51), 32451–32456

Inoue-Murayama, M., Yokoyama, C., Yamanashi, Y., & Weiss, A. (2018). Common marmoset (*Callithrix jacchus*) personality, subjective well-being, hair cortisol level and AVPR1a, OPRM1, and DAT genotypes. *Scientific Reports*, 8(1), 1–15. https://doi.org/10.1038/s41598-018-28112-7

Kim, H. S., Sherman, D. K., Mojaverian, T., et al. (2011). Gene–culture interaction: Oxytocin receptor polymorphism (OXTR) and emotion regulation. *Social Psychological and Personality Science*, 2(6), 665–672. https://doi.org/10.1177/1948550611405854

Kim, H. S., Sherman, D. K., Sasaki, J. Y., et al. (2010). Culture, distress, and oxytocin receptor polymorphism (OXTR) interact to influence emotional support seeking. *Proceedings of the National Academy of Sciences*, 107(36), 15717–15721. https://doi.org/10.1073/pnas.1010830107

King-Casas, B., Tomlin, D., Anen, C., Camerer, C. F., Quartz, S. R., & Montague, P. R. (2005). Getting to know you: Reputation and trust in a two-person economic exchange. *Science*, 308(5718), 78–83. https://doi.org/10.1126/science.1108062

Kirsch, P., Esslinger, C., Chen, Q., et al. (2005). Oxytocin modulates neural circuitry for social cognition and fear in humans. *Journal of Neuroscience*, 25 (49), 11489–11493. https://doi.org/10.1523/JNEUROSCI.3984-05.2005

Kiyonari, T., Yamagishi, T., Cook, K. S., & Cheshire, C. (2006). Does trust beget trustworthiness? Trust and trustworthiness in two games and two cultures: A research note. *Social Psychology Quarterly*, 69(3), 270–283. https://doi.org/10.1177/019027250606900304

Knafo, A., Israel, S., Darvasi, A., et al. (2008). Individual differences in allocation of funds in the dictator game associated with length of the arginine vaso-pressin 1a receptor RS3 promoter region and correlation between RS3 length and hippocampal mRNA. *Genes, Brain and Behavior*, 7(3), 266–275. https://doi.org/10.1111/j.1601-183X.2007.00341.x

Kong, D. T. (2015). A gene-environment interaction model of social trust: The 5-HTTLPR s-allele prevalence as a moderator for the democracy-trust linkage. *Personality & Individual Differences*, 87, 278–281. https://doi.org/10.1016/j.paid.2015.08.028

Kosfeld, M., Heinrichs, M., Zak, P. J., Fischbacher, U., & Fehr, E. (2005). Oxytocin increases trust in humans. *Nature*, 435(7042), 673–676. https://doi.org/10.1038/nature03701

Krueger, F., McCabe, K., Moll, J., et al. (2007). Neural correlates of trust. *Proceedings of the National Academy of Sciences*, 104(50), 20084–20089. https://doi.org/10.1073/pnas.0710103104

Krueger, F., Parasuraman, R., Iyengar, V., et al. (2012). Oxytocin receptor genetic variation promotes human trust behavior. *Frontiers in Human Neuroscience*, 6, Article 4. https://doi.org/10.3389/fnhum.2012.00004

Lesch, K. P., Meyer, J., Glatz, K., et al. (1997). The 5-HT transporter gene-linked polymorphic region (5-HTTLPR) in evolutionary perspective: Alternative biallelic variation in rhesus monkeys. *Journal of Neural Transmission*, 104 (11–12), 1259–1266. https://doi.org/10.1007/bf01294726

Liu, Y., & Wang, Z. X. (2003). Nucleus accumbens oxytocin and dopamine interact to regulate pair bond formation in female prairie voles. *Neuroscience*, 121(3), 537–544. https://doi.org/10.1016/S0306-4522(03)00555-4

Loup, F., Tribollet, E., Dubois-Dauphin, M., & Dreifuss, J. J. (1991). Localization of high-affinity binding sites for oxytocin and vasopressin in the human brain. An autoradiographic study. *Brain Research,* 555(2), 220–232. https://doi.org/10.1016/0006-8993(91)90345-V

Manuck, S. B., & McCaffery, J. M. (2014). Gene-environment interaction. *Annual Review of Psychology,* 65, 41–70. https://doi.org/10.1146/annurev-psych-010213-115100

Marek, S., Tervo-Clemmens, B., Calabro, F. J., et al. (2020). Towards reproducible brain-wide association studies. *bioRxiv.* https://doi.org/10.1101/2020.08.21.257758

McCabe, K., Houser, D., Ryan, L., Smith, V., & Trouard, T. (2001). A functional imaging study of cooperation in two-person reciprocal exchange. *Proceedings of the National Academy of Sciences,* 98(20), 11832–11835. https://doi.org/10.1073/pnas.211415698

Meyer-Lindenberg, A., Domes, G., Kirsch, P., & Heinrichs, M. (2011). Oxytocin and vasopressin in the human brain: Social neuropeptides for translational medicine. *Nature Reviews Neuroscience,* 12(9), 524–538. https://doi.org/10.1038/nrn3044

Mifune, N., & Li, Y. (2018). Trust in the faith game. *Psychologia,* 61(2), 70–88. https://doi.org/10.2117/psysoc.2019-B008

Nave, G., Camerer, C., & McCullough, M. (2015). Does oxytocin increase trust in humans? A critical review of research. *Perspectives on Psychological Science,* 10(6), 772–789. https://doi.org/10.1177/1745691615600138

Nishina, K., Takagishi, H., Fermin, A. S. R., et al. (2018). Association of the oxytocin receptor gene with attitudinal trust: Role of amygdala volume. *Social Cognitive and Affective Neuroscience,* 13(10), 1091–1097. https://doi.org/10.1093/scan/nsy075

Nishina, K., Takagishi, H., Inoue-Murayama, M., Takahashi, H., & Yamagishi, T. (2015). Polymorphism of the oxytocin receptor gene modulates behavioral and attitudinal trust among men but not women. *PLoS ONE,* 10(10), Article e0137089. https://doi.org/10.1371/journal.pone.0137089

Nishina, K., Takagishi, H., Takahashi, H., Sakagami, M., & Inoue-Murayama, M. (2019). Association of polymorphism of arginine-vasopressin receptor 1A (AVPR1a) gene with trust and reciprocity. *Frontiers in Human Neuroscience,* 13, Article 230. https://doi.org/10.3389/fnhum.2019.00230

Oskarsson, S., Dawes, C., Johannesson, M., & Magnusson, P. K. (2012). The genetic origins of the relationship between psychological traits and social trust. *Twin Research and Human Genetics,* 15(1), 21–33. https://doi.org/10.1375/twin.15.1.21

Putnam, R. D., Leonardi, R., & Nanetti, R. Y. (1994). *Making democracy work: Civic traditions in modern Italy.* Princeton University Press.

Reimann, M., Schilke, O., & Cook, K. S. (2017). Trust is heritable, whereas distrust is not. *Proceedings of the National Academy of Sciences,* 114(27), 7007–7012. https://doi.org/10.1073/pnas.1617132114

Riedl, R., & Javor, A. (2012). The biology of trust: Integrating evidence from genetics, endocrinology, and functional brain imaging. *Journal of*

Neuroscience, Psychology, and Economics, 5(2), 63–91. https://doi.org/10.1037/a0026318

Romano, A., Balliet, D., Yamagishi, T., & Liu, J. H. (2017). Parochial trust and cooperation across 17 societies. *Proceedings of the National Academy of Sciences*, 114(48), 12702–12707. https://doi.org/10.1073/pnas.1712921114

Rotter, J. B. (1967). A new scale for the measurement of interpersonal trust. *Journal of Personality*, 35(4), 651–665. https://doi.org/10.1111/j.1467-6494.1967.tb01454.x

Sasaki, J. Y., Kim, H. S., & Xu, J. (2011). Religion and well-being: The moderating role of culture and the oxytocin receptor (OXTR) gene. *Journal of Cross-Cultural Psychology*, 42(8), 1394–1405. https://doi.org/10.1177/0022022111412526

Savitz, J. B., & Ramesar, R. S. (2004). Genetic variants implicated in personality: A review of the more promising candidates. *American Journal of Medical Genetics Part B: Neuropsychiatric Genetics*, 131(1), 20–32. https://doi.org/10.1002/ajmg.b.20155

Shahrokh, D. K., Zhang, T. Y., Diorio, J., Gratton, A., & Meaney, M. J. (2010). Oxytocin-dopamine interactions mediate variations in maternal behavior in the rat. *Endocrinology*, 151(5), 2276–2286. https://doi.org/10.1210/en.2009-1271

Shalev, I., Israel, S., Uzefovsky, F., Gritsenko, I., Kaitz, M., & Ebstein, R. P. (2011). Vasopressin needs an audience: Neuropeptide elicited stress responses are contingent upon perceived social evaluative threats. *Hormones and Behavior*, 60(1), 121–127. https://doi.org/10.1016/j.yhbeh.2011.04.005

Simpson, J. A. (2007). Foundations of interpersonal trust. In A. W. Kruglanski & E. T. Higgins (Eds.), *Social psychology: Handbook of basic principles* (pp. 587–607). The Guilford Press.

Sturgis, P., Read, S., Hatemi, P. K., et al. (2010). A genetic basis for social trust? *Political Behavior*, 32(2), 205–230. https://doi.org/10.1007/s11109-009-9101-5

Takagishi, H. (2020). The role of oxytocin in prosocial behavior. *Psychology World*, 91, 13–16 (written in Japanese). https://psych.or.jp/publication/world091/pw05

Thibonnier, M., Graves, M. K., Wagner, M. S., Auzan, C., Clauser, E., & Willard, H. F. (1996). Structure, sequence, expression, and chromosomal localization of the human v1avasopressin receptor gene. *Genomics*, 31(3), 327–334. https://doi.org/10.1006/geno.1996.0055

Tost, H., Kolachana, B., Hakimi, S., et al. (2010). A common allele in the oxytocin receptor gene (OXTR) impacts prosocial temperament and human hypothalamic-limbic structure and function. *Proceedings of the National Academy of Sciences*, 107(31), 13936–13941. https://doi.org/10.1073/pnas.1003296107

Tribollet, E., Dubois-Dauphin, M., Dreifuss, J. J., Barberis, C., & Jard, S. (1992). Oxytocin receptors in the central nervous system: Distribution, development, and species differences. *Annals of the New York Academy of Sciences*, 652(1), 29–38. https://doi.org/10.1111/j.1749-6632.1992.tb34343.x

Walum, H., Waldman, I. D., & Young, L. J. (2016). Statistical and methodological considerations for the interpretation of intranasal oxytocin studies. *Biological Psychiatry*, 79(3), 251–257. https://doi.org/10.1016/j.biopsych.2015.06.016

Walum, H., Westberg, L., Henningsson, S., et al. (2008). Genetic variation in the vasopressin receptor 1a gene (AVPR1A) associates with pair-bonding behavior in humans. *Proceedings of the National Academy of Sciences*, 105(37), 14153–14156. https://doi.org/10.1073/pnas.0803081105

Wang, J., Qin, W., Liu, B., et al. (2014). Neural mechanisms of oxytocin receptor gene mediating anxiety-related temperament. *Brain Structure and Function*, 219(5), 1543–1554. https://doi.org/10.1007/s00429–013-0584-9

Wang, J., Qin, W., Liu, F., et al. (2016). Sex-specific mediation effect of the right fusiform face area volume on the association between variants in repeat length of AVPR1A RS3 and altruistic behavior in healthy adults. *Human Brain Mapping*, 37(7), 2700–2709. https://doi.org/10.1002/hbm.23203

Windle, R. J., Shanks, N., Lightman, S. L., & Ingram, C. D. (1997). Central oxytocin administration reduces stress-induced corticosterone release and anxiety behavior in rats. *Endocrinology*, 138(7), 2829–2834. https://doi.org/10.1210/endo.138.7.5255

Yamagishi, T. (2011). *Trust: The evolutionary game of mind and society*. Springer Science & Business Media. https://doi.org/10.1007/978-4-431-53936-0

Yamagishi, T., & Yamagishi, M. (1994). Trust and commitment in the United States and Japan. *Motivation and Emotion*, 18(2), 129–166. https://doi.org/10.1007/BF02249397

Yamagishi, T., Akutsu, S., Cho, K., Inoue, Y., Li, Y., & Matsumoto, Y. (2015). Two-component model of general trust: Predicting behavioral trust from attitudinal trust. *Social Cognition*, 33(5), 436–458. https://doi.org/10.1521/soco.2015.33.5.436

Yamagishi, T., Kikuchi, M., & Kosugi, M. (1999). Trust, gullibility, and social intelligence. *Asian Journal of Social Psychology*, 2(1), 145–161. https://doi.org/10.1111/1467-839X.00030

Yamagishi, T., Matsumoto, Y., Kiyonari, T., et al. (2017). Response time in economic games reflects different types of decision conflict for prosocial and proself individuals. *Proceedings of the National Academy of Sciences*, 114(24), 6394–6399. https://doi.org/10.1073/pnas.1608877114

Zak, P. J., & Knack, S. (2001). Trust and growth. *The Economic Journal*, 111(470), 295–321. https://doi.org/10.1111/1468-0297.00609

Zheng, S., Masuda, T., Matsunaga, M., et al. (2020). Oxytocin receptor gene (OXTR) and childhood adversity influence trust. *Psychoneuroendocrinology*, 121, Article 104840. https://doi.org/10.1016/j.psyneuen.2020.104840

PART V

Neuropathological Level of Trust

CHAPTER 16

Trust and Psychotic Disorders
Unraveling the Dynamics of Paranoia and Disturbed Social Interaction

Imke L. J. Lemmers-Jansen and Anne-Kathrin J. Fett

16.1 Introduction

Nonaffective psychotic disorders include schizophrenia, schizoaffective disorder, and psychotic, delusional, and schizophreniform disorders (i.e., the schizophrenia spectrum) and affect ~1% of the population (Insel, 2010). These disorders are characterized by heterogeneous symptoms, such as delusions (fixed false beliefs that are not amenable to change despite conflicting evidence, e.g., paranoia), hallucinations, disorganized thinking and speech, and abnormal motor behavior, referred to as positive symptoms; and avolition, anhedonia and diminished emotional expression, and the lack of interest in social interactions, referred to as negative symptoms (American Psychiatric Association, 2013). Although several of these symptoms may also occur in combination with other (psychiatric) disorders, and in the general, healthy, population, the focus of this chapter is on nonaffective psychotic disorders, which have been most extensively investigated. Crucially, many core symptoms have a strong social character and problems in social, interpersonal functioning are highly prevalent in individuals with psychotic disorders (American Psychiatric Association, 2013; Velthorst et al., 2017). The first changes in social behavior appear years before psychosis onset, with some studies reporting subtle impairments already in childhood (Velthorst et al., 2016, 2017). A further drop in social functioning precedes the first psychotic episode and the majority of affected individuals (~75%) experience chronically impaired social functioning over the following decades (Velthorst et al., 2017). Yet, effective interventions are still lacking. Consequently, there is great interest in the underlying mechanisms of social impairment and symptoms. Research has generally focused on social cognitive skills, which are necessary for the

Corresponding authors: Imke L.J. Lemmers-Jansen (imke.jansen@kcl.ac.uk) and Anne-Kathrin J. Fett (anne-kathrin.fett@city.ac.uk).

formation and maintenance of social relationships (Couture et al., 2006) and which are often impaired in psychosis (Pinkham, 2014). Particularly theory of mind (ToM), the ability to mentalize and to infer others' mental states, impacts on social outcomes (Fett et al., 2011). Misinterpretations of others' social signals may lead to profound distrust and suspiciousness (i.e., paranoia) (Freeman et al., 2002), and as a consequence to social with-drawal (Kirkpatrick et al., 2006). However, the latter might also stem from deficits in social motivation (Whitton & Lewandowski, 2019). Until recently, research into social cognition and social interactions in psychosis employed paradigms that required the interpretation of abstract and static social stimuli, for instance in stories or pictures. These studies yielded important insights but could not capture the interactive aspect of social behavior. In the last decade, interactive game-theoretical exchange para-digms have been adopted into psychosis research, where they offer an innovative and more direct way to study the underlying mechanisms of social dysfunction (Fett, Shergill, & Krabbendam, 2015).

This chapter will start with an overview of behavioral findings on trust in psychosis, and with a discussion of factors that influence trust, such as emotion recognition, attachment, and urbanicity. Studies in chronic and first-episode patients are included, as well as samples of individuals at clinical and genetic high risk for psychosis. Consequently, neural correlates of trust in psychosis are discussed, and brain regions with differential activation in patients are presented. Theoretical accounts for disturbed trust, including reward processing and social and nonsocial cognition are discussed. Finally, recommendations for future research are presented.

16.2   Overview of the Literature

Research on trust in psychosis mostly used the trust game (TG) in individuals with nonaffective chronic and early-stage psychosis, but also in genetic and clinical high-risk groups (Table 16.1). Individuals with psychosis (risk) were always in the role of the investor because the investor faces the question of whether to trust or not, depending on expectations of trustworthiness of the counterpart (trustee) (Colman, 2003). In the TG trust is operationalized as the amount invested by the investor and different elements of trust were investigated in repeated interactions (see also Chapter 2). During the first investment, referred to as baseline trust, trust is placed in an unknown trustee, yielding the purest measure of trust that is unconfounded by any behavioral cues or learning. When several repeated TG rounds are played with the same trustee, the impact of feedback learning on trust can be investigated.

Table 16.1. *Participant characteristics and trust measures of the reviewed studies*

Publication		Participants				Paradigm		
Author	N	Age (years) Mean (SD)	Gender, % Males	Symptoms Measure; Duration of Illness (DOI)	Medication	Game Description	Counterpart	Number of Trials
Campellone et al. (2016)	32 SZS (20 SZ, 12 SAD) 29 HC	SZS 47.5 (11.9) HC 46.2 (10.7)	49% SZS 48% HC	SCID M 23 years	29 medicated (26 atypical, 3 other) 3 medication free	Multi-round Invest 0–10 points, quadrupled Initial phase (congruent behavior and face and reversal (incongruent)	4 partners: 2 cooperative (smile or neutral face); 2 unfair (scowl or neutral face)	88 trials: Initial phase 40: 10 per partner Reversal phase 48: 12 per partner
Campellone et al. (2018)	64 SZS (34 SZ, 27 SAD, 3 SPD) 26 HC	SZS 23 (3.9) HC 25.2 (7.11)	73% SZS 62% HC	PANSS M 30 months	55 medicated CE 344.05 (351.9) 9 medication free	Multi-round Invest 0–10 points, quadrupled	4 partners: 2 cooperative (smile or neutral face); 2 unfair (scowl or neutral face)	40 trials: 10 per partner
Fett et al. (2012)	29 SZS (16 SZ, 4 SAD, 1 SPD, 5 UD, 3 PNOS) 24 GHR (13 sib, 2 off, 9 par) 35 HC	SZS 39.7 (8.4) GHR 42.3 (11.6) HC 41.3 (12.4)	43% SZS 21% HC	PANSS for SZS CAPE for GHR & HC	n.r.	Multi-round Invest £0–10, tripled	Real human (university students)	20 trials: Baseline condition: 5 no feedback Context condition: 5 with prior info, no feedback Feedback condition: 10 with feedback

Table 16.1. (cont.)

	Participants					Paradigm		
Author	N	Age (years) Mean (SD)	Gender, % Males	Symptoms Measure; Duration of Illness (DOI)	Medication	Game Description	Counterpart	Number of Trials
Fett et al. (2016)	39 EP adolescents (28 NAP, 11 AP) 100 HC of these 22 EP and 50 HC completed fMRI	EP 17 (1.2) HC 16 (1.5)	58% SZS 50% HC	PANSS M 1.3 years	37 medicated (28 antipsychotics, 5 antipsychotics & antidepressants, 2 antidepressants, 2 antipsychotics & benzodiazepines) 2 medication free	Multi-round Invest £0–10, tripled Associated with attachment	Preprogrammed: Cooperative and unfair	40 trials: 20 per partner
Fett, Mouchlianitis, et al. (2019)	22 EP (18 NAP, 4 AP) 25 HC Sample partly overlapping with Fett et al. (2016)	EP 17.6 (1.3) HC 16.8 (1.6)	100%	PANSS GPTS < 3 years	21 medicated (20 atypical, 1 typical & atypical) 1 medication free	Multi-round Invest £0–10, tripled	Preprogrammed: Cooperative and unfair	40 trials: 20 per partner
Gromann et al. (2013)	20 SZS 20 HC	SZ 33.7 (7.8) HC 32.2 (9.1)	100%	PANSS < 15 years	All 20 medicated All 20 atypical	Multi-round Invest £0–10, tripled	Preprogrammed: Cooperative and unfair	40 trials: 20 per partner
Gromann et al. (2014)	50 GHR 33 HC	GHR 33.9 (8.7) HC 33.4 (17.2)	42% GHR 57% HC	CAPE	All medication free	Multi-round Invest €0–10, tripled	Preprogrammed: Cooperative	20 trials

Study	Sample	Age	%	Measure	Medication	Task	Condition	Trials
Hanssen et al. (2020)	50 SZS 20 GHR 49 HC	SZS 36.2 (9.6) GHR 39.1 (13.3) HC 35.1 (9.9)	82% SZS 20% GHR 71% HC	PANSS	45 medicated (40 atypical, 5 typical) 5 medication free	Multi-round Invest £0-10 tripled	Preprogrammed: Cooperative human partner and cooperative computer partner (lottery)	40 trials: 20 per partner
Hanssen et al. (2021)	23 SZS (17 SZ, 4 SAD, 2 PSD) 25 HC Sample partly overlapping with Hanssen et al. (2020)	SZS 39.9 (9.1) HC 36.0 (7.3)	83% SZS 68% HC	PANSS	22 medicated (19 atypical, 3 typical) 1 medication free	Multi-round Invest £0-10, tripled Context manipulation about trustworthiness Associated with ESM measures	Preprogrammed: cooperative, regardless of context information (none, positive, negative)	60 trials: 20 per partner
Haut & MacDonald III (2010)	22 SZ 43 HC	SZ 38.4 (10.2) HC 30.8 (10.4)	41% SZ 54% HC	SAPS SANS BPRS	All 22 medicated	Trustworthiness and emotional ratings of neutral faces	Ratings of surprise, anger, happiness, attractiveness, fear, disgust, sadness, & trustworthiness	96 faces
Hooker et al. (2011)	23 SZS (15 SZ, 8 SAD) 35 HC	SZS 44.2 (10.3) HC 49.2 (7.7)	91% SZS 63% HC	PANSS M 26 years	21 medicated (18 atypical, 3 typical) 2 medication free	Social judgment task, rating trustworthiness of unfamiliar faces after affective prime	Each face was rated for trustworthiness after each of the three primes (negative [threat], neutral, and positive)	147 primes: 49 faces with 3 primes each
Jacob & Rao*	14 SZ 14 HC	SZ 33.5 (6.0) HC 24.4 (3.8)	n.r.	n.r.	n.r.	Multi-round Invest 4, 8, or 12 INR	Human and lottery Conditions n.r.	24 trials: 12 per condition

Table 16.1. (*cont.*)

Publication		Participants					Paradigm		
Author	N	Age (years) Mean (SD)	Gender, % Males	Symptoms Measure; Duration of Illness (DOI)	Medication	Game Description	Counterpart	Number of Trials
Keri et al. (2009)	50 SZ 50 HC	SZ 47.8 (7.3) HC 47.9 (9.0)	32% in both groups	PANSS HAM-D HAM-A RBANS	All 50 on stable medication typical or atypical, 8 with additional antidepressants CE 352.7 (135.8)	Sharing in writing information with the experimenter, and receiving it from the experimenter Associated with OXT	Sharing neutral information vs. an important secret	2 experiments on separate days
Lemmers-Jansen et al. (2018)	22 FEP 17 CHR 43 HC	FEP 19.9 (1.5) CHR 23.8 (2.4) HC 21.1 (2.7)	64% FEP 41% CHR 51% HC	PANSS	16 FEP medicated (13 atypical, 1 typical & atypical, 1 benzodiazepine, 1 serraline) 8 CHR medicated (6 antidepressant, 2 benzodiazepine) 15 medication free	Multi-round Invest €0–10 tripled	Preprogrammed: Cooperative and unfair	40 trials: 20 per partner
Lemmers-Jansen et al. (2020)	39 SZS (22 FEP, 17 CHR) 30 HC Sample partly overlapping with Lemmers-Jansen et al. (2018)	SZS 21.6 (2.8) HC 21.4 (3.0)	54% SZS 60% HC	PANSS	24 medicated (13 atypical, 1 typical & atypical, 3 benzodiazepine, 1 serraline, 6 antidepressant) 15 medication free	Multi-round Invest €0–10 tripled Associated with urban upbringing	Preprogrammed: Cooperative and unfair	40 trials: 20 per partner

| Sutherland et al. (2019) | 24 SZS (17 SZ, 7 SAD) 24 HC | SZS 51.9 (8.9) HC 45.6 (13.8) | 58% in both groups | SAPS SANS PDI | All 24 medicated (20 atypical, 2 typical, 2 atypical & typical, 14 with additional antidepressants) | Multi-round Invest $0–10 quadrupled Reliance on facial appearance and on fairness of returns | 4 conditions: untrustworthy/ trustworthy face x cooperative/ unfair returns | 32 trials: 8 per condition 1 of 8 trials was inconsistent with other trials |

Notes: *conference poster abstract; AP, affective psychosis; CAPE, community assessment of psychic experiences; CE, chlorpromazine equivalents; CHR, clinical high risk; DOI, duration of illness; EP, early psychosis; ESM, experience sampling method; FEP, first-episode psychosis; fMRI, functional magnetic resonance imaging; GHR, genetic high risk; GPTS, Green paranoid thought scale; HAM-A, Hamilton anxiety scale; HAM-D, Hamilton depression scale; HC, healthy controls; INR, Indian rupees; M, mean; n.r., not reported; NTR, treatment resistant; off, offspring; OXT, oxytocin; PANSS, positive and negative syndrome scale; par, parents; PDI, Peters et al. delusions inventory; PNOS, psychotic disorder not otherwise specified; PSD, psychotic disorder; RBANS, repeatable brief assessment of neuropsychological status; SAD, schizoaffective disorder; SAPS/SANS, scales for assessing positive and negative symptoms of schizophrenia; SCID, structured clinical interview for DSM-IV; SD, standard deviation; sib, siblings; SPD, schizophreniform disorder; SSRI, selective serotonin reuptake inhibitors; SZ, schizophrenia; SZS, schizophrenia spectrum; TR, treatment responsive; UD, undifferentiated type.

In the case of mutual cooperation, higher returns follow higher investments (e.g., trustworthy responses rewarding trust). In the case of defection, trust is not repaid and is followed by lower investments. Few studies investigated trust in psychosis through other means, such as trustworthiness ratings of faces. We will first review the behavioral evidence (Table 16.2), including studies on contextual and individual variables that influence trust, before discussing neuroimaging findings. In every section, we discuss findings across the psychosis continuum, first in chronic schizophrenia spectrum disorders, then in early (i.e., defined as illness duration of less than 3 years with one or more psychotic episodes) and first-episode psychosis (FEP), followed by findings in individuals at clinical and genetic high risk. Individuals at clinical high risk (CHR) are usually already in mental health care for various reasons, and often report positive psychotic symptoms, without meeting the diagnostic criteria for a schizophrenia spectrum disorder (SZS). Investigating these individuals informs us about the early prodromal stages of the disorder and risk mechanisms for conversion, without the confounding effects of factors related to illness duration. Healthy relatives of individuals with SZS have an increased genetic risk for psychosis (genetic high risk: GHR) yet are not affected by the disorder. Thus, their levels of trust are unconfounded by antipsychotic medication and other factors that are secondary to the clinical disorder, such as social stigma, which allows for the identification of familial risk-mechanisms for psychosis.

16.2.1 Baseline Trust

Eight studies reported findings on baseline trust in psychosis (Table 16.1). More than half of these studies found reduced baseline trust in those with SZS compared to controls, across all stages of the psychosis continuum: Two showed lower baseline trust in chronic SZS compared to controls (Fett et al., 2012; Fett, Shergill, et al., 2014); similar findings have been reported for adolescents and young adults with early psychosis (EP) and FEP (Fett et al., 2016; Lemmers-Jansen et al., 2018); and for those with CHR compared to FEP (Lemmers-Jansen et al., 2018, 2020) and in GHR (Fett et al., 2012), suggesting reduced baseline trust over the entire schizophrenia spectrum. However, others reported intact baseline trust in chronic SZS, EP, and GHR (Fett, Mouchlianitis, et al., 2019; Gromann et al., 2014; Hanssen et al., 2021). Thus, reduced trust could be part of a trait-like vulnerability for psychosis, rather than being secondary to disorder-related factors. However, the existing studies also suggest that symptoms further impact on trust in a state-like way.

Table 16.2. *Behavioral findings and symptom correlations in the reviewed studies on trust in psychosis*

| Publication | | Behavior | | |
Author (Year)	Baseline Trust	Repeated Investments	Correlation with Symptoms	Other Correlations
Campellone et al. (2016)	n.r.	SZS < HC trust in smiling and neutral trustworthy partners SZS > HC sensitivity to negative social interaction outcomes In the reversal condition, SZS did not reduce trust in smiling partners (now untrustworthy), reacting less to their behavior Both groups detected that formerly untrustworthy partners were now behaving in a trustworthy manner	n.r.	SZS and HC placed more trust in trustworthy than in untrustworthy social partners Both groups tended to trust smiling partners more than neutral partners across phases HC tended to trust scowling and neutral social partners more than SZS, regardless of their behavior
Campellone et al. (2018)	n.r.	SZS < HC trust over repeated interactions in cooperative, but not in unfair interactions	Higher negative symptoms associated with decreased trust and with avoiding TG interactions with negative outcomes	In SZS, greater trust during cooperative interactions was associated with greater real-world social functioning More anticipated pleasure was associated with increased trust in unfair interactions, only in HC Both groups placed more trust in smiling social partners No associations between medication and trust

397

Table 16.2. (cont.)

| Publication | | | Behavior | | |
Author (Year)	Baseline Trust	Repeated Investments	Correlation with Symptoms	Other Correlations
Fett et al. (2012)	SZS, GHR < HC	Feedback condition: SZS < HC in baseline trust and average investments Relatives' behavior was intermediate, although not significantly different from HC SZS engage less in trust-honoring behavior	In baseline and context condition: Results associated with subclinical negative symptoms in HC and marginally with positive psychotic symptoms in SZS and GHR	Prior positive information on the trustees' trustworthiness significantly increased trust of HC and relatives, but not SZS
Fett et al. (2016)	EP < HC	Cooperative interactions: - EP increased investments more than HC Unfair interactions: - EP reduced investments less	Negative symptoms associated with lower baseline trust and with lower average investments in both conditions	More attachment anxiety was associated with higher baseline trust
Fett, Mouchlianitis, et al. (2019)	No group differences EP = HC	No group differences in average investments during cooperative or unfair interactions	Higher PANSS positive and negative symptoms associated with lower baseline trust Persecutory delusions, PANSS positive and negative symptoms associated with lower investments during cooperation Negative symptoms associated with lower investments during unfair interactions	n.r.

398

Study				
Gromann et al. (2013)	SZS < HC	SZS had lower average investments during cooperative interactions No group differences in the unfair condition	n.r.	n.r.
Gromann et al. (2014)	No group differences GHR = HC	No significant differences in average investment between siblings and HC	n.r.	n.r.
Hanssen et al. (2020)	n.r.	HC increased investments over trials, SZS and GHR did not HC and SZS invested less in the TG compared to the lottery game, GHR more SZS increased investments less often and invested more often the same amounts in the TG and lottery game	Lower negative symptoms associated with higher investments in the trust than lottery game Higher negative symptoms showed the opposite, with higher investments in the lottery game than in the TG	n.r.
Hanssen et al. (2021)	Context effect found in HC but not in patients No group differences in all 3 contexts	No context: - SZS decreased investments, HC did not change investments over trials Negative context: - SZS decreased investments, HC increased investments Positive context: - SZS and HC did not show changes over trials	Higher paranoia interfered with learning over trials More negative symptoms were associated with lower investments in the positive context	Associations with ESM social measures, in SZS only: - Across contexts, higher investments associated with less time spent alone - Higher relationship quality associated with higher investments in the positive and negative context - Higher social exclusion with lower investments in no context condition

Table 16.2. (cont.)

Publication		Behavior			
Author (Year)	Baseline Trust	Repeated Investments	Correlation with Symptoms	Other Correlations
Haut & MacDonald III (2010)	n.r.	n.r.	Negative correlation between persecutory delusions and the trustworthiness–attractiveness correlation in SZ SZ with few persecutory delusions showed increased trustworthiness– attractiveness correlations, similar to controls Persecutory delusions did not predict trustworthiness ratings	No mean differences in ratings of emotional expressions of the faces between groups HC > SZ in positive correlation between ratings of trustworthiness and attractiveness No correlations between trust and emotion ratings of neutral faces
Hooker et al. (2011)	n.r.	n.r.	SZS with higher levels of suspiciousness/persecution rated faces as less trustworthy after the negative (but not neutral or positive affective prime Positive correlation between ratings after neutral and positive primes and disorganized symptoms Association between negative affect and judgments of trustworthiness varied with levels of suspiciousness/persecution	No effect of education, age, gender, or diagnosis on trustworthiness ratings SZS rated faces as less trustworthy than HC after the negative affective prime, but not after neutral or positive prime
Jacob & Rao* (2017)	n.r.	n.r.	n.r.	n.r.

400

Study				
Keri et al. (2009)	n.r.	n.r.	After trust-related interactions, higher negative symptoms resulted in lower OXT levels	In HC, higher OXT levels after trust-related interactions compared with the neutral condition. This was not found in SZ. No difference between SZ and HC in OXT levels after neutral interactions. Trust-related interactions did not provoke more anxiety in SZ compared with the neutral interactions. No relationship between OXT levels and medication (CE levels). No significant associations between medication and trust
Lemmers-Jansen et al. (2018)	FEP & CHR < HC	Cooperative interactions: FEP showed stronger increase of investment than HC. Unfair interactions: FEP showed less decrease of investment than HC. No mean investments reported	Cooperative interactions: higher negative symptoms associated with less learning over trials (i.e., less increase in investments) in FEP but not in CHR. Unfair interactions: higher positive symptoms associated with less decrease in investments in FEP and CHR, suggesting reduced learning	
Lemmers-Jansen et al. (2020)	FEP & CHR < HC	Cooperative interactions: no group effect. Unfair interactions: FEP & CHR adjusted their investments less than HC	Urbanicity-by-negative symptoms interactions on baseline trust	Interaction urbanicity X group X condition. FEP & CHR brought up in lower-urban areas adjusted their investments in response to positive feedback during cooperation more than FEP & CHR brought up in higher-urban areas. No such association in HC

Table 16.2. (*cont.*)

Publication		Behavior		
Author (Year)	Baseline Trust	Repeated Investments	Correlation with Symptoms	Other Correlations
Sutherland et al. (2019)	n.r.	Participants transferred more money to trustworthy than untrustworthy-looking partners, regardless of their returns SZS, unlike HC, failed to learn from partner behavior	n.r.	n.r.

Notes: * conference poster abstract; CE, chlorpromazine equivalents; CHR, clinical high risk; ESM, experience sampling method; EP, early psychosis; FEP, first-episode psychosis; GHR, genetic high risk; HC, healthy controls; n.r., not reported; NTR, treatment resistant; OXT, oxytocin; PANSS, positive and negative syndrome scale; SZ, schizophrenia; SZS, schizophrenia spectrum; TG, trust game; TR, treatment responsive.

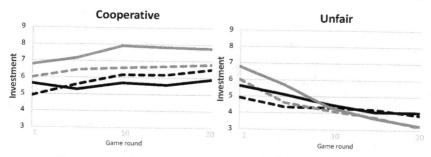

Figure 16.1   The development of trust across repeated interactions.
Changes in investments (£) over 20 repeated cooperative (left) and unfair interactions
(right). Black lines represent controls (dashed lines <19 years, solid lines >19 years), grey
lines represent SZS (dashed EP <19, solid chronic SZS >19).

In chronic, early, and first-episode psychosis, lower baseline trust has been associated with both higher positive and negative symptoms, albeit with some inconsistencies between studies (Fett, Mouchlianitis, et al., 2019; Fett et al., 2012, 2016). In sum, the evidence for reduced baseline trust is most consistent in chronic psychosis. Some work indicates that this pattern exists in GHR and early in the disorder, but the findings are not unequivocal, suggesting that differences in the early stages of the disorder may only emerge in the acutely ill. This tentatively supports a link between amplified suspiciousness, social withdrawal, and problematic social functioning.

16.2.2   Trust in Repeated Interactions

In repeated cooperative TG interactions with real and preprogrammed trustees, individuals with chronic SZS show significantly lower average trust compared to controls, as well as relatively stable levels of (reduced) trust over repeated interactions (Fett et al., 2012; Gromann et al., 2013; Hanssen et al., 2021). Low average trust might partly be a consequence of a lower set point in baseline trust; however, the findings that show flatter slopes over time suggest reduced responsiveness to positive social feedback (Figure 16.1, left panel, solid lines). Interestingly, SZS do not only have a lower tendency to trust but they also engage less in trust-honouring behavior, that is, they responded less often with stable or increasing investments to stable or increasing trustee returns in real social interactions (Fett et al., 2012). When the trustee was preprogrammed to play extremely unfair (i.e., punishing any increases in investor trust with decreased repayments), there were no group differences in average trust (Gromann et al., 2013) or in the decrease of trust over repeated trials (Figure 16.1, right panel, solid lines), suggesting an intact sensitivity to negative feedback. In fact, some studies even reported a stronger sensitivity to negative feedback (Campellone et al., 2016). In contrast to findings in chronic SZS, studies in EP and FEP suggest that individuals in the early stages of the disorder are able to override initial distrust in response to positive trustee reciprocity. Starting off with reduced initial investments, EP and FEP reach the same levels of trust as controls toward the end of the TG (Figure 16.1, left panel, dashed lines) (Fett et al., 2016; Lemmers-Jansen et al., 2018). Both studies also suggest that individuals with a beginning psychotic disorder react slightly less strongly to unfairness (Fett et al., 2016; Lemmers-Jansen et al., 2018) (see Figure 16.1, right panel); however, these differences did not always reach significance (Fett, Shergill, Gromann, & Krabbendam, 2015). The effects were independent of antipsychotic medication in FEP (Lemmers-Jansen et al., 2018); however, the impact of medication on trust has not yet been investigated in chronic SZS. Intermediate average levels of trust have been reported in GHR compared to controls and SZS, although not significantly differently from both groups (Fett et al., 2012; Gromann et al., 2014; Hanssen et al., 2020). Learning over trials with a subtly benevolent trustee was absent in GHR compared to controls, as also observed in SZS (Hanssen et al., 2020). As with the GHR group, CHR also tend to show intermediate levels of trust compared to controls and SZS, although not always significantly different (Lemmers-Jansen et al., 2018). The majority of evidence in the at-risk groups suggests that while baseline trust is diminished, learning from feedback is mostly intact when trustee feedback is obviously cooperative or unfair.

Reduced trust has most reliably been associated with higher negative symptoms in both cooperative and unfair interactions and across all stages of the disorder (Fett, Mouchlianitis, et al., 2019; Fett et al., 2012, 2016; Hanssen et al., 2020, 2021; Lemmers-Jansen et al., 2018). Higher negative symptoms were associated with lower trust in the TG, but not with lower investments in the nonsocial version of the game (Hanssen et al., 2020). In the early stages of the disorder, positive symptoms have been significantly associated with trust and in chronic SZS the associations were marginally significant; those with higher positive symptoms showed lower trust in cooperative interactions (Fett, Mouchlianitis, et al., 2019; Fett et al., 2012), as well as lower reductions of trust in unfair interactions (Lemmers-Jansen et al., 2018).

16.2.3 Factors Influencing Trust Behavior in Psychosis

A number of studies started to investigate factors that could explain reduced trust in SZS. Prior information indicating that the counterpart is trustworthy (i.e., reputation-based trust, see also Chapter 7) did not lead to higher baseline trust in SZS, while it did in GHR and controls (Fett et al., 2012; Hanssen et al., 2021). One study on social context processing in psychosis suggests that this finding does not reflect a specific bias or insensitivity to positive information, but rather a general insensitivity to explicit positive and negative social contextual information about others (Hanssen et al., 2021). However, others have shown that implicit social information does lead to changes in trust in SZS. Negative visual primes do affect perceptions of trustworthiness of others in SZS, particularly in individuals with higher paranoid delusions (Hooker et al., 2011), which suggests that an exaggerated sensitivity to negative social information might result from or contribute to these symptoms. Studies that investigated the effects of overt visual trustworthiness cues also showed an intact sensitivity in SZS, indicated by similar trustworthiness ratings of faces in SZS and controls (Haut & MacDonald III, 2010).

When the TG was combined with images of facial expressions, or video clips of the trustee both SZS and controls placed greater trust in trustworthy- than untrustworthy-looking trustees (Campellone et al., 2016, 2018; Sutherland et al., 2019), though SZS still trusted partners with positive facial expressions less than controls (Campellone et al., 2016, 2018). Trust in partners with a negative facial expression was either similar to controls (Campellone et al., 2018) or more reduced in SZS (Campellone et al., 2016), suggesting greater sensitivity to negative emotional displays in the latter. In two of the TGs, trustee behavior was either congruent or incongruent with the displayed facial expression. In incongruent trials, SZS failed to adjust their trust based on actual trustee reciprocity (Campellone et al., 2016; Sutherland et al., 2019). When trustworthy-looking partners behaved in an untrustworthy manner, SZS still trusted this partner (Campellone et al., 2016; Sutherland et al., 2019), whereas controls lowered their trust accordingly. Thus, in SZS but not controls, the social information provided by facial expressions interferes with the development of distrust in response to negative trustee feedback. However, when untrustworthy-looking partners were behaving in a trustworthy manner, SZS learned to trust them as controls did (Campellone et al., 2016).

Summarizing, SZS do not adjust their trust in response to explicit positive and negative contextual information. However, they do use implicit information about others' trustworthiness that is encoded in facial expressions to adjust their levels of trust, suggestive of intact perception and interpretation of these. Neither antipsychotic medication nor its dosage in chlorpromazine equivalents was associated with trust (Campellone et al., 2018). Only higher negative, but not positive symptoms were associated with lower trust in trustworthy-looking others (Campellone et al., 2016, 2018) and persecutory delusions did not predict trustworthiness ratings of faces (Haut & MacDonald III, 2010). Interestingly, and as previously suggested by others (Figure 16.1), a longer illness duration was associated with lower trust in trustworthy others, suggesting that the experience of having SZS for longer leads to greater difficulties with trust (Campellone et al., 2016).

Also, early social experiences that impact on attachment, that is, referring to the nature of social-emotional bonds with other people, have been suggested as a possible explanatory factor of disturbed trust and social functioning in psychosis (Palmier-Claus et al., 2019). Attachment in psychosis is often insecure (i.e., anxious and/or avoidant), meaning that social bonds are characterized by fear and negative feelings, such as dependence and rejection, which may lead to low trust in others. Surprisingly, the first study into the topic showed that only attachment anxiety, which is characterized by a positive view of others and a negative view of the self, was associated with higher rather than lower baseline trust, as well as higher trust during interactions with an unfair partner. In this context, higher trust might reflect the wish to affiliate and to be liked by the trustee. Attachment avoidance, which is characterized by a more negative view of others, in contrast, was unrelated to the levels of trust (Fett et al., 2016). Importantly, trust in the TG has been linked to real-world social functioning in psychosis. Greater trust in trustworthy and untrustworthy others has been associated with greater social networks in SZS (Campellone et al., 2016) and the ability to develop trust in a formerly untrustworthy social partner was associated with greater family functioning (Campellone et al., 2018), highlighting the importance of behavioral flexibility. Moreover, greater trust was also positively associated with anticipated pleasure in real life (Campellone et al., 2018), less time spent alone, higher friendship quality, and lower perceived social exclusion (Hanssen et al., 2021).

With regard to real-world implications of trust it has also been proposed that negative social characteristics of urban environments, which have been associated with an increased risk for the incidence of psychosis, could account for reduced trust in the disorder (Fett, Lemmers-Jansen,

& Krabbendam, 2019; Krabbendam et al., 2020). A first study showed that urban upbringing (i.e., spending the first 15 years of life in a densely populated urban environment) was unrelated to baseline trust and trust during unfair interactions. However, in interactions with a cooperative trustee, FEP and CHR who were brought up in less urban areas adjusted their levels of trust more than those who were brought up in more urban areas. This suggests that high urbanicity impacts on social reward learning in psychosis. With the additional risk factor of an urban upbringing, FEP resembled chronic SZS in trust behavior (Lemmers-Jansen et al., 2020).

Additionally, it has been argued that nonsocial cognitive functions might explain group differences in trust and the ability to develop trust in repeated social interactions. Most studies controlled statistically for cognitive ability but did not report on the effects. Those who did report on the associations showed mixed findings, with one study reporting that working memory performance was unrelated to levels of trust (Campellone et al., 2016), and two reporting slight reductions in effect sizes of the group differences in trust between SZS and controls due to general cognitive ability (Fett, Mouchlianitis, et al., 2019; Fett et al., 2012). And finally, exchanging trust-based messages has been associated with increased plasma levels of oxytocin (OXT), a hormone that is commonly associated with social affiliation (for a detailed discussion of OXT and trust see also Chapter 13), and which has been thought to be a social enhancer in SZS (Keri et al., 2009).

16.3   Neural Correlates of Trust in Psychosis

Eight studies conducted the TG during functional magnetic resonance imaging (fMRI) scanning (Table 16.3). These studies largely focused on the investigation of brain regions implicated in ToM and in reward anticipation and consumption during the investment and repayment phases. The first study in chronic SZS showed reduced activation in the right caudate during cooperative repayments and in the right temporoparietal junction (rTPJ) during cooperative and unfair repayments (Gromann et al., 2013). Less caudate activation was associated with higher levels of paranoia, suggesting that reduced social reward sensitivity might drive these symptoms or vice versa. Higher rTPJ activation during unfair repayments correlated with higher positive symptoms, which could suggest that SZS mentalized more or expended more effort when trying to understand or predict the unfair behavior of the trustee using ToM.

Table 16.3. *Neuroimaging studies on trust in psychosis*

Publication	fMRI Background				Summary
Author (Year)	Scanner	Software	fMRI Analyses	ROI	Neural Findings
Fett, Mouchlianitis, et al. (2019)	3 T Signa, General Electric (GE), Centre of Neuroimaging Sciences (CNS), IoPPN	FSL FEAT (FMRI Expert Analysis Tool) version 6.00	ROI Exploratory whole brain investment and repayment phase contrasted with control trials, informed human counterpart	5mm sphere: r caudate (TAL: 10,9,4) r TPJ (51,-54,27) mPFC (-3,64,20)	Interaction effect: HC showed greater caudate activation during cooperative and lower activation during unfair interactions vs. control condition. No such difference in EP. Similar finding in repayment phase Investment: trend EP < HC in r caudate during cooperation and r TPJ in both conditions Cooperative repayment > unfair repayment in EP in r TPJ During repayments, higher persecutory delusions were associated with lower r TPJ activation WAIS Vocabulary scores were significantly associated with caudate activation during cooperative repayment Whole brain - no group differences
Gromann et al. (2013)	3 T Signa, General Electric (GE), CNS, IoPPN	BrainVoyager QX, version 2.3	ROI Exploratory whole brain investment and repayment phase contrasted with control trials, informed human counterpart	5mm sphere: r caudate (TAL: 10,9,4) r TPJ (51,54,27) mPFC (-3,64,20)	Cooperative repayment SZS < HC in r caudate This activation correlated negatively with paranoia In HC caudate signal correlated with initial investment SZS < HC in r TPJ during both repayment phases TPJ correlated with positive symptoms Whole brain SZS < HC in r IPL and r MTG, during cooperative repayments SZS < HC in r IPL during unfair repayments

Study	Scanner	Software	Analysis	Coordinates	Results
Gromann et al. (2014)	3 T Philips Intera, Academic Medical Centre, Amsterdam	BrainVoyager QX, version 2.3.	ROI Exploratory whole brain investment and repayment phase contrasted with control trials, informed human counterpart	5mm sphere: r caudate (TAL: 16,17,6) l insula (-33,14,-1) r TPJ (51,-54,27) r STS (61,-56,7) mPFC (-3,64,20)	Investment GHR < HC in r caudate - Repayment GHR < HC in l insula Higher paranoia associated with less caudate activation Whole brain - Investment GHR < HC in r putamen, r caudate body, r SFG Repayment GHR < HC in l insula, l SFG, l subcallosal gyrus
Hanssen et al. (2021)	3 T Signa General Electric (GE), CNS, IoPPN	SPM 12	ROI Exploratory whole brain cue, investment and repayment phase contrasted with control trials, informed human counterpart	8 mm sphere: r caudate (MNI: 17,20,3) r TPJ (50,-56,27) mPFC (-3,64,24) l dlPFC (-43,18,29)	Cue phase SZS < HC in l dlPFC Investment - No group or context effects Repayment SZS < HC in r caudate - SZS > HC in mPFC (only uncorrected) - No significant associations with symptoms Associations with ESM measures - Higher perceived social relationship quality with higher mPFC activation - Lower perceived social exclusion associated with higher caudate activation in the positive context only (marginally significant) Whole brain - No group differences
Jacob & Rao* (2017)	n.r.	SPM 12	Whole brain decision phase	n.r.	Whole brain (uncorrected) - SZ < HC in right anterior and posterior cingulate gyri, right superior and middle frontal gyri, superior temporal gyrus, right supramarginal gyrus, and striate cortex - SZ > HC in posterior cingulate

Table 16.3. (*cont.*)

Publication	fMRI Background				Summary
Author (Year)	Scanner	Software	fMRI Analyses	ROI	Neural Findings
Lemmers-Jansen et al. (2018)	3 T Philips Achieva, Spinoza Center, Amsterdam	SPM 8	ROI Exploratory whole brain investment and repayment phase contrasted with control trials informed human counterpart	5mm sphere: r caudate (MNI: 16,17,7) 10mm sphere: r TPJ (51,-57,26) r STS (62,-58,5) l insula (-33,14,0) mPFC (-3,65,25)	Investment unfair condition: CHR > HC, FEP in r TPJ Interaction CHR > HC in r TPJ and mPFC, when investing in an unfair partner compared with a cooperative partner CHR & FEP: higher paranoia associated with increased TPJ activation CHR: stronger TPJ activation associated with higher paranoia, positive, and negative symptoms during unfair investments CHR higher paranoia, positive, and negative symptoms associated with stronger rTPJ activation during unfair investments Whole brain No significant group differences at p < 0.05 FWE cluster corrected

| Lemmers-Jansen et al. (2020) | 3 T Philips Achieva, Spinoza Center, Amsterdam | SPM 8 | ROI Exploratory whole brain investment and repayment phase contrasted with control trials informed human counterpart | 5mm sphere: r caudate (MNI: 10,9,5) l amygdala (-24,-2,-19) r amygdala (27,-1,-19) 10mm sphere: mPFC (-3,65,25) r TPJ (52,-57,26) pACC (-6,40,21) l insula (-32,20,-6) r insula (34,21,0) | The pACC and mPFC were activated in the investment phases, and the TPJ during repayments in both conditions. Bilateral insula was activated throughout the game, except during the cooperative investments. The caudate was only active during unfair investments. During repayments, FEP & CHR brought up in higher-urban areas showed increased activation of the right amygdala compared to the control condition of the task, whereas controls brought up in higher-urban areas showed decreased activation. No associations between ROI activation and symptoms. Whole brain. No significant group-by-urbanicity interactions |

Notes: *conference poster abstract; ACC, anterior cingulate cortex; CHR, clinical high risk; CNS, Centre of Neuroimaging Sciences; EP, early psychosis; dlPFC, dorsolateral prefrontal cortex; ESM, experience sampling method; FEP, first-episode psychosis; FSL, FreeSurfer FMRIB Software Library; FWE, family wise error; GHR, genetic high risk; HC, healthy controls; IoPPN, Institute of Psychiatry, Psychology and Neuroscience, King's College London; IPL, inferior parietal lobule; l, left; MFG, medial frontal gyrus; MNI, Montreal Neurological Institute coordinates; mPFC, medial prefrontal cortex; MTG, middle temporal gyrus; n.r., not reported; pACC, perigenual anterior cingulate cortex; r, right; ROI, region of interest; SFG, superior frontal gyrus; SPD, schizophreniform disorder; SPM, statistical parametric mapping; STS, superior temporal sulcus; SZ, schizophrenia; SZS, schizophrenia spectrum; T, Tesla; TAL, Talairach coordinates; TPJ, temporoparietal junction.

The caudate signal was only in controls associated with higher baseline trust, supporting the idea that for them trust is naturally rewarding (Gromann et al., 2013). A second study in chronic SZS probed context sensitivity in the TG. During the context presentation, which provided information about the trustee's trustworthiness, SZS showed reduced activation in the dorsolateral prefrontal cortex (dlPFC), suggesting reduced processing of this information, which was also supported by the absence of an effect of information about trustworthiness on trust. Corroborating earlier findings (Gromann et al., 2013), the study also showed less right caudate activation in SZS compared to controls during cooperative repayments (Hanssen et al., 2021). Importantly, higher caudate activation in the positive context was associated with real-life indices of social functioning, supporting the importance of social reward processing for relationship functioning (Hanssen et al., 2021). One small study that reported uncorrected whole brain analysis results suggested that lower activation of the superior frontal cortex in particular in SZS may suggest aberrant ToM, which could result in reduced trust (Jacob & Rao, 2017). However, behavioral outcomes to support such an interpretation were not reported. Others found reduced activation in the inferior parietal lobule (IPL) and the middle temporal gyrus during cooperative repayments, and in the IPL during unfair repayments in SZS compared to controls (Gromann et al., 2013), or no group differences at the whole brain level (Hanssen et al., 2021). In sum, in the TG chronic SZS is associated with patterns of mostly reduced brain activation relative to controls in hypothesis-driven regions of interest (ROIs) (Figure 16.2), with additional reduced frontal, temporal, parietal, and cingulate activation reported from whole brain analyses (Figure 16.3).

The findings in earlier stages of the disorder are more mixed, possibly due to the heterogeneity of the samples with regard to age and diagnoses. One study did not find differences in neural activation between FEP and controls in the predefined ROIs or on whole brain level (Lemmers-Jansen et al., 2018). Another showed reduced activation in EP in the right caudate and TPJ during investments and repayments, which was most pronounced during cooperative interactions (Fett, Mouchlianitis, et al., 2019). Neural activation in CHR was increased compared to controls and FEP in the rTPJ during investments toward an unfair trustee. These group differences in neural activation were not due to antipsychotic medication. Greater TPJ activation was at trend level associated with higher paranoia scores in both FEP and CHR, and in CHR also significantly associated with higher overall positive and negative symptoms (Lemmers-Jansen et al., 2018).

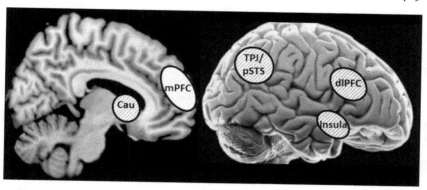

Figure 16.2   Brain regions tested in region of interest analyses during the trust game. Dashed areas indicate regions with reduced activation in psychosis compared to healthy control participants. The TPJ additionally showed increased activation in CHR. In the mPFC no significantly different activation was reported in psychosis (Cau, caudate; dlPFC, dorsolateral prefrontal cortex; mPFC, medial prefrontal cortex; pSTS, posterior superior temporal sulcus; TPJ, temporoparietal junction).

The results suggest that unfair interactions elicit ToM in CHR, particularly when symptoms are high. Interestingly, and similar to their family members with a clinical SZS diagnosis, healthy siblings also show patterns of reduced neural activation compared to controls in the caudate during investments, and in the left insula during repayments (Gromann et al., 2014). Reduced activation was also found at whole brain level during investments (right putamen, right caudate, and right superior frontal gyrus) and repayments (left insula, left superior frontal gyrus, and left subcallosal gyrus). Not many studies have investigated the effect of additional external factors on the neural mechanisms of trust in the earlier stages of psychosis. First, urban upbringing was associated with differential amygdala activation in FEP and CHR (grouped together) compared to controls. During investments, higher urbanicity was associated with reduced left amygdala activation and this effect was more pronounced in CHR and FEP than controls. During repayments, CHR and FEP brought up in more-urban areas showed increased right amygdala activation, whereas controls brought up in more-urban areas showed decreased activation, suggesting altered mechanisms of feedback learning (Lemmers-Jansen et al., 2020). Second, higher cognitive ability has been found to account partly for the group differences between EP and controls in caudate activation (Fett, Mouchlianitis, et al., 2019).

16.4   Theoretical Accounts of Disturbed Trust in Psychosis

Trust is thought to be driven by motivation, cognition, and affect (Krueger & Meyer-Lindenberg, 2019). Research in psychosis mostly focused on reward-related mechanisms, which are closely linked to motivation, and cognition, with a specific emphasis on social cognition in the domain of ToM (Figure 16.3). The investment phase of the TG, in which trust is placed in the trustee, and the repayment phase, in which the trustee's reciprocity is revealed and interpreted, have been associated with activation in ToM-related brain areas (King-Casas, 2005, 2008; Rilling et al., 2004; Van den Bos et al., 2011). Both TG phases have also been associated with activation in the dopamine-governed striatum (including the caudate) (King-Casas, 2005; Phan et al., 2010), which reflects reinforcement learning and the dynamic updating of trustworthiness beliefs based on trustee reciprocity (Chang et al., 2010), and the motivational salience and rewarding propensity of trust itself (Berridge & Robinson, 1998). In social interactions both mechanisms ensure that information about vital social cues and the interaction partner's actions are obtained to predict their future behavior and to adapt the own behavior accordingly.

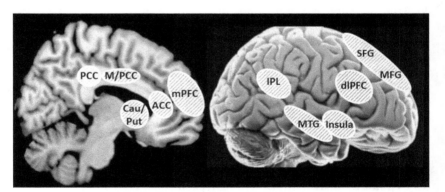

Figure 16.3   Outcomes of the whole brain analyses, showing reduced activation in psychosis.
Dashed areas indicate regions with reduced activation in psychosis compared to healthy control participants. Only the PCC showed increased activation in psychosis (ACC, anterior cingulate cortex; Cau, caudate; dlPFC, dorsolateral prefrontal cortex; IPL, inferior parietal lobule; MFG, medial frontal gyrus; M/PCC, medial part of the posterior cingulate cortex; mPFC, medial prefrontal cortex; PCC, posterior cingulate cortex; pSTS, posterior superior temporal sulcus; Put, putamen; SFG, superior frontal gyrus; TPJ, temporoparietal junction).

In addition, social expectations and beliefs about others (e.g., negative priors) influence social behavior (Delgado et al., 2005). These expectations are reflected in baseline trust. Several studies suggest that expectations of others are already more negative in the early stages of psychosis compared to controls and that the negative beliefs about others become more inflexible with illness duration (Fett et al., 2012, 2016; Gromann et al., 2013; Lemmers-Jansen et al., 2018, 2020). However, contradicting findings (Fett, Mouchlianitis, et al., 2019; Gromann et al., 2014) highlight the need for more research into possible modulators of prior social expectations in psychosis, including the rewarding value of trust itself, the impact of ToM and mentalizing about the signals that people send through nonverbal behavior and about the consequences of this behavior (e.g., how will the trustee react if I increase or decrease my trust), as well as mentalizing about others (e.g., why did the trustee reduce or increase their reciprocity toward me), and perceptions of risk and vulnerability. Reduced baseline trust has also been found in GHR and in CHR (Fett et al., 2012; Lemmers-Jansen et al., 2018), tentatively suggesting that it could be a vulnerability marker for psychosis, rather than the consequence of the disorder. Crucially, lower baseline trust sets the tone for less cooperative or mutually trusting relationships, which might be harder to overcome for individuals with SZS due to problems with reward learning.

16.4.1 *Reward Processing and Trust*

Dopaminergic neurotransmission plays a key role in learning (Schultz, 2016) and has been suggested to underlie the pathophysiology and core symptoms of psychosis (e.g., paranoia and reduced social motivation) (Deserno et al., 2016). In psychosis, aberrant dopaminergic firing in social situations may cause irrelevant social information to appear salient, while important social cues may be missed (Heinz & Schlagenhauf, 2010). In chronic SZS, problems with trust and reward learning in positive social interactions are evidenced by reduced positive reciprocity, by relatively low and stable levels of trust in the face of social cooperation (Campellone et al., 2016, 2018; Fett et al., 2012; Hanssen et al., 2020), and by diminished caudate activation during positive trustee reciprocity (i.e., cooperative repayments) (Gromann et al., 2013; Hanssen et al., 2021). This inability to establish trust during repeated cooperative interactions is socially and economically disadvantageous, leading to less beneficial outcomes in terms of relationship building, as well as monetary gains in the context of the TG. Interestingly, updating of trustworthiness beliefs in response to negative trustee reciprocity (i.e., punishment) and the associated neural reward response are intact (Campellone et al., 2016, 2018; Fett, Mouchlianitis, et al., 2019; Fett, Shergill, Gromann, & Krabbendam, 2015; Gromann et al., 2013), possibly facilitated by the congruence of trustee behavior with durable negative prior expectations about others' trustworthiness. This finding is consistent with work showing intact negative feedback learning in other social (Hanssen et al., 2018) and in nonsocial contexts (Hanssen et al., 2020; Waltz et al., 2007) and contradicts generalized problems with (social) salience and reward learning in SZS. Notably, the ability to establish trust during repeated cooperative social interactions appears to be still intact in the early stages of psychosis (Fett, Mouchlianitis, et al., 2019; Fett et al., 2016; Lemmers-Jansen et al., 2018).

Yet, while some neuroimaging evidence indicates normal reward processing in the caudate (Lemmers-Jansen et al., 2018, 2020), others already indicate a blunted neural reward response in EP (Fett, Mouchlianitis, et al., 2019). Such subtle reward-processing impairments might constitute a vulnerability or risk factor that underlies deficits in trust and impaired social interaction, as supported by findings of reduced trust (Fett et al., 2012; Hanssen et al., 2020) and a diminished neural reward response in GHR (Gromann et al., 2014). Possibly in EP, impaired reward processing is compensated through other (social) cognitive mechanisms, which deteriorate with illness duration, as cognition becomes more compromised (Fett et al., 2020). Moreover, with illness duration the preexisting reward-related vulnerabilities might be aggravated by environmental factors, such as urbanicity (a proxy for social/environmental stress, Krabbendam et al., 2020; Lemmers-Jansen et al., 2020), as suggested by altered amygdala activation (Lemmers-Jansen et al., 2020), and disorder-related mechanisms, such as chronic negative social experiences (e.g., stigma) (Van Zelst, 2009), or long-standing medication use (Huhtaniska et al., 2017), that can limit the ability or willingness to exert effort to overcome distrust and suspiciousness against others. Crucially, initial work shows that reduced trust and blunted caudate activation during positive social interactions are associated with real-world social outcomes, including reduced social engagement and higher feelings of social exclusion (Hanssen et al., 2021), highlighting the importance for patients' daily-life outcomes in social functioning.

Alternative explanations for reduced caudate activation in SZS in terms of prediction error signaling, where caudate activation should be reduced during expected as opposed to surprising trustee responses, appear less plausible. SZS is characterized by more negative prior expectations about others' trustworthiness, thus in contrast to the discussed findings, a stronger caudate signal would be expected in cooperative interactions. Another factor that may impact on trust and reward learning in SZS is antipsychotic anti-dopaminergic medication, which is taken by the majority of individuals with SZS (Table 16.1). Yet, there are several indications that this is not the case. Medication did not impact on trust and the associated neural mechanisms in at risk groups and FEP (Lemmers-Jansen et al., 2018), or on behavior in chronic SZS (Campellone et al., 2018), and healthy first-degree relatives show differential processing of social reward without any medication confounds (Gromann et al., 2014). Also, antipsychotics have been shown to normalize reward learning in nonsocial contexts (Nielsen et al., 2012), which implies that findings in medicated individuals may even underestimate effects that would be present in unmedicated SZS.

16.4.2   Social Cognition and Trust

The second core mechanism that is impaired in SZS and that has been hypothesized to play a role in disturbed trust and social interaction is social cognition (Krueger & Meyer-Lindenberg, 2019), specifically ToM (Fett et al., 2011). The two explanatory mechanisms are not mutually exclusive, but rather may have synergistic effects. For instance, positive social cues may not be interpreted correctly due to aberrant ToM, thus leading to a diminished experience of social reward, which precludes the formation of accurate beliefs about others and their intentions (Lewandowski et al., 2016; Rosenfeld et al., 2010). Without an accurate mental model of the trustee, trust is likely to remain limited or discordant with trustee behavior (Fett, Gromann, et al., 2014; Fett, Shergill, et al., 2014; Prevost et al., 2015). The current evidence suggests that this is the case during cooperative social interactions in chronic SZS (Fett et al., 2012; Gromann et al., 2013; Hanssen et al., 2021), but not in the earlier stages of the disorder (Fett et al., 2016; Lemmers-Jansen et al., 2018) (Figure 16.1). Impaired ToM in traditional social cognitive tasks is associated with reduced mPFC and rTPJ activation (Kronbichler et al., 2017). In the TG better ToM and a better mental model of the trustee have been associated with more tit-for-tat (Fett, Shergill, et al., 2014) and higher TPJ activation (Fett, Gromann, et al., 2014; Xiang et al., 2012). Along these lines, reduced rTPJ activation during repayments in chronic SZS could imply diminished mentalizing about the trustees' intentions and future behavior (Gromann et al., 2013). Reduced rTPJ activation in EP during investments could suggest reduced mentalizing about their own actions and consequences for the trustee or future reciprocity. The absence of differences in rTPJ activation between FEP and controls, and the reverse pattern in CHR, pinpoint the decline in ToM-related processing to after the first psychotic episode. Elevated rTPJ activation in EP during cooperative repayments (Fett, Mouchlianitis, et al., 2019) and during unfair investments in CHR (Lemmers-Jansen et al., 2018) could indicate hyper-ToM, that is, exaggerated mentalizing and attribution of specific intentions to others, and/or compensatory mentalizing strategies that counteract diminished social reward processing, although additional evidence will be needed to investigate this hypothesis.

In contrast to findings in traditional ToM paradigms all TG studies to date showed normal mPFC activation in SZS (Fett, Mouchlianitis, et al., 2019; Gromann et al., 2013; Hanssen et al., 2021; Jacob & Rao, 2017), and in one case elevated activation in CHR compared to controls (Lemmers-Jansen et al., 2018), consistent with meta-analytic evidence for stable patterns of increased neural activation during social cognition in CHR (Kozhuharova et al., 2020). Alternatively, it is possible that demands on the mPFC in the TG are relatively low, as suggested by meta-analytic work on the neural mechanisms of trust (Bellucci et al., 2017) and absent effects of brain stimulation to this area on levels of trust (Colzato et al., 2015). Finally, deficits in facial emotion recognition have robustly been found in nonaffective psychosis and could affect trust in social interactions where such cues play a role (Kohler et al., 2010). The current evidence is inconclusive, with some studies pointing toward normal emotion processing of facial trust cues and others pointing toward a hypersensitivity in SZS.

16.4.3 Nonsocial Cognition and Trust

Trust is not only based on social-emotional, but also rational cost-benefit calculations that require nonsocial cognitive abilities (e.g., attention/vigilance, working memory, and reasoning and problem solving) (Krueger & Meyer-Lindenberg, 2019; Millet & Dewitte, 2007), which are frequently impaired in SZS (Heinrichs & Zakzanis, 1998). Consequently, it is possible that aberrant trust and reward learning in SZS are at least partly explained by impairments in nonsocial cognition (Robison et al., 2020). To account for this, many studies controlled for cognitive ability statistically (Fett et al., 2016; Hanssen et al., 2020; Lemmers-Jansen et al., 2018, 2020). When cognitive ability was directly examined, a slight reduction of differences in trust between SZS and controls occurred, but group differences in rTPJ activation and caudate activation (during investments) remained stable (Fett, Mouchlianitis, et al., 2019; Fett et al., 2012; Gromann et al., 2013), suggesting a relative independence from ToM and reward-based mechanisms during decision making. Group differences between EP and controls in caudate activation during repayments became nonsignificant (Fett, Mouchlianitis, et al., 2019), suggesting that cognitive ability impedes reward computations during revelations of trustee reciprocity. In chronic SZS the effects remained stable. Possibly reward-processing impairments are more robust and therefore still visible when cognitive ability is accounted for (Gromann et al., 2013).

The second nonsocial cognitive ability that generated interest with respect to trust and psychosis is cognitive control (Krebs & Woldorff, 2017), the ability to pursue goal-directed behavior and regulate emotion and cognitive resources. Cognitive control is vital for behavioral flexibility and context-based decision making. It acts as a top-down modulator of bottom-up reward learning, for instance to adjust prepotent tendencies that influence trust (Delgado et al., 2005; Winecoff & Huettel, 2017) and is, among others, sub-served by the dlPFC (Winecoff & Huettel, 2017). Impaired processing of social context along with reduced dlPFC activation (Hanssen et al., 2021), supports the importance of cognitive control in impaired reputation-based trust in SZS (Mervis et al., 2017). Reduced dlPFC signaling has also been suggested to underlie social-motivational impairments in psychosis (Chung & Barch, 2016). However, in the context of the TG, no associations with negative symptoms emerged that could reflect these links with social motivation. Finally, it has been suggested that reasoning biases (Joyce et al., 2013) that have been observed in SZS such as "jumping to conclusions" (i.e., hasty decision making based on insufficient evidence) could explain reduced trust due to the tendency to hold on to negative prior expectations in the face of contradictory evidence based on trustee feedback (Fett et al., 2012, 2016; Gromann et al., 2013; Hanssen et al., 2018; Lemmers-Jansen et al., 2018, 2020). However, this still needs to be investigated.

16.4.4 Symptoms, Trust, and the Brain

Initially, in our work we were most interested in social reward processing as the underlying mechanism of distrust and paranoid delusions (Fett et al., 2012; Gromann et al., 2013), which reflect extreme suspiciousness and firm beliefs in others' ulterior motives. Lower baseline trust and trust during cooperation, as well as lower perceived trustworthiness in faces, have been associated with paranoia in early and chronic psychosis, albeit with marginal significance (Fett, Mouchlianitis, et al., 2019; Fett et al., 2012; Hooker et al., 2011). However, on the neural level lower caudate activation was only related to positive symptoms in chronic SZS (Gromann et al., 2013) and GHR (Gromann et al., 2014), and not in EP, FEP, or CHR (Fett, Mouchlianitis, et al., 2019; Lemmers-Jansen et al., 2018). Associations between negative symptoms, lower trust, and impaired reward learning have been more consistently found by most (Campellone et al., 2018; Fett et al., 2016; Hanssen et al., 2020, 2021; Keri et al., 2009; Lemmers-Jansen et al., 2018, 2020), but not all studies (e.g., Fett et al., 2012).

Again, despite a plausible connection between symptoms of reduced social motivation and the neural mechanisms of social reward processing, significant associations have rarely been reported (Fett, Mouchlianitis, et al., 2019). Symptom associations reported for the TPJ are also mixed. In chronic SZS higher rTPJ activation during unfair repayments has been linked to higher positive symptoms (Gromann et al., 2013). In FEP and CHR similar patterns emerged during unfair investments. In contrast, in EP higher paranoid delusions, but not positive or negative symptoms, were associated with lower rTPJ activation (Fett, Mouchlianitis, et al., 2019). In CHR, rTPJ activation was also associated with higher symptoms in other domains, thus associating higher general psychopathology with greater neural activity during social interactions. Whether higher versus lower rTPJ activation in the context of symptom associations represents underutilization of ToM versus hyper-ToM, as usually suggested (Kronbichler et al., 2017), needs further investigation. Overall, the pattern of correlations between symptoms and trust-related brain activation is inconsistent, as is often the case for studies that try to correlate neurobiological measures with symptoms (Mathalon & Ford, 2012). Possible explanations are the small samples, issues with reliability and validity of symptom assessment, medication and treatment response confounds. A more fine-grained approach that investigates specific aspects of the heterogeneous positive and negative symptom clusters (e.g., paranoia, avolition, disorganization) in a more reliable way and in larger samples might provide clearer answers in future (e.g., Le Heron et al., 2018).

16.5   Summary and Suggestions for Future Research

16.5.1   Summary

In this chapter we reviewed trust and its associated neural mechanisms in psychosis. The existing evidence suggests that reward mechanisms and (social) cognition may underlie disturbed social interaction in SZS, as recently proposed by others (Fulford et al., 2018). In line with this, whole brain analyses showing reduced frontal, temporal, parietal, and cingulate activation further support the role of disturbed processing in the salience, default mode, and central executive brain networks (Nekovarova et al., 2014). Processing of explicit social context (i.e., directly provided information about a person's trustworthiness) is impaired and might lead to a greater impact of negative prior expectations, along with intact processing of implicit social cues that are encoded in facial expressions and looks. Reduced (baseline) trust might also set the scene for more negative social interactions, which might be harder to overcome and could lead to social withdrawal and isolation in real life. Specifically, diminished reward sensitivity during cooperation and intact punishment sensitivity have been suggested to underpin reduced social motivation and paranoia. While the two mechanisms appear to influence the dynamics of social interactions, their relationship with symptoms remains unclear.

16.5.2   Methodological Considerations

Generally, the reviewed studies need to be considered as first insights into the mechanisms of (dis)trust and the dynamics of social interaction in psychosis. The research field is still young and existing studies have been largely (although not exclusively) conducted by our group and are partly based on overlapping samples (e.g., Fett, Mouchlianitis, et al., 2019; Fett et al., 2016 or Lemmers-Jansen et al., 2018, 2020). We mostly used a basic, social context-free version of a TG with a highly cooperative and unfair preprogrammed trustee, in which participants were told they were playing with real players via the Internet, with the exception of Fett et al. (2012), which included real human trustees. Using the same paradigm and ROIs, our studies generated comparable insights into the most basic mechanisms of trust and reward learning in social contexts across the psychosis continuum, ranging from at-risk groups to chronic SZS. However, different scanning sites and fMRI analysis methods, including the software packages SPM (Statistical Parametric Mapping), FSL (FreeSurfer FMRIB Software Library), and BrainVoyager, could account for some discrepancies in findings (Bowring et al., 2019). Several initial studies took basic work a step further and showed that the impact of implicit social cues (i.e., facial trustworthiness) on trust in psychosis is intact, while the impact of explicit social cues (i.e., trustee reputation) on trust is diminished (Hanssen et al., 2021; Hooker et al., 2011).

16.5.3   Suggestion for Future Research

The findings discussed in this chapter warrant replication and future research should broaden its focus to systematically scrutinize the impact of cognitive, affective, and illness-related mechanisms. Key factors of interest include disorder stage and duration, medication effects (e.g., duration and dosage), (social) cognitive ability (e.g., ToM, reasoning biases, nonsocial cognition), the impact of implicit and explicit social contextual cues in different modalities, and factors that have been associated with the incidence of psychosis and diminished trust, such as interpersonal trauma or urbanicity (Bell et al., 2019; Fett, Lemmers-Jansen, & Krabbendam, 2019; Krabbendam et al., 2020). With respect to our CHR samples, it needs to be noted that transition rates were low, suggesting that their psychotic experiences were transient or expressions of risk to other psychopathology than a psychotic disorder. For future research it will be important to look at larger CHR groups to be able to compare trust and its underlying mechanisms between those who convert to a psychotic disorder and those who do not. It is still unclear whether the issues with trust in SZS might be due to reward-learning impairments of a general nature (Hanssen et al., 2020; Wordecha et al., 2018) and further research is needed to investigate this issue and to evaluate the rewarding propensity of different social rewards (e.g., smiles, reputation-based or altruistic motives) and their associated neural mechanisms.

Also, the role of affective mechanisms in trust in psychosis has not yet been studied, leaving unexplored avenues open for investigation, through explicit ratings of the trustee or methods that do not rely on introspection (e.g., skin conductance or heart rate variability) (Krueger & Meyer-Lindenberg, 2019). Dynamic modeling approaches could be applied to examine the relative weighting of reciprocity as a function of strength and valence of prior expectations and experienced social reward (Chang et al.,

2010). Neuroimaging to date has predominantly relied on ROI-based approaches that were combined with exploratory whole brain analyses (Table 16.3). Future work needs to focus on larger-scale brain networks (Nekovarova et al., 2014) and (temporal) interactions between brain regions implicated in social learning, for instance by using dynamic causal modeling and network analysis.

Finally, it is important that future research examines the real-world implications of reduced trust and its amenability to change. Studies could investigate whether (social) cognitive training, noninvasive brain stimulation, or neuromodulation can enhance trust in SZS through activation of reward or ToM- related brain regions. For instance, OXT might help to improve trust and social functioning in SZS (Bradley et al., 2019), due to its modulatory effects on ToM (Bradley et al., 2019) or modification of the rewarding propensity of social interaction and enhanced activation of dopaminergic reward pathways; yet it has not been investigated in this context (Kosfeld et al., 2005; Shamay-Tsoory & Abu-Akel, 2016). Crucially, a better understanding of the mechanisms of reduced trust in psychosis and their amenability to change might be able to provide new targets for interventions that improve the social lives of individuals who are affected by SZS.

References

American Psychiatric Association. (2013). *Diagnostic and statistical manual of mental disorders (DSM-5®)*. American Psychiatric Association. http://doi.org/10.1176/appi.books.9780890425596

Bell, V., Robinson, B., Katona, C., Fett, A.-K. J., & Shergill, S. (2019). When trust is lost: The impact of interpersonal trauma on social interactions. *Psychological Medicine*, 49(6), 1041–1046. http://doi.org/10.1017/S0033291718001800

Bellucci, G., Chernyak, S. V., Goodyear, K., Eickhoff, S. B., & Krueger, F. (2017). Neural signatures of trust in reciprocity: A coordinate-based meta-analysis. *Human Brain Mapping*, 38(3), 1233–1248. http://doi.org/10.1002/hbm.23451

Berridge, K. C., & Robinson, T. E. (1998). What is the role of dopamine in reward: Hedonic impact, reward learning, or incentive salience? *Brain Research Reviews*, 28(3), 309–369. http://10.1016/s0165-0173(98)00019-8

Bowring, A., Maumet, C., & Nichols, T. E. (2019). Exploring the impact of analysis software on task fMRI results. *Human Brain Mapping*, 40(11), 3362–3384. http://doi.org/10.1002/hbm.24603

Bradley, E. R., Brustkern, J., De Coster, L., et al. (2019). Victory is its own reward: Oxytocin increases costly competitive behavior in schizophrenia.

Psychological Medicine, 50(4), 674–682. http://doi.org/10.1017/S0033291719000552

Campellone, T. R., Fisher, A. J., & Kring, A. M. (2016). Using social outcomes to inform decision making in schizophrenia: Relationships with symptoms and functioning. *Journal of Abnormal Psychology*, 125(2), 310–321. http://doi.org/10.1037/abn0000139

Campellone, T. R., Truong, B., Gard, D., & Schlosser, D. A. (2018). Social motivation in people with recent-onset schizophrenia spectrum disorders. *Journal of Psychiatric Research*, 99, 96–103. http://doi.org/10.1016/j.jpsychires.2018.01.006

Chang, L. J., Doll, B. B., Van 't Wout, M., Frank, M. J., & Sanfey, A. G. (2010). Seeing is believing: Trustworthiness as a dynamic belief. *Cognitive Psychology*, 61(2), 87–105. http://doi.org/10.1016/j.cogpsych.2010.03.001

Chung, Y. S., & Barch, D. M. (2016). Frontal-striatum dysfunction during reward processing: Relationships to amotivation in schizophrenia. *Journal of Abnormal Psychology*, 125(3), 453–469. http://10.1037/abn0000137

Colman, A. M. (2003). Cooperation, psychological game theory, and limitations of rationality in social interaction. *Behavioral and Brain Sciences*, 26(2), 139–153. http://doi.org/10.1017/S0140525X03000050

Colzato, L. S., Sellaro, R., Van den Wildenberg, W. P., & Hommel, B. (2015). tDCS of medial prefrontal cortex does not enhance interpersonal trust. *Journal of Psychophysiology*, 29, 131–134. http://doi.org/10.1027/0269-8803/a000144

Couture, S. M., Penn, D. L., & Roberts, D. L. (2006). The functional significance of social cognition in schizophrenia: A review. *Schizophrenia Bulletin*, 32(Suppl. 1), S44–S63. http://doi.org/10.1093/schbul/sbl029

Delgado, M. R., Frank, R. H., & Phelps, E. A. (2005). Perceptions of moral character modulate the neural systems of reward during the trust game. *Nature Neuroscience*, 8(11), 1611–1618. http://10.1038/nn1575

Deserno, L., Schlagenhauf, F., & Heinz, A. (2016). Striatal dopamine, reward, and decision making in schizophrenia. *Dialogues in Clinical Neuroscience*, 18 (1), 77–89. www.ncbi.nlm.nih.gov/pmc/articles/PMC4826774

Fett, A.-K. J., Gromann, P. M., Giampietro, V., Shergill, S. S., & Krabbendam, L. (2014). Default distrust? An fMRI investigation of the neural development of trust and cooperation. *Social Cognitive and Affective Neuroscience*, 9 (4), 395–402. http://doi.org/10.1093/scan/nss144

Fett, A.-K. J., Lemmers-Jansen, I. L. J., & Krabbendam, L. (2019). Psychosis and urbanicity: A review of the recent literature from epidemiology to neurourbanism. *Current Opinion in Psychiatry*, 32(3), 232–241. http://doi.org/10.1097/YCO.0000000000000486

Fett, A.-K. J., Mouchlianitis, E., Gromann, P. M., Vanes, L., Shergill, S. S., & Krabbendam, L. (2019). The neural mechanisms of social reward in early psychosis. *Social Cognitive and Affective Neuroscience*, 14(8), 861–870. http://doi.org/10.1093/scan/nsz058

Fett, A.-K. J., Shergill, S. S., Gromann, P. M., et al. (2014). Trust and social reciprocity in adolescence: A matter of perspective-taking. *Journal of Adolescence*, 37(2), 175–184. http://10.1016/j.adolescence.2013.11.011

Fett, A.-K. J., Shergill, S., Gromann, P., & Krabbendam, L. (2015). Trust vs. paranoia: The dynamics of social interaction in early and chronic psychosis. *Schizophrenia Bulletin*, 41(Suppl. 1), S1–S341. http://doi.org/10.1093/schbul/sbvo10

Fett, A.-K. J., Shergill, S., Joyce, D., et al. (2012). To trust or not to trust: The dynamics of social interaction in psychosis. *Brain*, 135(3), 976–984. http://10.1093/brain/awr359

Fett, A.-K. J., Shergill, S., Korver-Nieberg, N., Yakub, F., Gromann, P., & Krabbendam, L. (2016). Learning to trust: Trust and attachment in early psychosis. *Psychological Medicine*, 46(7), 1437–1447. http://10.1017/S0033291716000015

Fett, A.-K. J., Shergill, S. S., & Krabbendam, L. (2015). Social neuroscience in psychiatry: Unravelling the neural mechanisms of social dysfunction. *Psychological Medicine*, 45(6), 1145–1165. http://10.1017/s0033291714002487

Fett, A.-K. J., Velthorst, E., Reichenberg, A., et al. (2020). Long-term changes in cognitive functioning in individuals with psychotic disorders: Findings from the Suffolk County mental health project. *JAMA Psychiatry*, 77(4), 387–396. http://doi.org/10.1001/jamapsychiatry.2019.3993

Fett, A.-K. J., Viechtbauer, W., Penn, D. L., Van Os, J., & Krabbendam, L. (2011). The relationship between neurocognition and social cognition with functional outcomes in schizophrenia: A meta-analysis. *Neuroscience & Biobehavioral Reviews*, 35(3), 573–588. http://doi.org/10.1016/j.neubiorev.2010.07.001

Freeman, D., Garety, P. A., Kuipers, E., Fowler, D., & Bebbington, P. E. (2002). A cognitive model of persecutory delusions. *British Journal of Clinical Psychology*, 41(4), 331–347. http://doi.org/10.1348/014466502760387461

Fulford, D., Campellone, T., & Gard, D. E. (2018). Social motivation in schizophrenia: How research on basic reward processes informs and limits our understanding. *Clinical Psychology Review*, 63, 12–24. https://doi.org/10.1016/j.cpr.2018.05.007

Gromann, P., Heslenfeld, D., Fett, A.-K. J., Joyce, D., Shergill, S., & Krabbendam, L. (2013). Trust versus paranoia: Abnormal response to social reward in psychotic illness. *Brain*, 136, 1968–1675 awt076. http://doi.org/10.1093/brain/awt076

Gromann, P., Shergill, S., De Haan, L., et al. (2014). Reduced brain reward response during cooperation in first-degree relatives of patients with psychosis: An fMRI study. *Psychological Medicine*, 44(16), 3445–3454. http://doi.org/10.1093/scan/nsz058

Hanssen, E., Fett, A.-K. J., White, T. P., Caddy, C., Reimers, S., & Shergill, S. S. (2018). Cooperation and sensitivity to social feedback during group interactions in schizophrenia. *Schizophrenia Research*, 202, 361–368. http://doi.org/10.1016/j.schres.2018.06.065

Hanssen, E., Krabbendam, L., Robberegt, S., & Fett, A.-K. J. (2020). Social and non-social reward learning reduced and related to a familial vulnerability in schizophrenia spectrum disorders. *Schizophrenia Research*, 215, 256–262. http://doi.org/10.1016/j.schres.2019.10.019

Hanssen, E., Van Buuren, M., Van Atteveldt, N., Lemmers-Jansen, I. L. J., & Fett, A.-K. J. (2021). Neural, behavioural and real-life correlates of social context sensitivity and social reward learning during interpersonal interactions in the schizophrenia spectrum. *Australian & New Zealand Journal of Psychiatry*, 1–12. http://doi.org/10.1177/00048674211010327

Haut, K. M., & MacDonald III, A. W. (2010). Persecutory delusions and the perception of trustworthiness in unfamiliar faces in schizophrenia. *Psychiatry Research*, 178(3), 456–460. http://doi.org/10.1016/j.psychres.2010.04.015

Heinrichs, R. W., & Zakzanis, K. K. (1998). Neurocognitive deficit in schizophrenia: A quantitative review of the evidence. *Neuropsychology*, 12(3), 426–445. http://doi.org/10.1037/0894-4105.12.3.426

Heinz, A., & Schlagenhauf, F. (2010). Dopaminergic dysfunction in schizophrenia: Salience attribution revisited. *Schizophrenia Bulletin*, 36(3), 472–485. http://doi.org/10.1093/schbul/sbq031

Hooker, C. I., Tully, L. M., Verosky, S. C., Fisher, M., Holland, C., & Vinogradov, S. (2011). Can I trust you? Negative affective priming influences social judgments in schizophrenia. *Journal of Abnormal Psychology*, 120 (1), 98–107. http://doi.org/10.1037/a0020630

Huhtaniska, S., Jääskeläinen, E., Hirvonen, N., et al. (2017). Long-term antipsychotic use and brain changes in schizophrenia: A systematic review and meta-analysis. *Human Psychopharmacology: Clinical and Experimental*, 32 (2), Article e2574. http://doi.org/10.1002/hup.2574

Insel, T. R. (2010). Rethinking schizophrenia. *Nature*, 468(7321), 187–193. http://10.1038/nature09552

Jacob, A., & Rao, N. (2017). SA69. Neural basis of trust deficits in schizophrenia: An fMRI investigation. *Schizophrenia Bulletin*, 43(Suppl. 1), S138. http://doi.org/10.1093/schbul/sbx023.068

Joyce, D. W., Averbeck, B. B., Frith, C. D., & Shergill, S. S. (2013). Examining belief and confidence in schizophrenia. *Psychological Medicine*, 43(11), 2327–2338. http://doi.org/10.1017/S0033291713000263

Keri, S., Kiss, I., & Kelemen, O. (2009). Sharing secrets: Oxytocin and trust in schizophrenia. *Social Neuroscience*, 4(4), 287–293. http://doi.org/10.1080/17470910802319710

King-Casas, B. (2005). Getting to know you: Reputation and trust in a two-person economic exchange. *Science*, 308, 78–83. http://dx.doi.org/10.1126/science.1108062

King-Casas, B., Sharp, C., Lomax-Bream, L., Lohrenz, T., Fonagy, P., & Montague, P. R. (2008). The rupture and repair of cooperation in borderline personality disorder. *Science*, 321, 806–810. http://doi.org/10.1126/science.1156902

Kirkpatrick, B., Fenton, W. S., Carpenter, W. T., & Marder, S. R. (2006). The NIMH-MATRICS consensus statement on negative symptoms. *Schizophrenia Bulletin*, 32(2), 214–219. http://doi.org/10.1093/schbul/sbj053

Kohler, C. G., Walker, J. B., Martin, E. A., Healey, K. M., & Moberg, P. J. (2010). Facial emotion perception in schizophrenia: A meta-analytic review. *Schizophrenia Bulletin*, 36(5), 1009–1019. http://doi.org/10.1093/schbul/sbn192

Kosfeld, M., Heinrichs, M., Zak, P. J., Fischbacher, U., & Fehr, E. (2005). Oxytocin increases trust in humans. *Nature*, 435(7042), 673–676. http://doi.org/10.1038/nature03701

Kozhuharova, P., Saviola, F., Ettinger, U., & Allen, P. (2020). Neural correlates of social cognition in populations at risk of psychosis: A systematic review. *Neuroscience & Biobehavioral Reviews*, 108, 94–111. https://doi.org/10.1016/j.neubiorev.2019.10.010

Krabbendam, L., Van Vugt, M., Conus, P., et al. (2020). Understanding urbanicity: How interdisciplinary methods help to unravel the effects of the city on mental health. *Psychological Medicine*, 1–12. http://doi.org/10.1017/S0033291720000355

Krebs, R. M., & Woldorff, M. G. (2017). Cognitive control and reward. In T. Egner (Ed.), *The Wiley handbook of cognitive control* (pp. 422–439). Wiley-Blackwell. http://doi.org/10.1002/9781118920497.ch24

Kronbichler, L., Tschernegg, M., Martin, A. I., Schurz, M., & Kronbichler, M. (2017). Abnormal brain activation during theory of mind tasks in schizophrenia: A meta-analysis. *Schizophrenia Bulletin*, 43(6), 1240–1250. http://doi.org/10.1093/schbul/sbx073

Krueger, F., & Meyer-Lindenberg, A. (2019). Toward a model of interpersonal trust drawn from neuroscience, psychology, and economics. *Trends in Neurosciences*, 42(2), 92–101. http://doi.org/10.1016/j.tins.2018.10.004

Le Heron, C., Apps, M. A. J., & Husain, M. (2018). The anatomy of apathy: A neurocognitive framework for amotivated behaviour. *Neuropsychologia*, 118, 54–67. http://doi.org/10.1016/j.neuropsychologia.2017.07.003

Lemmers-Jansen, I. L., Fett, A.-K. J., Hanssen, E., Veltman, D. J., & Krabbendam, L. (2018). Learning to trust: Social feedback normalizes trust behavior in first-episode psychosis and clinical high risk. *Psychological Medicine*, 49(5), 780–790. http://doi.org/10.1017/S003329171800140X

Lemmers-Jansen, I. L., Fett, A.-K. J., Van Os, J., Veltman, D. J., & Krabbendam, L. (2020). Trust and the city: Linking urban upbringing to neural mechanisms of trust in psychosis. *Australian & New Zealand Journal of Psychiatry*, 54(2), 138–149. https://doi.org/10.1177/0004867419865939

Lewandowski, K. E., Whitton, A. E., Pizzagalli, D. A., Norris, L. A., Ongur, D., & Hall, M.-H. (2016). Reward learning, neurocognition, social cognition, and symptomatology in psychosis. *Frontiers in Psychiatry*, 7, Article 100. http://doi.org/10.3389/fpsyt.2016.00100

Mathalon, D. H., & Ford, J. M. (2012). Neurobiology of schizophrenia: Search for the elusive correlation with symptoms. *Frontiers in Human Neuroscience*, 6, Article 136. http://doi.org/10.3389/fnhum.2012.00136

Mervis, J. E., Capizzi, R. J., Boroda, E., & MacDonald, A. W. (2017). Transcranial direct current stimulation over the dorsolateral prefrontal cortex in schizophrenia: A quantitative review of cognitive outcomes. *Frontiers in Human Neuroscience*, 11, Article 44. http://doi.org/10.3389/fnhum.2017.00044

Millet, K., & Dewitte, S. (2007). Altruistic behavior as a costly signal of general intelligence. *Journal of Research in Personality*, 41(2), 316–326. http://doi.org/10.1016/j.jrp.2006.04.002

Nekovarova, T., Fajnerova, I., Horacek, J., & Spaniel, F. (2014). Bridging disparate symptoms of schizophrenia: A triple network dysfunction theory. *Frontiers in Behavioral Neuroscience*, 8, Article 171. http://doi.org/10.3389/fnbeh.2014.00171

Nielsen, M. O., Rostrup, E., Wulff, S., et al. (2012). Improvement of brain reward abnormalities by antipsychotic monotherapy in schizophrenia. *Archives of General Psychiatry*, 69(12), 1195–1204. http://doi.org/10.1001/archgenpsychiatry.2012.847

Palmier-Claus, J., Korver-Nieberg, N., Fett, A.-K. J., & Couture, S. (2019). Attachment and social functioning in psychosis. In K. Berry, S. Bucci, & A. N. Danquah (Eds.), *Attachment theory and psychosis: Current perspectives and future directions* (pp. 84–95). Routledge. https://doi.org/10.4324/9781315665573

Phan, K. L., Sripada, C. S., Angstadt, M., & McCabe, K. (2010). Reputation for reciprocity engages the brain reward center. *Proceedings of the National Academy of Sciences*, 107(29), 13099–13104. http://doi.org/10.1073/pnas.1008137107

Pinkham, A. E. (2014). Social cognition in schizophrenia. *Journal of Clinical Psychiatry*, 75(Suppl. 2), 14–19. http://doi.org/10.4088/JCP.13065su1.04

Prevost, M., Brodeur, M., Onishi, K. H., Lepage, M., & Gold, I. (2015). Judging strangers' trustworthiness is associated with theory of mind skills. *Frontiers in Psychiatry*, 6, Article 52. http://doi.org/10.3389/fpsyt.2015.00052

Rilling, J. K., Sanfey, A. G., Aronson, J. A., Nystrom, L. E., & Cohen, J. D. (2004). The neural correlates of theory of mind within interpersonal interactions. *NeuroImage*, 22(4), 1694–1703. http://doi.org/10.1016/j.neuroimage.2004.04.015

Robison, A. J., Thakkar, K. N., & Diwadkar, V. A. (2020). Cognition and reward circuits in schizophrenia: Synergistic, not separate. *Biological Psychiatry*, 87(3), 204–214. http://doi.org/10.1016/j.biopsych.2019.09.021

Rosenfeld, A. J., Lieberman, J. A., & Jarskog, L. F. (2010). Oxytocin, dopamine, and the amygdala: A neurofunctional model of social cognitive deficits in schizophrenia. *Schizophrenia Bulletin*, 37(5), 1077–1087. http://doi.org/10.1093/schbul/sbq015

Schultz, W. (2016). Dopamine reward prediction-error signalling: A two-component response. *Nature Reviews Neuroscience*, 17(3), 183–195. http://doi.org/10.1038/nrn.2015.26

Shamay-Tsoory, S. G., & Abu-Akel, A. (2016). The social salience hypothesis of oxytocin. *Biological Psychiatry*, 79(3), 194–202. http://doi.org/10.1016/j.biopsych.2015.07.020

Sutherland, C. A., Rhodes, G., Williams, N., et al. (2019). Appearance-based trust processing in schizophrenia. *British Journal of Clinical Psychology*, 59(2), 139–153. http://doi.org/10.1111/bjc.12234

Van den Bos, W., Van Dijk, E., Westenberg, H., Rombout, S. A. R. B., & Crone, E. A. (2011). Changing brains, changing perspectives: The neurocognitive development of reciprocity. *Psychological Science*, 22(1), 60–70. http://doi.org/10.1177%2F0956797610391102

Van Zelst, C. (2009). Stigmatization as an environmental risk in schizophrenia: A user perspective. *Schizophrenia Bulletin*, 35(2), 293–296. http://doi.org/10.1093/schbul/sbn184

Velthorst, E., Fett, A.-K. J., Reichenberg, A., et al. (2017). The 20-year longitudinal trajectories of social functioning in individuals with psychotic disorders. *American Journal of Psychiatry*, 174(11), 1075–1085. http://doi.org/10.1176/appi.ajp.2016.15111419

Velthorst, E., Reichenberg, A., Kapara, O., et al. (2016). Developmental trajectories of impaired community functioning in schizophrenia. *JAMA Psychiatry*, 73(1), 48–55. http://doi.org/10.1001/jamapsychiatry.2015.2253

Waltz, J. A., Frank, M. J., Robinson, B. M., & Gold, J. M. (2007). Selective reinforcement learning deficits in schizophrenia support predictions from computational models of striatal-cortical dysfunction. *Biological Psychiatry*, 62(7), 756–764. http://doi.org/10.1016/j.biopsych.2006.09.042

Whitton, A. E., & Lewandowski, K. E. (2019). Reward processing and social functioning in psychosis. In K. E. Lewandowski & A. A. Moustafa (Eds.), *Social cognition in psychosis* (pp. 177–200). Academic Press. http://doi.org/10.1016/B978-0-12-815315-4.00007-0

Winecoff, A. A., & Huettel, S. (2017). Cognitive control and neuroeconomics. In T. Egner (Ed.), *The Wiley handbook of cognitive control* (pp. 408–421). Wiley. http://doi.org/10.1002/9781118920497.ch23

Wordecha, M., Jarkiewicz, M., Kossowski, B., Lee, J., & Marchewka, A. (2018). Brain correlates of recognition of communicative interactions from biological motion in schizophrenia. *Psychological Medicine*, 48(11), 1862–1871. http://doi.org/10.1017/S0033291717003385

Xiang, T., Ray, D., Lohrenz, T., Dayan, P., & Montague, P. R. (2012). Computational phenotyping of two-person interactions reveals differential neural response to depth-of-thought. *PLoS Computational Biology*, 8(12), Article e1002841. http://doi.org/10.1371/journal.pcbi.1002841

CHAPTER 17

Trust and Personality Disorders
Phenomenology, Determinants, and Therapeutical Approaches

Stefanie Lis, Miriam Biermann, and Zsolt Unoka

17.1 Introduction

Impairment of interpersonal relationships is a central feature of many mental disorders, including personality disorders (PDs). In general, a mental disorder often negatively impacts social relationships. A disorder may cause many changes in everyday life, like financial problems due to unemployment after prolonged periods of illness or changes in the reciprocity of emotional support in a relationship when the patient is overwhelmed by symptoms. These may increase the burden for the patients themselves and members of their social network. Beyond such factors that might be relevant in general for both somatic and mental disorders, many mental disorders have been linked to changes in social-emotional processing. Among the most widely investigated functions is the ability to correctly and confidently recognize social-emotional cues such as another's cognitive and affective mental state indicated by a facial expression, a voice, or even a body posture. While such alterations may affect interpersonal behaviors and in consequence the smoothness of social interactions across different social domains, the building and maintaining of social relationships relies additionally on an individual's ability to trust social interaction partners.

In the current chapter, we will start with a short introduction to the definition and classification of PDs and subsequently provide an overview of methodological approaches used to study trust as one domain of interpersonal functioning in PDs. We report findings elucidating the specific importance of issues with trust in PDs and present the limited neurobiological findings to date. We describe trust as a target concept in psychotherapeutic and pharmacological interventions and, finally, outline implications for future research. However, studies on the impairments of

Corresponding author: Stefanie Lis (stefanie.lis@zi-mannheim.de).

trust in PDs are sparse. Thus, we will focus on borderline personality disorder (BPD) as an example of a PD because, among PDs, most of the published research on trust is about BPD patients.

17.2 Trust and the Diagnosis of Personality Disorders

17.2.1 Definition of Personality Disorders

The *Diagnostic and Statistical Manual* (DSM-5), which is one established diagnostic system for mental disorders, defines a PD as an "enduring pattern of inner experience and behavior that deviates markedly from the expectations of the individual's culture resulting in distress and functional impairments" (American Psychiatric Association [APA], 2013, p. 645). Prevalence in the general populations is reported in the range of, for example, 7.8% in community samples worldwide (Winsper et al., 2020) and 12%–17% in Western countries (Volkert et al., 2018). Prevalence rates vary across different PDs (e.g. Winsper et al., 2020) and are markedly higher in the context of psychiatric disorders (see, e.g., Friborg et al., 2013, 2014; Martinussen et al., 2017).

The DSM-5 comprises two approaches to define PDs. The categorical approach conceptualizes PDs as distinct clinical syndromes and defines the diagnostic criteria for 10 specific PDs (section II). The alternative dimensional approach aims to characterize PDs by impairments of personality functioning and maladaptive personality traits (section III). Personality functioning comprises two domains, that is, self-functioning and interpersonal functioning. The maladaptive personality traits are assumed to be extreme variants of traits underlying personality in general. Overall, 25 personality facets are defined that are allocated to five trait domains, that is, negative affectivity, detachment, antagonism, disinhibition, and psychoticism. For both a categorical and a dimensional diagnosis of PDs, PD features have to be pervasive and inflexible, occurring across different domains of personal or social situations and being stable over time with an onset in adolescence or early adulthood (APA, 2013).

Based on phenomenological similarities, but not consistently validated, PD categories are assumed to form three clusters: Cluster A includes the paranoid, schizoid, and schizotypal PDs, cluster B the antisocial, borderline, histrionic, and narcissistic PDs, and cluster C the avoidant, dependent, and obsessive-compulsive PDs. The behavior of individuals with a PD is characterized as odd or eccentric in cluster A, as dramatic, emotional, or erratic in cluster B, and as anxious or fearful in cluster C (APA, 2013).

However, the different PDs are not exclusive categories, and even PDs from different clusters often co-occur within an individual. The issue of assigning unequivocally one specific PD diagnosis to an individual is avoided in the dimensional approach. Please note that only the categories of the antisocial, avoidant, borderline, narcissistic, obsessive-compulsive, and schizotypal PDs can be derived from the dimensional approach.

17.2.2   Trust as Part of the Diagnostic Criteria for Personality Disorders

In the categorical approach to PD diagnosis, issues with trust are explicitly emphasized as part of the psychopathology only for the paranoid PDs (cluster A). Here, diagnostic criterion A describes paranoid PDs as defined by "a pervasive distrust and suspiciousness of others such that their motives are interpreted as malevolent" (APA, 2013, p. 649). Related behaviors of the patients are specified for example as he or she "suspects, without sufficient basis, that others are exploiting, harming, or deceiving him or her," as being "preoccupied with unjustified doubts about the loyalty or trustworthiness of friends or associates," as being "reluctant to confide in others because of unwarranted fear that the information will be used maliciously against him or her," or as having "recurrent suspicions, without justification, regarding fidelity of spouse or sexual partner." The importance of alterations in trust are less obvious for the other PDs.

Based on the five-factor model of general personality structure that describes trust as a facet of the personality trait "agreeableness (vs. antagonism)," Widiger and Costa (2012) outlined changes in trust for most categories of PDs. Exceptions are the schizoid, the avoidant, and the obsessive-compulsive PDs. In the majority of PDs, that is, for the paranoid, the schizotypal, the antisocial, the borderline, and the narcissistic PDs, the authors suggested alterations in form of reduced trust (see also, e.g., for BPD Furnham & Crump, 2014 and for avoidant personality disorder Wilberg et al., 1999). In contrast, they linked the histrionic and dependent PDs to excessive trust (see also Furnham, 2014). However, a recent study by Mike et al. (2018) suggests, based on self- and informant-based assessments with a personality questionnaire, that trust toward others is also reduced in obsessive-compulsive PD.

In the dimensional model of PDs of the DSM-5, impaired interpersonal functioning – as one domain of personality functioning – is defined as the dysfunction of empathy and intimacy. Intimacy comprises deep and durable connections with others as well as the desire and capacity for closeness. Trusting in others forms an essential facet of close interpersonal relationships (Rempel et al., 1985). In this line of thinking, the ability to trust may form a prerequisite for the experience of intimacy. Thus, a lack of trust might be one factor resulting in issues in experiencing intimacy in social relations across different PDs, suggesting trust issues as one mechanism underlying this domain of psychopathology. The role of trust issues for impairments of intimacy is stated explicitly only for two PDs in the dimensional approach: Marked impairments in developing close relationships associated with mistrust and anxiety characterize the schizotypal PD, while close relationships for the BPD are described as intense, unstable, conflicted, and marked by mistrust. Without being clearly linked to issues with trust, a "reluctance to get involved with people unless being certain of being liked, a diminished mutuality within intimate relationships because of fear of being shamed or ridiculed" (APA, 2013, p. 765) describes impairments in intimacy for the avoidant PD, suggesting a lack in trust toward the behaviors of others as an underlying mechanism. Similarly, the desire to be in control of people, tasks, and situations and an inability to delegate tasks in obsessive-compulsive PD points to a lack of trust as an essential component in this PD.

Moreover, the dimensional model allows to diagnose and describe a PD exclusively based on personality functioning together with specified traits, but without the assignment of a specific PD category. The personality trait relevant for trust issues is "detachment." It comprises "suspiciousness" as one component among others on the personality facet level. Suspiciousness refers to "expectations of – and sensitivity to – signs of interpersonal ill intent or harm, doubts about loyalty and fidelity of others, feelings of being mistreated, used, and/or persecuted by others" (APA, 2013, p. 779).

In sum, the descriptions of many of the PDs explicitly refer or implicitly suggest issues with trust as an essential part of psychopathology. In contrast to this relevance, empirical studies on trust in PDs are sparse.

17.3 Empirical Findings on Trust in Personality Disorders

17.3.1 Definition of Trust

The construct "trust" is studied in various disciplines ranging from economy and psychology to neurosciences (see also Chapters 1–4). Depending on the single discipline, the definition of this concept varies, and with that the applied measurement approach. Nevertheless, there is consent that trust is a multifaceted construct with many dimensions. Essential aspects are the differentiation between trust and reciprocity, trust and distrust as well as trust propensity and trust dynamics (see also Chapters 10 and 12). In the context of PDs, some aspects might be of particular importance that we will discuss in the following paragraphs.

While trust might be conceptualized as an unspecific and generalized expectation about the beneficent behavior of others, some approaches stress its dependency on the specific social interaction partner and the specific situation (Bauer & Freitag, 2017). Mayer et al. (1995) proposed a model of trust that differentiated between trust as a situational state and trust propensity, that is, an individual's stable personality feature. People high in trust propensity are more likely to actually trust others. This underlines the need to assess trust in PDs within different contexts to investigate whether issues with trust are – as assumed for the maladaptive personality traits – indeed an overarching pattern in interpersonal contacts. The situation dependency of trust is emphasized by the fact that trust is particularly challenged in situations of uncertainty during which a social counterpart may act in a way that benefits or harms another and with that makes the trusting individual vulnerable. In consequence, trust comprises an individual's willingness to accept vulnerability in interpersonal encounters.

Trust may develop and be maintained in different ways. These comprise trust in the form of a personality trait, a moral commitment, or a cognitive bias that characterizes the trustor. Other approaches emphasize the relevance of interpersonal encounters such as the influence of preceding experiences with social partners, shared features between trustor and trustee such as being part of the same group (in-group bias) as well as "third-party" reputation. Thus, trust may affect not only the reciprocity of interpersonal encounters, but also an individual's ability for social learning (see, e.g., Landrum et al., 2015). Indeed, alterations in social learning play a role in models characterizing interpersonal impairments in PDs. Moreover, experiences with others in the past might be of particular importance in some PDs. The experience of adverse events during childhood and adolescence (ACE) has been reported in several PDs such as paranoid, antisocial, and borderline PDs (Natsuaki et al., 2009; White et al., 2019). Moreover, the experience of trauma with a high degree of betrayal is a strong predictor of BPD personality traits (Yalch & Levendosky, 2019). These are examples suggesting an important role of ACE on the willingness to trust or to be vulnerable in PDs.

Jones and Shah (2016) emphasized the distinction of three different components of trust: trusting beliefs, trusting intentions, and trusting actions. They showed a differential relevance of these components during the course of social contacts. Trusting beliefs differentially characterize individuals in regard to their appraisal of another one's trustworthiness that is formed by observing, interpreting, and attributing motives that may result in a positive expectation toward the trustee's actions. Thereby, trusting beliefs are influenced by different features of the trustees, that is, their ability, benevolence, and integrity (Mayer et al., 1995). Trusting intentions refer to an individual's willingness to be vulnerable. Finally, trusting actions are the behaviors indicating that people rely on others. While trusting beliefs are most important during first contacts with others, they become less influential with augmenting information about the context or the interaction partner.

17.3.2 Assessing Trust in Personality Disorders

In line with the complex construct of trust, there exist many different approaches to measure trust in PDs. Examples are approaches that focus on an individual's view of oneself in regard to trustfulness and trustworthiness measured by self-evaluations of general trust beliefs or hypothetical behaviors in theoretical scenarios, the appraisal of others as trustworthy, or the behavioral correlates of trust measured during real or simulated social encounters. These different approaches target different facets of trust, are related to specific strengths and weaknesses, and may provide seemingly inconsistent findings. While all of them allow additionally for self-reports or behavioral indices to use neurobiological methods to take the involved neuronal processes into account, this is nearly never done (for an exception see the study by Fertuck et al., 2019 and see Section 17.3.3).

Self-reports of trustfulness and trustworthiness reflect particularly the self-image of an individual with the well-known problems linked to self-report measures particularly in case of a negative self-image. To our knowledge, in the context of PDs, questionnaires on trait and state trust have been rarely applied. Visual appraisal paradigms where participants are asked to assess the trustworthiness of a stranger based on static or dynamic facial expressions or short movie clips ("thin slice paradigm") have been used more often. These tasks focusing on first impressions vary in the extent of additionally available information about the judged person. Finally, due to the increasing impact of approaches from the behavioral economy, a larger body of studies exist that investigated trusting behavior with exchange games. However, the informative significance of these studies in regard to impairments of trust in PDs varies, since they exist in a variety of settings. These capture trust to a different extent in contrast to, for example, reciprocity, cooperative behavior, altruism, and risk-taking (see also Chapters 5 and 10). For example, during a trust game (TG) the measured processes differ on whether a person takes the role of the trustor or the trustee and whether they comprise single exchanges as in one-shot TGs or repeated interactions with the same co-player as in multi-round games. Moreover, they refer to a restricted domain of social interactions, that is, sharing real or virtual monetary units.

17.3.3   Empirical Findings

Only recently, Poggi et al. (2019) reviewed empirical findings on trust in PDs. Their analyses revealed a significant lack of studies on trust in most PDs, with BPD being an exception. In many areas, BPD is the most researched among PDs, which may relate to the clinical relevance of this PD. Although the prevalence rate of BPD (1.9%) is in the middle range among specific PDs (0.78%–4.32%; Volkert et al., 2018) sufferers use more therapy sessions, have more medical consultations, emergency department visits, and hospitalizations, and spent more days in hospitals than those with other PDs and major depression (Bender et al., 2001). Nevertheless, Poggi et al. (2019) concluded that different PDs might be associated to different pattern of trust impairments: They suggested that BPD is primarily linked to a negatively biased misinterpretation of social situations, while mistrust plays a role for aggressive behaviors in narcissistic PD.

Self-Reports of Trust. Surprisingly, to our knowledge, studies that evaluate explicit self-reports of general trust in PDs are sparse. The personality inventory for DSM-5, a self-report questionnaire for the assessment of maladaptive personality traits as defined in the dimensional approach of PDs of the DSM-5, includes the facet of suspiciousness with items that explicitly measure general trust (e.g. item 131: "People are basically trustworthy"; APA, 2013). Nevertheless, there are only a small number of studies on trust in PDs that report related findings. Eikenaes et al. (2013) could show that avoidant personality disorder is linked to higher levels of mistrust compared with social phobia. A recent study by Torres-Sot et al. (2019) suggests that trustfulness may not selectively be impaired in specific PDs: The authors found no differences between patients with BPD and other PDs in self-reports of the personality facet suspiciousness.

A recent study by Botsford et al. (2019) applied a self-report questionnaire that asks participants to judge their trust behavior in different social situations. BPD patients reported lower trust behaviors compared with participants of a nonclinical control group and patients with a major depressive disorder, while no differences were observed in comparison to participants with a social anxiety disorder. When analyzing self-reports of trust behavior in two different domains, BPD patients reported fewer trusting behaviors in the domain of "entrusting known people with material items." In contrast, for situations related to "entrusting unknown people with one's well-being," only patients with a depressive disorder differed from the other groups with reporting a higher willingness for trust behaviors. It seems worth noting that many studies investigated sensitivity to social rejection in BPD. These revealed that BPD patients more anxiously expect to be rejected by others compared with patients with avoidant PDs, anxiety disorders, social phobia, and mood disorders (Staebler et al., 2011). These findings suggest a lack of trust or a lack of positive expectations toward being socially included by others, pointing to an association between trust and rejection sensitivity (see also Poggi et al., 2019). So far, there are no empirical data explicitly relating rejection sensitivity and trust beliefs to each other. However, some studies could confirm a relationship between rejection sensitivity and facial trustworthiness appraisals in BPD. While studies are widely missing that apply comparable approaches in other PDs, these findings suggest changes in interpersonal trust beliefs that seem to be situation-specific, at least when assessed from the perspective of the individual.

Beyond the importance of holding the complexity of the construct trust in mind, it seems essential to take the variability of the mechanism underlying specific personality traits into account. Grandiose narcissism, that is, the tendency of people to achieve and preserve high self-esteem, is one example. While narcissists are, in general, considered to be less trusting, different facets of narcissism seem to be linked to opposite changes in trust beliefs (Kwiatkowska et al., 2018). A high level of communal narcissism that is characterized by using communal means to preserve a high self-esteem was related to increased trust beliefs. In contrast, antagonistic narcissism characterized by competition with others was linked to lower trust beliefs. Although this study relied on the measurement of narcissistic personality traits in the general population in contrast to a clinical sample of individuals with a narcissistic PD, it emphasizes the need to take potential heterogeneity in facets of personality traits into account. Different facets may engage different mechanisms to achieve the same overall goal, for example in the case of narcissism and self-enhancement. Heterogeneity in trust between individuals with the same

PD might also explain variability in treatment efficacy: Already in 1993, Alden and Capreol found that a subgroup of patients with avoidant PD that was associated with distrustful behavior profited less from skill training involving interpersonal contacts in contrast to a graduated exposure intervention during behavior therapy.

Trustworthiness Appraisal. An experimental approach to investigate impairments in trust is the use of facial trustworthiness appraisal tasks. Most studies focused on BPD, while to our knowledge there is only one study in other PDs. Richell et al. (2005) investigated psychopathic offenders and their findings revealed no changes in the appraisal of trustworthiness when compared with offenders without psychopathic features.

In contrast, but in line with the often-reported negative evaluations of others (Barnow et al., 2009), BPD patients assessed unknown others as less trustworthy (Fertuck et al., 2013, 2018, 2019; Miano et al., 2013; Nicol et al., 2013). However, these studies revealed consistently that the differences observed in BPD patients compared with healthy control participants are caused by an evaluation bias, but not a change in evaluative processes specific for trust: The patients' ratings indicated lower trustworthiness ratings independently of the trustworthiness expressed in the presented facial stimuli.

Many studies in healthy individuals have linked first impression trustworthiness appraisals with the displayed facial emotion associating an angry expression with untrustworthiness and a happy expression with trustworthiness (e.g. Krumhuber et al., 2007; Oosterhof & Todorov, 2009). Richell et al. (2005) found a comparable association in their study on psychopathy. Considering that facial emotion recognition is impaired in many mental disorders including some PDs, one may ask whether alterations in trustworthiness appraisals in PDs are specific for impairments of trust, or whether they reflect unspecific changes in social judgments in general. Fertuck et al. (2019) addressed this question in BPD. They showed that appraisals of low trustworthiness are – at least in BPD – not caused by an increased responsiveness to threat: BPD patients assessed facial stimuli as less trustworthy while they rated the fearfulness of faces comparable to healthy control participants. They confirmed that both social judgments, that is, the appraisal of trustworthiness and fearfulness in facial expression, rely on different cognitive functions implemented in distinct neural structures. Most importantly, changes in trustworthiness appraisal were not linked to altered amygdala activation. This contradicted the assumption that issues with trust correspond to a subcortical threat response. In contrast, they were linked to reduced activation of prefrontal regions including the insula and the lateral prefrontal cortex. The attenuated engagement of these brain areas was linked to the BPD patients' response bias, that is, patients who assessed the facial stimuli as less trustworthy showed stronger deficits in the engagement of prefrontal regions during trustworthiness appraisals. This first study on trust in PDs taking advantage of brain imaging methods emphasizes the usefulness of neurobiological approaches to gain a deeper understanding of the cognitive and affective processes that may or may not underlie alterations of trust in PDs. The findings exclude a hypersensitivity to threat as a mechanism of reduced interpersonal trust in BPD.

Since trust and mistrust are not opposite poles of a continuum but different functional systems (see also Chapter 9), further studies have to investigate whether changes in interpersonal trust in PDs may instead be linked to a hyposensitivity for positive social cues. Several studies revealed that the appraisal of positive emotions is impaired in BPD (Fenske et al., 2015; Izurieta Hidalgo et al., 2016; Reichenberger et al., 2017; Thome et al., 2016). Thus, a negative bias linked to deficits in the appraisal of positive social cues may contribute to the appraisal of others as less trustworthy in this PD. A recent study by Richetin et al. (2018) revealed lower trustworthiness ratings of low intense happy facial expressions in individuals high in BPD features. This relationship was mediated by negative emotions anticipated for an experience of social rejection. In contrast, the level to which participants expected to be socially rejected did not affect this association, suggesting that trust beliefs or expectations about the behavior of others are not relevant for altered trustworthiness appraisals in BPD. However, findings from Miano et al. (2013) suggest that facial trustworthiness appraisals are not only driven by negative emotions, but also by rejection sensitivity. Rejection sensitivity is a personality disposition determined by the interplay between a cognitive and affective component, that is, between the expectation and anxiety of being rejected. The authors found rejection sensitivity to mediate the relation between BPD features and reduced facial trustworthiness appraisals.

Moreover, the affective context has been shown to affect the strength of alterations in facial trustworthiness appraisals in PDs. In an affective priming paradigm, the negatively biased judgment of facial trustworthiness in BPD patients was exaggerated by precedence of negative pictures displaying, for example, weapons, snakes, or assaults (Masland & Hooley, 2019). These findings are in line with a more naturalistic approach by

Miano et al. (2017): When asked to judge the trustworthiness of their romantic partner, female BPD patients assessed their partner only as less trustworthy compared with healthy individuals following a conversation about threatening topics such as personal fears and potential reasons for a break-up of the relationship, but not after a conversation about an emotionally neutral topic.

In a recent study, Hepp et al. (2018) changed the perspective and focused on how healthy individuals assess facial trustworthiness of patients with BPD as one example of a PD. They showed that the patients were evaluated as less trustworthy based on their facial expression. Since social interactions can be understood as dynamic sequences of actions during which the behavior of the interaction partner affects subsequent actions, the authors identified an important factor that might determine a disadvantageous course of an exchange independently of the patients' real behavior. A reduced positive affect display was responsible for the reduced trustworthiness appraisals (Hepp et al., 2019). In contrast, a negative affect was linked to lower likeability, but not trustworthiness. However, the importance of a smile for evaluating trustworthiness may depend on context information about the depicted character. Healthy participants assessed the trustworthiness of a face consistently as lower when combined with information about the individual's social behaviors tailored to patterns typical for different PDs (Reed et al., 2018, 2019). However, manipulating the emotional expression of the face revealed that the trustworthiness-enhancing effect of a smile may even be reversed depending on the context information: Depending on the specific features of behaviors associated with an antisocial PD, smiling faces were evaluated as less trustworthy compared with faces with a neutral expression (Reed et al., 2020).

These findings confirm the importance of emotional social cues in judging trustworthiness and emphasize the need to investigate trust in PDs while taking its interplay with emotion processing and the dynamics of a social interaction into account.

Trusting Behavior. Like studies on trustworthiness appraisals in strangers, several studies applied exchange games such as the TG to study trust behavior in PDs (see reviews in BPD [Jeung et al., 2016] and in mental disorders including PDs [Lis & Kirsch, 2016]). All of these studies rely on behavioral indices. Only one study used neurobiological methods. King-Casas et al. (2008) used functional magnetic resonance imaging (fMRI) to study the exchange behavior during a multi-round TG in BPD. While this has been one of the most cited and most influential studies in this research field, it has to be emphasized that in the strict sense it does not inform us about trust in BPD. Since the BPD patients took the role of the trustee in this multi-round TG, possible conclusions refer more to reciprocity than trust. Nevertheless, this study shows clearly the advantages of applying brain imaging methods to gain further insights into the mechanism underlying alterations of interpersonal impairments in PDs.

Most of the studies on trusting behavior have been conducted in patients with BPD. They seem to support consistently general issues with trust behavior in BPD. However, the picture might be more complex and dependent on specific features of the context. In an one-shot TG measuring trust propensity, Botsford et al. (2019) found reduced investments during hypothetical exchanges in BPD patients compared with healthy control participants. The findings revealed no differences between groups in the mechanism to adjust interpersonal trust: All participants adjusted their behavior to the specific trustee, that is, they invested a higher amount when imagining a close friend or romantic partner as co-player compared to interacting with an unknown person.

Several studies applied multi-round exchange games to study the dynamics of trust behavior. They focused on the influence of a variation of emotional social cues and the fairness of the co-players' behavior while taking the course of the exchange into account.

Findings on the effects of emotional facial expression on trust behavior suggest that BPD patients are less likely to trust a co-player solely based on emotional facial cues. Franzen et al. (2011) showed that healthy controls (HCs) and BPD patients adapted their investments to a similar extent to the valence of the co-player's emotional expression. However, in contrast to HCs, the BPD patients additionally differentiated their co-players based on the fairness of their actual behavior and adjusted their investments accordingly in case of unfair co-players even in the presence of emotional cues. Polgar et al. (2014) identified a comparable behavioral pattern when participants took the role of the responder during an ultimatum game: While healthy subjects accepted in general more offers when the partner displayed a happy facial expression, this was only true for BPD patients in the case of fair offers. Thus, emotional social cues seem to be less sufficient to guide the BPD patients' trust behavior compared with healthy individuals, pointing toward a stronger importance of the fairness of another's actual behavior.

Findings on trust dynamics in BPD point to alterations in interaction behavior primarily during the formation of trust. Unoka et al. (2009)

showed that reduced investments during a multi-round TG were caused by impairments in building trust, that is, in a lack of increasing the amount of invested monetary units over the course of the game. This finding was supported by a study of Liebke et al. (2018): Differences in investments between BPD patients and HCs were observed during phases of the trustee's cooperative behavior, but not in response to the trustee's rupture of cooperation or subsequent attempts to repair it. Correspondingly, Abramov et al. (2020) found trust impairments during interaction with a new and cooperative co-player in individuals high in BPD features. Moreover, they even showed a stronger increase of trust after trust violations compared with people low in BPD features. The mechanism underlying these changes in formation of trust might be altered social norms in BPD. The behavioral changes could arise when the co-player's behavior is not experienced as fair, that is, when higher repayments are required to satisfy an individual's idea of fairness. This interpretation is supported by higher rejection rates of offers in exchange games in BPD that are already accepted, that is, considered to be fair, by healthy control participants (De Panfilis et al., 2019; Thielmann et al., 2014).

A study by King-Casas et al. (2008) suggests that BPD patients may refuse to take the first step to repair a social relationship when they experience a behavior as unfair. King-Casas et al. applied a TG during which BPD patients and HC participants took the role of the trustee. The trustor was always a healthy participant. Over 10 consecutive rounds, dyads with a BPD trustee showed less cooperation. This was due to exchange rounds during which the trustor signaled low trust by transferring a very low number of monetary units. In these exchanges, healthy trustees often repaid a high sum, encouraging the investor to be more cooperative during the subsequent trials. However, BPD trustees responded with a low repayment that was interpreted as an inability to "repair" the cooperation. In this case, the patients even risked a complete break-down of the cooperation as a consequence (see also Thielmann et al., 2014). Such behavior is comprehensible taking the exaggerated concerns about injustice into account that have been reported for individuals high in BPD features (Lis et al., 2018). King-Casas et al. suggested as the underlying mechanism alterations in the perception of violations of social norms caused by negative expectations during social interactions in BPD. They based their interpretation on brain activation patterns simultaneously measured by magnetic resonance tomography. Bilateral activation in the anterior insula strongly reflected the height of the investment in healthy participants with a stronger engagement of this brain region linked to lower investments. In contrast, the blood oxygen level-dependent (BOLD) response revealed a lack in the modulation of insula engagement in BPD. These differences between groups were seen specifically in response to the trustor's investment. The insula activation varied with the height of the repayment comparably in both groups, with higher engagement linked to lower repayments.

First findings in BPD suggest that alterations in trust dynamics might be modulated by the social context. Impairments in the formation of trust in BPD were particularly strong in a context of accepting social situations: Trust formation was attenuated following the experience of social acceptance, but not following social rejection (Liebke et al., 2018). Moreover, the strength of the alteration depended on the extent to which a feedback violated the patients' expectations: The more positive the feedback of social acceptance in relation to the negative expectations of social rejection, the more attenuated was the trust formation during a subsequent TG. While this effect is at first glance counter-intuitive, an unexpected feedback of social acceptance might be inconsistent with the patients' negative self-image and, in consequence, activate schemas of distrust that influence subsequent interaction behavior even toward strangers who have not met before (see Section 17.4.1; see also Winter et al., 2017).

Studies on trust behavior in PDs other than BPD are widely missing. However, several studies have focused on the relation between trust and personality traits in the general population. For example, Engelmann et al. (2019) investigated the association between an antisocial personality profile and trust behavior. Based on different variations of a TG, they concluded that an antisocial personality is linked to reduced trusting behavior except when there is an opportunity to punish a co-player. Simultaneously, individuals high in antisocial personality trait were shown to be less trustworthy themselves and punished more strongly even at their own costs when their trust was not reciprocated. Another example is studies on trust and paranoid ideation. They suggest a cognitive bias in individuals high in paranoid ideation: They tend to over-attribute harmful intent instead of self-interest as the explanation for unfair behaviors (Ellett & Chadwick, 2007). Thus, distrust predicted competitive instead of cooperative strategies in the Prisoners' Dilemma in those high in paranoid ideation (Raihani & Bell, 2017, 2018). For further details on paranoia and psychosis see Chapter 16.

Taken together, experimental studies suggest alterations in trust behavior caused by changes in how trust behavior is adjusted to context and may be associated to underlying mechanisms that vary between different PDs.

Summary of Empirical Studies. In sum, empirical studies supporting deficits of trust are widely missing for PDs other than BPD. This emphasizes the need for further studies. Moreover, only a very small number of studies have applied brain imaging methods to study neuronal correlates although those that did confirm that this might be a promising approach to understand issues with trust in PDs. At first glance, the findings might seem to be inconsistent for BPD. Some studies suggest reduced trust based on findings from self-reports, as well as from experimental studies on trustworthiness appraisals and trust behavior, while others do not. However, corresponding to the complex construct of trust a clearer picture arises when taking the specific measurement approaches and modulating factors into account. While overall findings suggest that BPD patients assess themselves as less trusting and others as less trustworthy, behavioral indices strongly suggest that the actual behavior often resembles that of healthy participants or clinical controls. One exception seems to be that BPD patients are less willing to form trust during repeated exchanges with the same person. So far, empirical findings contradict the assumption that a hypersensitivity to threat linked to a stronger responsiveness of subcortical brain regions such as the amygdala might be the underlying mechanism. However, negative expectations toward being socially accepted in contrast to being socially rejected, altered norms regarding fairness and injustice, a stronger responsiveness to a negative context as well as a reduced integration of positive social cues during social judgments may predispose BPD patients to issues with trust. To decide whether this pattern of determinants of trust and mistrust is specific for BPD or can be observed in other PDs or even mental disorders in general, further studies are needed that apply comparable assessments of the different aspects of trust in different mental disorders.

17.4   Trust as Target Construct in Therapeutic Approaches

As for social relationships in general, trust significantly influences the interpersonal interactions between patient and therapist during the treatment process and in consequence the efficacy of an intervention (Birkhauer et al., 2017). In BPD as one example of a PD, trust was identified by clinicians and patients as crucial for both the establishment and maintenance of the therapeutic relationship (Langley & Klopper, 2005). Botsford et al. (2019) found a particularly strong association between self-reports of interpersonal trust in BPD patients and the quality of the therapeutic alliance compared with patients with social anxiety disorder and major depression.

Beyond this general relevance of trust during the treatment process, impairments of trust form target constructs in psychotherapeutic approaches to PDs and are currently discussed as targets in psychopharmacological treatments.

17.4.1 Psychotherapeutic Interventions

Psychotherapeutic interventions are currently regarded as the primary intervention for PDs and the number of controlled, randomized studies investigating their efficacy in different PDs has been steadily increasing during the last few years (e.g. Johnson et al., 2018; Simonsen et al., 2019). Among the variety of different and mostly highly complex approaches are – with a cognitive behavioral tradition – dialectical behavior therapy (DBT), schema therapy, and standard cognitive behavioral therapy and – with a psychodynamic background – mentalization-based treatment and transference-focused psychotherapy. Although trust is a relevant topic in all approaches, we will focus on mentalization-based treatment and schema therapy since they target trust issues most explicitly.

Nevertheless, it should be mentioned that, for example, the biopsychosocial model of BPD in DBT assumes an invalidating environment to be crucial in the development of this PD (Linehan, 1993). Invalidation of intense emotional experiences is assumed to lead to mistrust in one's thoughts, feelings, and bodily sensations in a first step and, with constant repetition, to turn into distrust and uncertainty regarding identity and self-image. In DBT, patients learn to trust themselves and others by validating their thoughts and emotions and those of others (Salsman & Linehan, 2006). The therapist himself works in DBT with commitment and validation strategies (such as radical authenticity) that strengthen the therapeutic relationship by building trust, providing a model for the patient's interactions with others. Trust issues are also important in transference-focused psychotherapy since it relies on the psychoanalytic object relations theory of BPD. It postulates as important features of BPD the propensity to evaluate others as persecutory or idealized and a paranoid view of others (see for theory and empirical background also Fertuck et al., 2018).

In most psychotherapeutic approaches, issues in interpersonal relationships are assumed to develop as a consequence of dysfunctional interactions between caregivers and the patient's neurobiological vulnerabilities. Attachment theory suggests that individuals develop specific attachment styles based on their social relationships with significant others during early life that influence interpersonal relationships throughout life (Bowlby, 1977). Correspondingly, an individual's attachment style, that is, a specific behavioral pattern during social interactions, has been proposed as a relevant construct to understand PDs. Thereby, an insecure attachment style is assigned particular importance as a risk factor for the development of a PD and a modulating factor for trust (Bakermans-Kranenburg & Van IJzendoorn, 2009; Bartholomew et al., 2001; Beech & Mitchell, 2009; Fossati et al., 2015; Levy et al., 2015, 2018; Zhang et al., 2017).

Epistemic Trust and Mentalization-Based Therapy. One of the core concepts of mentalization-based therapy (MBT) is a lack of "epistemic trust." Epistemic trust is trust in the authenticity and personal relevance of interpersonally transmitted information that allows an individual to learn from others in a changing social and cultural world (Wilson & Sperber, 2012). Impairments of epistemic trust are assumed to result in a reduced openness to social communications and, in consequence, to an inability of learning through interpersonal experiences (Fonagy et al., 2015). The first sign of the development of children's epistemic mistrust was identified as early as at the age of 16–18 months. At the age of 4, children develop selective trust and mistrust and are able to differentiate between an accurate and an error-prone informant, that is, they become vigilant toward the source of information (Koenig & Harris, 2005; Sperber et al., 2010).

Epistemic vigilance is the self-protective suspicion toward information coming from others that may be potentially damaging, deceptive, or inaccurate and constitutes a part of healthy cognitive development (Fonagy et al., 2014). Traumatizing, neglecting, insensitive parenting in combination with some genetic predisposition is assumed to lead to epistemic hypervigilance and mistrust, which is conceived as a common factor in psychopathology (Fonagy et al., 2017). In their theory of natural pedagogy, Gergely and Csibra (2013) identified communicative tools they named "ostensive cues." These activate the pedagogic stance in the listener. In the pedagogic stance, the listener assumes that the informant's teaching is significant, relevant to him/her, and socially generalizable. Fonagy et al. (2015) claim that ostensive cues trigger epistemic trust, and a secure attachment style is a sufficient condition for generating epistemic trust. They propose that the misuse of ostensive cues and the pedagogic stance by a caregiver transmits destructive information as culturally relevant generalizable knowledge. Epistemic mistrust and hypervigilance block the learning process and lead to rigidity and isolation from communication. This is assumed to be one of the main characteristics of PDs, specifically BPD (Fonagy et al., 2017). Kamphuis and Finn (2019) draw our attention to the existence of "epistemic hypovigilance" (or naive trust). They emphasize that many clients "vacillate between states of epistemic hypovigilance and hypervigilance." (Kamphuis & Finn, 2019, p. 665). Flexible use of epistemic trust and vigilance is needed for adaptive social learning, which is the prerequisite of healthy personality development.

According to Fonagy et al. (2019), the aim of the treatment of PDs is to facilitate epistemic trust and lower epistemic hypervigilance. They suggest that this is a common factor in all successful psychotherapies. Thereby, the therapist and patient have to solve the paradoxical situation of epistemic mistrust caused by the patient's mistrust in the authenticity and personal relevance of interpersonally transmitted knowledge in the therapeutic context (Fonagy & Allison, 2014). According to the epistemic mistrust theory of BPD, the psychotherapist has to expect that patients are unlikely to accept statements and information of the therapist purely based on trust. Instead, the patient might check how far they cohere with his/her own beliefs due to epistemic hypervigilance. In the worst case, patients might outright reject the therapist's intervention and hinder achieving the therapeutic goals. To overcome this issue, Fonagy et al. (2014) propose three distinct processes of communication to lower epistemic hypervigilance and induce epistemic trust. They comprise teaching and learning content about the working of the patient's mind, strengthening the patient's capacity for mentalization and social cognition, and facilitating the reemergence of social learning by systematic and coherent use of the two previous processes (Fonagy et al., 2017).

Although most often used in the treatment of BPD, MBT has been more recently developed into a more comprehensive approach to understand and treat a broader range of PDs. Correspondingly, MBT has been shown to positively affect trust in BPD and in other PDs (Johnson et al., 2018). For example, MBT induced a higher level of trust in adolescents with avoidant PD, even if the generalizability to persons outside the therapy was limited (Bo et al., 2019).

Although a theoretical link between a lack of epistemic trust and the level of BPD has been drawn, so far an association between the level of epistemic trust and MBT outcome has not been confirmed (Orme et al., 2019). One reason might be that reliable and valid measures of epistemic vigilance and epistemic trust across different contents and social partners are needed to investigate whether psychotherapeutic interventions enhance the flexibility of epistemic trust and vigilance and in turn reduce the severity of PD pathology. It seems worthwhile to mention that, for example, BPD patients participate in experimental research, and the published results show that, most of the time, they followed the instructions of the experimenter. This implies that they assessed the provided information as relevant, they learned it and behaved accordingly. This suggests that hypervigilance might be of particular importance toward attachment-related issues, figures, and interpersonal situations such as social rejection.

Early Maladaptive Schema and Schema Therapy. "Early maladaptive schemas" and "modes" are among the core concepts of schema therapy (ST). In general, a schema is defined as a cognitive structure that organizes experiences based on interactions with the environment (Arbib, 2003). The ST approach postulates the existence of 18 different maladaptive schemas that develop based on an individual's predisposition when specific emotional needs are not met during childhood or adolescence (Young et al., 2006). These schemas reflect beliefs about an individual him/herself and others and may result in maladaptive coping strategies. Schemas can be understood as internal working models that comprise schematic representations of interpersonal experiences. Based on repeated experiences, an internal working model develops that is specific to each of the emotional needs and attachment figures. If later on in life a need is frustrated, the person will predict the other's reaction based on this internal working model as it represents expectations of others' reactions to the self's needs. When events lead to a predominance of a specific schema and the related coping strategies, it determines an individual's emotional and cognitive state as well as his/her behavior, and any contradicting evidence is rejected, questioned, or ignored. The predominance of a schema results in a specific state, that is, the schema mode. In contrast to schemas that represent trait-like features of an individual, schema modes are state-dependent and may vary from moment to moment.

Each PD has been assumed to be associated with elevated levels of specific early maladaptive schemas (Jovev & Jackson, 2004; Nordahl et al., 2005; Petrocelli et al., 2001). A recent study identified the schema of mistrust/abuse to be of particular importance in BPD, differentiating this personality disorder from others (Bach & Farrell, 2018). This schema comprises the expectation that social partners will take advantage of the individual or that they will abuse and cheat motivated by intentions to harm or as a consequence of unjustified negligence.

In the case of a secure internal working model and adaptive schemas, the individual predicts that the other will help to satisfy a frustrated need. In other words, the trustor is optimistic about the trustee's intentions and abilities and expects the trustee to be trustworthy. Thus, the risk of trusting is low, and trusting is well grounded (Lockwood & Perris, 2012; Louis et al., 2018; Mikulincer, 1998). In the case of insecure internal working models and maladaptive schemas, the individual will predict that the other will not help to satisfy the frustrated need. For example, in the case of a high level of the abandonment/instability schema the individual may expect that those available for support will be unstable or unreliable, will leave since they favor another person, or even die. Although this schema is not explicitly related to mistrust, it implies a high risk when trusting. In other words, the trustor is pessimistic about the trustee's intentions and abilities and expects the trustee to be untrustworthy. Thus, the risk of trusting is high, and trusting is not well grounded (Mikulincer, 1998; Young et al., 2006). In consequence, the potential trustor might avoid expressing his/her vulnerable state and needs to the trustee and try to cope alone as in the avoidant/detached coping mode. Alternatively, the trustor might shift into the overcompensator coping mode in which he/she tries to control the trustee by monitoring or constraining his/her behavioral options (McLeod, 2020). In sum, the level of early maladaptive schemas calibrates the level of risk of trusting others in different domains of social life related to specific core emotional needs.

The target of schema therapy is the modification of early maladaptive schemas and schema modes by helping the patients to identify, validate, express, and satisfy their core emotional needs in interpersonal relationships and replace maladaptive coping strategies (Young et al., 2006). Schema therapists monitor the therapeutic relationship. They activate early traumatizing or neglecting episodic memories of situations during which the patient's core needs were not met. In imagination or chair work, the therapy aims to rescript the experiences during childhood and adolescence by using a technique called limited reparenting. The aim of rescripting is to create an experience during which the patient's core need is met. This is intended to become the experiential base for a newly formed adaptive schema that may predict that the risk of trusting others to satisfy the emotional need is low.

A growing number of randomized controlled trials on the efficacy of schema therapy indicate beneficial effects on the reduction of symptom severity, recovery rates, and low dropout rates in BPD and other PDs (Bamelis et al., 2014; Jacob & Arntz, 2013). However, future studies are needed that investigate whether different elevated maladaptive schemas result indeed in higher mistrust associated with the related core emotional needs and whether limited reparenting as the core schema therapeutic intervention reduces mistrust mediated by a modification of maladaptive schemas. Finally, it is theoretically and empirically important to understand the associations between early maladaptive schema and epistemic hypervigilance. One may expect that early maladaptive schemas and epistemic hypervigilance are closely associated, particularly in regard to whether schema-related core emotional need will be satisfied.

17.4.2   Psychopharmacological Interventions

Great hope had been placed in a treatment of trust issues in mental disorders with the "pro-social" peptide oxytocin. However, during the last few years, the findings of an increasing number of studies draw a complex picture that contradicts a simple and stable beneficial effect of oxytocin on trust (Declerck et al., 2020); see also Chapter 14). This let Erdozain and Penagarikano (2019) state that oxytocin is not "the miraculous molecule" that works in a "one size fits all" manner.

In the domain of PDs, alterations in the oxytocin system have been extensively studied in BPD (for a review on oxytocin and BPD see Bertsch & Herpertz, 2018). Bartz et al. (2011) were the first to investigate the effect of oxytocin on interpersonal trust in BPD. Contrary to an expected beneficial effect, oxytocin had no effect on trust behavior toward a cooperatively acting virtual partner in an assurance game. In contrast, the patients reported to expect less cooperation by their co-players and even expected to behave less cooperatively themselves in a hypothetical scenario during which the co-player would behave fairly. These effects were stronger in patients with an anxious attachment style and high rejection sensitivity.

A subsequent study by Ebert et al. (2013) observed even a decrease in actual trust behavior during a TG in BPD. The adverse effect of oxytocin on trust was particularly strong in patients with a higher level of childhood traumatization. Similar findings were reported by Ramseyer et al. (2019): They found a negative effect on nonverbal synchrony after administration of oxytocin in BPD that was also accentuated in those patients with higher levels of childhood traumatization. In contrast, a study by Domes et al. (2019) suggests beneficial effects of oxytocin on affective empathy and approach motivation in BPD patients: Under oxytocin, affective empathy and approach motivation toward positive pictures increased in BPD patients up to a level corresponding to performance of healthy individuals under placebo. However, this effect was not specific for positive stimuli, but was also observed – with an even higher intensity – for empathy and approach motivation toward negative pictures. These findings emphasize that issues with trust in BPD cannot simply be beneficially influenced by elevating a reduced oxytocin level. In contrast, studies on the effects of oxytocin in BPD suggest some caution around the usefulness of this substance for targeting issues with trust at least in this PD. One reason might be that oxytocin may affect the salience of social cues, and trigger positive or negative social emotions based on the social repertoire of the individual and/or the social context (e.g., Bartz et al., 2011; Shamay-Tsoory & Abu-Akel, 2016).

Studies on the effects of oxytocin in other PDs are sparse and to our knowledge none of these investigated its effect on trust (e.g. see review in antisocial personality disorder by Gedeon et al., 2019).

Approaches to improve trust with substances other than oxytocin are widely missing. Roberts et al. (2018) tested the effects of acetaminophen (paracetamol) on trust in BPD. They based their choice of substance on the assumption that its dampening effect on negative and positive affect might improve trust in BPD. They found an increase of trust behavior measured with one-shot TGs, specifically in those participants with a high level of BPD features. While these findings might point to alternative pharmacological pathways to target trust issues in PDs, further studies are required that confirm the efficacy in clinical samples of PDs with a broader assessment of the different facets of trust.

17.5 Summary and Implications

Clinical descriptions and empirical findings support the prominent role of trust for the understanding and treatment of interpersonal dysfunction in PDs. However, in contrast to the relevance of trust in diagnostic and therapeutical approaches, empirical studies on trust impairments and the underlying mechanism are still sparse. In contrast to other PDs, the increasing body of findings in BPD already draws a complex but consistent picture, forming the basis for a successful treatment of interpersonal dysfunction in this clinical sample. However, trust is a complex and dynamic phenomenon and even in BPD there are still many unanswered questions that have to be addressed in the future. With the growing relevance of a dimensional concept of PDs, the long history of studies on the relation between trust and personality traits based on samples derived from the general population may allow for a fast progress during the next few decades. Since a review of these studies would have exceeded the scope of the current chapter and the validity of their findings for clinical samples has still to be confirmed, we have only briefly referred the reader to some exemplary studies.

Nevertheless, studies on trust in healthy individuals inform us about important factors that may modulate trust and contribute to the understanding of its changes in PDs. To bridge the gap between the relevance of trust in diagnostic and therapeutical approaches and the number of empirical studies on trust impairments, further studies are needed. Beyond a differentiated description of trust impairments taking their stability across time and context into account, future research has to identify the mechanism responsible for dysfunctions of interpersonal functioning in the domain of trust. Due to the lack of experimental studies, today one may only speculate about the relevance of cognitive functions such as theory of mind, reward processing, or emotion regulation for impairments of trust in most PDs. This is in contrast to other mental disorders such as psychosis for which the relevance of these domains of cognitive and social-cognitive functioning for issues with trust has already been demonstrated (see also Chapter 16). Last but not least, future studies have to take advantage of the growing availability of brain imaging methods. By studying the neuronal correlates of trust, we may deepen our understanding of the mechanism underlying alterations of trust in PDs. Methods such as fMRI, magnetencephalography, or functional near-infrared spectroscopy allow measurement of the involvement of different brain regions with high temporal or high spatial resolution. Particularly, the combination of the different methodologies may allow localizing of fast processes in distinct brain areas and their complex interplay in neuronal networks. So far, these potentials have not been used to study trust in PDs.

Among the factors already confirmed to contribute to issues with trust in PDs are environmental factors such as adverse experiences during childhood and adolescence. These might lead to personality dispositions such as rejection sensitivity, justice sensitivity, risk aversion, reduced optimism and affect an individual's attachment style. Issues with trust may arise or be exaggerated by an interaction with a biological vulnerability and result in altered social-cognitive processing such as how people use social-emotional cues to guide their behavior.

Moreover, some recent studies emphasized that the link between personality traits and trust might be dynamic. While honesty-humility has been linked in many studies to high levels of trust, Pfattheicher and Bohm

(2018) could show that increasing self-uncertainty results, particularly in those high in honesty-humility, in a reduction of trust by decreasing positive expectations toward others. Depending on unexpected behaviors of others in our life, we may switch between adapting trust in personal relations toward sociopolitical relations or vice versa with the aim of counteracting anxiety evoked by uncertainty and preserving our social-safety system (Murray et al., 2020). These aspects might be of particular importance in the context of PDs when self-confidence is low as in dependent PDs. Indeed, patients with an avoidant PD named the development of trust in themselves as one of the core themes of treatment (Sorensen et al., 2019). Correspondingly, patients suffering from avoidant PD have not only problems in trusting others, but also in trusting themselves (Millon & Davis, 1996; Rettew, 2000). However, so far, the interplay between self- and other-related trust and its relevance for PD is a topic still to be investigated.

Finally, we have to keep in mind that many of the patients with PDs that participate in empirical studies may receive psychotropic medication and often suffer from other mental disorders. Studies on how this may affect trust or mistrust in PDs are widely missing.

Since clinical phenomenology, self-reports, and social behaviors often diverge, we need further empirical studies. While it might be plausible to infer issues with trust based upon phenomenological descriptions of interpersonal behavior or patients' reports, the underlying mechanism might not necessarily be an impairment of trust. One example of a mental disorder that is characterized by exaggerated approach behavior even toward strangers is Williams syndrome (Riby et al., 2014). While this behavior suggests alterations in trust, a study by Ng et al. (2015) suggested that it is not an overgeneralization of trustworthiness appraisals that explains the behavior of these patients. This emphasizes the need for further studies to deepen our understanding of trust issues in PDs and other mental disorders to successfully target this domain of interpersonal functioning in therapeutic interventions.

References

Abramov, G., Miellet, S., Kautz, J., Grenyer, B. F. S., & Deane, F. P. (2020). The paradoxical decline and growth of trust as a function of borderline personality disorder trait count: Using discontinuous growth modelling to examine trust dynamics in response to violation and repair. *PLoS ONE*, 15(7), Article e0236170. https://doi.org/10.1371/journal.pone.0236170

Alden, L. E., & Capreol, M. J. (1993). Avoidant personality disorder: Interpersonal problems as predictors of treatment response. *Behavior Therapy*, 24(3), 357–376.

American Psychiatric Association. (2013). *Diagnostic and statistical manual of mental disorders* (5th ed.). American Psychiatric Association.

Arbib, M. A. (2003). Schema theory. In M. A. Arbib & F. Jones (Eds.), *The handbook of brain theory and neural networks* (pp. 1427–1443). MIT Press.

Bach, B., & Farrell, J. M. (2018). Schemas and modes in borderline personality disorder: The mistrustful, shameful, angry, impulsive, and unhappy child. *Psychiatry Research*, 259, 323–329. https://doi.org/10.1016/j.psychres.2017.10.039

Bakermans-Kranenburg, M. J., & Van IJzendoorn, M. H. (2009). The first 10,000 adult attachment interviews: Distributions of adult attachment representations in clinical and non-clinical groups. *Attachment & Human Development*, 11(3), 223–263. https://doi.org/10.1080/14616730902814762

Bamelis, L. L., Evers, S. M., Spinhoven, P., & Arntz, A. (2014). Results of a multicenter randomized controlled trial of the clinical effectiveness of schema therapy for personality disorders. *American Journal of Psychiatry*, 171(3), 305–322. http://doi.org/10.1176/appi.ajp.2013.12040518

Barnow, S., Stopsack, M., Grabe, H. J., et al. (2009). Interpersonal evaluation bias in borderline personality disorder. *Behaviour Research and Therapy*, 47(5), 359–365. https://doi.org/10.1016/j.brat.2009.02.003

Bartholomew, K., Kwong, M. J., & Hart, S. D. (2001). Attachment. In W. J. Livesley (Ed.), *Handbook of personality disorders* (pp. 196–230). The Guilford Press.

Bartz, J., Simeon, D., Hamilton, H., et al. (2011, Oct). Oxytocin can hinder trust and cooperation in borderline personality disorder. *Social Cognitive and Affective Neuroscience*, 6(5), 556–563. https://doi.org/10.1093/scan/nsq085

Bauer, P. C., & Freitag, M. (2017). Measuring trust. In E. M. Uslaner (Ed.), *The Oxford handbook of social and political trust*. Oxford University Press. https://10.1093/oxfordhb/9780190274801.013.1

Beech, A. R., & Mitchell, I. (2009). Attachment difficulties. In M. McMurran & R. C. Howard (Eds.), *Personality, personality disorder, and violence: An evidence-based approach* (pp. 213–228). John Wiley & Sons.

Bender, D. S., Dolan, R. T., Skodol, A. E., et al. (2001, Feb). Treatment utilization by patients with personality disorders. *American Journal of Psychiatry*, 158(2), 295–302. https://doi.org/10.1176/appi.ajp.158.2.295

Bertsch, K., & Herpertz, S. C. (2018). Oxytocin and borderline personality disorder. *Current Topics in Behavioral Neurosciences*, 35, 499–514. https://doi.org/10.1007/7854_2017_26

Birkhauer, J., Gaab, J., Kossowsky, J., et al. (2017). Trust in the health care professional and health outcome: A meta-analysis. *PLoS ONE*, 12(2), Article e0170988. https://doi.org/10.1371/journal.pone.0170988

Bo, S., Bateman, A., & Kongerslev, M. T. (2019). Mentalization-based group therapy for adolescents with avoidant personality disorder: Adaptations and findings from a practice-based pilot evaluation. *Journal of Infant, Child & Adolescent Psychotherapy*, 18, 249–262. https://doi.org/10.1080/15289168 .2019.1625655

Botsford, J., Schulze, L., Bohlander, J., & Renneberg, B. (2019, Dec 30). Interpersonal trust: Development and validation of a self-report inventory and clinical application in patients with borderline personality disorder. *Journal of Personality Disorders*, 1–22. https://doi.org/10.1521/pedi_2019_ 33_462

Bowlby, J. (1977). The making and breaking of affectional bonds: II. Some principles of psychotherapy: The Fiftieth Maudsley Lecture (expanded version). *The British Journal of Psychiatry*, 130(5), 421–431.

De Panfilis, C., Schito, G., Generali, I., et al. (2019). Emotions at the border: Increased punishment behavior during fair interpersonal exchanges in borderline personality disorder. *Journal of Abnormal Psychology*, 128(2), 162–172. https://doi.org/10.1037/abn0000404

Declerck, C. H., Boone, C., Pauwels, L., Vogt, B., & Fehr, E. (2020). A registered replication study on oxytocin and trust. *Nature Human Behaviour*, 4(6), 646–655. https://doi.org/10.1038/s41562–020-0878-x

Domes, G., Ower, N., von Dawans, B., et al. (2019). Effects of intranasal oxytocin administration on empathy and approach motivation in women with borderline personality disorder: A randomized controlled trial. *Translational Psychiatry*, 9(1), Article 328. https://doi.org/10.1038/ s41398–019-0658-4

Ebert, A., Kolb, M., Heller, J., Edel, M. A., Roser, P., & Brune, M. (2013). Modulation of interpersonal trust in borderline personality disorder by intranasal oxytocin and childhood trauma. *Social Neuroscience*, 8(4), 305–313. https://doi.org/10.1080/17470919.2013.807301

Eikenaes, I., Hummelen, B., Abrahamsen, G., Andrea, H., & Wilberg, T. (2013). Personality functioning in patients with avoidant personality disorder and social phobia. *Journal of Personality Disorders*, 27(6), 746–763. https://doi .org/10.1521/pedi_2013_27_109

Ellett, L., & Chadwick, P. (2007). Paranoid cognitions, failure, and focus of attention in college students. *Cognition Emotion*, 21, 558–576. https://doi .org/10.1080/02699930600758155

Engelmann, J. B., Schmid, B., De Dreu, C. K. W., Chumbley, J., & Fehr, E. (2019). On the psychology and economics of antisocial personality. *Proceedings of the National Academy of Sciences of the United States of America*, 116(26), 12781–12786. https://doi.org/10.1073/pnas.1820133116

Erdozain, A. M., & Penagarikano, O. (2019). Oxytocin as treatment for social cognition, not there yet. *Frontiers in Psychiatry*, 10, Article 930. https://doi .org/10.3389/fpsyt.2019.00930

Fenske, S., Lis, S., Liebke, L., Niedtfeld, I., Kirsch, P., & Mier, D. (2015). Emotion recognition in borderline personality disorder: Effects of emotional information on negative bias. *Borderline Personality Disorder and Emotion Dysregulation*, 2, Article 10. https://doi.org/10.1186/s40479–015-0031-z

Fertuck, E. A., Fischer, S., & Beeney, J. (2018). Social cognition and borderline personality disorder: Splitting and trust impairment findings. *Psychiatric Clinics of North America*, 41(4), 613–632. https://doi.org/10.1016/j.psc.2018.07.003

Fertuck, E. A., Grinband, J., Mann, J. J., et al. (2019). Trustworthiness appraisal deficits in borderline personality disorder are associated with prefrontal cortex, not amygdala, impairment. *NeuroImage Clinical*, 21, Article 101616. https://doi.org/10.1016/j.nicl.2018.101616

Fertuck, E. A., Grinband, J., & Stanley, B. (2013, May 30). Facial trust appraisal negatively biased in borderline personality disorder. *Psychiatry Research*, 207 (3), 195–202. https://doi.org/10.1016/j.psychres.2013.01.004

Fonagy, P., & Allison, E. (2014). The role of mentalizing and epistemic trust in the therapeutic relationship. *Psychotherapy (Chic)*, 51(3), 372–380. https://doi.org/10.1037/a0036505

Fonagy, P., Luyten, P., & Allison, E. (2015). Epistemic petrification and the restoration of epistemic trust: A new conceptualization of borderline personality disorder and its psychosocial treatment. *Journal of Personality Disorders*, 29(5), 575–609. https://doi.org/10.1521/pedi.2015.29.5.575

Fonagy, P., Luyten, P., Allison, E., & Campbell, C. (2017). What we have changed our minds about: Part 2. Borderline personality disorder, epistemic trust and the developmental significance of social communication. *Borderline Personality Disorder and Emotion Dysregulation*, 4, Article 9. https://doi.org/10.1186/s40479-017-0062-8

(2019). Mentalizing, epistemic trust and the phenomenology of psychotherapy. *Psychopathology*, 52(2), 94–103. https://doi.org/10.1159/000501526

Fonagy, P., Luyten, P., Campbell, C., & Allison, L. (2014, Dec). *Epistemic trust, psychopathology and the great psychotherapy debate*. http://www.societyforpsychotherapy.org/epistemic-trust-psychopathology-and-the-great-psychotherapy-debate

Fossati, A., Krueger, R. F., Markon, K. E., Borroni, S., Maffei, C., & Somma, A. (2015). The DSM-5 alternative model of personality disorders from the perspective of adult attachment: A study in community-dwelling adults. *The Journal of Nervous and Mental Disease*, 203(4), 252–258. https://doi.org/10.1097/NMD.0000000000000274

Franzen, N., Hagenhoff, M., Baer, N., et al. (2011). Superior "theory of mind" in borderline personality disorder: An analysis of interaction behavior in a virtual trust game. *Psychiatry Research*, 187(1–2), 224–233. https://doi.org/10.1016/j.psychres.2010.11.012

Friborg, O., Martinsen, E. W., Martinussen, M., Kaiser, S., Overgard, K. T., & Rosenvinge, J. H. (2014). Comorbidity of personality disorders in mood disorders: A meta-analytic review of 122 studies from 1988 to 2010. *Journal of Affective Disorders*, 152–154, 1–11. https://doi.org/10.1016/j.jad.2013.08.023

Friborg, O., Martinussen, M., Kaiser, S., Overgard, K. T., & Rosenvinge, J. H. (2013). Comorbidity of personality disorders in anxiety disorders: A meta-analysis of 30 years of research. *Journal of Affective Disorders*, 145(2), 143–155. https://doi.org/10.1016/j.jad.2012.07.004

Furnham, A. F. (2014). A bright side, facet analysis of histrionic personality disorder: The relationship between the HDS Colourful factor and the NEO-PI-R facets in a large adult sample. *Journal of Social Psychology*, 154 (6), 527–536. https://doi.org/10.1080/00224545.2014.953026

Furnham, A. F., & Crump, J. D. (2014). A bright side facet analysis of borderline personality disorder. *Borderline Personality Disorder and Emotion Dysregulation*, 1, Article 7. https://doi.org/10.1186/2051-6673-1-7

Gedeon, T., Parry, J., & Vollm, B. (2019). The role of oxytocin in antisocial personality disorders: A systematic review of the literature. *Frontiers in Psychiatry*, 10, Article 76. https://doi.org/10.3389/fpsyt.2019.00076

Gergely, G., & Csibra, G. (2013). Natural pedagogy. In M. R. Banaji & S. A. Gelman (Eds.), *Navigating the social world: What infants, children, and other species can teach us* (pp. 127–132). Oxford University Press. https://doi.org/10.1093/acprof:oso/9780199890712.003.0023

Hepp, J., Gebhardt, S., Kieslich, P. J., Storkel, L. M., & Niedtfeld, I. (2019). Low positive affect display mediates the association between borderline personality disorder and negative evaluations at zero acquaintance. *Borderline Personality Disorder and Emotion Dysregulation*, 6, Article 4. https://doi.org/10.1186/s40479-019-0103-6

Hepp, J., Storkel, L. M., Kieslich, P. J., Schmahl, C., & Niedtfeld, I. (2018). Negative evaluation of individuals with borderline personality disorder at zero acquaintance. *Behaviour Research and Therapy*, 111, 84–91. https://doi.org/10.1016/j.brat.2018.09.009

Izurieta Hidalgo, N. A., Oelkers-Ax, R., Nagy, K., et al. (2016). Time course of facial emotion processing in women with borderline personality disorder: An ERP study. *Journal of Psychiatry and Neuroscience*, 41(1), 16–26. http://www.ncbi.nlm.nih.gov/pubmed/26269211

Jacob, G. A., & Arntz, A. (2013). Schema therapy for personality disorders: A review. *International Journal of Cognitive Therapy*, 6(2), 171–185. https://doi.org/10.1521/ijct.2013.6.2.171

Jeung, H., Schwieren, C., & Herpertz, S. C. (2016). Rationality and self-interest as economic-exchange strategy in borderline personality disorder: Game theory, social preferences, and interpersonal behavior. *Neuroscience & Biobehavioral Reviews*, 71, 849–864. https://doi.org/10.1016/j.neubiorev.2016.10.030

Johnson, B. N., Clouthier, T. L., Rosenstein, L. K., & Levy, K. N. (2018). Psychotherapy for personality disorders. In V. Zeigler-Hill & T. K. Shackelford (Eds.), *Encyclopedia of personality and individual differences* (pp. 1–20). Springer. https://doi.org/10.1007/978-3-319-28099-8_925-1

Jones, S. L., & Shah, P. P. (2016). Diagnosing the locus of trust: A temporal perspective for trustor, trustee, and dyadic influences on perceived trustworthiness. *Journal of Applied Psychology*, 101(3), 392–414. https://doi.org/10.1037/apl0000041

Jovev, M., & Jackson, H. J. (2004). Early maladaptive schemas in personality disordered individuals. *Journal of Personality Disorders*, 18(5), 467–478. https://doi.org/10.1521/pedi.18.5.467.51325

Kamphuis, J. H., & Finn, S. E. (2019). Therapeutic assessment in personality disorders: Toward the restoration of epistemic trust. *Journal of Personality Assessment*, 101(6), 662–674. https://doi.org/10.1080/00223891.2018 .1476360

King-Casas, B., Sharp, C., Lomax-Bream, L., Lohrenz, T., Fonagy, P., & Montague, P. R. (2008). The rupture and repair of cooperation in borderline personality disorder. *Science*, 321(5890), 806–810. https://doi.org/10.1126/ science.1156902

Koenig, M. A., & Harris, P. L. (2005). The role of social cognition in early trust. *Trends in Cognitive Sciences*, 9(10), 457–459. https://doi.org/10.1016/j.tics .2005.08.006

Krumhuber, E., Manstead, A. S., Cosker, D., Marshall, D., Rosin, P. L., & Kappas, A. (2007). Facial dynamics as indicators of trustworthiness and cooperative behavior. *Emotion*, 7(4), 730–735. https://doi.org/10.1037/ 1528-3542.7.4.730

Kwiatkowska, M., Jułkowski, T., Rogoza, R., & Żemojtel-Piotrowska, M. (2018). Narcissism and trust: Differential impact of agentic, antagonistic, and communal narcissism. *Personality and Individual Differences*, 137, 139–143. https://doi.org/10.1016/j.paid.2018.08.027

Landrum, A. R., Eaves, B. S., Jr., & Shafto, P. (2015). Learning to trust and trusting to learn: A theoretical framework. *Trends in Cognitive Sciences*, 19 (3), 109–111. https://doi.org/10.1016/j.tics.2014.12.007

Langley, G. C., & Klopper, H. (2005). Trust as a foundation for the therapeutic intervention for patients with borderline personality disorder. *Journal of Psychiatric and Mental Health Nursing*, 12(1), 23–32. https://doi.org/10 .1111/j.1365-2850.2004.00774.x

Levy, K. N., Johnson, B. N., Clouthier, T. L., Scala, J., & Temes, C. M. (2015). An attachment theoretical framework for personality disorders. *Canadian Psychology/Psychologie Canadienne*, 56(2), 197–207. https://psycnet.apa.org/ doi/10.1037/cap0000025

Levy, K. N., Kivity, Y., Johnson, B. N., & Gooch, C. V. (2018). Adult attachment as a predictor and moderator of psychotherapy outcome: A meta-analysis. *Journal of Clinical Psychology*, 74(11), 1996–2013. https://doi.org/ 10.1002/jclp.22685

Liebke, L., Koppe, G., Bungert, M., et al. (2018, Oct). Difficulties with being socially accepted: An experimental study in borderline personality disorder. *Journal of Abnormal Psychology*, 127(7), 670–682. https://doi.org/10.1037/ abn0000373

Linehan, M. M. (1993). *Cognitive-behavioral treatment of borderline personality disorder*. The Guilford Press.

Lis, S., & Kirsch, P. (2016). Neuroeconomic approaches in mental disorders. In C. Montag & M. Reuter (Eds.), *Neuroeconomics* (pp. 311–330). Springer.

Lis, S., Schaedler, A., Liebke, L., et al. (2018, Apr). Borderline personality disorder features and sensitivity to injustice. *Journal of Personality Disorder*, 32(2), 192–206. https://doi.org/10.1521/pedi_2017_31_292

Lockwood, G., & Perris, P. (2012). A new look at core emotional needs. In M. Van Vreeswijk, J. Broersen, & M. Nadort (Eds.), *The Wiley-Blackwell handbook of schema therapy: Theory, research, and practice* (pp. 41–66). John Wiley & Sons. https://doi.org/10.1002/9781119962830.ch3

Louis, J. P., Wood, A. M., Lockwood, G., Ho, M.-H. R., & Ferguson, E. (2018). Positive clinical psychology and Schema Therapy (ST): The development of the Young Positive Schema Questionnaire (YPSQ) to complement the Young Schema Questionnaire 3 Short Form (YSQ-S3). *Psychological Assessment*, 30(9), 1199–1213. https://psycnet.apa.org/doi/10.1037/pas0000567

Martinussen, M., Friborg, O., Schmierer, P., et al. (2017). The comorbidity of personality disorders in eating disorders: A meta-analysis. *Eating and Weight Disorders – Studies on Anorexia, Bulimia and Obesity*, 22(2), 201–209. https://doi.org/10.1007%2Fs40519-016-0345-x

Masland, S. R., & Hooley, J. M. (2019). When trust does not come easily: Negative emotional information unduly influences trustworthiness appraisals for individuals with borderline personality features. *Journal of Personality Disorders*, 34(3), 394–409. https://doi.org/10.1521/pedi_2019_33_404

Mayer, R. C., Davis, J. H., & Schoorman, F. D. (1995). An integrative model of organizational trust. *Academy of Management Review*, 20, 709–734. https://psycnet.apa.org/doi/10.2307/258792

McLeod, C. (2020). Trust. In E. N. Zalta (Ed.), *The Stanford encyclopedia of philosophy*. Metaphysics research lab. https://plato.stanford.edu/archives/fall2020/entries/trust/

Miano, A., Fertuck, E. A., Arntz, A., & Stanley, B. (2013). Rejection sensitivity is a mediator between borderline personality disorder features and facial trust appraisal. *Journal of Personality Disorders*, 27(4), 442–456. https://doi.org/10.1521/pedi_2013_27_096

Miano, A., Fertuck, E. A., Roepke, S., & Dziobek, I. (2017). Romantic relationship dysfunction in borderline personality disorder: A naturalistic approach to trustworthiness perception. *Personality Disorders*, 8(3), 281–286. https://doi.org/10.1037/per0000196

Mike, A., King, H., Oltmanns, T. F., & Jackson, J. J. (2018). Obsessive, compulsive, and conscientious? The relationship between OCPD and personality traits. *Journal of Personality*, 86(6), 952–972. https://doi.org/10.1111/jopy.12368

Mikulincer, M. (1998). Attachment working models and the sense of trust: An exploration of interaction goals and affect regulation. *Journal of Personality and Social Psychology*, 74(5), 1209–1224. https://doi.org/10.1037/0022-3514.74.5.1209

Millon, T., & Davis, R. O. (1996). *Disorders of personality: DSM-IV and beyond* (2nd ed.). John Wiley & Sons.

Murray, S. L., Lamarche, V., Seery, M. D., Jung, H. Y., Griffin, D. W., & Brinkman, C. (2020). The social-safety system: Fortifying relationships in the face of the unforeseeable. *Journal of Personality and Social Psychology*, 120 (1), 99–130. https://doi.org/10.1037/pspi0000245

Natsuaki, M. N., Cicchetti, D., & Rogosch, F. A. (2009). Examining the developmental history of child maltreatment, peer relations, and externalizing problems among adolescents with symptoms of paranoid personality disorder. *Development and Psychopathology*, 21(4), 1181–1193. https://doi .org/10.1017/S0954579409990101

Ng, R., Fillet, P., DeWitt, M., Heyman, G. D., & Bellugi, U. (2015). Reasoning about trust among individuals with Williams syndrome. *American Journal on Intellectual and Developmental Disabilities*, 120(6), 527–541. https://doi.org/ 10.1352/1944-7558-120.6.527

Nicol, K., Pope, M., Sprengelmeyer, R., Young, A. W., & Hall, J. (2013). Social judgement in borderline personality disorder. *PLoS ONE*, 8(11), Article e73440. https://doi.org/10.1371/journal.pone.0073440

Nordahl, H. M., Holthe, H., & Haugum, J. A. (2005). Early maladaptive schemas in patients with or without personality disorders: Does schema modification predict symptomatic relief? *Clinical Psychology & Psychotherapy*, 12(2), 142–149. https://doi.org/10.1002/cpp.430.

Oosterhof, N. N., & Todorov, A. (2009). Shared perceptual basis of emotional expressions and trustworthiness impressions from faces. *Emotion*, 9(1), 128–133. https://doi.org/10.1037/a0014520

Orme, W., Bowersox, L., Vanwoerden, S., Fonagy, P., & Sharp, C. (2019). The relation between epistemic trust and borderline pathology in an adolescent inpatient sample. *Borderline Personality Disorder and Emotion Dysregulation*, 6, Article 13. https://doi.org/10.1186/s40479-019-0110-7

Petrocelli, J. V., Glaser, B. A., Calhoun, G. B., & Campbell, L. F. (2001). Early maladaptive schemas of personality disorder subtypes. *Journal of Personality Disorders*, 15(6), 546–559. https://doi.org/10.1521/pedi.15.6.546.19189

Pfattheicher, S., & Bohm, R. (2018). Honesty-humility under threat: Self-uncertainty destroys trust among the nice guys. *Journal of Personality and Social Psychology*, 114(1), 179–194. https://doi.org/10.1037/pspp0000144

Poggi, A., Richetin, J., & Preti, E. (2019). Trust and rejection sensitivity in personality disorders. *Current Psychiatry Reports*, 21(8), 1–9. https://doi.org/ 10.1007/s11920-019-1059-3

Polgar, P., Fogd, D., Unoka, Z., Siraly, E., & Csukly, G. (2014). Altered social decision making in borderline personality disorder: An Ultimatum Game study. *Journal of Personality Disorders*, 28(6), 841–852. https://doi.org/10 .1521/pedi_2014_28_142

Raihani, N. J., & Bell, V. (2017). Paranoia and the social representation of others: A large-scale game theory approach. *Scientific Reports*, 7(1), Article 4544. https://doi.org/10.1038/s41598-017-04805-3

(2018). Conflict and cooperation in paranoia: A large-scale behavioural experiment. *Psychological Medicine*, 48(9), 1523–1531. https://doi.org/10.1017/S0033291717003075

Ramseyer, F., Ebert, A., Roser, P., Edel, M. A., Tschacher, W., & Brune, M. (2019). Exploring nonverbal synchrony in borderline personality disorder: A double-blind placebo-controlled study using oxytocin. *British Journal of Clinical Psychology*, 59(2), 186–207. https://doi.org/10.1111/bjc.12240

Reed, L. I., Best, C. K., & Hooley, J. M. (2018). Cooperation with characters: How a partner's personality disorder decreases cooperation in two economic games. *Personality and Individual Differences*, 126, 33–37. https://doi.org/10.1016/j.paid.2018.01.008

Reed, L. I., Harrison, E. G., Best, C. K., & Hooley, J. M. (2019). Bargaining with characters: How personality pathology affects behavior in the ultimatum and dictator games. *Personality and Individual Differences*, 140, 65–69. https://doi.org/10.1016/j.paid.2018.05.035

Reed, L. I., Meyer, A. K., Okun, S. J., Best, C. K., & Hooley, J. M. (2020). In smiles we trust? Smiling in the context of antisocial and borderline personality pathology. *PLoS ONE*, 15(6), Article e0234574. https://doi.org/10.1371/journal.pone.0234574

Reichenberger, J., Eibl, J. J., Pfaltz, M., et al. (2017, Feb). Don't praise me, don't chase me: Emotional reactivity to positive and negative social-evaluative videos in patients with borderline personality disorder. *Journal of Personality Disorders*, 31(1), 75–89. https://doi.org/10.1521/pedi_2016_30_238

Rempel, J. K., Holmes, J. G., & Zanna, M. P. (1985). Trust in close relationships. *Journal of Personality and Social Psychology*, 49(1), 95–112. https://psycnet.apa.org/doi/10.1037/0022-3514.49.1.95

Rettew, D. C. (2000). Avoidant personality disorder, generalized social phobia, and shyness: Putting the personality back into personality disorders. *Harvard Review of Psychiatry*, 8(6), 283–297. https://psycnet.apa.org/doi/10.1093/hrp.8.6.283

Riby, D. M., Kirk, H., Hanley, M., & Riby, L. M. (2014). Stranger danger awareness in Williams syndrome. *Journal of Intellectual Disability Research*, 58(6), 572–582. https://doi.org/10.1111/jir.12055

Richell, R. A., Mitchell, D. G. V., Peschardt, K. S., et al. (2005). Trust and distrust: The perception of trustworthiness of faces in psychopathic and non-psychopathic offenders. *Personality and Individual Differences*, 38(8), 1735–1744. https://doi.org/10.1016/j.paid.2004.11.017

Richetin, J., Poggi, A., Ricciardelli, P., Fertuck, E. A., & Preti, E. (2018). The emotional components of rejection sensitivity as a mediator between borderline personality disorder and biased appraisal of trust in faces. *Clinical Neuropsychiatry*, 15, 200–205. www.researchgate.net/publication/327931236_The_emotional_components_of_rejection_sensitivity_as_a_mediator_between_Borderline_Personality_Disorder_and_biased_appraisal_of_trust_in_faces

Roberts, I. D., Krajbich, I., Cheavens, J. S., Campo, J. V., & Way, B. M. (2018). Acetaminophen reduces distrust in individuals with borderline personality disorder features. *Clinical Psychological Science*, 6, 145–154. https://doi.org/10.1177%2F2167702617731374

Salsman, N., & Linehan, M. M. (2006). Dialectical-behavioral therapy for borderline personality disorder. *Primary Psychiatry*, 13(5), 51–58. https://doi.org/10.1177/2167702617731374

Shamay-Tsoory, S. G., & Abu-Akel, A. (2016). The social salience hypothesis of oxytocin. *Biological Psychiatry*, 79(3), 194–202. https://doi.org/10.1016/j.biopsych.2015.07.020

Simonsen, S., Bateman, A., Bohus, M., et al. (2019). European guidelines for personality disorders: Past, present and future. *Borderline Personality Disorder and Emotion Dysregulation*, 6, Article 9. https://doi.org/10.1186/s40479-019-0106-3

Sorensen, K. D., Wilberg, T., Berthelsen, E., & Rabu, M. (2019). Lived experience of treatment for avoidant personality disorder: Searching for courage to be. *Frontiers in Psychology*, 10, Article 2879. https://doi.org/10.3389/fpsyg.2019.02879

Sperber, D., Clément, F., Heintz, C., et al. (2010). Epistemic vigilance. *Mind & Language*, 25(4), 359–393. https://doi.org/10.1111/j.1468-0017.2010.01394.x

Staebler, K., Helbing, E., Rosenbach, C., & Renneberg, B. (2011). Rejection sensitivity and borderline personality disorder. *Clinical Psychology & Psychotherapy*, 18(4), 275–283. https://doi.org/10.1002/cpp.705

Thielmann, I., Hilbig, B. E., & Niedtfeld, I. (2014). Willing to give but not to forgive: Borderline personality features and cooperative behavior. *Journal of Personality Disorders*, 28(6), 778–795. https://doi.org/10.1521/pedi_2014_28_135

Thome, J., Liebke, L., Bungert, M., et al. (2016). Confidence in facial emotion recognition in borderline personality disorder. *Personality Disorders*, 7(2), 159–168. https://doi.org/10.1037/per0000142

Torres-Sot, J. F., Moya-Faz, F. J., Giner-Alegría, C. A., & Oliveras-Valenzuela, M. A. (2019). The PID-5 Inventory, the dimensional profile of DSM-5 to guide diagnosis and therapeutic needs in personality disorders. *Anales de Psicología*, 35, 47–57. https://doi.org/10.6018/analesps.35.1.333191

Unoka, Z., Seres, I., Aspan, N., Bodi, N., & Keri, S. (2009). Trust game reveals restricted interpersonal transactions in patients with borderline personality disorder. *Journal of Personality Disorders*, 23(4), 399–409. https://doi.org/10.1521/pedi.2009.23.4.399

Volkert, J., Gablonski, T. C., & Rabung, S. (2018). Prevalence of personality disorders in the general adult population in Western countries: Systematic review and meta-analysis. *British Journal of Psychiatry*, 213(6), 709–715. https://doi.org/10.1192/bjp.2018.202

White, C. N., Conway, C. C., & Oltmanns, T. F. (2019). Stress and personality disorders. In K. Harkness & E. P. Hayden (Eds.), *The Oxford handbook of stress and mental health.* Oxford University Press. https://doi.org/10.1093/oxfordhb/9780190681777.013.8

Widiger, T. A., & Costa, P. T. (2012). Integrating normal and abnormal personality structure: The five-factor model. *Journal of Personality,* 80(6), 1471–1506. https://doi.org/10.1111/j.1467-6494.2012.00776.x.

Wilberg, T., Urnes, Ø., Friis, S., Pedersen, G., & Karterud, S. (1999). Borderline and avoidant personality disorders and the five-factor model of personality: A comparison between DSM-IV diagnoses and NEO-PI-R. *Journal of Personality Disorders,* 13(3), 226–240. https://doi.org/10.1521/pedi.1999.13.3.226

Wilson, D., & Sperber, D. (2012). *Meaning and relevance.* Cambridge University Press. https://doi.org/10.1017/CBO9781139028370

Winsper, C., Bilgin, A., Thompson, A., et al. (2020). The prevalence of personality disorders in the community: A global systematic review and meta-analysis. *British Journal of Psychiatry,* 216(2), 69–78. https://doi.org/10.1192/bjp.2019.166

Winter, D., Bohus, M., & Lis, S. (2017). Understanding negative self-evaluations in borderline personality disorder: A review of self-related cognitions, emotions, and motives. *Current Psychiatry Reports,* 19(3), Article 17. https://doi.org/10.1007/s11920-017-0771-0

Yalch, M. M., & Levendosky, A. A. (2019). Influence of betrayal trauma on borderline personality disorder traits. *Journal of Trauma & Dissociation,* 20(4), 392–401. https://doi.org/10.1080/15299732.2019.1572042

Young, J. E., Klosko, J. S., & Weishaar, M. E. (2006). *Schema therapy: A practitioner's guide.* The Guilford Press.

Zhang, Q., Zhang, L., & Li, C. (2017). Attachment, perceived parental trust and grandiose narcissism: Moderated mediation models. *Personality and Individual Differences,* 104, 470–475. https://doi.org/10.1016/j.paid.2016.09.013

CHAPTER 18

Trust and Lesion Evidence
Lessons from Neuropsychology on the Neuroanatomical Correlates of Trust

Hannah E. Wadsworth and Daniel Tranel

18.1   Introduction

On the face of it, trust seems like a relatively straightforward concept: belief in the reliability, truth, or ability of someone or something. But the act of trusting another person can quickly become complicated, for example when it involves relying on someone when the outcome is uncertain (i.e., strategic uncertainty [Houser et al., 2010]). Understanding when to trust in a social, interpersonal setting and establishing judgments of trustworthiness are complex processes that are critical and essential for human life. Appropriate judgments in trustworthiness lead to the formation of cooperative, mutually beneficial relationships that facilitate personal success, a sense of achievement, increased well-being, and good quality of life. However, difficulty forming accurate judgments about trustworthiness often leads to adverse outcomes such as exploitation (e.g., if one is too trusting) or loss of positive, helpful relationships (e.g., if one does not reciprocate trust). These important social and personal repercussions are at the foundation of trust and reciprocity decisions. The process becomes even more complex because to assess another person's trustworthiness, one must engage in numerous interactions with a variety of others to gauge who reciprocates trust and whose behavior violates social norms. Each individual must then adjust to their understanding of those in their interpersonal circle and their own behavior to account for their judgments of trustworthiness. Given this intricate and important practice, understanding the cognitive processes underlying the ability to accurately form trustworthiness judgments is essential to understanding human behavior in social settings and interpersonal relationships.

This work was supported in part by grant 2P50MH094258 from the National Institute of Mental Health and a grant from the Kiwanis Neuroscience Research Foundation. Corresponding authors: Hannah E. Wadsworth (hannah-wadsworth@uiowa.edu) and Daniel Tranel (daniel-tranel@uiowa.edu).

Perhaps the most compelling example of social trust was encountered by the world population at the exact time this chapter was written. The pandemic of COVID-19 (caused by the novel coronavirus SARS-CoV-2) has created a social trust imperative that has not been faced in modern times. With the highly contagious and rapidly spreading SARS-CoV-2, and the deadly COVID-19 disease it causes, the population has required unprecedented levels of social distancing, self-isolation, and quarantining. Social systems and individuals are extremely reliant on trusting that healthcare providers and everyday citizens who are out in public are not sick. Moreover, we are also trusting that those who have been exposed are taking the necessary precautions to slow the spread of the virus by staying home and avoiding contact with others as much as possible. We are reliant on everyone to take basic precautionary steps, even if not sick or with known exposure, including wearing face coverings, staying six feet apart, and limiting unnecessary contact with other people. We trust our political and scientific leaders to tell the truth. Life or death stakes depend on this social trust and the compliance with social norms, including protecting the health of high-risk groups and not overwhelming the healthcare system. Lack of trust in leadership can be devastating (Editors of *The New England Journal of Medicine*, 2020).

A first step in appreciating processes of trust is realizing that the ability to actively engage in judgments of trustworthiness requires the activation of several cognitive systems including multiple levels of social, emotional/ psychological, and reward-processing networks. Neuropsychology is uniquely positioned to examine these processes and the associated neuro-anatomical correlates related to trust. The study of patients with discrete, focal brain lesions can not only help to uncover neuroanatomical regions that are necessary for normal trust behavior, but can also help determine where the psychological processes related to trust can be "carved at the joints" – that is, where the normal process of trust behavior can be fractionated and selectively impaired (Caramazza, 1992). Neuropsychology also furnishes important measurement approaches and tools, providing the foundation for the development of instruments for measuring a highly complex behavior such as "trust" in ways that are reliable and valid.

In this chapter, we will first review the trust game (TG) (Berg et al., 1995), a widely used experimental measure developed to understand the way people approach trusting a stranger. Then, we will go on to review several brain structures that are believed to be associated with the cognitive and emotional processes that are germane to the different stages of trust behavior. In each section, we will describe how abilities may change when those regions are damaged through a review of lesion studies, followed by how these findings and support from functional magnetic resonance imaging (fMRI) literature speak to the broader understanding of the neural correlates of trust.

18.2   The Trust Game

The TG (Berg et al., 1995) is an economic decision-making game that was specifically designed to measure trust (see also Chapter 2). The TG covers reasonably well the gambit of different processes subsumed under the construct of "trust" (see Section 18.1). It is typically used to help understand behavior when people approach trusting someone new, how behavior changes in response to the other person's actions, and what areas of the brain are involved during the complex cognitive process of trusting (see also Chapter 2). The TG is an important and unique measure in the study of trust and differs from other economic decision-making games. Specifically, other such tasks, like the prisoner's dilemma game, the Iowa gambling task (Bechara et al., 1994), the ultimatum game (Guth et al., 1982), and the cups task (Levin et al., 2007; Levin & Hart, 2003; Weller et al., 2007), are typically focused on risk assessment, risk/betrayal aversion, cooperation, and uncertainty (Weller et al., 2009). While clearly all of these factors are useful in understanding integral pieces of the trust process, the TG is the only economic decision-making task that measures the entirety of the trust process and how it can evolve over time with multiple interactions.

Specifically, the TG is an economic exchange between two players, the first player (aka the *investor*) who invests money with the other player (aka the *trustee*), who can choose whether or not to reciprocate the investment (Figure 18.1). Take this example: The investor is provided with an endowment of $20, and then decides to invest the entirety of that endowment to the trustee. The investor and the trustee will then see the investment triple to $60. At that point, the trustee decides how to split the money between the two players, giving the trustee the opportunity to exhibit trust or distrust in the investor. The trustee can demonstrate trust in the investor by reciprocating in kind (returning a fair amount of money, e.g., $30), in the hope that the investor will reciprocate and invest a high proportion of their endowment in the next round. Or the trustee can demonstrate distrust in the investor by keeping a large portion of the money (aka "defecting"), suggesting that the trustee does not believe the

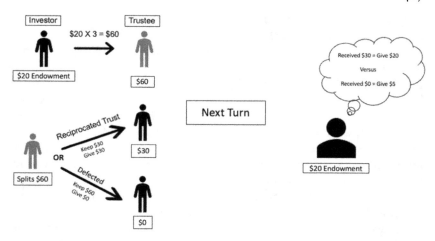

Figure 18.1   The trust game.
The figure depicts the steps of the trust game and the actions of each player. In the first trial, the investor (depicted throughout the figure in black) is given an initial endowment of $20. The investor chooses to entrust the full endowment to the trustee (depicted throughout the figure in gray). The investment is then tripled, leaving the trustee with $60 to divide between themselves and the investor. The trustee can either choose to reciprocate the investor's initial trust by dividing the money fairly OR defect by dividing the money unfairly. The decision that the trustee makes can then influence the investor's decision on the next trial when they are again provided with a new $20 endowment.

investor will provide a fair portion of the endowment in the next round. Once the decision is made, a new trial begins with a new endowment available to the investor. Both players are able to see the amount of money available for each decision, the actions of both players, and the amount of money earned by each player throughout the game (running totals are displayed for both players). See Figure 18.1 for a figural depiction of the TG.

Given the structure of the game, the amount of money earned by each player is dependent on both parties: the investor (the initial amount invested in the trustee) and the trustee (how the money is split). Mutual trust leads to economic gains for both players, whereas lack of trustworthiness (misplaced trust or distrust) results in a less successful exchange (lower monetary gains for both players). Although various fields of study have speculated at length about the kinds of "rational behavior" that would be expected in this situation, it turns out that most normal healthy adults tend to invest approximately 50% or more of the initial endowment, signaling to the trustee that they are trusting, and the trustee tends to reciprocate trust in the investor (King-Casas et al., 2005; Koscik & Tranel, 2011; Krueger et al., 2008).

The TG requires multiple types of processing, including economic decision making, assessment of uncertainty and risk, mentalizing/perspective taking, inhibition, and judgments about appropriateness of social behavior. Each of these is present to various degrees at various points during the game: at the initial investment decision (subsequently seen by the trustee), when the trustee chooses to reciprocate (or defect), and at the time the investor sees the trustee's decision and then decides how much to invest in the next round. Not surprisingly, this complex task requires multifold cognitive and emotional process, and several brain regions are activated when participants are engaged in this game. Many studies have used the TG as a means to explore the neuroanatomical correlates of trust. Next, we will review the structures that are consistently found to be implicated in the process of trust. At the beginning of each section, we will review available lesion literature to explain how the trust process is interrupted when regions of interest are damaged. This will then be supported with fMRI research that has demonstrated activation in certain brain areas when participants are engaged in this and other trust tasks.

18.3   Insula

The insula is an area of cortex located deep beneath the lateral sulcus and frontoparietal opercula (Figure 18.2). The insula, a key component of the so-called limbic system, is known to be important for many aspects of emotional processing. Although the insula is frequently implicated in processing negative emotions, such as pain, distress, and disgust (Kross et al., 2007; Ostrowsky et al., 2002; Phillips et al., 1997), research suggests that the insula is also integral in processing positive emotions (Berntson et al., 2011; Damasio et al., 2000). The insula is also strongly implicated in processing social emotions including empathy and social rejection (Eisenberger et al., 2003; Lamm & Singer, 2010; Singer et al., 2006). Moreover, the insula is associated with risk tracking and risk prediction (Bossaerts, 2010; Preuschoff et al., 2008), betrayal aversion (Aimone et al., 2014), and uncertainty (Critchley et al., 2001). Additionally, it is known that conscious interoception, or the sense and understanding of what is happening inside one's body, can potentially influence decision making (Bechara & Damasio, 2005; Damasio, 1996), and this process is regulated, in part, by the insula (Bar-on et al., 2003; Clark et al., 2008; Craig, 2002). Finally, the insula is involved in economic decision-making tasks such as

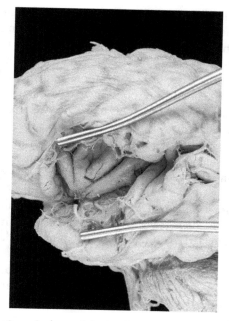

Figure 18.2　A photo of the insular cortex in left hemisphere.

the prisoner's dilemma (Gabay et al., 2019; Singer et al., 2004), the ultimatum game (Cheng et al., 2017; Sanfey et al., 2003), the cups task (Xue et al., 2010), and the Iowa gambling task (D'Acremont et al., 2009; Krawitz et al., 2010).

18.3.1　Lesion Studies

Belfi et al. (2015) investigated interpersonal trust in participants with damage to the insula. The authors studied 11 neurological patients with focal insula lesions (7 left, 4 right), 15 focal brain-damaged comparisons with lesions outside the insula, amygdala, and medial prefrontal cortex, and 31 neurologically healthy comparisons. All participants engaged in multiple rounds of the TG, first playing 20 rounds as the trustee, then an additional 20 rounds as the investor. The participants were told they were playing against the "other player" though all played against a computer programmed to mirror the participants' behavior (tit-for-tat or responding in kind). Behavioral results showed that the healthy comparisons responded, as expected, in the typical tit-for-tat style. However, participants with insula damage responded quite differently. As the investor, the participants with insula damage tended to respond in a benevolent manner, expressing trust in their partner even when their partner had betrayed their trust – meaning they made risky choices by investing more money, even when these decisions were not rewarded. As the trustee, those with insula damage tended to respond in a malevolent manner, betraying their partners even when their partners had expressed trust, also reflecting a risky choice as it jeopardizes future investments and economic gains for both players. It is possible that this risky choice behavior would extend to other domains besides trust, and this is a question for future research. Those in the brain-damaged comparison group responded differently than those with insula damage and healthy comparisons. As investors, they behaved in a tit-for-tat manner less frequently than healthy comparisons, but more frequently than those with insula damage. In contrast, as the trustee, brain-damaged comparisons behaved similarly to healthy comparisons.

These results provide evidence that the insula is important for complex social decision making including accurately assessing trustworthiness, the recognition of risky and socially inappropriate decisions, and creating and maintaining mutually beneficial social interactions. More specifically, this study supported previous research that showed increased insula activation when participants provided a risky investment that was subsequently not rewarded. Furthermore, the greater the insula activation, the more likely the participant would make a safer investment the following turn. The theory presented suggested that insula activation may indicate a risky decision and be implicated in risk judgment. If that risky decision results in a poor outcome, it was thought that the insula signals to the participant that they should not make a similar decision. Belfi et al. (2015) demonstrated that those with insula lesions made benevolent investments and malevolent returns repeatedly, even when the investment was not reciprocated. This suggests that those with insula lesions may not understand that they are making a risky decision and do not respond to the behaviors of their partner. Collectively, these findings provide strong support for the involvement of the insula in the cognitive and emotional process of trust.

18.3.2   Functional Imaging Studies

King-Casas et al. (2008) paired 55 participants with a diagnosis of borderline personality disorder (as the trustee) with 38 healthy participants (as the investor) and compared the interactions with two groups of healthy comparisons (as both trustees and investors). The authors found that the bilateral anterior insula was implicated in response to small investments in trustees. A small investment from an investor suggests that trust has been ruptured (i.e., the amount of the investment is not reciprocated after the money was tripled, therefore the investor decided to provide less money in the next round). When this happens, it is in the best interests of both parties to repair the relationship and recreate a mutually beneficial relationship. To initiate a repair in the presence of a low investment, the trustee is required to "coax" the investor by providing a high rate of return on the investment. Coaxing engenders trust from the investor and pays dividends for five rounds into the future. In healthy participants, activation in the bilateral anterior insula is notable when a trustee is faced with a small investment amount. This was in contrast with those with borderline personality disorder, who did not show anterior insula activation, and behaviorally these participants were half as likely to engage in coaxing behavior, though when they did coax, it was to a smaller magnitude than their healthy counterparts. Finally, both groups (borderline personality disorder and healthy) had increased anterior insula activation when the decision was made to return a small amount to the investor. These findings suggest that the insula is activated during consideration of the social appropriateness of behavior within the self and others. In persons with borderline personality disorder, characterized by impaired social interactions and negative expectations of others, diminished activity in the insula in response to a low offer from an investor suggests that the participants do not perceive or recognize the low offers are a response to a violation of social norms committed by themselves.

In another study using a brief version of the TG, Van den Bos et al. (2009) studied participants' ability to focus on the other person. Specifically, the investigators' goal was to study the neural correlates of mentalizing how different outcomes would affect the other player and how cooperative intentions of the other player benefit the participant. In this version of the TG (fixed choice), the first participant is given a choice to either split up the money in a predetermined way (e.g., participant 1 gets $8 and participant 2 gets $6), or pass on the choice to the second player, allowing that participant to make the decision to divide the money but also introducing the possibility that both players could receive more. Participant 2 can then choose a mutually beneficial fixed choice (e.g., participant 1 gets $11 and participant 2 gets $10), or a personally beneficial option (e.g., participant 1 gets $5 while participant 2 gets $17), thus introducing risk for the first participant. In this study, the 18 participants were told that previous participants had completed the first set of choices at an earlier time (predetermined series of choices by a computer); hence, all participants were actually assigned to make a reciprocal choice as the second player. Each participant was told that their choices affected how much both people were paid for participating in the experiment and that all participants would receive compensation upon the completion of the study. The predetermined choices fell into a risk-level category (high vs. low) for the first player, and a benefit category (high vs. low) for the second player. For additional characterization of participants, each person was identified as either prosocial (tendency to prioritize outcomes for others) or proself (tendency to prioritize outcomes for themselves) based on a self-report questionnaire.

Results from this study showed that the rate of reciprocity was highest when the risk for the first player was high *and* the benefit for the second player was high, suggesting that participants took into account conse-quences for others *and* themselves when making trust decisions. In terms of insula involvement, the researchers found that activation was sensitive to norm violations. Specifically, when someone had rated themselves as prosocial, they had greater activation in the insular cortices when choosing to award themselves more money. In contrast, those who rated themselves as proself had greater activation when they chose to reciprocate. These results are consistent with the theory that the insula becomes activated when a personal norm and social expectation is violated. A practical implication of these findings relates back to the current COVID-19 pandemic. Given the high risk for others including the possibility of death if they contract SARS-CoV-2, and the high benefit for oneself by avoiding SARS-CoV-2, these findings suggest that people would work to self-isolate. However, other factors including economic concerns, isolation hardship and fatigue, and perceived low health risk (particularly in younger age groups) have led a subset of people to stop self-isolating and at times go so far as to mount armed protests against stay-at-home orders. One caveat to this study is that for those who participated in proself behavior, these participants may have been motivated by selfishness *or* social efficiency, as the personally beneficial option is the socially optimal option. As such further research is needed in this area.

Kang et al. (2011) explored the influence of physical temperature on trust and insula activation in two small experiments. The authors explored the influence of temperature on trust as the insular cortex is central to temperature processing (Brooks et al., 2002; Craig et al., 2000; Moulton et al., 2005). In the initial behavioral experiment, 30 college students simply held either a cold or warm pack in their hand for 10 seconds prior to completion of the TG. Participants were randomly assigned to the temperature of the pack and they were asked to complete a consumer product review on the pack in order to disguise the role of temperature priming in the experiment. For the TG paradigm, participants were assigned to the investor role in the TG and were told they were playing real people at other sites (all answers were computer generated). In this first study, the investigators found that participants who were exposed to cold packs later invested significantly less money than those who were exposed to warm packs. In a follow-up study, 16 participants were exposed to a cold and warm pack before participating in the TG (order of exposure was counterbalanced and with neutral room temperature intervals in between temperature trials). It was found that cold temperature activated the bilateral insula above neutral temperatures, but warm temperature did not. During the TG, the left anterior insula had greater activation after exposure to the cold temperature pack than those who had the warm temperature pack. These findings support the notion that increased insular activation by interoception (noticing the feeling/physical discomfort of being cold) plays a role in decision making and trust.

Finally, a recent meta-analysis of anterior insula involvement in social norm compliance in both the single trial TG and the ultimatum game (Bellucci et al., 2018) showed that the right anterior insula was the only structure consistently activated in both tasks across multiple studies. More specifically, it was found that the decision to trust activated the right dorsal anterior insula, while the decision to reciprocate trust activated the right ventral anterior insula. A previous meta-analysis (Bellucci et al., 2017) of neural signatures of the TG found anterior insula activation both during the decision to trust in the one-trial TG and during the decision to reciprocate in the multi-round game. The latter is suggestive of experience of aversive feelings by the trustee.

It is clear that the insula is an important component of recognizing social norm violations. Interestingly, it is also activated when participants view trustworthy (Killgore et al., 2013; Singer et al., 2004) and untrustworthy faces (Todorov, 2008; Todorov et al., 2008; Winston et al., 2002). Haas et al. (2015) collected imaging data from 82 healthy participants, along with levels of the "tendency to trust" on a self-report measure. The participants were then presented with 36 neutral-expression pictures of faces and asked to rate their trustworthiness on a 7-point Likert scale. A positive association was found between the trustworthy rating of neutral faces, self-report level of trust, and gray matter volume in the bilateral anterior insula. Said another way, those who rated faces as more trustworthy and reported higher baseline levels of trust, tended to have greater gray matter volume in both anterior insular cortices. These findings may suggest that the anterior insula is involved in evaluating social situations and stimuli, and in turn influencing social decision making.

18.4   Amygdala

The amygdala is an almond-shaped gray matter structure located in the medial temporal lobes, anterior to the hippocampus, and belonging to the so-called limbic system (Figure 18.3). It has been well studied in both animals and humans, and is known to be involved in social, emotional, and reward processing. Classic studies by Kluver and Bucy in the 1930s (Kluver & Bucy, 1937, 1939) explored behavior in monkeys after large bitemporal lesions, noting dramatically decreased social inhibition and increased social affiliation. Later studies found that when the amygdala is selectively lesioned, monkeys lose a normal level of cautiousness and distrust when approaching people, predators, and new or frightening objects (Machado et al., 2009; Mason et al., 2006). Focal bilateral lesions to the amygdala in humans are very rare, making it challenging to study the effects of such damage. However, many studies have been done with participants who have intractable temporal lobe epilepsy and undergo selective ablation surgeries such as unilateral amygdalohippocampectomies. Some studies have found impaired fear conditioning (LaBar et al., 1995) in these patients. Other studies have suggested greater dysfunction of social cognition associated with damage to the right amygdala when compared to the left (Adolphs et al., 2001).

One very compelling opportunity to study focal bilateral amygdala damage is in patients who have Urbach-Wiethe disease (also known as lipoid proteinosis), an extremely rare genetic disease that can result in the calcification of the amygdala, bilaterally (Meletti et al., 2014; Thornton et al., 2008). Our group has conducted extensive research on patient SM, who has complete, focal bilateral amygdala lesions due to Urbach-Wiethe disease (Tranel & Hyman, 1990). Patient SM has contributed extensively to the human neuropsychological literature on amygdala function (Buchanan et al., 2009). In several early studies, we showed that SM has a very specific impairment in her ability to recognize fear in facial expressions (Adolphs et al., 1994). In fact, another study from our group (Adolphs et al., 1998) examined social judgments in three participants with complete bilateral amygdala damage, including SM. Additionally, the

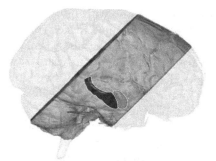

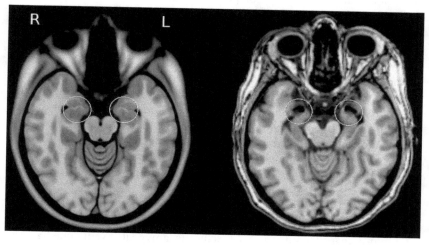

Figure 18.3   Illustration of the amygdala.
Top illustration of the amygdala depicted in gray, next to the hippocampus shown in black. Bottom image is a magnetic resonance imaging cross-section of healthy amygdalae in the left image, and patient SM's damaged amygdalae in the right image.

study included social judgments by seven participants with unilateral amygdala damage, and both bilateral and unilateral lesion groups were compared to those with damage in other regions of the brain and a healthy, nonbrain-damaged group.

The amygdala lesion group and the brain-damaged comparison group were shown 100 pictures of faces to rate on a scale of approachability and trustworthiness. These pictures consisted of 50 faces that healthy comparisons assigned the most negative ratings, and 50 faces that received the most positive ratings. Those with bilateral amygdala damage rated the 50 negative pictures consistently more positive than either healthy or brain-damaged comparisons. Those with unilateral amygdala damage did not differ from either healthy or brain-damaged comparisons. These results found an overall positive bias, rating these unfamiliar faces as more approachable and trustworthy even when healthy comparisons rated the faces as very unapproachable and trustworthy. During this study, SM spontaneously made comments that in real life, she would not know how to judge if a person were untrustworthy. This is consistent with SM's tendency to approach and engage in physical contact with strangers rather indiscriminately. From other studies, we also know that SM does not understand the concept of personal space, nor does she experience discomfort when standing too close or even touching a stranger (Adolphs, 2010; Kennedy et al., 2009). Finally, studies from other investigators provided further indication that the amygdala is involved in processing trustworthiness in faces (Haas et al., 2015; Said et al., 2009).

Later studies with SM examined her ability to discriminate fear in faces if her visual attention was specifically directed to the eye regions of faces (Adolphs et al., 2005). When told to fixate on the eyes, the area of the face most important to recognize fear, her ability to discriminate fear from other emotions improved (temporarily). These results suggest that the amygdala plays a role in vigilance, ambiguity/uncertainty resolution, tracking emotions and arousal, and implementing selective cortical processing of relevant stimuli (Adolphs, 2010).

In the TG specifically, Koscik and Tranel (2011) compared TG performances in three groups: 32 individuals with unilateral amygdala damage, 48 brain-damaged comparisons (excluding amygdala, ventromedial prefrontal, and insular cortex damage), and 59 neurologically normal comparisons. All participants completed a multi-round version of the TG: 20 rounds each as the trustee and the investor, respectively. Despite the deliberate impression that participants were engaging with another human (referred to as the "other player"), opponents were in reality simulated to respond in a tit-for-tat manner. Behavioral results showed that participants with amygdala damage behaved benevolently, both as the investor and as the trustee, meaning they responded with trust in the other player even when their trust had been betrayed. In contrast, brain-damaged comparisons behaved ambivalently toward the other player, and healthy comparisons responded with a tit-for-tat strategy or responded in kind.

The authors pose that a damaged amygdala interferes with the ability to appropriately evaluate social situations and extract information about how others are behaving. By not accurately evaluating betrayals of trust and instead responding positively, it places these individuals at risk for

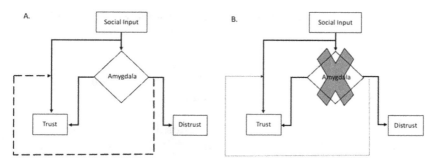

Figure 18.4   The role of the amygdala in trust.
(A) In this model, people trust others as a default mode of behavior. The amygdala serves to
evaluate incoming social stimuli to either enhance trust-related behaviors for positive
evaluations, or to distrust the individual for negative evaluations. Dashed lines indicate
inhibitory processes. (B) Amygdala lesions knock out the evaluative process, resulting in
default trust and lack of negative evaluations.
Adapted model from Koscik and Tranel (2011).

exploitation. This is consistent with the role of the amygdala in fear
processing, and findings that patients with amygdala damage do not alter
their behavior in the presence of aversive stimuli (Feinstein et al., 2016).
More specifically, it has been proposed that the amygdala evaluates incoming stimuli to determine whether or not to trust another person, with the
default behavior being to trust. Therefore, distrust is dependent on the
amygdala to evaluate incoming stimuli as negative, but damage to the
amygdala removes that process, leaving trust as the default (Figure 18.4)
(see also Chapter 9 for more information on distrust).

18.5   Prefrontal Cortex

The frontal lobes, and more specifically the prefrontal cortices, are the last
area of the brain to fully develop. With the development of the prefrontal
cortex, many important and adaptive cognitive changes occur, including
maturation of judgment, social comportment, social awareness, and consideration of the thoughts and needs of others. Therefore, in considering
the role the prefrontal cortex plays in the process of trust, it is helpful to
start with examining changes seen as children and adolescents mature into
adulthood.

It has been established that theory-of-mind, or the ability to consider
that others have different perspectives and the ability to consider what
those perspectives may be, develops around ages 4–5 (Wellman et al.,

2001). However, higher-order skills required for more complex tasks, such as the ability to take multiple perspectives, continue to develop throughout childhood and into late adolescence (Dumontheil et al., 2010). Improvements in mentalizing and sensitivity to others' perspectives are thought to drive increases in trust and cooperation (Dumontheil et al., 2010; Eisenberg et al., 2005), which in turn involve the prefrontal cortices. To examine the relationship between improvements in mentalizing, perspective taking, and trust, Crone (2013) studied the TG in groups of early adolescence, late adolescence, and early adulthood (the four age groups included 9–10, 12–13, 15, and 18–20) (see also Chapter 11).

The participants acted as the trustee with an anonymous investor who provided a variety of high- and low-risk trials. The author found that reciprocity increased generally between ages 9 and 16 but overall increased with age when the risk to the investor was high (i.e., when the investor gave a large amount of money, older adolescents reciprocated with a higher amount more often). In all participants, there was increased activation in the dorsolateral prefrontal cortex (dlPFC) when receiving trust in comparison to distrust from the investor. Additionally, increased activation in the dlPFC was associated with the choice to defect or betray the trust of an investor in older adolescents and early adults. In contrast, younger adolescents showed activation in the dlPFC regardless of whether they decided to defect or reciprocate investor trust. Studies prior to this one had established that the dlPFC is involved in perspective taking, bargaining (Rilling & Sanfey, 2011), self-referential processing (Denny et al., 2012), inhibition of selfish impulses, and increased cognitive control (Bunge et al., 2005; Steinbeis et al., 2012).

Crone (2013) noted supporting evidence that perspective-taking abilities, cognitive capacities, and inhibition of selfish impulses improve with maturity in adolescence and early adulthood. Finally, research also demonstrates that the dlPFC is activated in young adolescents when those participants are thinking about themselves (Pfeifer et al., 2007). Therefore, it has been postulated that reciprocity decisions in younger adolescence may rely more heavily on self-oriented strategizing in social dilemmas when compared to older adolescence and adulthood. This in turn appears to activate the dlPFC during reciprocity decisions. Crone's (2013) results further supported an earlier study (Van den Bos et al., 2011) that found that advanced social perspective-taking behavior during the TG was associated with increased involvement of the right dlPFC in older adolescents and young adults. In contrast, younger adolescents had greater activity in the anterior medial prefrontal cortex (amPFC), a region that is typically associated with self-oriented processing and mentalizing.

Another study examining how trust and brain activation mature through adolescence into middle adulthood was done by Fett et al. (2014). In this study, 45 healthy participants between the ages of 12 and 49 completed two iterations of the TG, one with a fair, trustworthy partner and one with an unfair, untrustworthy partner. During cooperative, reciprocal decisions, activation in the orbitofrontal cortex decreased with age. However, increased activation was noted in the medial frontal and precentral gyrus. The authors suggest changes in activation reflect mentalizing, cognitive control, and increased sensitivity to social signals.

In considering healthy adults, it is instructive to revisit the study reported by Van den Bos et al. (2009; see Section 18.3.2 on the insula for more details about the study). The authors found that the anterior medial PFC (amPFC) was more activated when participants decided to defect (or betray trust) than when they chose to reciprocate. This result is consistent with the understanding that the amPFC is implicated in the evaluation of reward and self-referential processing, despite the fact that this area was not sensitive to changing magnitude of personal gain. Furthermore, the authors found that the right dlPFC was activated when participants reciprocated trust, even when the external incentive was low. Recall that the study design included high benefit versus low benefit paradigms: In the low benefit paradigm, reciprocating a trust decision only provided participants a small amount of money above what they would have earned if the investor had made an untrusting decision (7 coins vs. 10 coins); however, in this paradigm, defecting would provide a significantly higher amount of money than if they reciprocated (10 coins vs. 17 coins). These results suggest that the right dlPFC is important for cognitive control and inhibition of self-oriented impulses.

Another frontal region that should be highlighted in the trust process is the ventromedial prefrontal cortex (vmPFC), which is known to be involved in social/interpersonal and personal decision making, as well as reciprocity and cooperation. The vmPFC has been examined extensively in the literature, including a long tradition of research on patients with focal vmPFC lesions by our group. Our early research showed that patients with focal vmPFC lesions have largely intact performances on intellectual and most neuropsychological measures, while at the same time exhibiting severe impairments in real-life decision making (Bechara et al., 1994; Damasio et al., 1991). Specifically, research participant EVR has been the subject of frequent study in our lab (Koenigs & Tranel, 2006; Reber & Tranel, 2019). EVR is unable to learn from his mistakes and anticipate the consequences of his actions, despite a fully intact ability to verbally solve social problems and ethical dilemmas. His impairments are notable during real-world, online decision making, and are apparent in tasks like the Iowa gambling task. EVR has consistently demonstrated the clear inability to make choices that will be to his advantage in the future, over the long run. These results were later extended, and it has been shown that patients with ventromedial prefrontal damage have a "myopia for the future" or are insensitive to future consequences, whether positive or negative, and instead are guided by immediate prospects (Bechara et al., 2000).

In direct relation to vmPFC damage and impaired ability to judge trustworthiness, a study done by Moretto et al. (2013) studied performances of participants with vmPFC lesions on a single trial of the TG. Participants were recruited into one of three groups, 10 with focal vmPFC lesions, 10 brain-damaged comparisons (damage outside the frontal lobes and amygdala), and 10 neurologically healthy comparisons. All participants engaged in two paradigms, one in which they were led to believe the other player was a human (labeled the "TG") and a second in which they were told they were playing with a computer (labeled the "risk game"). The participants completed several one-trial rounds of both games, both as the investor and trustee. It was found that participants with vmPFC lesions took the same amount of risk when playing a human opponent as when playing a computer. In contrast, the healthy and brain-damaged participants were less willing to invest when they believed they were interacting with a human rather than a computer. Furthermore, participants with vmPFC lesions showed reduced reciprocity when in the role of trustee, compared to healthy and brain-damaged participants. These findings suggest that patients with vmPFC damage have an inability to anticipate potential betrayals and are driven by immediate prospects – so that patients with vmPFC lesions have increased willingness to take social risks that may eventually invite exploitation and are more likely to damage mutually beneficial relationships.

Finally, returning to the judgment of trustworthiness in neutral, unfamiliar faces, Haas et al. (2015) found that higher levels of trust and higher ratings of trustworthiness in faces were associated with increased gray matter volume in the bilateral vmPFC (and anterior insula; see Section 18.3). These findings are consistent with the understanding that the vmPFC is involved in coding social value.

18.6   Other Neural Regions Associated with Trust

In addition to the insula, amygdala, and parts of the prefrontal cortex, other neuroanatomical areas appear frequently in research on the neural correlates of trust. These areas are reviewed briefly below, with the understanding that most of this research comes from functional neuroimaging as such regions generally have not been the subject of focal lesion studies.

18.6.1 Temporoparietal Junction

The temporoparietal junction (TPJ) is aptly named as it is located where the temporal and parietal lobes meet at the posterior end of the lateral sulcus. This area is thought to work together with aspects of the frontal lobe (e.g., anterior prefrontal cortex), and is thought to be important for mentalizing and perspective taking (Frith & Frith, 2003). In the previously reviewed 2009 study by Van den Bos et al. (see Sections 18.3.2 and 18.5 for more study details), it was found that the right hemisphere TPJ had greater activation in the trustee when the risk for the investor was high (in comparison to a low-risk condition). It was thought that this pattern of activation supported the idea that the right TPJ is associated with reflection on the consequences of one's actions on other people, and in turn reorienting attention from the self to the other. It was also noted that individuals who were classified as proself had greater activation in the right TPJ when reciprocating, whereas those who were classified as prosocial had greater activation when defecting. The authors postulate that this pattern of activation could be a reflection of having to shift attention from typical goal-directed behavior to behaviors that are out of character for them. A follow-up study by Crone's group (Van den Bos et al., 2011) examined brain activation in early adolescence through early adulthood (62 healthy volunteers ages 12–22). Behaviorally, it was found that with increasing age came greater consideration for the consequences for another individual, as reflected in increased reciprocity on high-risk trials and decreased reciprocity on low-risk trials. These findings were accompanied by increased activity in the left TPJ with increasing age, which was thought to demonstrate improved abilities in perspective taking, inferring the intentions of others, and shifting attention from the self to others.

Crone (2013) also found gradually increased activation in the TPJ (bilaterally) with increased age during the TG. These findings supported the previous notion that this region is associated with thinking about others' intentions and theory-of-mind tasks. Finally, Fett et al. (2014) found increased activation in the left TPJ regardless of whether the participant (adolescents in this study) was playing a fair or unfair partner. According to the authors, this may be an indication that the left TPJ is involved in the mentalizing process at the time of deciding how much to trust someone and attempting to predict their behavior.

18.6.2   Striatum/Caudate and Cingulate Cortex

The caudate is a gray matter structure located deep in the brain and is part of the striatum (STR) and basal ganglia complex. Considerable research has shown that the caudate and STR are often implicated in reward processing. The cingulate is a large structure that is located dorsally to the corpus callosum and is considered part of the limbic system. The anterior cingulate cortex (ACC) in particular is associated with emotion processing, decision making, and impulse control. In our review, these two structures have been combined into a single section, as patterns of activation have been found to be correlated. King-Casas et al. (2005) found that activation of the head of the caudate in trustees was strongest immediately before the participant chose to make a trusting decision, and notably less strong before a selfish decision. Therefore, this activation was labeled "intention to trust." When the "intention to trust" was activated in the trustee's brain, it was significantly correlated with activation in the middle cingulate cortex (MCC) in the investor's brain, notably while the investor was making a decision to reciprocate. The activation in the caudate of the trustee and the following activation in the MCC of the investor were also strongly correlated with activation in the ACC of the trustee when they saw the subsequent decision of the investor. The authors suggest that this pattern of activation may signal that the head of the caudate receives information about the fairness of a social partner's decision and reciprocation of trust.

Van den Bos et al. (2009) found that the ventral STR (vSTR) had greater activation when prosocial particpants reciprocated, and when proself participants defected. The authors noted this pattern is consistent with reward processing in both groups, postulating that activation in the vSTR in those who are prosocial represents the positive experience of cooperation and mutual benefit. It was also found that the ACC and the right dlPFC were activated when social impulse control was required, particularly when reciprocating even when the benefit of trust was low. Additionally, greater activation in the ACC was seen in prosocial individuals when reciprocating, and then when proself individuals defected.

Finally, in Fett et al.'s developmental study (2014), it was reported that during cooperative interactions, activation in the caudate decreased with increased age. This is thought to be associated with a shift from self-focused thought to other focused thought. Additionally, the investigators reported increased activity in the ACC with increased age and responses to unfair behavior from their partner. The authors propose that based on these results the ACC may play a role in conflict monitoring.

18.7 Summary

Understanding the process of trust is a highly compelling challenge for cognitive neuroscience and neuropsychology. As trust plays such an important role in basic human interaction, including warm and supportive interpersonal relationships, sense of achievement, and quality of life, it stands to reason that natural curiosity about this fundamental human process has driven research into trust. This is supported by the fact that so many branches of academia have delved into the topic, from economics to psychology, from philosophy to neuroscience, and the body of literature on "trust" is expansive. From a neuropsychological perspective, placing focus on the cognitive, emotional, and social aspects of the overall process is important in understanding how people make trust decisions that in turn guide their behavior.

It is clear that the process of trusting is a complex act that requires multiple layers of social, emotional/psychological, and reward processing. In order to adequately employ these processes, we are reliant on several systems of the brain. Most notably, neuropsychological studies have shown that damage to the insula, amygdala, and prefrontal cortex significantly impairs the ability to trust at appropriate times and reciprocate trust when warranted. Other regions like the TPJ, the STR, and the cingulate cortex have also been implicated in the trust process, though no lesion studies are available to examine behavior when these structures are damaged.

The neuropsychology of trust is not just an academic exercise – this line of work is incredibly valuable to the overall domains of human health and disease. Millions of people around the world live with neurological diseases, some of which result in brain lesions (e.g., stroke, tumor, epilepsy). It is well established that when these lesions are in certain brain regions, they result in a variety of impairments. Documenting the type of impairment that arises when a specific area is damaged has helped develop our scientific understanding of the neuroanatomical correlates of cognition. Through this understanding, we are able to provide assistance with disease prognosis and treatment planning, and we work with patients and families to manage their deficits. This understanding of the relationship between neurological disease and cognition is continually growing and improving.

Further classification of which structures are involved in trust decisions and how behaviors change when these structures are damaged is crucial to furthering our knowledge of human cognition, emotions, and social relationships.

Specifically, individuals who have discrete, bilateral lesions to the insula, amygdala, or parts of the prefrontal cortex (i.e., vmPFC) often perform relatively well on traditional neuropsychological evaluations. This has been shown in patients like SM and EVR (Feinstein et al., 2016; Reber & Tranel, 2019). However, it is also well documented that these individuals have debilitating impairments in real life despite intact intellect, memory, and attention – for example, the patients have trouble maintaining employment, and are highly susceptible to scams. By digging deeper into these complex problems to describe and quantify impairments and behaviors, providers can provide more informed prognoses and recommendations. With greater individualized plans, treatment teams can better anticipate needs and provide resources to patients and their families. In turn, the hope is to improve patient safety and increase quality of life.

One limitation of lesion studies is limited racial, ethnic, and socioeconomic status (SES) diversity, which may hinder generalizability. Patients with focal lesions, especially bilateral lesions to specific structures such as the amygdala, are rare, and it is challenging to recruit participants from a variety of backgrounds and then compare performances across demographic groups. Therefore, lesion studies are limited by the number and diversity of the participants who are available and willing to participate in research. That said, lesion registries, such as the one at the University of Iowa, are active and growing and multisite research is providing more opportunities for research with a more diverse sample of lesion patients. It will be important for future research to replicate findings in larger, more diverse groups. Replication is particularly important across groups of varying SES, as environmental factors may fundamentally change how people initially approach trust decisions and how they integrate information about the other person's behavior in future decisions.

Finally, although we understand the basic process of trust and some important brain structures involved in that process, the next steps are to expand our knowledge and develop a sense of the trust network. In other words, we seek better understanding of the specifics of the cognitive and emotional process, starting with the presentation of the trust decision and extending through the action taken. This should include additional lesion research for regions that are thought to be important in this process such as the STR and the cingulate cortex. Understanding this full process and how individuals behave when different aspects of the network are disrupted will continue to hone our knowledge of the functional neuroanatomy of trust behavior. Greater and more specific knowledge of the function of these structures and networks, as well as the dysfunction that arises from disruption, will aid in our ability to manage behavior, provide resources, and support patients who have lesions to this system.

References

Adolphs, R. (2010). What does the amygdala contribute to social cognition? *Annals of the New York Academy of Sciences*, 1191(1), 42–61. https://doi.org/10.1111/j.1749-6632.2010.05445.x

Adolphs, R., Gosselin, F., Buchanan, T. W., Tranel, D., Schyns, P., & Damasio, A. R. (2005). A mechanism for impaired fear recognition after amygdala damage. *Nature*, 433(7021), 68–72. https://doi.org/10.1038/nature03086

Adolphs, R., Tranel, D., & Damasio, A. R. (1998). The human amygdala in social judgment. *Nature*, 393(6684), 470–474. https://doi.org/10.1038/30982

Adolphs, R., Tranel, D., & Damasio, H. (2001). Emotion recognition from faces and prosody following temporal lobectomy. *Neuropsychology*, 15(3), 396–404. https://doi.org/10.1037/0894-4105.15.3.396

Adolphs, R., Tranel, D., Damasio, H., & Damasio, A. R. (1994). Impaired recognition of emotion in facial expressions following bilateral damage to the human amygdala. *Nature*, 372(6507), 669–672. https://doi.org/10.1038/246170a0

Aimone, J. A., Houser, D., & Weber, B. (2014). Neural signatures of betrayal aversion: An fMRI study of trust. *Proceedings of the Royal Society B: Biological Sciences*, 281(1782), Article 20132127. https://doi.org/10.1098/rspb.2013.2127

Bar-on, R., Tranel, D., Denburg, N. L., & Bechara, A. (2003). Exploring the neurological substrate of emotional and social intelligence. *Brain*, 126(8), 1790–1800. https://doi.org/10.1093/brain/awg177

Bechara, A., & Damasio, A. R. (2005). The somatic marker hypothesis: A neural theory of economic decisions. *Games and Economic Behavior*, 52, 336–372. https://doi.org/10.1016/j.geb.2004.06.010

Bechara, A., Damasio, A. R., Damasio, H., & Anderson, S. W. (1994). Insensitivity to future consequences following damage to human prefrontal cortex. *Cognition: International Journal of Cognitive Science*, 50(1–3), 7–15. https://doi.org/10.1016/0010-0277(94)90018-3

Bechara, A., Tranel, D., & Damasio, H. (2000). Characterization of the decision making deficit of patients with ventromedial prefrontal cortex lesions. *Brain*, 123(11), 2189–2202. https://doi.org/10.1093/brain/123.11.2189

Belfi, A. M., Koscik, T. R., & Tranel, D. (2015). Damage to the insula is associated with abnormal interpersonal trust. *Neuropsychologia*, 71, 165–172. https://doi.org/10.1016/j.neuropsychologia.2015.04.003

Bellucci, G., Chernyak, S. V., Goodyear, K., Eickhoff, S. B., & Krueger, F. (2017). Neural signatures of trust in reciprocity: A coordinate-based meta analysis. *Human Brain Mapping*, 38, 1233–1248. https://doi.org/10.1002/hbm.23451

Bellucci, G., Feng, C., Camilleri, J., Eickhoff, S. B., & Krueger, F. (2018). The role of the anterior insula in social norm compliance and enforcement: Evidence from coordinate-based and functional connectivity meta-analyses. *Neuroscience and Biobehavioral Reviews*, 92, 378–389. https://doi.org/10.1016/j.neubiorev.2018.06.024

Berg, J., Dickhaut, J., & McCabe, K. (1995). Trust, reciprocity, and social history. *Games and Economic Behavior*, 10, 122–142. https://doi.org/10.1006/game.1995.1027

Berntson, G. G., Norman, G. J., Bechara, A., Tranel, D., & Cacioppo, J. T. (2011). The insula and evaluative processes. *Psychological Science*, 22(1), 80–86. https://doi.org/10.1177/0956797610391097

Bossaerts, P. (2010). Risk and risk prediction error signals in anterior insula. *Brain Structure and Function*, 214(5–6), 645–653. https://doi.org/10.1007/s00429

Brooks, J. C., Nurmikko, T. J., Bimson, W. E., Singh, K. D., & Roberts, N. (2002). fMRI of thermal pain: Effects of stimulus laterality and attention. *NeuroImage*, 15(2), 293–301. https://doi.org/10.1006/nimg.2001.0974

Buchanan, T. W., Tranel, D., & Adolphs, R. (2009). The human amygdala in social functioning. In P. W. Whalen & L. Phelps (Eds.), *The human amygdala* (pp. 289–320). Oxford University Press.

Bunge, S. A., Wallis, J. D., Parker, A., et al. (2005). Neural circuitry underlying rule use in humans and nonhuman primates. *Journal of Neuroscience*, 25(45), 10347–10350. https://doi.org/10.1523/JNEUROSCI.2937-05.2005

Caramazza, A. (1992). Is cognitive neuropsychology possible? *Journal of Cognitive Neuroscience*, 4(1), 80–95. https://doi.org/10.1162/jocn.1992.4.1.80

Cheng, X., Zheng, L., Li, L., Zheng, Y., Guo, X., & Yang, G. (2017). Anterior insula signals inequalities in a modified Ultimatum Game. *Neuroscience*, 348, 126–134. https://doi.org/10.1016/j.neuroscience.2017.02.023

Clark, L., Bechara, A., Damasio, H., Aitken, M. R., Sahakian, B. J., & Robbins, T. W. (2008). Differential effects of insular and ventromedial prefrontal cortex on risky decision making. *Brain*, 131(5), 1311–1322. https://doi.org/10.1093/brain/awn066

Craig, A. D. (2002). Interoception: The sense of the physiological condition of the body. *Nature Reviews Neuroscience*, 3(8), 655–666. https://doi.org/10.1016/S0959-4388(03)00090-4

Craig, A. D., Chen, K., Bandy, D., & Reiman, E. M. (2000). Thermosensory activation of insular cortex. *Natural Neuroscience*, 3(2), 184–190. https://doi.org/10.1038/72131

Critchley, H. D., Mathias, C. J., & Dolan, R. J. (2001). Neural activity in the human brain relating to uncertainty and arousal during anticipation. *Neuron*, 29(2), 537–545. https://doi.org/10.1016/S0896-6273(01)00225-2

Crone, E. A. (2013). Considerations of fairness in the adolescent brain. *Child Development Perspectives*, 7(2), 97–103. https://doi.org/10.1111/cdep.12022

D'Acremont, M., Lu, Z. L., Li, X., Van der Linden, M., & Bechara, A. (2009). Neural correlates of risk prediction error during reinforcement learning in humans. *NeuroImage*, 47(4), 1929–1939. https://doi.org/10.1016/j.neuroimage.2009.04.096

Damasio, A. R. (1996). The somatic marker hypothesis and the possible function of the prefrontal cortex. *Philosophical Transactions of the Royal Society B*, 351 (1346), 1413–1420. https://doi.org/10.1098/rstb.1996.0125

Damasio, A. R., Grabowski, T. J., Bechara, A., et al. (2000). Subcortical and cortical brain activity during the feeling of self-generated emotions. *Nature Neuroscience*, 3(10), 1049–1056. https://doi.org/doi.org/10.1038/79871

Damasio, A. R., Tranel, D., & Damasio, H. (1991). Somatic markers and guidance of behavior. In H. S. Levin, H. Eisenberg, & A. Benton (Eds.), *Frontal lobe function and dysfunction* (pp. 217–228). Oxford University Press.

Denny, B. T., Kober, H., Wager, T. D., & Ochsner, K. N. (2012). A meta-analysis of functional neuroimaging studies of self- and other judgments reveals a spatial gradient for mentalizing in the medial prefrontal cortex. *Journal of Cognitive Neuroscience*, 24(8), 1742–1752. https://doi.org/10.1162/jocn_a_00233

Dumontheil, I., Apperly, I. A., & Blakemore, S.-J. (2010). Online usage of theory of mind continues to develop in late adolescence. *Developmental Science*, 13 (2), 331–338. https://doi.org/10.1111/j.1467-7687.2009.00888.x

Editors of *The New England Journal of Medicine*. (2020). Dying in a leadership vacuum. *The New England Journal of Medicine*, 383(15), 1479–1480. https://doi.org/10.1056/NEJMe2029812

Eisenberg, N., Cumberland, A., Guthrie, I. K., Murphy, B. C., & Shepard, S. A. (2005). Age changes in prosocial responding and moral reasoning in adolescence and early adulthood. *Journal of Research on Adolescence*, 15(3), 235–260. https://doi.org/10.1111/j.1532-7795.2005.00095.x

Eisenberger, N. I., Lieberman, M. D., & Williams, K. D. (2003). Does rejection hurt? An fMRI study of social exclusion. *Science*, 302(5643), 290–292. https://doi.org/10.1126/science.1089134

Feinstein, J., Adolphs, R., & Tranel, D. (2016). A tale of survival from the world of patient SM. In D. G. Amaral & R. Adolphs (Eds.), *Living without an amygdala* (pp. 1–38). The Guilford Press.

Fett, A. K. J., Gromann, P. M., Giampietro, V., Shergill, S. S., & Krabbendam, L. (2014). Default distrust? An fMRI investigation of the neural development of trust and cooperation. *Social Cognitive and Affective Neuroscience*, 9 (4), 395–402. https://doi.org/10.1093/scan/nss144

Frith, U., & Frith, C. D. (2003). Development and neurophysiology of mentalizing. *Philosophical Transactions of the Royal Society B*, 358(1431), 459–473. https://doi.org/10.1098/rstb.2002.1218

Gabay, A. S., Kempton, M. J., Gilleen, J., & Mehta, M. A. (2019). MDMA increases cooperation and recruitment of social brain areas when playing trustworthy players in an iterated prisoner's dilemma. *Journal of*

Neuroscience, 39(2), 307–320. https://doi.org/10.1523/JNEUROSCI.1276-18.2018

Guth, W., Schmittberger, R., & Schwarze, B. (1982). An experimental analysis of ultimatum bargaining. *Journal of Economic Behavior and Organization*, 3(4), 367–388. https://doi.org/10.1016/0167-2681(82)90011-7

Haas, B. W., Ishak, A., Anderson, I. W., & Filkowski, M. M. (2015). The tendency to trust is reflected in human brain structure. *NeuroImage*, 107, 175–181. https://doi.org/10.1016/j.neuroimage.2014.11.060

Houser, D., Schunk, D., & Winter, J. (2010). Distinguishing trust from risk: An anatomy of the investment game. *Journal of Economic Behavior and Organization*, 74(1–2), 72–81. https://doi.org/10.1016/j.jebo.2010.01.002

Kang, Y., Williams, L. E., Clark, M. S., Gray, J. R., & Bargh, J. A. (2011). Physical temperature effects on trust behavior: The role of insula. *Social Cognitive and Affective Neuroscience*, 6(4), 507–515. https://doi.org/10.1093/scan/nsq077

Kennedy, D. P., Gläscher, J., Tyszka, J. M., & Adolphs, R. (2009). Personal space regulation by the human amygdala. *Nature Neuroscience*, 12, 1226–1227. https://doi.org/10.1038/nn.2381

Killgore, W. D., Schwab, Z. J., Tkachernko, O., et al. (2013). Emotional intelligence correlates with functional responses to dynamic changes in facial trustworthiness. *Social Neuroscience*, 8(4), 334–346. https://doi.org/10.1080/17470919.2013.807300

King-Casas, B., Sharp, C., Lomax-Bream, L., Lohrenz, T., Fonagy, P., & Montague, P. R. (2008). The rupture and repair of cooperation in borderline personality disorder. *Science*, 321(5890), 806–810. https://doi.org/10.1126/science.1156902

King-Casas, B., Tomlin, D., Anen, C., Camerer, C. F., Quartz, S. R., & Montague, P. R. (2005). Getting to know you: Reputation and trust in a two-person economic exchange. *Science*, 308(5718), 78–83. https://doi.org/10.1126/science.1108062

Kluver, H., & Bucy, P. C. (1937). "Psychic blindness" and other symptoms following bilateral temporal lobectomy in rhesus monkeys. *American Journal of Physiology*, 119, 352–353.

(1939). Preliminary analysis of functions of the temporal lobes in monkeys. *Archives of Neurology & Psychiatry*, 42, 979–997. https://doi.org/10.1001/archneuropsych.193902270240017001

Koenigs, M., & Tranel, D. (2006). Pseudopsychopathy: A perspective from cognitive neuroscience. In D. H. Zald & S. L. Rauch (Eds.), *The orbitofrontal cortex* (pp. 597–619). Oxford University Press.

Koscik, T. R., & Tranel, D. (2011). The human amygdala is necessary for developing and expressing normal interpersonal trust. *Neuropsychologia*, 49(4), 602–611. https://doi.org/10.1016/j.neuropsychologia.2010.09.023

Krawitz, A., Fukunaga, R., & Brown, J. W. (2010). Anterior insula activity predicts the influence of positively framed messages on decision making.

Cognitive, Affective, & Behavioral Neuroscience, 10, 392–405. https://doi.org/10.3758/CABN.10.3.392

Kross, E., Egner, T., Ochsner, K., Hirsch, J., & Downey, G. (2007). Neural dynamics of rejection sensitivity. *Journal of Cognitive Neuroscience, 19*(6), 945–956. https://doi.org/10.1162/jocn.2007.19.945

Krueger, F., Grafman, J., & McCabe, K. (2008). The neural correlates of the economic game playing. *Philosophical Transactions of the Royal Society B: Biological Sciences, 363,* 3859–3874. https://doi.org/10.1098/rstb.2008.0165

LaBar, K. S., LeDoux, J. E., Spencer, D. D., & Phelps, E. A. (1995). Impaired fear conditioning following unilateral temporal lobectomy in humans. *Journal of Neuroscience, 15*(10), 6846–6855. https://doi.org/10.1523/JNEUROSCI.15-10-06846.1995

Lamm, C., & Singer, T. (2010). The role of anterior insular cortex in social emotions. *Brain Structure and Function, 214*(5–6), 579–591. https://doi.org/10.1007/s00429-010-0251-3

Levin, I. P., & Hart, S. S. (2003). Risk preference in young children: Early evidence of individual differences in reaction to potential gains and losses. *Journal of Behavioral Decision Making, 16*(5), 397–413. https://doi.org/10.1002/bdm.453

Levin, I. P., Weller, J. A., Pederson, A., & Harshman, L. (2007). Age-related differences in adaptive decision making: Sensitivity to expected value in risky choice. *Judgment and Decision Making, 2*(4), 225–233.

Machado, C. J., Kazama, A. M., & Bachevalier, J. (2009). Impact of amygdala, orbital frontal, or hippocampal lesions on threat avoidance and emotional reactivity in nonhuman primates. *Emotion, 9*(2), 147–163. https://doi.org/10.1037/a0014539

Mason, W. A., Capitanio, J. P., Machado, C. J., Mendoza, S. P., & Amaral, D. G. (2006). Amygdalectomy and responsiveness to novelty in rhesus monkeys (Macaca mulatta): Generality and individual consistency of effects. *Emotion, 6*(1), 73–81. https://doi.org/10.1037/1528-3542.6.1.73

Meletti, S., Cantalupo, G., Santoro, F., et al. (2014). Temporal lobe epilepsy and emotion recognition without amygdala: A case study of Urbach-Wiethe disease and review of the literature. *Epileptic Disorders, 16*(4), 518–527. https://doi.org/10.1684/epd.2014.0696

Moretto, G., Sellitt, M., & di Pellegrino, G. (2013). Investment and repayment in a trust game after ventromedial prefrontal damage. *Frontiers in Human Neuroscience, 7,* 1–10. https://doi.org/10.3389/fnhum.2013.00593

Moulton, E. A., Keaser, M. I., Gullapalli, R. P., & Greenspan, J. D. (2005). Regional intensive and temporal patterns of functional MRI activation distinguishing noxious and innocuous contact heat. *Journal of Neurophysiology, 93*(4), 2183–2193. https://doi.org/10.1152.jn.01025.2004

Ostrowsky, K., Magnin, M., Ryvlin, P., Isnard, J., Guenot, M., & Mauguiere, F. (2002). Representation of pain and somatic sensation in the human insula:

A study of response to direct electrical cortical stimulation. *Cerebral Cortex*, 12(4), 376–385. https://doi.org/10.1093/crecor/12.4.376

Pfeifer, J. H., Lieberman, M. D., & Dapretto, M. (2007). "I know you but what am I?!": Neural bases of self- and social knowledge retrieval in children and adults. *Journal of Cognitive Neuroscience*, 19(8), 1323–1337. https://doi.org/10.1162/jocn.2007.19.8.1323

Phillips, M. L., Young, A. W., Senior, C., et al. (1997). A specific neural substrate for perceiving facial expressions of disgust. *Nature*, 389, 495–498. https://doi.org/10.1038/39051

Preuschoff, K., Quartz, S. R., & Bossaerts, P. (2008). Human insula activation reflects risk prediction errors as well as risk. *Journal of Neuroscience*, 28(11), 2745–2752. https://doi.org/10.1523/JNEUROSCI.4268-07.2008

Reber, J., & Tranel, D. (2019). Frontal lobe syndromes. In J. Grafman & M. D'Esposito (Eds.), *The frontal lobes (handbook of clinical neurology)* (pp. 147–164). Elsevier.

Rilling, J. K., & Sanfey, A. G. (2011). The neuroscience of social decision making. *Annual Review of Psychology*, 62, 23–48. https://doi.org/10.1146/annurev.psych.121208.131647

Said, C. P., Baron, S. G., & Todorov, A. (2009). Nonlinear amygdala response of face trustworthiness: Contributions of high and low spatial frequency information. *Journal of Cognitive Neuroscience*, 21(3), 519–528. https://doi.org/10.1162/jocn.2009.21041

Sanfey, A. G., Rilling, J. K., Aronson, J. A., Nystrom, L. E., & Cohen, J. D. (2003). The neural basis of economic decision making in the ultimatum game. *Science*, 300(5626), 1755–1758. https://doi.org/1126/science.1082976

Singer, T., Kiebel, S. J., Winston, J. S., Dolan, R. J., & Firth, C. D. (2004). Brain responses to the acquired moral status of faces. *Neuron*, 41(4), 653–662. https://doi.org/10.1016/S0896-6273(04)00014-5

Singer, T., Seymour, B., O'Doherty, J. P., et al. (2006). Empathic neural responses are modulated by the perceived fairness of others. *Nature*, 439, 466–469. https://doi.org/10.1038/nature04271

Steinbeis, N., Bernhardt, B. C., & Singer, T. (2012). Impulse control and underlying functions in the left DLPFC mediate age-related and age-independent individual differences in strategic social behavior. *Neuron*, 73(5), 1040–1051. https://doi.org/10.1016/j.neuron.2011.12.027

Thornton, H. B., Nel, D., Thornton, D., Van Honk, J., Baker, G. A., & Stein, D. J. (2008). The neuropsychiatry and neuropsychology of lipoid proteinosis. *Journal of Neuropsychiatry and Clinical Neurosciences*, 20(1), 86–92. https://doi.org/10.1176/jnp.2008.20.1.86

Todorov, A. (2008). Evaluating faces on trustworthiness: An extension of systems for recognition of emotions signaling approach/avoidance behaviors. *Annals of the New York Academy of Sciences*, 1124(1), 208–224. https://doi.org/10.1196/annals.1440.012

Todorov, A., Baron, S. G., & Oosterhof, N. N. (2008). Evaluating face trust-worthiness: A model based approach. *Social Cognitive and Affective Neuroscience*, 3(2), 119–127. https://doi.org/10.1093/scan/nsn009

Tranel, D., & Hyman, B. T. (1990). Neuropsychological correlates of bilateral amygdala damage. *Archives of Neurology*, 47(3), 349–355. https://doi.org/10.1001/archneur.1990.00530030131029

Van den Bos, W., Van Dijk, E., Westenberg, M., Rombouts, S. A. R. B., & Crone, E. A. (2009). What motivates repayment? Neural correlates of reciprocity in the Trust Game. *Social Cognitive and Affective Neuroscience*, 4(3), 294–304. https://doi.org/10.1093/scan/nsp009

(2011). Changing brains, changing perspectives: The neurocognitive development of reciprocity. *Psychological Science*, 22(1), 60–70. https://doi.org/10.1177/0956797610391102

Weller, J. A., Levin, I. P., & Bechara, A. (2009). Do individual differences in Iowa Gambling Task performance predict adaptive decision making for risky gains and losses? *Journal of Clinical and Experimental Neuropsychology*, 32(2), 141–150. https://doi.org/10.1080/13803390902881926

Weller, J. A., Levin, I. P., Shiv, B., & Bechara, A. (2007). Neural correlates of adaptive decision making for risky gains and losses. *Psychological Science*, 18(11), 958–964. https://doi.org/10.1111/j.1467-9280.2007.02009.x

Wellman, H. M., Cross, D., & Watson, J. (2001). Meta-analysis of theory-of-mind development: The truth about false belief. *Child Development*, 72(3), 655–684. https://doi.org/10.1111/1467-8624.00304

Winston, J. S., Strange, B. A., O'Doherty, J. P., & Dolan, R. J. (2002). Automatic and intentional brain responses during evaluation of trustworthi-ness of faces. *Nature Neuroscience*, 5, 277–283. https://doi.org/10.1038/nn816

Xue, G., Lu, Z., Levin, I. P., & Bechara, A. (2010). The impact of prior risk experiences on subsequent risky decision making: The role of the insula. *NeuroImage*, 50(2), 709–716. https://doi.org/10.1016/j.neuroimage.2009.12.097

Index

accumbens, nucleus, 161, 296, 316, 341, 347, 371

affiliation, 159, 321, 329, 347, 353, 407, 474

agreeableness, 27, 29, 83, 190, 225, 432

anger, 126, 128, 131–132, 134, 136, 224, 239, 328

anthropomorphism, 64, 68–70, 85

anxiety, 128, 131–132, 138, 140, 142–143, 259–260, 329, 348, 355, 372, 375–376, 406, 433, 437, 439, 445, 453

assurance, 128, 341, 450

attachment, 15, 19–20, 39, 273, 325, 347, 352, 390, 406, 445–446, 448, 450, 452

attitude, 16, 21, 27, 82, 87, 90, 104–105, 109, 113, 128, 136, 160, 189, 192, 243, 323, 327, 369–376, 378

attribution, 81, 86, 418

aversion, betrayal, 43–44, 101, 106–107, 110–112, 115–118, 134–136, 139, 239, 244–245, 296–297, 318, 350, 466, 468

aversion, inequity, 106, 126, 196–197, 238–239

Bayesian, 41, 206

belief, 41, 43, 50, 92, 102, 132–133, 155, 200, 202–204, 206, 238, 240, 242, 244, 246–253, 255–257, 464

benevolence, 57, 59, 63–64, 70, 188–189, 340, 348, 435

bias, 28, 44, 86, 90, 126, 134, 159–160, 162, 164–166, 168–169, 171, 198, 200, 225, 227, 247, 321, 372–373, 405, 419, 422, 434, 438–439, 443, 476

bonding, 155, 162, 164–166, 168, 170–171, 192, 254, 315, 352, 355, 372, 376, 406

calibration, 80, 88–89, 92

capital, social, 47, 369

caudate, 60, 113, 159, 161, 163, 201, 247–248, 260, 272, 278–279, 284, 286, 296, 300, 341, 351, 407, 412, 414–416, 419–420, 482

cognition, social, 62, 136, 138, 140, 143, 158, 161, 164, 206, 228, 278, 316, 324–325, 328, 353, 372, 390, 414, 417–418, 422, 447, 474

cortex
  anterior cingulate, 58, 61, 113, 116, 159, 165, 203–204, 242–243, 245–251, 253, 257, 260, 272, 279, 297–298, 482
  dorsolateral prefrontal, 61, 91, 116, 159, 242, 278, 412, 478
  lateral prefrontal, 244, 300, 302
  medial prefrontal, 113–114, 136, 138, 140–141, 143, 158–159, 165, 203–204, 206, 242, 245–250, 253, 257, 261, 272, 278–279, 281, 297–298, 301, 316, 344, 412, 419, 469, 478–479
  middle cingulate, 260, 482
  orbitofrontal, 60, 113, 195, 202, 204, 206, 244, 278, 316, 326, 479
  posterior cingulate, 142, 165, 203, 253, 278
  ventrolateral prefrontal, 138, 248, 285, 297–298, 301–302
  ventromedial prefrontal, 136, 138, 142–143, 159, 165, 226, 228–229, 240, 242, 247, 249–250, 252, 302, 479–480, 484

culture, 30, 39–40, 44, 59, 81, 287, 431

depression, 142, 259–260, 436, 445

development
  adolescent, 113, 247, 249, 274, 276, 278–279, 281, 283, 285, 396, 447, 477–478, 481
  adulthood, 15, 23, 113, 247, 249, 273, 275, 277–279, 281–282, 285–286, 373, 396, 431, 467, 477–479, 481
  age, 80–81, 228, 246–247, 249, 269, 271–281, 283, 285–286, 353, 355, 373, 412, 446, 472, 478–479, 481–482
  childhood, 22, 26, 39, 273, 276–277, 281, 354, 446, 477

digitalization, 55

dilemma, social, 125, 131–132, 297, 325, 478
disorder
  autism spectrum disorder, 259–260, 300, 324, 355
  borderline personality, 46, 142, 221, 259–260, 324, 355, 431–432, 434, 436, 438–445, 447–451, 470
  personality, 259, 430–437, 439–440, 444–453, 471
  post-traumatic stress, 259–260
  psychiatric, 248, 259–260, 348, 389, 431
dopamine, 59, 161, 195, 202, 342–344, 346–348, 351, 354, 356, 370, 377, 414–415, 417, 423

economics, 36, 42–43, 47, 101, 104, 112, 117, 125, 221, 236, 243–244, 293, 369–370, 483
electroencephalography, 92, 112, 294, 339
emotion, anticipatory, 133
emotion, immediate, 62, 125
emotion, incidental, 125–127, 130–133, 135
emotion, integral, 125, 133, 136, 139, 141
endowment, 46, 57–58, 114, 125, 185, 237, 240, 246, 293, 339, 356, 466–467

fear, 60, 110, 115, 117, 131–132, 141, 223, 245, 326, 375–376, 406, 432–433, 474, 476–477
functional connectivity, 114, 138, 142, 204–205, 248, 252–253, 258, 296, 299–302

game
  dictator, 107, 127, 131, 135, 139, 224, 240, 255, 303, 348–349, 352, 356
  investment, 40, 49, 91, 101, 114, 185, 370
  prisoner's dilemma, 40, 45, 224, 227, 351
  public goods, 45, 130, 162, 224, 240, 270
  theory, 17, 36, 42–43, 257
  ultimatum, 128, 143, 160, 228, 240, 255, 258, 345, 441, 466
gender, 49, 80, 247, 260, 269, 271, 282–287, 323, 327, 329, 344, 353, 355
gene
  arginine vasopressin receptor 1A, 370, 376–377, 379
  dopamine D4 receptor, 370, 377, 379
  genotype, 323, 373–376, 378
  oxytocin receptor, 59, 317, 320–321, 323–324, 327–328, 370, 372–376, 379
  serotonin transporter, 370, 378
guilt, 37, 43, 50, 128, 131–132, 197, 238–240, 242–243, 253

hippocampus, 195, 327, 371, 474
honesty, 132, 142, 164, 190, 199, 203, 225, 228, 452

hormone, 253–254, 259, 315–316, 376, 407
human factors, 77
hyperscanning, 161, 295
hypothalamus, 316, 371, 376

inequality, 24, 41, 239–240, 242–243, 247–248, 251–253
institution, 38, 47–49, 59, 103, 105–106, 108, 117, 270
insula, 46, 58, 61, 91, 137–141, 143, 165, 195, 228, 242–246, 248–253, 257, 259, 296, 316, 340, 352, 413, 439, 442, 468–473, 479–480, 483–484
insula, anterior, 143, 296–298, 302, 340–341, 350
integrity, 23, 57, 59, 63–64, 70, 188–189, 198, 270, 340, 435
intelligence, artificial, 77, 89

junction, temporoparietal, 136, 138, 140–142, 159, 162, 167, 169, 194, 206, 227, 229, 242–243, 245–246, 248–250, 253, 260, 266, 272, 278–279, 281, 284–286, 297–298, 300, 302, 407, 412, 417, 419–420, 481, 483

learning, feedback, 165, 326, 390, 413, 416
learning, reinforcement, 161, 164, 194–195, 199–200, 202, 204, 206, 296, 340–341, 346, 414
lesion, 115, 227, 252, 294, 339–340, 465–466, 468–470, 474, 479–481, 483–484
lobule, inferior parietal, 203, 206, 253, 412

mentalizing, 58, 60–61, 65–70, 137, 139–140, 159, 197, 200, 204–205, 240, 242–243, 246, 248, 251, 272–273, 275–276, 278–279, 281, 286, 298, 468, 471, 478, 481–482
meta-analysis, 25, 43–44, 49, 58, 66, 91, 113, 132, 137, 139, 157, 226, 246, 251, 275, 277, 282–284, 287, 296, 322, 324, 350, 473
midbrain, 195, 326, 377
motivation, 18–19, 21, 27, 63, 78, 132, 139, 189, 229, 238, 242, 245–247, 249–252, 255, 257, 284, 298, 329, 341, 346–347, 390, 414–415, 419–421, 450

network
  action-perception, 301
  brain, 137
  central-executive, 62, 253, 297–302, 341
  cingulo-opercular, 253
  default-mode, 166, 253, 297–301, 316, 326, 341

network (cont.)
  functional, 253, 258
  large-scale, 297–298, 300–302, 339, 341–342
  neural, 138, 167, 228, 253, 258, 338, 340
  resting-state, 205
  reward, 62, 297–298, 300–301, 341
  salience, 297–302, 340–341, 350
neuroeconomics, 112–114, 125, 136
neuromodulator, 339, 342, 344, 354–355, 371
neuropeptide, 248, 315–316, 328–329, 338,
  347, 371
neuroscience, social, 50, 134, 168–169, 206,
  236, 304, 356

oxytocin, 59, 115–116, 163, 248, 254–255, 259,
  294, 315–317, 320–324, 326, 338, 347,
  352–353, 370–377, 407, 450–451

polymorphism, 116, 317, 355, 370–371, 373,
  376, 378
precuneus, 162, 253, 278, 285, 301
prediction, error, 42, 124, 133, 159, 165, 194,
  260, 416
probability, 44, 102, 104–107, 114, 117–118,
  128, 135, 192–193, 224, 244, 324, 372
psychiatry, 46, 142
psychopathology, 221, 259, 261, 420, 422,
  432–433, 446
psychopathy, 132, 438
psychosis, 260, 389–390, 396–397, 404–407,
  412, 414–416, 418–423, 443, 452
punishment, 132, 197, 236, 240, 300, 416, 421

reliability, 64, 70, 79, 84–85, 92, 171, 191, 299,
  303, 323, 340, 420, 464
resting-state, 205, 252–253, 294, 299
risk, preference, 57, 101, 104–105, 107,
  113–114, 192, 244
risk, social, 101, 104–118, 133, 135, 140, 254,
  277, 285–287, 339, 347, 349–350, 355, 480

schizophrenia, 300, 325, 348, 354, 389, 396,
  403–407, 413, 415–416, 418–423
self-report, 27, 29, 60, 90, 92, 127, 132, 168,
  224–225, 242, 270, 321–322, 326, 346,
  348, 435–436, 444, 453, 472–473

serotonin, 378
status, socioeconomic, 23, 248, 484
stimulation, 118, 140, 158, 227, 242, 347, 352,
  418, 423
strain-test, 16, 27
strategy, 36, 46, 66, 130, 199, 204, 206, 283,
  298, 301, 341, 348, 476
striatum, 60, 159, 195, 297, 414, 466
striatum, dorsal, 61, 91, 296–298, 326,
  341
striatum, ventral, 136, 138, 143, 166, 195, 201,
  205, 240, 242, 246, 248, 251, 257, 261,
  296–298, 341, 347, 482
sulcus, superior temporal, 58, 136, 138,
  140–141, 162, 205, 248, 278
system
  central nervous, 316, 376
  mesocorticolimbic, 316
  neurotransmitter, 316, 338, 342, 352, 356,
    377–378

testosterone, 59, 254, 294, 328, 338
theory of mind, 124, 136, 227, 240, 298, 372,
  390, 407, 413–415, 417–420, 422–423,
  452, 487
therapy, 356, 436, 438, 445–449
trust
  calculus-based, 298, 301, 341
  identification-based, 298, 341
  impression-based, 340, 343–344, 349
  knowledge-based, 298, 341
  network, 138, 248, 340, 484
  propensity, 87, 90, 190, 205, 295, 300–303,
    317, 321, 338, 340, 434, 441

uncertainty, 18, 60, 102, 104–106, 108, 113,
  115, 117–118, 190–191, 222, 243–244,
  297, 301, 317, 344, 434, 445, 453, 464,
  466, 468, 476
utility, 43, 113–114, 196, 239, 243–245

vasopressin, 59, 316, 376–377
vulnerability, 17, 102, 236, 270, 396, 415–416,
  434, 452

World Value Survey, 47

9 781108 726702